Oncology of CNS Tumors

Oncology of CNS Tumors

Editor: Matthew Martin

AMERICAN
MEDICAL PUBLISHERS
www.americanmedicalpublishers.com

AMERICAN
MEDICAL PUBLISHERS
www.americanmedicalpublishers.com

Cataloging-in-Publication Data

Oncology of CNS tumors / edited by Matthew Martin.
p. cm.
Includes bibliographical references and index.
ISBN 979-8-88740-350-2
1. Central nervous system--Tumors. 2. Central nervous system--Tumors--Diagnosis.
3. Central nervous system--Tumors--Treatment. 4. Oncology. 5. Neurology. I. Martin, Matthew.
RC280.N43 O53 2023
616.994 8--dc23

American Medical Publishers,
41 Flatbush Avenue,
1st Floor, New York,
NY 11217, USA

ISBN 979-8-88740-350-2 (Hardback)

Contents

Preface

In my initial years as a student, I used to run to the library at every possible instance to grab a book and learn something new. Books were my primary source of knowledge and I would not have come such a long way without all that I learnt from them. Thus, when I was approached to edit this book; I became understandably nostalgic. It was an absolute honor to be considered worthy of guiding the current generation as well as those to come. I put all my knowledge and hard work into making this book most beneficial for its readers.

The spinal cord and the brain together form the central nervous system (CNS). A CNS tumor develops when healthy cells in the brain or spinal cord start growing uncontrollably forming a mass. CNS tumors may be malignant or benign. Malignant tumors grow rapidly and can spread to other parts of the body, whereas benign tumors grow slowly and do not spread to other parts of the body. Astrocytoma, diffuse intrinsic pontine glioma (DIPG or the brain stem glioma), ependymoma, germ cell tumor, medulloblastoma, primitive neuroectodermal tumor (PNET), and optic pathway glioma are a few types of CNS tumors. Diagnosis of CNS cancer is done using tests and procedures including neurological examination, imaging tests such as CT scan and MRI, and biopsy. Treatment options include radiation therapy, radiosurgery, chemotherapy, and targeted drug therapy. The results of various researches and advanced studies related to CNS tumors have been included in this book. It includes some of the vital pieces of work being conducted across the globe, on various topics related to CNS oncology. This book will help the readers in keeping pace with the rapid changes in this field.

I wish to thank my publisher for supporting me at every step. I would also like to thank all the authors who have contributed their researches in this book. I hope this book will be a valuable contribution to the progress of the field.

Editor

1

Gene Expression Profiling Stratifies IDH-Wildtype Glioblastoma With Distinct Prognoses

Yu-Qing Liu [1,2], *Fan Wu* [1,2], *Jing-Jun Li* [1,2], *Yang-Fang Li* [1,2], *Xing Liu* [1,2], *Zheng Wang* [2,3] *and Rui-Chao Chai* [1,2*]

[1] *Department of Molecular Neuropathology, Beijing Neurosurgical Institute, Beijing, China,* [2] *Chinese Glioma Genome Atlas Network, Beijing, China,* [3] *Department of Neurosurgery, Beijing Tiantan Hospital, Capital Medical University, Beijing, China*

***Correspondence:**
Rui-Chao Chai
chairuichao_glia@163.com;
chairuichao@bjtth.org

Objectives: In the present study, we aimed to determine the candidate genes that may function as biomarkers to further distinguish patients with isocitrate dehydrogenase (IDH)-wildtype glioblastoma (GBM), which are heterogeneous with respect to clinical outcomes.

Materials and Methods: We selected 41 candidate genes associated with overall survival (OS) using univariate Cox regression from IDH-wildtype GBM patients based on RNA sequencing (RNAseq) expression data from the Chinese Glioma Genome Atlas (CGGA, $n = 105$) and The Cancer Genome Atlas (TCGA, $n = 139$) cohorts. Next, a seven-gene-based risk signature was formulated according to Least Absolute Shrinkage and Selection Operator (LASSO) regression algorithm in the CGGA RNAseq database as a training set, while another 525 IDH-wildtype GBM patient TCGA datasets, consisting of RNA sequencing and microarray data, were used for validation. Patient survival in the low- and high-risk groups was calculated using Kaplan-Meier survival curve analysis and the log-rank test. Uni-and multivariate Cox regression analysis was used to assess the prognosis value. Gene oncology (GO) and gene set enrichment analysis (GSEA) were performed for the functional analysis of the seven-gene-based risk signature.

Results: We developed a seven-gene-based signature, which allocated each patient to a risk group (low or high). Patients in the high-risk group had dramatically shorter overall survival than their low-risk counterparts in three independent cohorts. Univariate and multivariate analysis showed that the seven-gene signature remained an independent prognostic factor. Moreover, the seven-gene risk signature exhibited a striking prognostic validity, with AUC of 78.4 and 73.9%, which was higher than for traditional "age" (53.7%, 62.4%) and "GBM sub-type" (57.7%, 52.9%) in the CGGA- and TCGA-RNAseq databases, respectively. Subsequent bioinformatics analysis predicted that the seven-gene signature was involved in the inflammatory response, immune response, cell adhesion, and apoptotic process.

Conclusions: Our findings indicate that the seven-gene signature could be a potential prognostic biomarker. This study refined the current classification system of IDH-wildtype GBM and may provide a novel perspective for the research and individual therapy of IDH-wildtype GBM.

Keywords: glioma, GBM, IDH wildtype, risk signature, biomarker, prognosis

INTRODUCTION

Glioblastoma (GBM, WHO grade IV) is the most common and malignant primary intracranial tumor and is associated with a poor prognosis, with a median survival rate of 14–16 months, despite the use of intensive treatments, including surgery, radiotherapy, and chemotherapy (1–4). Isocitrate dehydrogenase (IDH) mutations are one of the most common and earliest detectable genetic alterations in diffuse gliomas, and evidence supports this mutation as a driver of glioma genesis (5). Based on the updated 2016 edition of World Health Organization (WHO) classification of central nervous system (CNS) tumors, GBM could be classified into IDH-wildtype, and IDH-mutant GBM, wherein the former (IDH-wildtype GBM) is associated with a worse prognosis (6, 7). IDH-mutant GBM accounts for about 12% of all GBM, with an occurrence rate in secondary GBM of 84.6%, while its counterpart in primary GBM is rare (5.0%) (8, 9).

Previous studies have indicated that a six-gene signature could further stratify the prognosis of IDH-mutant glioma using gene expression profiling (10). Given that IDH-wildtype and IDH-mutant GBM are regarded as distinct entities despite their similar histology (11), further stratification of patients with IDH-mutant or IDH-wildtype GBM could be a promising approach for the diagnosis and treatment of GBM. The methylation status of the methylguanine methyltransferase (MGMT) promoter has been reported to have predictive value for both IDH-mutant and IDH-wildtype GBM (12, 13). Our recent study presented a comprehensive somatic mutation landscape of secondary GBM and provided a protocol for MET-targeted therapy for precision neuro-oncology (14). A handful of recent studies have assessed the molecular spectrum of IDH-mutant GBM on the basis of genome-wide DNA methylation analysis, copy-number profiling, and gene expression profiling, respectively (11, 15). Nevertheless, the systematical investigation of IDH-wildtype GBM (88%), which is overwhelmingly more common than for IDH-mutant GBM, as well as being heterogeneous with respect to clinical outcomes, remains to be discussed completely.

In the present study, we aimed to further analyze and stratify IDH-wildtype GBM assessed by whole-genome expression profile analysis. We identified a seven-gene-based risk signature for IDH-wildtype GBM in the CGGA-RNAseq cohort, which was then validated in TCGA-RNAseq and TCGA-microarray cohorts. Furthermore, the prognostic value of our signature and underlying biological functions correlated with this signature were also systemically investigated. By improving our understanding of the molecular basis of IDH-wildtype GBM, we expect to develop a superior stratification of these tumors according to the risk signature and supply additional therapeutic targets for the treatment of for IDH-wildtype GBM.

TABLE 1 | Clinicopathological characteristics of patients in the CGGA RNAseq, TCGA RNAseq, and TCGA microarray cohorts.

Characteristics		CGGA RNAseq cohort	TCGA RNAseq cohort	TCGA microarray cohort
		GBM-IDH wildtype (*n* = 105)	GBM-IDH wildtype (*n* = 139)	GBM-IDH wildtype (*n* = 386)
Age (years)	Median (range)	52 (8–81)	62 (24–89)	61 (19–89)
	Age≥45	35 (33.3%)	11 (7.9%)	43 (11.1%)
	Age<45	70 (66.7%)	128 (92.1%)	343 (88.9%)
Gender	Male	68 (64.8%)	89 (64.0%)	239 (61.9%)
	Female	37 (35.2%)	50 (36.0%)	147 (38.1%)
GBM sub-type	Proneural	5 (4.8%)	24 (17.3%)	72 (18.7%)
	Neural	10 (9.5%)	5 (3.6%)	70 (18.1%)
	Classical	41 (39.0%)	85 (61.1%)	108 (28.0%)
	Mesenchymal	49 (46.7%)	25 (18.0%)	115 (29.8%)
	NA	0 (0.00%)	0 (0.00%)	21 (5.4%)
MGMT promoter methylation status	Methylated	37 (35.2%)	43 (30.9%)	122 (31.6%)
	Unmethylated	65 (61.9%)	67 (48.2%)	151 (39.1%)
	NA	3 (2.9%)	29 (20.9%)	113 (29.3%)
TERT promoter status	Wildtype	49 (46.7%)	NA	NA
	Mutation	33 (31.4%)	NA	NA
	NA	23 (21.9%)	NA	NA
EGFR	Wildtype	NA	104 (74.8%)	NA
	Mutation	NA	34 (24.5%)	NA
	NA	NA	1 (0.7%)	NA
TP53	Wildtype	NA	106 (76.3%)	NA
	Mutation	NA	32 (23.0%)	NA
	NA	NA	1 (0.7%)	NA
Chr 7 gain/Chr 10 loss	Combined	NA	93 (66.9%)	NA
	No combined	NA	42 (30.2%)	NA
	NA	NA	4 (2.9%)	NA

CGGA, Chinese Glioma Genome Atlas; TCGA, The Cancer Genome Atlas; MGMT, methylguanine methyltransferase; TERT, telomerase reverse transcriptase; NA, not applicable; Chr, chromosome.

MATERIALS AND METHODS

Samples and Data Collection

This study collected 630 GBM samples from three cohorts: the CGGA-RNA sequencing (RNAseq, $n = 105$), TCGA-RNAseq ($n = 139$), and TCGA-microarray ($n = 386$) cohorts. The clinical and molecular information of the cases in the CGGA-RNAseq cohort were obtained from the CGGA database@@uline (http://www.cgga.org.cn/) and were used as the training set (16). Each case with newly diagnosed GBM was treated by the CGGA group. All tissues were diagnosed histologically by two or more neuropathologists, independently. The overall survival (OS) was calculated from the date of diagnosis until the death of the patient or the end of the clinical follow-up. The study protocol was approved by the Ethics Committee of the Beijing Tiantan Hospital. Another 525 GBM were included from TCGA-RNAseq and TCGA-microarray cohorts (https://tcga-data.nci.nih.gov/tcga/) (17, 18) as validation sets. The characteristics of the patient in the three cohorts are provided in **Table 1**.

Gene Oncology (GO), Kyoto Encyclopedia of Genes and Genomes (KEGG), and Gene Set Enrichment Analysis (GSEA)

GO and KEGG pathway analyses were performed in DAVID (http://david.abcc.ncifcrf.gov/home.jsp) for the functional annotation of the genes correlated positively and negatively with the risk score in the two cohorts (19). GO was used to analyze the main function of the differential expression genes. KEGG was performed to analyze pathway enrichment. GSEA was performed to determine whether the gene sets were statistically different between the two groups (high-risk score vs. low-risk score) using GSEA v3 software (http://www.broadinstitute.org/gsea/index.jsp) (20).

Statistical Analysis

Univariate Cox regression analysis was performed to select genes associated with the OS in the CGGA-RNAseq and TCGA-RNAseq cohorts, respectively. Next, the risk associated genes (HR >1) and protective genes (HR<1) were both overlapped between the two cohorts. Ultimately, a total of 41 OS-correlated genes, consisting of 34 risk associated genes and 7 protective genes, were selected to perform further gene signature selection and risk-based classification in the training dataset. A risk signature was formulated according to Least Absolute Shrinkage and Selection Operator (LASSO) regression algorithm (21–25). The penalty parameter λ was chosen based on a 50-fold cross validation within the training dataset, which produced the minimum mean cross-validated error for the Cox model. Accordingly, seven genes and their regression coefficients were achieved. The risk score was then calculated in the training and validation datasets using the following equation:

$$Risk\ score = \sum_{i=1}^{n} Coef_i \times Expr_i$$

where $Coef_i$ is the coefficient and $Expr_i$ is the z-score-transformed relative expression value of each selected gene. Based on the median risk value (23, 26), patients in CGGA-RNAseq, TCGA-RNAseq, and TCGA microarray databases were divided into high- and low-risk groups. Kaplan-Meier survival curves were calculated and the log rank tests were conducted to assess the prognostic significance (13, 27). Differences in clinicopathologic features between the groups were determined using the Student's t- or Chi-square tests. Multivariate Cox regression analyses were used to confirm independent prognostic factors. All statistical analyses were performed using SPSS version 16.0 software (SPSS Inc., Chicago, IL). P-value < 0.05 was considered as statistically significant.

RESULTS

Screening for Critical Genes Stratified for IDH-Wildtype GBM Through Gene Expression

To stratify IDH-wildtype GBM based on the whole genome expression profiling, we firstly selected genes associated with overall survival (OS) using univariate Cox regression from IDH-wildtype GBM patients in the CGGA ($n = 105$) and TCGA cohorts ($n = 139$), respectively. Next, the OS-related genes in the two cohorts were divided into two groups: protective genes (HR<1) and risk associated genes (HR >1). The protective genes and risk associated genes were then overlapped between the two cohorts, respectively. Finally, 41 candidate genes, including 34 risk associated genes and 7 protective genes, were selected (**Figure 1A**). The functional annotations of the 41 candidate genes were enriched in GO terms for biological processes including "Innate immune response," "Glial cell-derived neurotrophic factor receptor signaling pathway," and "Cellular response to lipopolysaccharide" (**Figure 1B**).

Identification of a Seven-Gene Risk Signature for IDH-Wildtype GBM

Given the prognostic importance of these 41 candidate genes, we attempted to develop a gene expression-based signature that could further stratify IDH-wild type GBM derived from these genes. To this end, using LASSO regression algorithm, seven genes, including 4 protective (*ZNF419*, *FOXG1*, *STARD7*, and *ZBTB16*) genes and 3 risk associated genes (*CD180*, *SDK1*, and *CYP21A2*), were selected as active covariates to assess their prognostic value, thereby obtaining the risk scores for the patients in the training cohort (**Figures 2A–C**).

According to their median risk score, patients were assigned to either a low- or high-risk group. In GBM with IDH-wildtype, Kaplan-Meier analysis showed that patients in the high-risk group ($n = 53$) had a lower OS than patients in the low-risk group ($n = 52$) in the training cohort (median OS = 8.47 vs. 17.13 months; $P < 0.0001$; **Figure 3A**). Furthermore, we validated the prognostic value of the risk score in the TCGA-RNAseq cohort. Consequently, we found that OS differed significantly between the high-risk ($n = 70$) and low-risk groups ($n = 69$) in IDH-wildtype GBM patients in the TCGA cohort (median OS = 9.27 vs. 15.57 months; $P = 0.0003$; **Figure 3F**).

Moreover, given that glioma sub-types are stratified according to the MGMT promoter methylation status, wherein telomerase reverse transcriptase (TERT) status showed distinct tumor characteristics and OS outcomes, we investigated the prognostic value of risk score in these populations. A similar trend was observed in these patients, although no significant difference was found in the unmethylated MGMT promoter or TERT mutation patients (most likely due to the small sample size) (**Figures 3B–E,G,H**). In summary, our results indicated that the high-risk group was markedly correlated with an unfavorable prognosis in patients with IDH-wildtype GBM.

To further validate the prognostic value of the seven-gene-based risk signature in other cohorts, we computed the risk scores for each patient in the TCGA microarray databases with the same formula. Patients were divided into low- and high-risk groups according to their median risk value. The survival analysis suggested that patients in the high-risk group ($n = 193$) had a lower OS than patients in the low-risk group ($n = 193$; median OS = 12.4 vs. 15.57 months; $P = 0.0097$; **Figure 3I**). For the

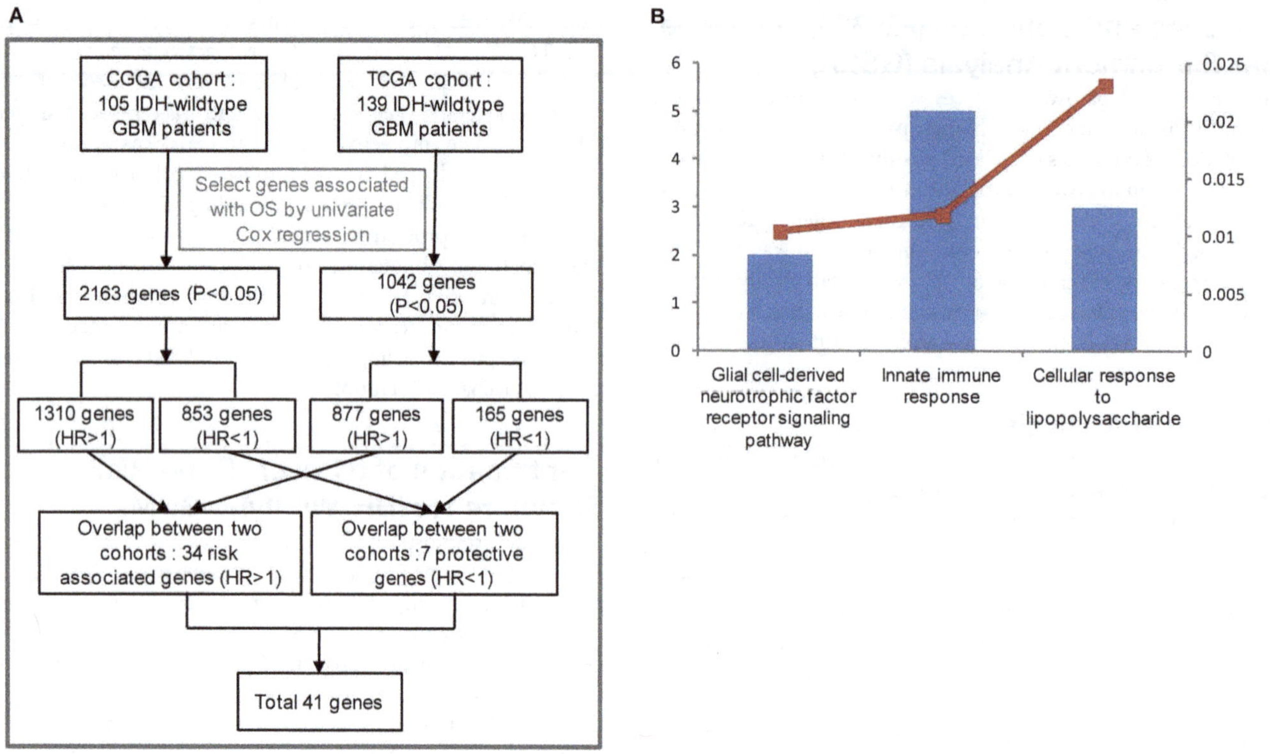

FIGURE 1 | Functional analysis of 41 candidate genes associated with overall survival (OS). **(A)** Flowchart of data analysis for the search of OS-correlated critically important genes. The GBM IDH-wild type patients from the CGGA (105) and TCGA cohorts (139) were analyzed. As a result, 2,163 and 1,042 genes associated with OS were selected by univariate Cox regression, respectively. Among the 2,163 genes for the CGGA cohort, 1,310 genes were considered to be risk associated genes (HR >1) and 853 genes were identified to be protective genes (HR<1). As for the 1,042 genes from the TCGA cohort, 877 genes (HR >1), and 165 genes (HR<1) were regarded as risk associated and protective genes, respectively. The risk associated and protective genes were then overlapped between the CGGA and TCGA cohorts, respectively. As a result, 41 candidate genes associated with OS were obtained by combining 34 risk associated genes with 7 protective genes. **(B)** Functional annotation of 41 candidate genes using GO terms of biological processes. The left bar represents the gene number and the right bar represents the *P*-value. CGGA, Chinese Glioma Genome Atlas; TCGA, The Cancer Genome Atlas; HR, hazard ratio; OS, overall survival.

group with a methylated MGMT promoter, compared to the low-risk patients, the OS of high-risk patients was also significantly lower ($P = 0.0219$; **Figure 3J**). On the other hand, there were no significant differences between patients with a methylated MGMT promoter ($P > 0.05$; **Figure 3K**).

Subsequently, we explored whether the prognostic value of the seven-gene signature could be extended to IDH-mutant GBM and lower grade glioma (LGG, WHO grade II-III), by calculating a risk score using the same formula in the CGGA and TCGA cohorts. A Kaplan-Meier analysis showed that there was no significant difference between the low- and high-risk groups in IDH-mutant GBM from the CGGA-RNAseq and TCGA-microarray datasets (**Figures S1A,B**). According to the WHO 2016 update to the classification strategy, LGG were categorized into three subtypes (IDH-wildtype LGG, LGG-IDHmut- non-codel and LGG-IDHmut-codel) based on the status of IDH mutation and 1p/19q codeletion (7). The results showed that the survival time of the high-risk group was remarkably shorter than that of the low-risk group in LGG-IDHmut-non-codel (**Figure S1D**), whereas there was no significant difference in IDH-wildtype LGG and LGG-IDHmut-codel between the two risk groups in the CGGA-RNAseq cohort (**Figures S1C,E**). Furthermore, we found there was no significant difference in the survival of the high- and low-risk groups in all three subtypes of LGG from the TCGA-RNAseq cohort (**Figures S1F–H**). In summary, these results indicated that the seven-gene signature could not predict the prognosis of patients with IDH-mutant GBM and LGG, identified as an exclusive prognostic marker for IDH-wildtype GBM.

Seven-Gene Signature Is an Independent Prognostic Factor for IDH-Wildtype GBM

We further evaluated the prognostic value of the seven-gene signature for IDH-wildtype GBM patients. Uni- and multivariate Cox regression analyses of the clinical features and seven-gene-based risk score for OS were performed to determine the prognostic significance of the seven-gene signature in IDH-wildtype GBM patients from the CGGA datasets. The results showed that the seven-gene signature was independently associated with OS by adjusting for clinicopathological factors (age, gender, GBM sub-type, radiotherapy, chemotherapy, MGMT promoter methylation status, and TERT status; $P < 0.001$; **Figure 4A**). Consistently, the seven-gene risk signature was validated as an independent indicator after

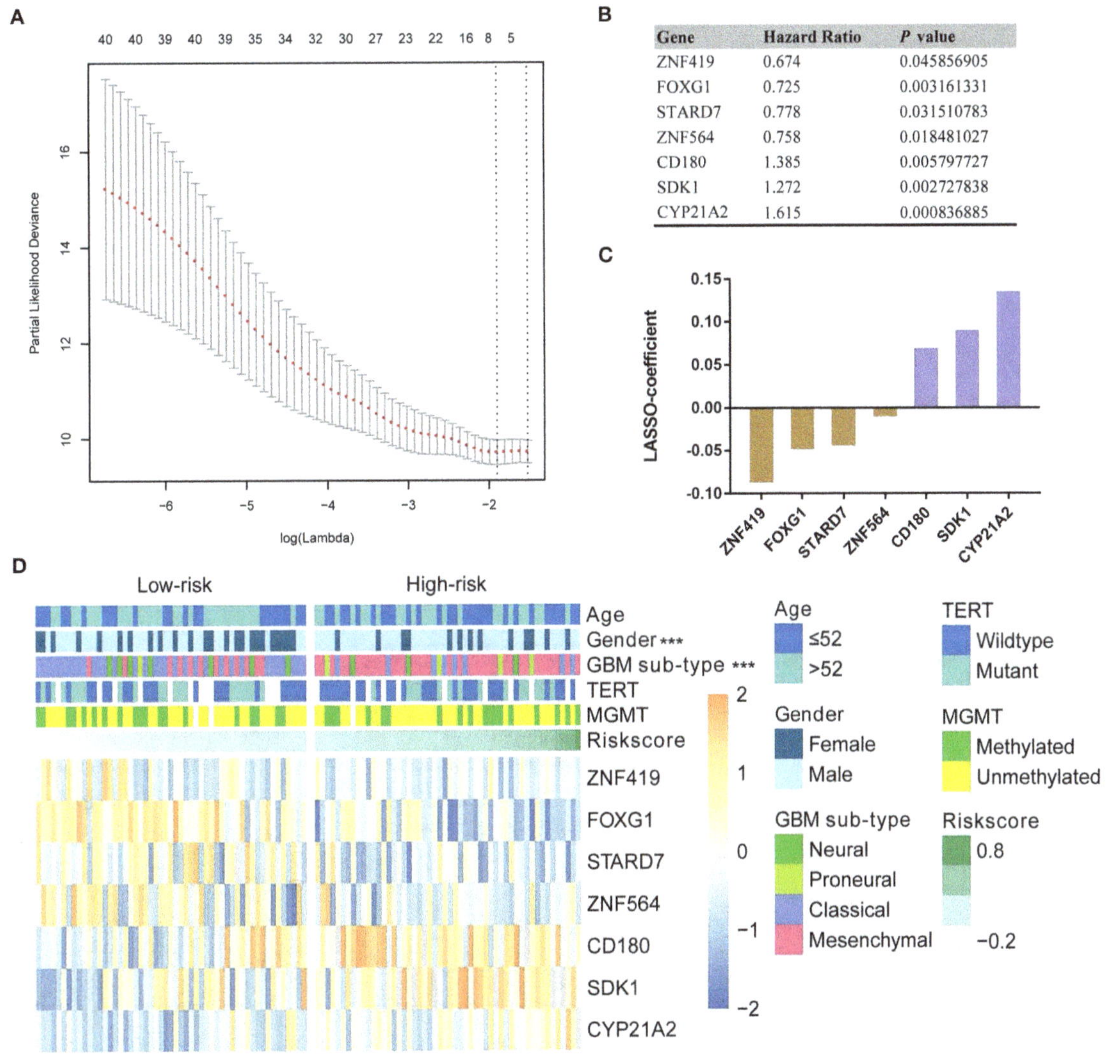

Gene	Hazard Ratio	*P* value
ZNF419	0.674	0.045856905
FOXG1	0.725	0.003161331
STARD7	0.778	0.031510783
ZNF564	0.758	0.018481027
CD180	1.385	0.005797727
SDK1	1.272	0.002727838
CYP21A2	1.615	0.000836885

FIGURE 2 | Identification of a seven-gene risk signature for OS by LASSO regression analysis in CGGA GBM-IDH wildtype datasets. **(A)** Partial likelihood deviance as a function of the regularization parameter λ in the CGGA GBM-IDH wildtype dataset. The red point denotes the λ value along the regularization paths, and the gray error bars represent the confidence intervals for the cross-validated error rate. The horizontal row of numbers above the plot denotes the gene number in each condition upon shrinkage and selection based on linear regression. The left vertical dotted line denotes the minimum error, and the right vertical dotted line represents the largest λ value. The gene expression analyses of seven genes selected and their regression coefficients by LASSO are shown in **(B,C)**, respectively. **(D)** Heat map showing the association between the risk scores and clinicopathological features based on the seven-gene risk signature. CGGA, Chinese Glioma Genome Atlas; LASSO, Least Absolute Shrinkage and Selection Operator; MGMT, methylguanine methyltransferase; TERT, telomerase reverse transcriptase; TCGA, The Cancer Genome Atlas; HR, hazard ratio.

multivariate Cox regression analyses in the TCGA cohort ($P < 0.001$; **Figure 4B**).

Prognostic Validity of the Seven-Gene Signature for IDH-Wildtype GBM

Subsequently, we determined the specificity and sensitivity of the risk score in the prediction of 1-year survival by calculating the area under the curve (AUC) of the risk score and the pathologic features using the receiving operator characteristic (ROC) curve. As shown in **Figures 4C,D**, the seven-gene signature showed a striking prognostic validity, with an AUC of 78.4 and 73.9%, which were higher those found for the traditional "age" (53.7%, 62.4%) and "GBM sub-type" (57.7%, 52.9%) in the CGGA- and TCGA-RNAseq databases, respectively. These data indicate that the seven-gene signature could be used as a potential prognostic marker of IDH-wildtype GBM.

Association of the Seven-Gene Signature With Other Clinicopathological Features of IDH-Wildtype GBM

To evaluate the performance of the identified signature as a classifier, we classified the CGGA dataset into low- and high-risk groups using the median risk score as a cutoff point, and found a significant difference in several clinical characteristics

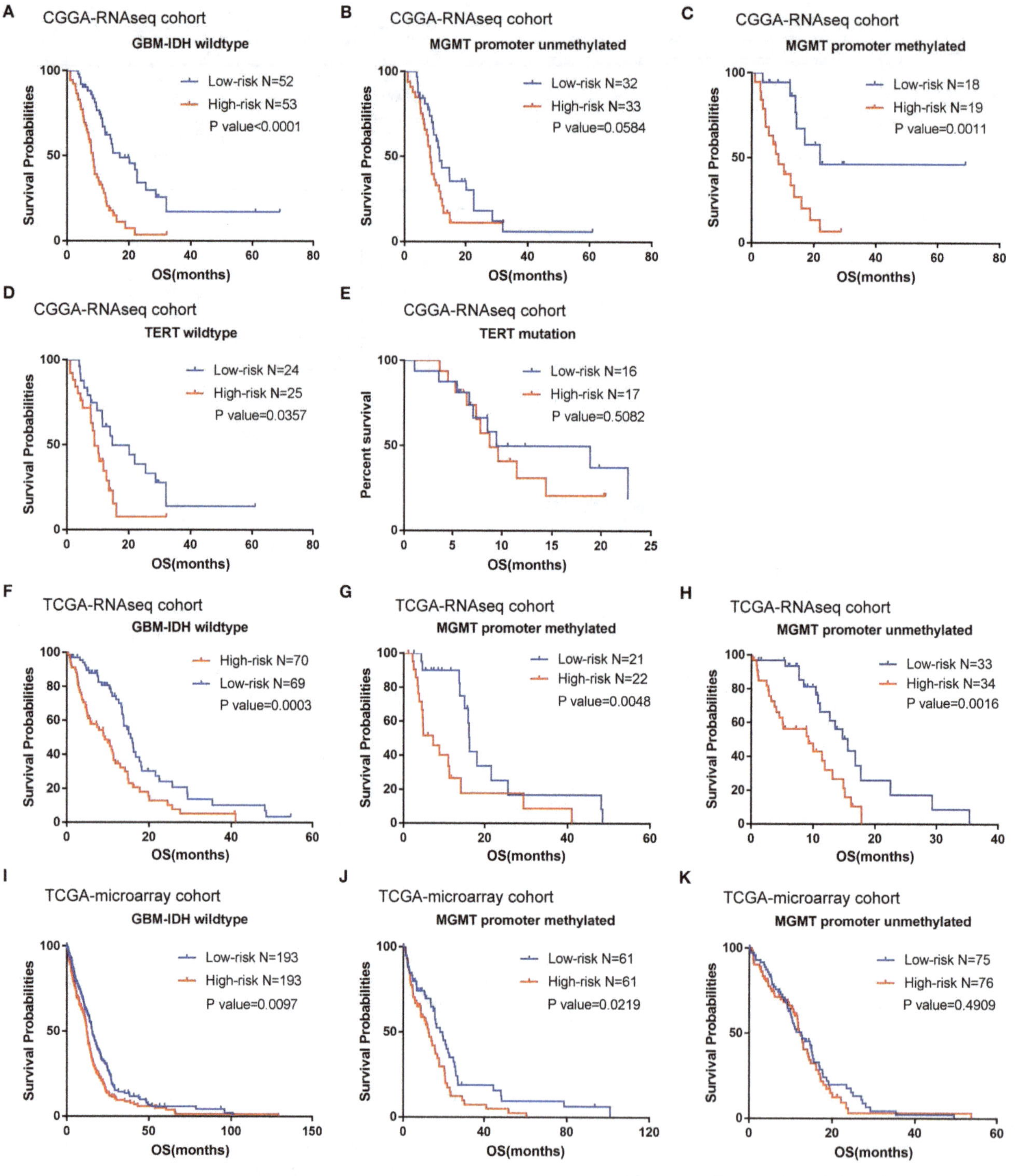

FIGURE 3 | Prognostic significance of the seven-gene signature-based risk scores in GBM-IDH wildtype samples from CGGA and TCGA-RNAseq datasets. **(A–E)** Prognosis efficiency of the seven-gene risk signature in the total GBM-IDH wildtype **(A)**, and MGMT promoter unmethylated **(B)** and methylated **(C)**, TERT promoter wildtype **(D)**, and mutation samples **(E)** from the CGGA-RNAseq datasets, respectively. **(F–H)** Prognosis efficiency of the seven-gene risk signature in TCGA GBM-IDH wildtype datasets **(F)** and MGMT promoter unmethylated **(G)** and methylated **(H)** of GBM-IDH wildtype from the TCGA-RNAseq datasets, respectively. **(I–K)** Prognosis efficiency of the seven-gene risk signature in IDH wildtype GBM from TCGA-microarray datasets **(I)** and MGMT promoter unmethylated **(J)** and methylated **(K)** from the CGGA GBM-IDH wildtype datasets, respectively. The *P*-value shown in each panel were determined using a log-rank test between the two groups. $P < 0.05$ was considered as statistically significant. CGGA, Chinese Glioma Genome Atlas; GBM, glioblastoma; OS, overall survival; TCGA, The Cancer Genome Atlas; IDH, isocitrate dehydrogenases.

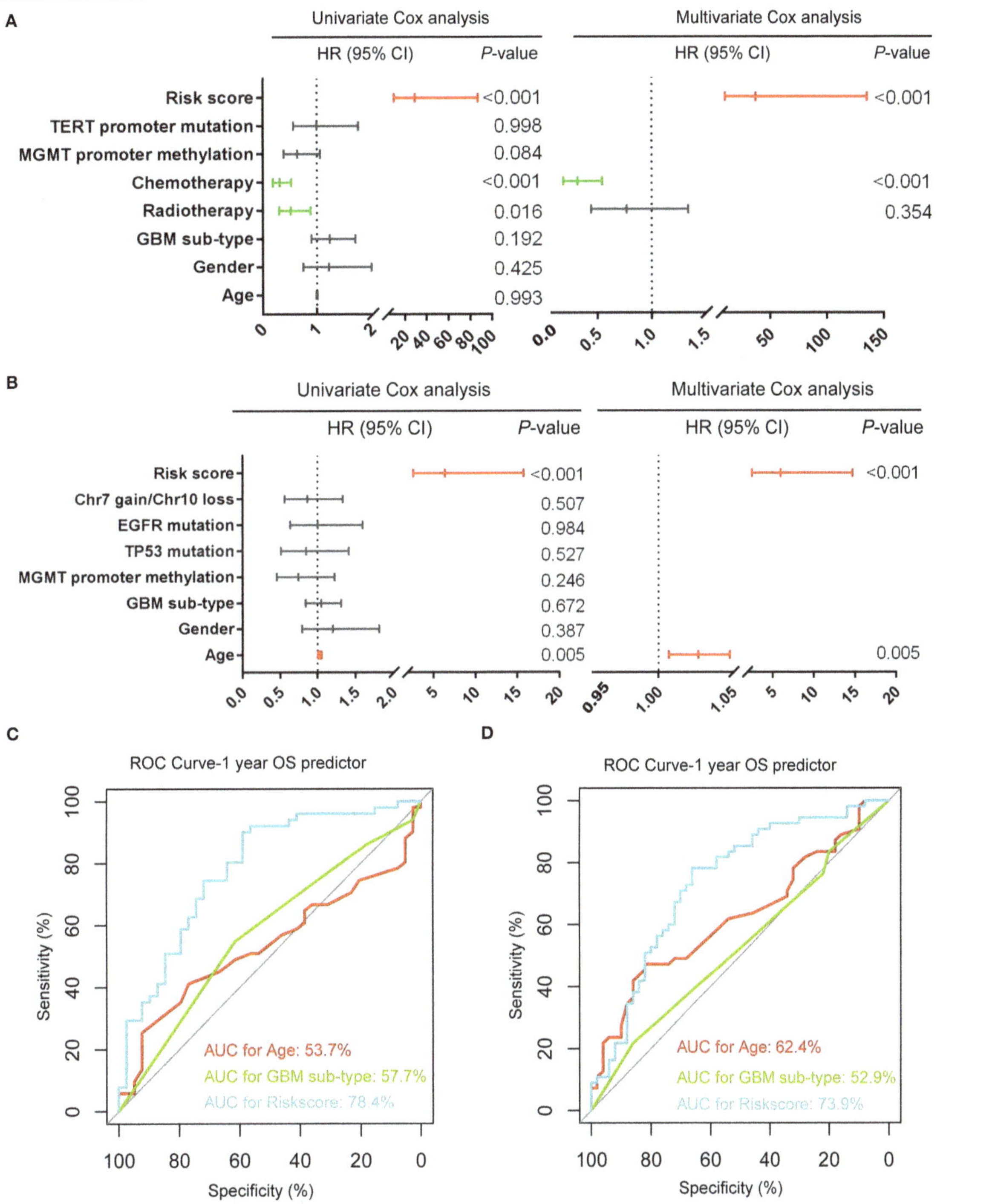

FIGURE 4 | Prognostic validity of the seven-gene signature-based risk scores in GBM-IDH wildtype samples from CGGA and TCGA-RNAseq datasets. **(A,B)** Uni-and multivariate Cox regression analysis of the clinical features and seven-gene-based risk score for OS in GBM-IDH wildtype from CGGA **(A)** and TCGA **(B)** datasets. Variables with prognostic significance in univariate Cox regression analysis were included in further multivariate Cox analysis. Gender (female and male); GBM sub-type (neural, proneural, mesenchymal, and classical); MGMT promoter methylation status (methylated and unmethylated); TERT promoter status (mutant and wildtype); TP53 status (mutant and wildtype); EGFR status (mutant and wildtype); Chr7 gain/Chr10 loss status (combined and not combined); radiotherapy (yes and no); chemotherapy (yes and no); risk score (low and high). **(C,D)** Comparison between the seven-gene signature and traditional risk factors such as age and GBM sub-type in terms of sensitivity and specificity for predicting 1-year survival in the CGGA **(C)** and TCGA **(D)** datasets, respectively. CI, confidence interval; CGGA, Chinese Glioma Genome Atlas; HR, hazard ratio; OS, overall survival; ROC, receiver operating characteristic.

between the two groups (**Figure 2D**). We found that male patients accounted for a large proportion, 75.5% of the total, of the high-risk group, compared to a proportion of male patients of 53.8% in the low-risk group ($P < 0.001$). As shown in **Table S1**, the classical and mesenchymal subtypes were found in 61.5 and 23.1%, 17.0 and 69.8% of low-risk and high-risk groups, respectively ($P < 0.001$) (**Table S1**).

In the TCGA-RNAseq cohort, patients were divided into low- and high-risk groups based on their median risk value. A marked difference was found in several molecular features between the two groups (**Figure S2**). The combination of "gain of chromosome 7" and "loss of chromosome 10" was found in 78.3 and 55.7% of patients in the low-risk and high-risk groups, respectively ($P < 0.001$). Moreover, we found that 30.4 and 18.6% of samples in the low- and high-risk groups, respectively, were found to harbor mutations in the epidermal growth factor receptor (EGFR) gene ($P = 0.029$) (**Table S2**). In conclusion, for the CGGA and TCGA cohorts, in comparison with the low-risk group, the high-risk group tended to consist of patients with a worse prognosis.

A previous study identified four clinically relevant subtypes (neural, proneural, classical, mesenchymal) of GBM using integrated genomic analysis (28). Here, we investigated the association between the seven-gene signature and subtype, and found that patients with mesenchymal GBM had a higher risk score than those with classical GBM in the CGGA ($P < 0.0001$; **Figure S3A**) and TCGA cohorts ($P < 0.05$; **Figure S3E**). On the other hand, there was no significant correlation between the risk signature and other features, such as age, MGMT status, TERT status, and P53 status in the CGGA (**Figures S3B–D**) and TCGA cohorts (**Figures S3F–H**).

Functional Annotation of the Seven-Gene Signature

To investigate the potentially altered functional features correlated with the seven-gene signature, GO and KEGG analyses were conducted based on 589 high-risk score positively-related genes ($P < 0.05$) and 152 negatively-related genes ($P < 0.05$) using Pearson correlation analysis. GO enrichment showed that the top five involved biological processes, that is upregulated gene- in the high-risk group, were "inflammatory response," "immune response," "cell adhesion," "innate immune response," and "apoptotic process." In contrast, downregulated genes in the high-risk group were closely associated with neurogenesis functions, such as "brain development," "nervous system development," "axon guidance," and "ion transmembrane transport" (**Figure 5A**).

Moreover, KEGG pathway analysis showed that positively-related genes in the high-risk group were primarily enriched in biological processes for "TNF signaling pathway," "cytokine-cytokine receptor interaction," "leukocyte transendothelial migration," "toll-like receptor signaling pathway," and "chemokine signaling pathway," whereas the negatively correlated genes were enriched in biological terms including "GABAergic synapse," "Rap1 signaling pathway," and "glioma" (**Figure 5B**).

In addition, GSEA analyses were performed for validation, showing that the high-risk groups were positively associated with inflammatory response ($P < 0.001$) and TNFα signaling via NFκB ($P = 0.019$), IL2-STAT5 signaling ($P < 0.001$), K-ras signaling ($P < 0.001$), and apoptosis ($P < 0.001$; **Figures 5C–H**). Consistently, these results were validated in the TCGA cohort (**Figure S4**).

DISCUSSION

In the current study, we studied various candidate genes with potential functions as biomarkers for the stratification of IDH-wildtype GBM with distinct prognoses using whole-genome expression data. We first screened 41 candidate genes, closely associated with OS of IDH-wildtype GBM, by combining the CGGA-RNAseq and TCGA-RNAseq datasets. We then created a seven-gene-based risk signature for IDH-wildtype GBM in the CGGA-RNAseq cohort, which was subsequently validated in the TCGA-RNAseq and TCGA-microarray cohorts. Moreover, the seven-gene risk signature, identified as an independent prognostic significance for IDH1-wildtype GBM, exhibited a greater prognostic value than other factors, underscoring the superiority of a gene expression profile-based signature (29, 30). Finally, bioinformatics analysis was used to predict that the seven-gene signature was involved in the inflammatory response, immune response, cell adhesion, and apoptotic process. To summarize, our seven-gene-based signature refined the current classification system of IDH-wildtype GBM and contributed to improving our understanding of the carcinogenesis and development of IDH-wildtype GBM.

In this study, we established a seven-gene-based signature based on the diversity of genes, including protective (*ZNF419, FOXG1, STARD7*, and ZBTB16) and risk associated (*CD180, SDK1*, and *CYP21A2*) genes, which could classify IDH-wildtype GBM into low- and high-risk groups to distinguish between the clinical outcomes. Among these genes, several had been previously studied in various tumors. Some studies have suggested that FoxG1 functions as an oncogene by promoting proliferation, as well as inhibiting differential responses in glioblastoma, by downregulating FoxO/Smad signaling (31). Moreover, low FoxG1 and high Olig-2 labeling indices define a prognostically favorable subset in IDH-mutant gliomas (32). ZBTB16 (Zinc Finger and BTB Domain Containing 16), is a transcription factor involved in the regulation of diverse biological processes, including cell proliferation, differentiation, organ development, stem cell maintenance, and innate immune cell development. A number of recent studies have now implicated PLZF in cancer progression as a tumor suppressor (33). CYP21A2 (21-hydroxylase) is a steroidogenic enzyme crucial for the synthesis of mineralocorticoids and glucocorticoids, and was identified as the most frequently mutated gene in esophageal squamous cell carcinoma by whole exome sequencing (34, 35).

The 2016 WHO classification made a clear difference between GBM that were IDH-mutant and those that were IDH-wildtype, and IDH-wildtype GBM carried a worse prognosis. Consistently, in the cohorts used in this study, the median OS of the

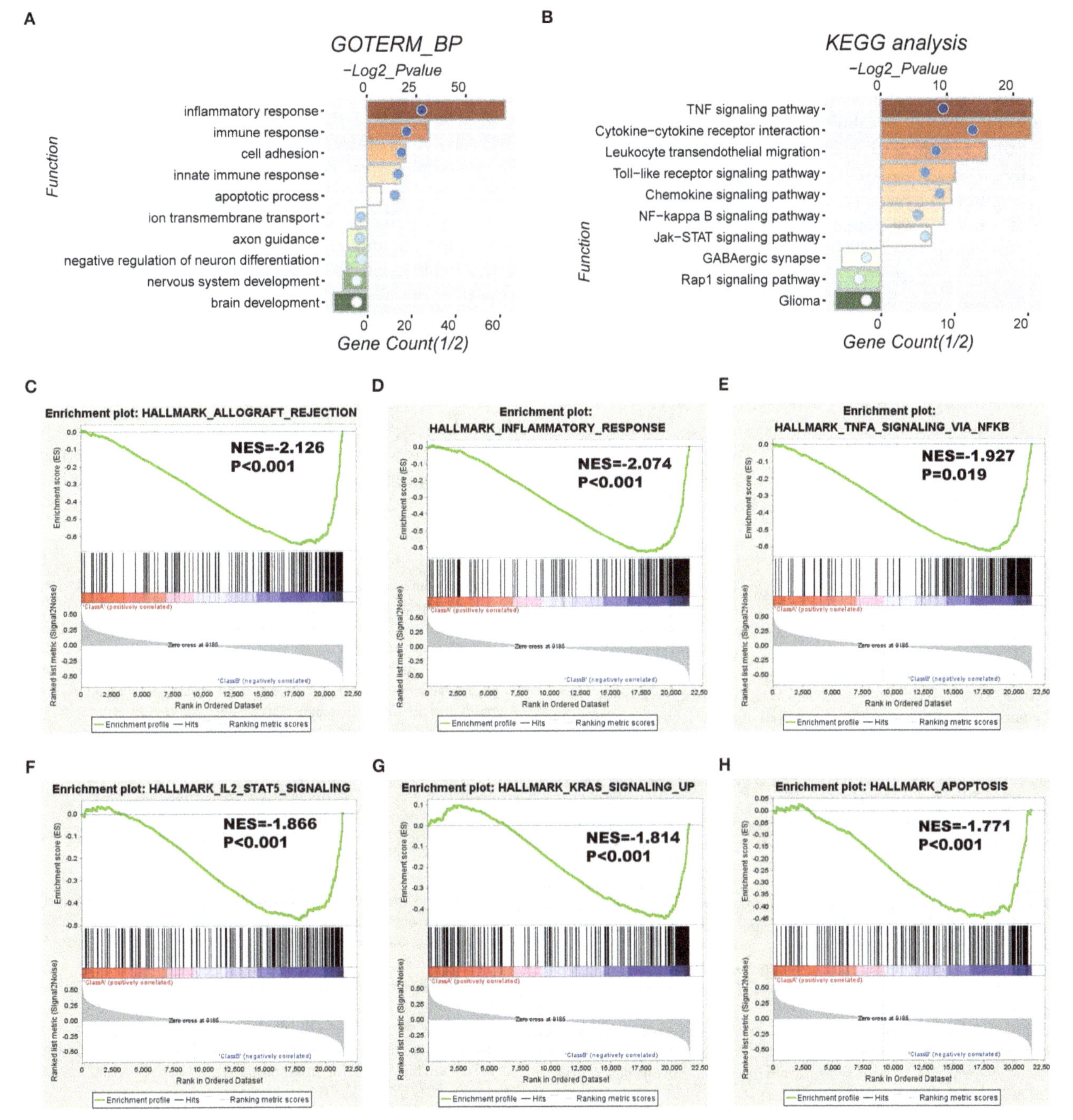

FIGURE 5 | Functional characteristics correlated with the seven-gene signature in CGGA-RNAseq datasets. **(A,B)** Functional annotation of genes positively (red bar chart) or negatively (green bar chart) correlated with the risk score using the GO terms of biological processes **(A)** and the KEGG pathway **(B)**. Orange and green bars represent the *P*-value, and the blue dots represent the 1/2 gene count. **(C–H)** Gene set enrichment analysis (GSEA) shows that a higher risk score was positively associated with the inflammatory response, immune response-related signaling pathways, and apoptosis. NES, normalized enrichment score.

IDH-wildtype GBM are 11.5, 13.3, and 13.83 months in the CGGA-RNAseq cohort, TCGA-RNAseq cohort and TCGA-microarray cohort, respectively, while, those of the IDH-mutant GBM are 18.5 months (CGGA-RNAseq cohort), 34.13 months (TCGA-RNAseq cohort), and 35.9 months (TCGA microarray cohort). However, we observed that the survival of patients with IDH-wildtype GBM varies from <3 months to more than 3 years, and the similar findings have also been reported in the previous study (3). Therefore, to further stratify IDH-wildtype GBM becomes important and meaningful.

In this study, we determined a seven-gene-based risk signature, a useful tool for risk stratification, to distinguish between prognoses for IDH-wildtype GBM in three independent cohorts. The median OS of patients with low- and high-risk are significantly different in the CGGA-RNAseq (17.13 vs. 8.47 months), TCGA-RNAseq (15.57 vs. 9.27 months) and TCGA-microarray cohorts (15.57 vs. 12.4 months). This is very meaningful to the post-operative management of these patients with IDH-wildtype GBM. Our previous study presented a gene signature based on GBM stem-like cell relevant genes for primary GBM (36). In addition, several previous studies have found a local immune signature for GBM, indicating the relationship between prognosis and the local immune response (19). Meanwhile, the strength of our study was based on the systematical expression profiling, the robust nature of risk score method (37), and validation across multi-platforms and multi-populations. Although the predictive value of the seven-gene signature was confirmed in distinct datasets, a prospective study with a larger sample size will be needed to assess its clinical relevance.

In conclusion, our results indicate that the seven-gene signature could be a potential prognostic biomarker, providing a novel perspective for research and treatment of IDH-wildtype GBM.

AUTHOR CONTRIBUTIONS

Y-QL and R-CC designed the study. Y-QL and FW reviewed the literature, created the figures and tables, and were responsible for the writing and critical editing of the manuscript. J-JL, Y-FL, XL, and ZW contributed to the data collection and analysis, as well as the critical revision of the manuscript. R-CC supervised the critical revision of the manuscript.

FUNDING

The authors represent the Chinese Glioma Cooperative Group (CGCG). This work was supported by grants from the National Natural Science Foundation of China (grant numbers 81903078, 81672479, 81702460, and 81773208).

REFERENCES

1. Ricard D, Idbaih A, Ducray F, Lahutte M, Hoang-Xuan K, Delattre JY. Primary brain tumours in adults. *Lancet.* (2012) 379:1984–96. doi: 10.1016/S0140-6736(11)61346-9
2. Brat DJ, Verhaak RG, Aldape KD, Yung WK, Salama SR, Cooper LA, et al. Comprehensive, integrative genomic analysis of diffuse lower-grade gliomas. *N Engl J Med.* (2015) 372:2481–98. doi: 10.1056/NEJMoa1402121
3. Jiang T, Mao Y, Ma W, Mao Q, You Y, Yang X, et al. CGCG clinical practice guidelines for the management of adult diffuse gliomas. *Cancer Lett.* (2016) 375:263–73. doi: 10.1016/j.canlet.2016.01.024
4. Chai RC, Wu F, Wang QX, Zhang S, Zhang KN, Liu YQ, et al. m(6)A RNA methylation regulators contribute to malignant progression and have clinical prognostic impact in gliomas. *Aging.* (2019) 11:1204–25. doi: 10.18632/aging.101829
5. Agnihotri S, Aldape KD, Zadeh G. Isocitrate dehydrogenase status and molecular subclasses of glioma and glioblastoma. *Neurosurg Focus.* (2014) 37:E13. doi: 10.3171/2014.9.FOCUS14505
6. Yan H, Parsons DW, Jin G, McLendon R, Rasheed BA, Yuan W, et al. IDH1 and IDH2 mutations in gliomas. *N Engl J Med.* (2009) 360:765–73. doi: 10.1056/NEJMoa0808710
7. Louis DN, Perry A, Reifenberger G, von Deimling A, Figarella-Branger D, Cavenee WK, et al. The 2016 world health organization classification of tumors of the central nervous system: a summary. *Acta Neuropathol.* (2016) 131:803–20. doi: 10.1007/s00401-016-1545-1
8. Watanabe T, Nobusawa S, Kleihues P, Ohgaki H. IDH1 mutations are early events in the development of astrocytomas and oligodendrogliomas. *Am J Pathol.* (2009) 174:1149–53. doi: 10.2353/ajpath.2009.080958
9. Kloosterhof NK, Bralten LB, Dubbink HJ, French PJ, van den Bent MJ. Isocitrate dehydrogenase-1 mutations: a fundamentally new understanding of diffuse glioma? *Lancet Oncol.* (2011) 12:83–91. doi: 10.1016/S1470-2045(10)70053-X
10. Cheng W, Ren X, Zhang C, Cai J, Han S, Wu A. Gene expression profiling stratifies IDH1-mutant glioma with distinct prognoses. *Mol Neurobiol.* (2017) 54:5996–6005. doi: 10.1007/s12035-016-0150-6
11. Korshunov A, Casalini B, Chavez L, Hielscher T, Sill M, Ryzhova M, et al. Integrated molecular characterization of IDH-mutant glioblastomas. *Neuropathol Appl Neurobiol.* (2019) 45:108–18. doi: 10.1111/nan.12523
12. Arita H, Yamasaki K, Matsushita Y, Nakamura T, Shimokawa A, Takami H, et al. A combination of TERT promoter mutation and MGMT methylation status predicts clinically relevant subgroups of newly diagnosed glioblastomas. *Acta Neuropathol Commun.* (2016) 4:79. doi: 10.1186/s40478-016-0351-2
13. Chai RC, Liu YQ, Zhang KN, Wu F, Zhao Z, Wang KY, et al. A novel analytical model of MGMT methylation pyrosequencing offers improved predictive performance in patients with gliomas. *Mod Pathol.* (2018) 32:4–15. doi: 10.1038/s41379-018-0143-2
14. Hu H, Mu Q, Bao Z, Chen Y, Liu Y, Chen J, et al. Mutational landscape of secondary glioblastoma guides MET-targeted trial in brain tumor. *Cell.* (2018)175:1665–78 e1618. doi: 10.1016/j.cell.2018.09.038
15. Wu F, Chai RC, Wang Z, Liu YQ, Zhao Z, Li GZ, et al. Molecular classification of IDH-mutant glioblastomas based on gene expression profiles. *Carcinogenesis.* (2019) 40:853–60. doi: 10.1093/carcin/bgz032
16. Wu F, Zhao Z, Chai R, Liu Y, Wang K, Wang Z, et al. Expression profile analysis of antisense long non-coding RNA identifies WDFY3-AS2 as a prognostic biomarker in diffuse glioma. *Cancer Cell Int.* (2018) 18:107. doi: 10.1186/s12935-018-0603-2
17. Brennan CW, Verhaak RG, McKenna A, Campos B, Noushmehr H, Salama SR, et al. The somatic genomic landscape of glioblastoma. *Cell.* (2013) 155:462–77. doi: 10.1016/j.cell.2013.09.034
18. Zhang C, Cheng W, Ren X, Wang Z, Liu X, Li G, et al. Tumor purity as an underlying key factor in Glioma. *Clin Cancer Res.* (2017) 23:6279–91. doi: 10.1158/1078-0432.CCR-16-2598
19. Cheng W, Ren X, Zhang C, Cai J, Liu Y, Han S, et al. Bioinformatic profiling identifies an immune-related risk signature for glioblastoma. *Neurology.* (2016) 86:2226–34. doi: 10.1212/WNL.0000000000002770
20. Subramanian A, Tamayo P, Mootha VK, Mukherjee S, Ebert BL, Gillette MA, et al. Gene set enrichment analysis: a knowledge-based approach for interpreting genome-wide expression profiles. *Proc Natl Acad Sci USA.* (2005) 102:15545–50. doi: 10.1073/pnas.0506580102
21. Gao J, Kwan PW, Shi D. Sparse kernel learning with LASSO and Bayesian inference algorithm. *Neural Netw.* (2010) 23:257–64. doi: 10.1016/j.neunet.2009.07.001
22. Qian Z, Li Y, Fan X, Zhang C, Wang Y, Jiang T, et al. Molecular and clinical characterization of IDH associated immune signature in lower-grade gliomas. *Oncoimmunology.* (2018) 7:e1434466. doi: 10.1080/2162402X.2018.1434466

23. Chai RC, Li YM, Zhang KN, Chang YZ, Liu YQ, Zhao Z, et al. RNA processing genes characterize RNA splicing and further stratify lower-grade glioma. *JCI Insight.* (2019) 5:130591. doi: 10.1172/jci.insight.130591
24. Chai RC, Zhang KN, Chang YZ, Wu F, Liu YQ, Zhao Z, et al. Systematically characterize the clinical and biological significances of 1p19q genes in 1p/19q non-codeletion glioma. *Carcinogenesis.* (2019) 40:1229–39. doi: 10.1093/carcin/bgz102
25. Liu YQ, Chai RC, Wang YZ, Wang Z, Liu X, Wu F, et al. Amino acid metabolism-related gene expression-based risk signature can better predict overall survival for glioma. *Cancer Sci.* (2019) 110:321–33. doi: 10.1111/cas.13878
26. Chai RC, Chang YZ, Wang QW, Zhang KN, Li JJ, Huang H, et al. A novel DNA methylation-based signature can predict the responses of MGMT promoter unmethylated glioblastomas to temozolomide. *Front Genet.* (2019) 10:910. doi: 10.3389/fgene.2019.00910
27. Chai RC, Zhang KN, Liu YQ, Wu F, Zhao Z, Wang KY, et al. Combinations of four or more CpGs methylation present equivalent predictive value for MGMT expression and temozolomide therapeutic prognosis in gliomas. *CNS Neurosci Ther.* (2018) 25:314–22. doi: 10.1111/cns.13040
28. Verhaak RG, Hoadley KA, Purdom E, Wang V, Qi Y, Wilkerson MD, et al. Integrated genomic analysis identifies clinically relevant subtypes of glioblastoma characterized by abnormalities in PDGFRA, IDH1, EGFR, and NF1. *Cancer Cell.* (2010) 17:98–110. doi: 10.1016/j.ccr.2009.12.020
29. Gravendeel LA, Kouwenhoven MC, Gevaert O, de Rooi JJ, Stubbs AP, Duijm JE, et al. Intrinsic gene expression profiles of gliomas are a better predictor of survival than histology. *Cancer Res.* (2009) 69:9065–72. doi: 10.1158/0008-5472.CAN-09-2307
30. Freije WA, Castro-Vargas FE, Fang Z, Horvath S, Cloughesy T, Liau LM, et al. Gene expression profiling of gliomas strongly predicts survival. *Cancer Res.* (2004) 64:6503–10. doi: 10.1158/0008-5472.CAN-04-0452
31. Wang L, Wang J, Jin T, Zhou Y, Chen Q. FoxG1 facilitates proliferation and inhibits differentiation by downregulating FoxO/Smad signaling in glioblastoma. *Biochem Biophys Res Commun.* (2018) 504:46–53. doi: 10.1016/j.bbrc.2018.08.118
32. Schafer S, Behling F, Skardelly M, Koch M, Ott I, Paulsen F, et al. Low FoxG1 and high Olig-2 labelling indices define a prognostically favourable subset in isocitrate dehydrogenase (IDH)-mutant gliomas. *Neuropathol Appl Neurobiol.* (2018) 44:207–23. doi: 10.1111/nan.12447
33. Stopsack KH, Gerke T, Tyekucheva S, Mazzu YZ, Lee GM, Chakraborty G, et al. Low expression of the androgen-induced tumor suppressor gene PLZF and lethal prostate cancer. *Cancer Epidemiol Biomarkers Prev.* (2019) 28:707–14. doi: 10.1158/1055-9965.EPI-18-1014
34. Neunzig J, Milhim M, Schiffer L, Khatri Y, Zapp J, Sanchez-Guijo A, et al. The steroid metabolite 16(beta)-OH-androstenedione generated by CYP21A2 serves as a substrate for CYP19A1. *J Steroid Biochem Mol Biol.* (2017) 167:182–91. doi: 10.1016/j.jsbmb.2017.01.002
35. Deng J, Weng X, Ye J, Zhou D, Liu Y, Zhao K. Identification of the germline mutation profile in esophageal squamous cell carcinoma by whole exome sequencing. *Front Genet.* (2019) 10:47. doi: 10.3389/fgene.2019.00047
36. Chai R, Zhang K, Wang K, Li G, Huang R, Zhao Z, et al. A novel gene signature based on five glioblastoma stem-like cell relevant genes predicts the survival of primary glioblastoma. *J Cancer Res Clin Oncol.* (2018) 144:439–47. doi: 10.1007/s00432-017-2572-6
37. Yan W, Zhang W, You G, Zhang J, Han L, Bao Z, et al. Molecular classification of gliomas based on whole genome gene expression: a systematic report of 225 samples from the Chinese Glioma Cooperative Group. *Neuro Oncol.* (2012) 14:1432–40. doi: 10.1093/neuonc/nos263

2

A Risk Classification System With Five-Gene for Survival Prediction of Glioblastoma Patients

Yulin Wang [1], *Xin Liu* [2], *Gefei Guan* [3], *Weijiang Zhao* [4*] *and Minghua Zhuang* [1*]

[1] *Department of Neurosurgery, The First Affiliated Hospital of Shantou University Medical College, Shantou, China,*
[2] *Department of Stomatology, The First Affiliated Hospital of Shantou University Medical College, Shantou, China,*
[3] *Department of Neurosurgery, The First Hospital of China Medical University, Shenyang, China,* [4] *Center for Neuroscience, Shantou University Medical College, Shantou, China*

***Correspondence:**
Weijiang Zhao
neuromancn@aliyun.com
Minghua Zhuang
281902113@qq.com

Objective: Glioblastoma (GBM) is the most common and fatal primary brain tumor in adults. It is necessary to identify novel and effective biomarkers or risk signatures for GBM patients.

Methods: Differentially expressed genes (DEGs) between GBM and low-grade glioma (LGG) in TCGA samples were screened out and weight correlation network analysis (WGCNA) was performed to confirm WHO grade-related genes. Five genes were selected via multivariate Cox proportional hazards regression analysis and were used to construct a risk signature. A nomogram composed of the risk signature and clinical characters (age, radiotherapy, and chemotherapy experience) was established to predict 1, 3, 5-year survival rate for GBM patients.

Results: One hundred ninety-four DEGs in blue gene module were found to be positively related to WHO grade via WGCNA. Five genes (DES, RANBP17, CLEC5A, HOXC11, POSTN) were selected to construct a risk signature for GBM via R language. This risk signature was identified to independently predict the outcome of GBM patients, as well as stratified by IDH1 status, MGMT promoter status, and radio-chemotherapy. The nomogram was established which combined the risk signature with clinical factors. The results of c-index, ROC curve and calibration plot revealed the nomogram showing a good accuracy for predicting 1, 3, or 5-year survival of GBM patients.

Conclusion: The risk signature with five genes could serve as an independent factor for predicting the prognosis of patients with GBM. Moreover, the nomogram with the risk signature and clinical traits proved to perform better for predicting 1, 3, 5-year survival rate.

Keywords: glioblastoma (GBM), WGCNA, risk signature, nomogram, prognosis

INTRODUCTION

Glioblastoma (GBM) is the most common and aggressive type of primary brain tumor in adult. Despite comprehensive regimens including maximum surgical resection, radiation therapy and chemotherapy, the prognosis of GBM is notoriously poor, with a median survival of 14 months and the 5-year survival rate remaining at ~5% (1). While intervention of these multimodal treatments cannot eradicate this devastating disease, therapeutic resistance and GBM recurrence were inevitable. Although temozolomide (TMZ) has been proven to prolong the survival of GBM patients as a first-line chemotherapeutic agent, recent studies show that an amount of patients with GBM develop resistance to TMZ during treatment (2), and the recurrence rate of GBM was up to 90% (3). These awful therapeutic outcomes were mainly attributed to glioma stem cells (GSCs) and heterogeneity in GBM (4, 5). Likewise, several new drugs, such as monoclonal antibody targeting epidermal growth factor receptor variant III (EGFRvIII), have been proven to show therapeutic efficiency in some cancers, but not in glioma (6). Since only 30% of GBM cases contain EGFRvIII, this means a majority of GBM patients fail to benefit from EGFRvIII-targeted therapy (7, 8). Therefore, it becomes particularly important to search for novel molecular biomarkers that precisely predict the prognosis and to choose appropriate individualized treatment strategies for patients with GBM.

With the progress of genetics and molecular biology, an increasing number of molecular biomarkers were discovered in glioma, for instance, IDH mutation, MGMT methylation, TERT promoter mutation, EGFR and P53 (9). As is known to all, IDH1/2 mutation and MGMT promoter methylation are two important biomarkers in glioma. IDH mutation mainly exists in low grade glioma and secondary GBM, and associates with prognosis and GBM subtype (10). Moreover, IDH phenotype was also reported to be potent to form a glioma CpG island methylator phenotype (G-CIMP) and to be related to genomic methylation and gene mutation, such as P53 and TERT mutation (10). MGMT promoter methylation accounts for ~40% of GBM samples and associates with favorable prognosis of patients receiving radiotherapy and chemotherapy (11). Interestingly, it has been observed that IDH-mutated gliomas frequently carry MGMT promoter methylation and are sensitive to temozolomide (12). These findings indicate that there are cross talks among these key molecular biomarkers and a single gene cannot completely represent the characters of the glioma, as well as GBM. This may partially explain that GBM patients fail to take more advantages from some targeted small molecule inhibitors application (13). Therefore, risk signatures with correlative biomarkers have been developed, which have shown better performance in GBM treatment and survival prediction (14, 15). In this study, we developed a risk signature with five genes associated with survival of GBM patients. On this basis, a nomogram including the risk signature and clinical factors was established and it proved to be effective in predicting the clinical outcome of patients with GBM.

MATERIALS AND METHODS

Data of Glioma Patients in the Study

Gene expression and survival data of glioma in TCGA were downloaded from GlioVis (http://gliovis.bioinfo.cnio.es/) (16). six hundred twenty samples from TCGA GBMLGG (RNA-seq) were selected for screening differentially expressed genes between GBM and low-grade glioma (LGG). Five hundred twenty-five samples from TCGA GBM (HG-UG133A) were used to construct a clinical survival prediction model and internal validation.

Identification of Differentially Expressed Genes Between GBM and LGG

Based on 470 lower grade glioma (LGG, World Health Organization [WHO] grade II and III) (17, 18) and 150 GBM samples in TCGA GBMLGG dataset, R language (edgeR package, R version 3.51) was performed to identify differentially expressed genes (DEGs). Genes with $|\log_2(\text{fold-change})| > 1$ and false discovery rate (FDR) < 0.05 were considered as DEGs for further analysis.

Weighted Correlation Network Analysis for Discovering Grade-Related Gene Modules

To select glioma grade-related genes from DEGs, we performed weight correlation network analysis (WGCNA) (19). The expression data of DEGs and clinical data (WHO grade, age, gender, IDH status, survival time, and status) were imported and analyzed by R package WGCNA. The genes were classified into several gene modules using an appropriate soft-thresholding power which was calculated by the pickSoftThreshold function (20). The minimum gene size in each module was set as 10. The module eigengenes were calculated and similar modules were clustered and merged according to the module dissection threshold. The correlations between gene modules and clinical traits were calculated and visualized through a heatmap. In this research, we chose the module which is positively related to WHO grade for further study.

Construction and Evaluation of Risk Signature With Selected Genes

Univariate Cox proportional hazards regression analysis was applied to assess the relationship between the expression of DEGs and the overall survival (OS) of patients with GBM in TCGA GBMLGG (RNA-seq) and HG-UG133A platform, respectively. Common genes with $P < 0.05$ were sorted out and presented as a Venn diagram by R. We then performed multivariate Cox proportional hazards models and filtered the common genes by step function in R. A risk score formula was designed according to the multivariate Cox regression analysis results (18), as follows:

$$\text{Risk score} = (\text{expr}_{\text{gene1}} \times \text{Coef}_{\text{gene1}}) + (\text{expr}_{\text{gene2}} \times \text{Coef}_{\text{gene2}}) + \ldots + (\text{expr}_{\text{genen}} \times \text{Coef}_{\text{genen}})$$

The patients were divided into low-risk and high-risk groups according to the median risk score value. KM survival analysis and time-dependent receiver operating characteristic (ROC) curve analysis were used to evaluate the prognostic value.

Bioinformatics Analysis

DEGs between low-risk and high-risk groups with FDR < 0.05 were filtered by R language (edgeR package) and used for Gene ontology (GO) and KEGG pathway analysis via DAVID website (https://david.ncifcrf.gov/) (21). GO terms (FDR <0.05) and KEGG pathways (*P*-value <0.05) were screened out and visualized via R package ggplot2. Gene set enrichment analysis (GSEA, http://software.broadinstitute.org/gsea/index.jsp) were used to confirm the GO terms and KEGG pathways in the low-risk and high-risk groups (22). Normalized enrichment score (NES) and FDR were calculated to verify the statistical difference for GSEA analysis.

Construction and Evaluation of Clinical Survival Prediction Model

By combining with clinical data, a nomogram of clinical survival prediction model was established by using the package of "rms" in R. Samples from TCGA HG-UG133A platform were divided into training cohort (accounting for 70%) and validation cohort (accounting for 30%) by randomly using R package "caret." The inclusion criteria for data extraction in the predictive model were patients diagnosed with WHO grade IV glioma (GBM).

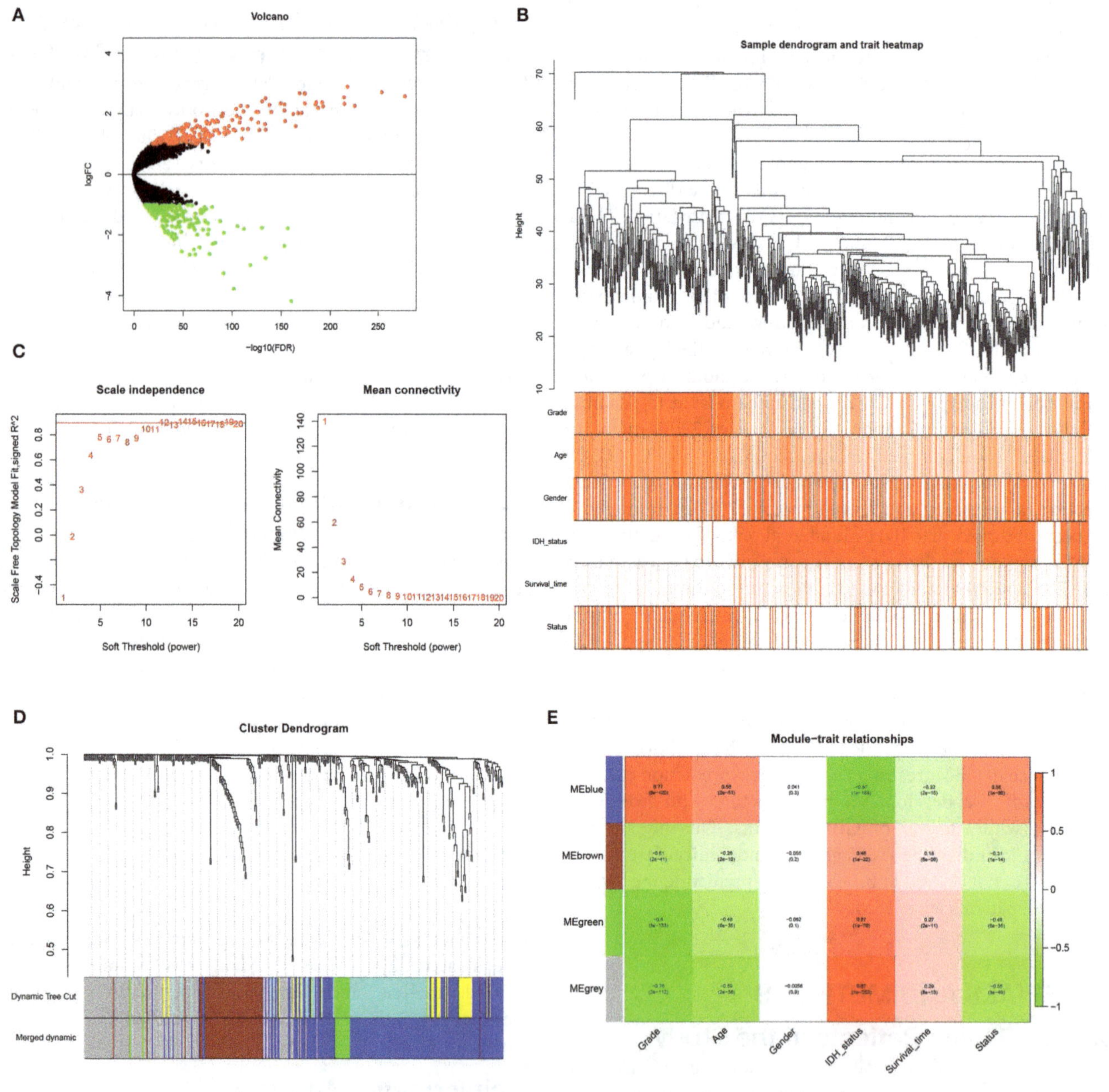

FIGURE 1 | Identification of WHO grade-related genes in glioma. **(A)** Volcano plot showed the distribution of DEGs. **(B)** Sample clusters showed basic clinical information of glioma patients. **(C)** The soft threshold power was calculated and 10 was selected as the power value. **(D)** Similar modules were merged and four modules were generated. **(E)** Heatmap exhibited the relationships between gene modules and clinical traits by Pearson correlation.

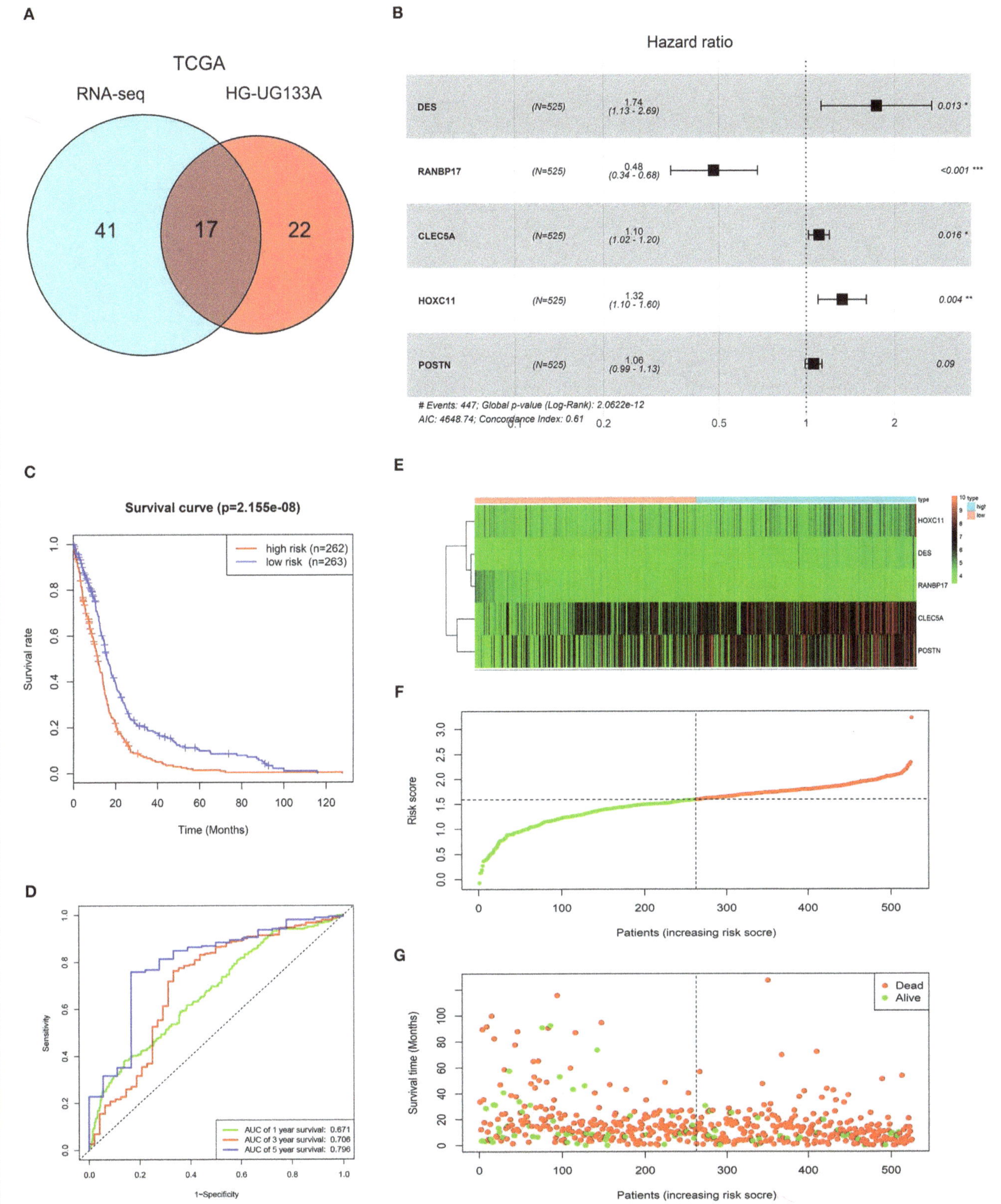

FIGURE 2 | Characteristics of the risk signature with five genes. **(A)** Venn diagram showed 17 common genes correlated with overall survival ($P < 0.05$) between TCGA GBMLGG (RNA-seq) and HG-UG133A platforms. **(B)** Multivariable Cox regression analysis was performed and five genes (DES, RANBP17, CLEC5A, HOXC11, POSTN) were selected to construct the risk signature. **(C)** Difference of overall survival between low-risk and high-risk groups ($P < 0.0001$). **(D)** ROC analysis of 1, 3, 5-year survival according to the five-gene risk signature. **(E)** The expression levels of the five genes (DES, RANBP17, CLEC5A, HOXC11, POSTN) in the signature. **(F)** The distribution of the five-gene signature risk score for each patient. **(G)** The survival time of each patient with GBM and their survival status.

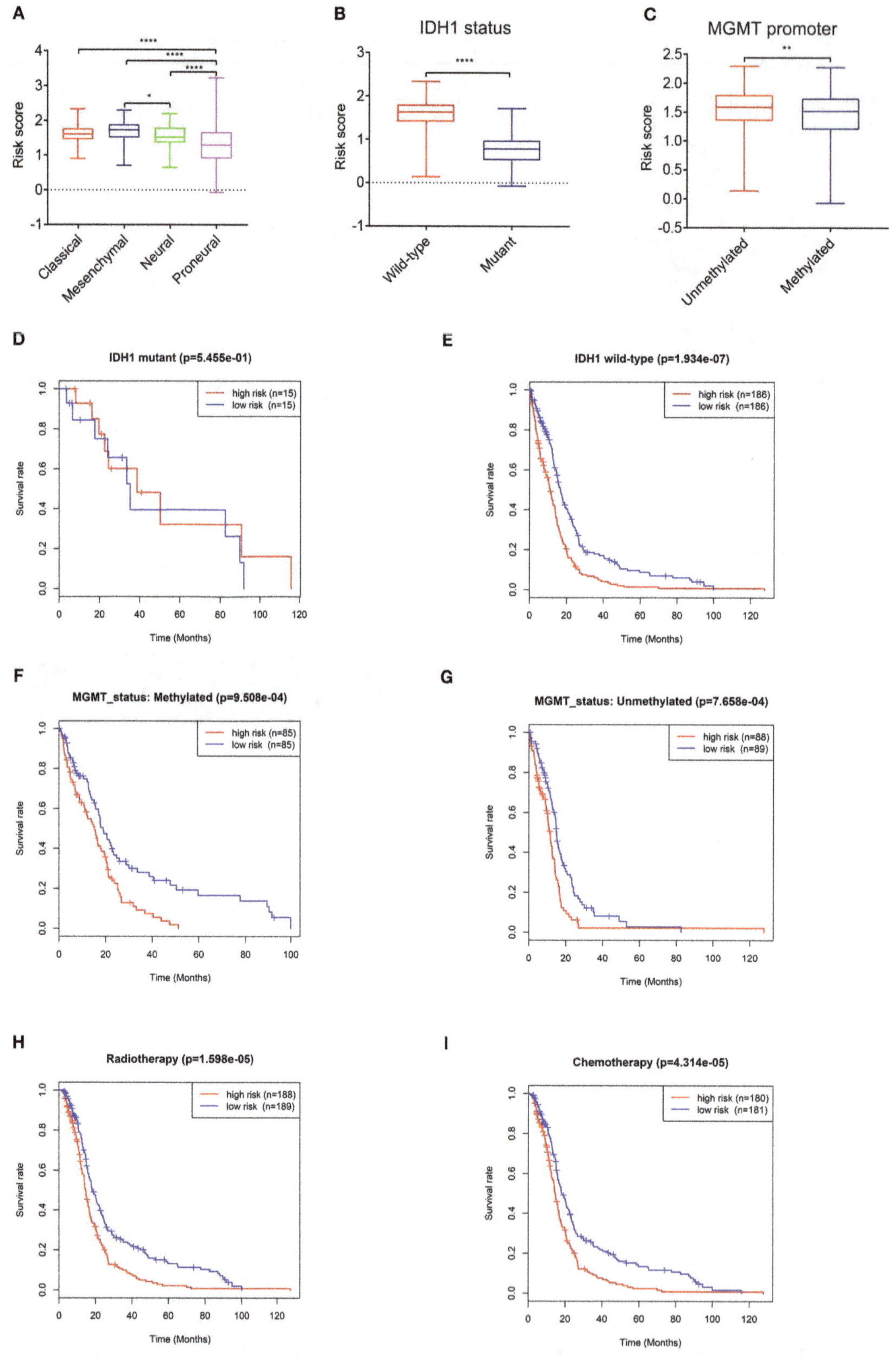

FIGURE 3 | Expression and prognostic significance of the risk signature in different cohorts. Association between the risk signature and different cohorts stratified by molecular subtype **(A)**, IDH1 **(B)**, and MGMT status **(C)** (*$P < 0.05$, **$P < 0.01$, ****$P < 0.0001$). Prognostic significance of the risk signature in different cohorts stratified by IDH1 status **(D,E)**, MGMT status **(F,G)**, radiotherapy **(H)**, and chemotherapy **(I)**.

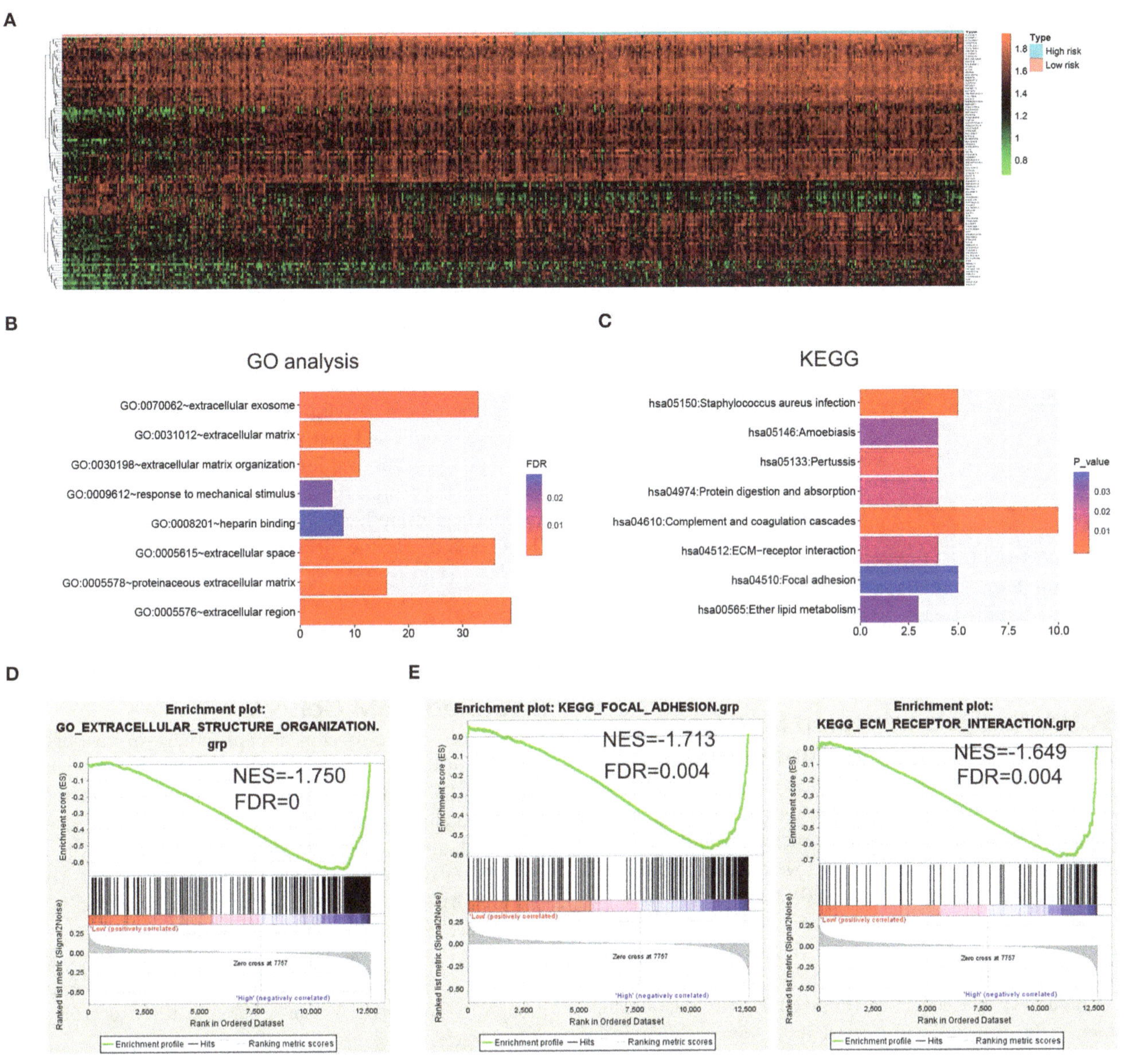

FIGURE 4 | Biological functions and KEGG pathways related to the risk signature with five genes. **(A)** Heatmap showed the DEGs between the high-risk group and the low-risk group (FDR < 0.05). GO analysis **(B)** and KEGG pathway analysis **(C)** via DAVID based on the DEGs. **(D,E)** GSEA was performed to confirm the GO term (extracellular structure organization) and KEGG pathways (ECM receptor interaction and focal adhesion).

The exclusion criteria included patients with incomplete data such as survival status and time, radiotherapy, and chemotherapy records. The training cohort was used to construct the nomogram of clinical survival prediction model, and the validation cohort was applied for internal validation. Concordance index (C-index), ROC curve analysis and calibration curve were used to measure the performance of the nomogram, which were conducted by R.

Statistical Analysis

Risk scores of the samples in GBM subtype, IDH1 status, and MGMT promoter were presented as mean ± standard deviation and calculated by Graphpad Prism 8.0. Statistical differences between and among groups were examined by two tailed *t*-test and one-way analysis of variance (ANOVA) followed by Dunnett's post-test, respectively. Kaplan-Meier survival analysis and Cox proportion hazards regression model were conducted with R and R package. $P < 0.05$ was regarded as statistically significant.

RESULTS

Identification of Differentially Expressed Genes Between GBM and LGG

GBM is one of the devastating malignancies with poor prognosis. To better construct a survival prediction signature for patients with GBM, we searched for differentially expressed genes

TABLE 1 | Demographics and clinicopathologic characteristics of patients in training cohort and validation cohort.

Characteristic	Training cohort (n = 364)		Validation cohort (n = 155)	
	No. of patients	%	No. of patients	%
RISK SCORE				
Median	1.5332		1.5356	
Range	0.1301 to 2.2929		−0.0730 to 3.2246	
AGE, YEARS				
Median	59		57	
Range	15–89		11–89	
RADIOTHERAPY				
Yes	260	71.4286	118	76.1290
No	104	28.5714	37	23.8710
CHEMOTHERAPY				
Yes	246	67.5824	115	74.1935
No	118	32.4176	40	25.8065

between GBM and LGG in TCGA GBMLGG (RNA-seq) dataset. Genes with $|\log_2 FC| > 1$ and FDR < 0.05 were chosen as DEGs. Four hundred eight genes (including 211 up-regulated genes and 197 down-regulated genes) were identified (**Figure 1A; Supplementary Table 1**).

WGCNA Analysis Revealed Blue Gene Module Was Related to Glioma Grade

To identify genes associated with clinical traits, we collected the RNA-seq data of DEGs and clinical information (WHO grade, age, gender, IDH status, survival time and status), and performed WGCNA analysis. Firstly, the samples were clustered and basic clinical traits were displayed (**Figure 1B**). A soft threshold power was then calculated and 10 was selected as the power value to produce a hierarchical clustering tree (**Figure 1C**). The module dissection threshold was set at 0.15 to merge similar modules and 4 modules were generated (**Figure 1D**). The relationships between gene modules and clinical traits were confirmed by Pearson correlation and exhibited in a heatmap (**Figure 1E**). Among the modules, blue gene module contained 194 genes and was the most positively related to WHO grade ($r = 0.77$, $P < 0.0001$). In addition, the blue gene module was also correlated with age ($r = 0.56$), IDH status ($r = -0.87$), survival time ($r = -0.32$), and survival status ($r = 0.56$). Therefore, genes in the blue module were used for further study.

Construction of the Risk Signature With Five-Gene in GBM Cohorts

To select prognosis related genes, we performed univariate Cox proportional hazards regression analysis to analyze the genes in blue module in TCGA GBMLGG (RNA-seq) and HG-UG133A platforms. Seventeen overlapped genes significantly correlated with overall survival ($P < 0.05$) between the two platforms were obtained (**Figure 2A; Supplementary Table 2**). Next, multivariable Cox regression analysis was implemented to filter and optimize the genes for constructing risk signature. Five genes (DES, RANBP17, CLEC5A, HOXC11, POSTN) were screened out, among which RANBP17 was defined as protective with HR < 1, whereas others were defined as risky with HR > 1 (**Figure 2B**). The risk-score formula was constructed as follows: risk score = (0.5536 × expression level of DES) + (−0.7340 × expression level of RANBP17) + (0.0995 × expression level of CLEC5A) + (0.2810 × expression level of HOXC11) + (0.0566 × expression level of POSTN). The risk score for each patient in TCGA HG-UG133A platform was calculated (mean ±SD, 1.5290 ± 0.4039; Quartiles were 1.3257 at 25%, 1.5936 at 50%, and 1.7968 at 75%, respectively) and all the 525 patients were divided into high-risk or low-risk groups based on the median cutoff value of the scores. As shown in **Figure 2C**, GBM patients with high risk scores indicated poor prognosis. The AUC for the five-gene signature risk score model at 1, 3, and 5-year survival were 0.671, 0.706, and 0.796, respectively (**Figure 2D**). The results indicated that the risk signature can better predict 1, 3, and 5-year survival for GBM patients. With the increase of risk score, the expression level of RANBP17 was down-regulated, and the expression level of the other 4 genes were up-regulated (**Figures 2E,F**). In the mean-time, the number of alive patients decreased (**Figure 2G**).

Application of the Risk Signature in Stratified GBM Cohorts

To further explore its clinical application, we investigated the relationship between the risk score and glioma subtype, IDH1 and MGMT promoter status, respectively. The mesenchymal subtype inclined to have higher risk scores than neural and proneural subtype (**Figure 3A**). The risk scores of patients with IDH1 mutant type were lower than IDH1 wild type (**Figure 3B**). This result was in accordance with the conclusion that IDH1 mutant in glioma was related to better patient prognosis (23). For MGMT promoter, the risk scores decreased in patients with methylated status ($P < 0.01$, **Figure 3C**), though the average risk scores between the two groups didn't differ largely.

The relationships between the risk score and patient prognosis stratified by IDH1, MGMT promoter status were also explored. There was no significant statistical difference between high-risk group and low-risk group in GBM patients with IDH1 mutant (**Figure 3D**). This result might be mainly due to the insufficient number of patients. In IDH1 wild-type cohort, patients with low risk scores exhibited longer survival time than high risk group (**Figure 3E**). In terms of MGMT promoter, no matter of methylated or unmethylated state, the high-risk group indicated dismal prognosis compared with the low-risk group (**Figures 3F,G**). Furthermore, in consideration of the importance of radio- and chemo-therapy in the treatment of glioma, we analyzed the association between the risk score and the response to standard radio- and chemo-therapy. The patients with low risk scores exhibited favorable prognosis in either radiotherapy or chemotherapy (**Figures 3H,I**). These results revealed that the risk signature could serve as an independent factor for predicting the prognosis of patients with GBM.

TABLE 2 | Multivariate analysis of the training cohort and validation cohort for overall survival.

Variable	Training cohort			Validation cohort		
	P	HR	95% CI	*P*	HR	95% CI
Risk score	<0.0001	2.4617	1.7110–3.5417	0.0043	1.9083	1.2246–2.9738
Age (years)	0.0004	1.0177	1.0079–1.0276	0.001	1.0244	1.0098–1.0392
Radiotherapy yes vs. no	<0.0001	0.4230	0.3139–0.5701	0.0013	0.4827	0.3099–0.7518
Chemotherapy yes vs. no	0.0011	0.6274	0.4740–0.8304	0.0159	0.5825	0.3755–0.9036

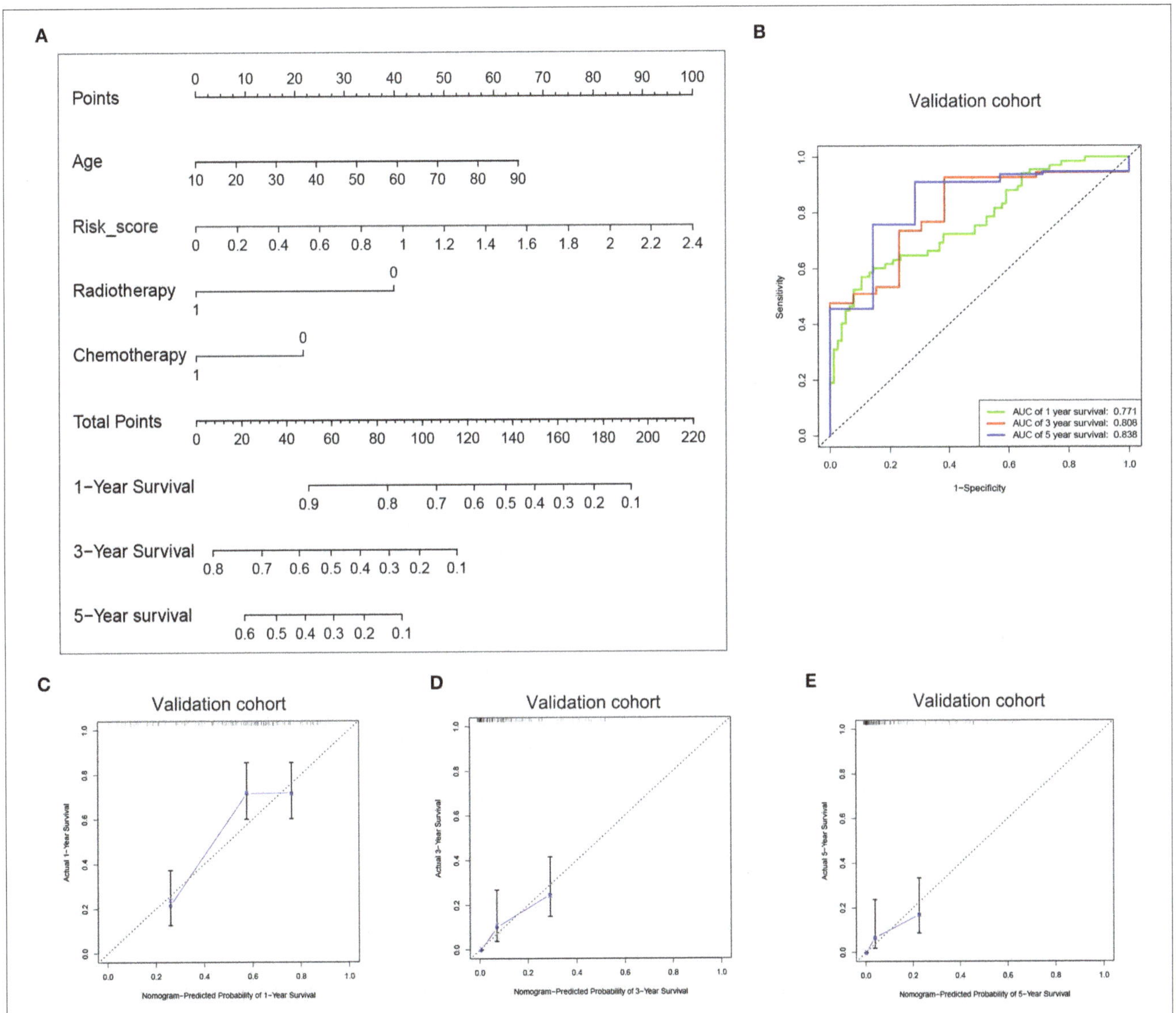

FIGURE 5 | Construction of the nomogram based on the risk signature with five-gene. **(A)** The nomogram was constructed for predicting 1, 3, 5-year survival rate of GBM patients. **(B)** ROC curve was used to evaluate the efficiency of the clinical predictive model. **(C–E)** The calibration curves for predicting patient survival at 1, 3, and 5 years in the validation cohort.

Functional Analysis of the Five Genes in the Risk Signature

To further investigate the functional roles and KEGG pathways associated with the risk signature, we first screened out the DEGs between the high-risk group and low-risk group. Ninety-five genes with FDR < 0.05 were selected for GO and KEGG pathway analysis via DAVID (**Figure 4A; Supplementary Table 3**). We discovered that the five-gene risk signature was functionally associated with extracellular matrix related terms, including extracellular exosome, extracellular matrix, and extracellular matrix organization (FDR < 0.05, **Figure 4B**). Correspondingly, several KEGG pathways ($P < 0.05$) such as ECM-receptor interaction and focal adhesion pathways were also obtained (**Figure 4C**). To further confirm these results, the samples were divided into high-risk and low-risk groups according to the median of risk scores, and GSEA were applied. Similar GO terms and KEGG pathways were observed via GSEA analysis (**Figures 4D,E**). Collectively, these results revealed that the five-gene risk signature was correlated to extracellular matrix and cell adhesion functions, which play vital roles in glioma invasion and progression (24, 25).

Construction of a Clinical Survival Prediction Model via the Risk Signature Combined With Clinicopathologic Features

Since the risk signature had a better performance in predicting the prognosis of GBM patients, we explored its clinical significance combining with clinical characters (age, radiotherapy, and chemotherapy experience). Firstly, the samples in the TCGA HG-UG133A platform were divided into training cohort (364 cases) and validation cohort (155 cases) randomly (**Table 1**). Then, multivariable Cox regression analysis was performed to assess the selected variable's contribution in predicting prognosis of GBM patients. The results indicated that the factors, such as risk score, age, acceptance of radiotherapy and chemotherapy, were correlated with patients' survival significantly both in training cohort and validation cohort (**Table 2**). A clinical survival prediction model was constructed based on the data in training cohort and presented in a nomogram for predicting 1, 3, 5-year survival (**Figure 5A**). C-index, ROC curve and calibration plot were used to evaluate the efficiency of the clinical predictive model. The C-indexes in training cohort and validation cohort were 0.729 and 0.708, respectively. The area under the curves (AUC) of the nomogram for 1, 3, 5-year-survival were 0.771, 0.808, and 0.838 in validation cohort, respectively (**Figure 5B**). In the training set, the area under the curves (AUC) for 1, 3, 5-year-survival were 0.796, 0.79, and 0.851, respectively (**Supplementary Figure 1A**). The calibration plot for the probability of survival at 1, 3, or 5-years showed an optimal agreement between the prediction and observation, both in the validation cohort (**Figures 5C–E**) and training cohort (**Supplementary Figures 1B–D**). These results above revealed that the nomogram demonstrated a good accuracy for predicting 1, 3, or 5-year survival of GBM patients.

DISCUSSION

So far, GBM is still a lethal disease without efficient therapeutic regimens. The failure to develop new treatments ascribes to a lack of validation of novel molecular targets, which are often performed in animal models and directly translated to human trials (26). Thus, exploration and validation novel molecular targets are not only necessary, but also very urgent. In the present study, we identified DEGs between GBM and LGG in TCGA data, and confirmed 17 genes significantly correlated with prognosis. Finally, five genes (DES, RANBP17, CLEC5A, HOXC11, POSTN) were selected to construct a risk signature for GBM. Among the five genes, POSTN is an ECM protein and is involved in various cellular processes, including epithelial-mesenchymal transition (EMT) and cell migration (27). POSTN is highly expressed in glioma tissues and has been considered as a biomarker of glioma malignancy and recurrence (28, 29). It has also been reported that POSTN recruits M2 tumor-associated macrophages and promotes glioma stem cells (GSCs) growth (30). CLEC5A is a spleen tyrosine kinase-coupled receptor, which is abundantly expressed in monocytes, macrophages and neutrophils, and critical for inflammation response (31, 32). A recent study has shown that CLEC5A is upregulated in GBM significantly and is associated with poor prognosis (33). Furthermore, downregulation of CLEC5A can inhibit the capabilities of proliferation, migration, and invasion, and promotes apoptosis and G1 arrest in GBM cell lines (33). These results are consistent with our findings that the expression level of CLEC5A increased with the ascent of risk scores and CLEC5A was a risk factor in GBM. Although few have been reported about the other three genes in glioma, they have vital functions and might serve as potential targets for GBM. For instance, DES encodes the intermediate filament protein desmin, which is expressed in cardiac, skeletal, and smooth muscle cells, and its mutations can cause isolated cardiomyopathies and cardiac conduction diseases (34, 35). A recent study demonstrated that desmin loss is observed in 92% malignant mesothelioma samples, 76% malignant effusions, 29% benign mesothelial hyperplasia tissues, but not in the reactive effusions (36). Thus, desmin may serve as a useful biomarker in the discrimination between reactive mesothelial proliferation and malignant mesothelioma. As a RanGTP-binding protein, RANBP17 belongs to the importin beta family and is preferentially expressed in the testis (37, 38). RANBP17 is upregulated in dilated cardiomyopathy and ischemic cardiomyopathy samples, and may regulate the transport of different cargos in specific cardiomyopathies through enhancing the transcriptional activation of the EA2 transcription factors E12 and E47 (39). HOXC11 belongs to homeobox superfamily that are responsible for encoding transcription factors regulating development (40). HOXC6 and HOXC11 have been shown to induce differentiation of GOTO neuroblastoma cells into Schwannian cells via transcription activation of S100β (41). Moreover, HOXC11 is found to be closely correlated with the survival of patients with renal cell cancer, cervical cancer or breast cancer, and serves as a therapeutic target (40, 42). This risk signature comprised of the five genes was identified to significantly correlate with the survival of GBM patients, as well as stratified by IDH1 status, MGMT promoter status, and radiochemotherapy. In addition, GO and KEGG pathway analysis were applied via DAVID and GSEA, and elucidated that the five-gene risk signature was mainly related to extracellular matrix and cell adhesion function. EMC organization and cell adhesion are indispensable biological processes in tumor development and progression (43, 44), indicating the essential value of our signature.

Nomograms have been applied extensively and exhibit favorable effects on predicting clinical risk signatures and outcomes in some cancers (45, 46). For better clinical application, we combined the risk signature with clinical factors (age, radiotherapy, and chemotherapy experience) and established a nomogram, which was validated to have better performance for predicting the outcomes of patients with GBM. The nomogram contained four items, and predicted the 1, 3, 5-year survival rate based on the sum of the score in each item. This clinical prediction model aimed at precisely predicting the prognosis of GBM patients and corresponded to the idea of individual treatment. However, there were some deficiencies in this study. Firstly, the sample size was limited. Five hundred nineteen samples were incorporated, and 364 cases were used for constructing model. The second limitation was that the samples were downloaded from TCGA, and it didn't contain information about extent of tumor resection, which is a key factor closely related to survival time in patients with GBM (47). A collection of detailed clinical records and further validation should be carried out in future study. Despite the above shortcomings, this study still has its advantages and innovations. Firstly, we performed an accurate and widely used method, WGCNA (48), and confirmed genes associated with glioma grade, which is an clinical indicator directly associated with the prognosis of glioma patients. Secondly, the risk signature with five genes was proven to be an independent prognostic biomarker in GBM via Kaplan-Meier survival analysis and multivariable Cox regression analysis. In addition, on the basis of the risk signature and other clinical factors (age, radiotherapy, and chemotherapy experience), the nomogram can predict the 1, 3, 5-year survival rate precisely, thus providing evidences of treatment for GBM patients. Altogether, our study indicated the potential value of our model for predicting the survival of GBM patients.

AUTHOR CONTRIBUTIONS

YW: conceptualization and writing-original draft. YW and GG: methodology. YW and XL: project administration. MZ: supervision. WZ and MZ: writing-review and editing.

REFERENCES

1. Delgado-Lopez PD, Corrales-Garcia EM. Survival in glioblastoma: a review on the impact of treatment modalities. *Clin Transl Oncol.* (2016) 18:1062–71. doi: 10.1007/s12094-016-1497-x
2. Dai S, Yan Y, Xu Z, Zeng S, Qian L, Huo L, et al. SCD1 confers temozolomide resistance to human glioma cells via the Akt/GSK3beta/beta-catenin signaling axis. *Front Pharmacol.* (2017) 8:960. doi: 10.3389/fphar.2017.00960
3. Hager J, Herrmann E, Kammerer S, Dinc N, Won SY, Senft C, et al. Quick-weller: impact of resection on overall survival of recurrent glioblastoma in elderly patients. *Clin Neurol Neurosurg.* (2018) 174:21–5. doi: 10.1016/j.clineuro.2018.08.033
4. Hombach-Klonisch S, Mehrpour M, Shojaei S, Harlos C, Pitz M, Hamai A, et al. Glioblastoma and chemoresistance to alkylating agents: involvement of apoptosis, autophagy, and unfolded protein response. *Pharmacol Ther.* (2018) 184:13-41. doi: 10.1016/j.pharmthera.2017.10.017
5. Auffinger B, Spencer D, Pytel P, Ahmed AU, Lesniak MS. The role of glioma stem cells in chemotherapy resistance and glioblastoma multiforme recurrence. *Expert Rev Neurother.* (2015) 15:741-52. doi: 10.1586/14737175.2015.1051968
6. Raucher D, Dragojevic S, Ryu J. Macromolecular drug carriers for targeted glioblastoma therapy: preclinical studies, challenges, and future perspectives. *Front Oncol.* (2018) 8:624. doi: 10.3389/fonc.2018.00624
7. Chistiakov DA, Chekhonin IV, Chekhonin VP. The EGFR variant III mutant as a target for immunotherapy of glioblastoma multiforme. *Eur J Pharmacol.* (2017) 810:70-82. doi: 10.1016/j.ejphar.2017.05.064
8. Paff M, Alexandru-Abrams D, Hsu FP, Bota DA. The evolution of the EGFRvIII (rindopepimut) immunotherapy for glioblastoma multiforme patients. *Hum Vaccin Immunother.* (2014) 10:3322-31. doi: 10.4161/21645515.2014.983002
9. Ludwig K, Kornblum HI. Molecular markers in glioma. *J Neurooncol.* (2017) 134:505-12. doi: 10.1007/s11060-017-2379-y
10. Karsy M, Guan J, Cohen AL, Jensen RL, Colman H. New molecular considerations for glioma: IDH, ATRX, BRAF, TERT, H3 K27M. *Curr Neurol Neurosci Rep.* (2017) 17:19. doi: 10.1007/s11910-017-0722-5
11. Chen R, Smith-Cohn M, Cohen AL, Colman H. Glioma subclassifications and their clinical significance. *Neurotherapeutics.* (2017) 14:284-97. doi: 10.1007/s13311-017-0519-x
12. Abe H, Natsumeda M, Kanemaru Y, Watanabe J, Tsukamoto Y, Okada M, et al. MGMT expression contributes to temozolomide resistance in H3K27M-mutant diffuse midline gliomas and MGMT silencing to temozolomide sensitivity in IDH-mutant gliomas. *Neurol Med Chir.* (2018) 58:290-5. doi: 10.2176/nmc.ra.2018-0044
13. Brandes AA, Carpentier AF, Kesari S, Sepulveda-Sanchez JM, Wheeler HR, Chinot O, et al. A Phase II randomized study of galunisertib monotherapy or galunisertib plus lomustine compared with lomustine monotherapy in patients with recurrent glioblastoma. *Neuro Oncol.* (2016) 18:1146–56. doi: 10.1093/neuonc/now009
14. Gao WZ, Guo LM, Xu TQ, Yin YH, Jia F. Identification of a multidimensional transcriptome signature for survival prediction of postoperative glioblastoma multiforme patients. *J Transl Med.* (2018) 16:368. doi: 10.1186/s12967-018-1744-8
15. Capper D, von Deimling A, Brandes AA, Carpentier AF, Kesari S, Sepulveda-Sanchez JM, et al. Biomarker and histopathology evaluation of patients with recurrent glioblastoma treated with galunisertib, lomustine, or the combination of galunisertib and lomustine. *Int J Mol Sci.* (2017) 18:E995. doi: 10.3390/ijms18050995
16. Bowman RL, Wang Q, Carro A, Verhaak RG, Squatrito M. GlioVis data portal for visualization and analysis of brain tumor expression datasets. *Neuro Oncol.* (2017) 19:139-41. doi: 10.1093/neuonc/now247
17. Dworkin M, Mehan W, Niemierko A, Kamran SC, Lamba N, Dietrich J, et al. Increase of pseudoprogression and other treatment related effects in low-grade glioma patients treated with proton radiation and temozolomide. *J Neurooncol.* (2018) 142:69-77. doi: 10.1007/s11060-018-03063-1
18. Qian Z, Li Y, Fan X, Zhang C, Wang Y, Jiang T, et al. Molecular and clinical characterization of IDH associated immune signature in lower-grade gliomas. *Oncoimmunology.* (2018) 7:e1434466. doi: 10.1080/2162402x.2018.1434466
19. Langfelder P, Horvath S. WGCNA: an R package for weighted correlation network analysis. *BMC Bioinformatics.* (2008) 9:559. doi: 10.1186/1471-2105-9-559

20. Zhang X, Feng H, Li Z, Li D, Liu S, Huang H, et al. Application of weighted gene co-expression network analysis to identify key modules and hub genes in oral squamous cell carcinoma tumorigenesis. *Onco Targets Ther.* (2018) 11:6001-21. doi: 10.2147/ott.s171791
21. Huang da W, Sherman BT, Lempicki RA. Systematic and integrative analysis of large gene lists using DAVID bioinformatics resources. *Nat Protoc.* (2009) 4:44-57. doi: 10.1038/nprot.2008.211
22. Subramanian A, Tamayo P, Mootha VK, Mukherjee S, Ebert BL, Gillette MA, et al. Gene set enrichment analysis: a knowledge-based approach for interpreting genome-wide expression profiles. *Proc Natl Acad Sci USA.* (2005) 102:15545-50. doi: 10.1073/pnas.0506580102
23. Seliger C, Luber C, Gerken M, Schaertl J, Proescholdt M, Riemenschneider MJ, et al. Use of metformin and survival of patients with high-grade glioma. *Int J Cancer.* (2019) 144:273-80. doi: 10.1002/ijc.31783
24. Gritsenko PG, Friedl P. Adaptive adhesion systems mediate glioma cell invasion in complex environments. *J Cell Sci.* (2018) 131:jcs216382. doi: 10.1242/jcs.216382
25. Ferrer VP, Moura Neto V, Mentlein R. Glioma infiltration and extracellular matrix: key players and modulators. *Glia.* (2018) 66:1542–65. doi: 10.1002/glia.23309
26. Caponegro MD, Moffitt RA, Tsirka SE. Expression of neuropilin-1 is linked to glioma associated microglia and macrophages and correlates with unfavorable prognosis in high grade gliomas. *Oncotarget.* (2018) 9:35655–65. doi: 10.18632/oncotarget.26273
27. Park SY, Piao Y, Jeong KJ, Dong J, de Groot JF. Periostin (POSTN) regulates tumor resistance to antiangiogenic therapy in glioma models. *Mol Cancer Ther.* (2016) 15:2187-97. doi: 10.1158/1535-7163.Mct-15-0427
28. Mikheev AM, Mikheeva SA, Trister AD, Tokita MJ, Emerson SN, Parada CA, et al. Periostin is a novel therapeutic target that predicts and regulates glioma malignancy. *Neuro Oncol.* (2015) 17:372-82. doi: 10.1093/neuonc/nou161
29. Tian B, Zhang Y, Zhang J. Periostin is a new potential prognostic biomarker for glioma. *Tumour Biol.* (2014) 35:5877-83. doi: 10.1007/s13277-014-1778-3
30. Zhou W, Ke SQ, Huang Z, Flavahan W, Fang X, Paul J, et al. Periostin secreted by glioblastoma stem cells recruits M2 tumour-associated macrophages and promotes malignant growth. *Nat Cell Biol.* (2015) 17:170-82. doi: 10.1038/ncb3090
31. Chen ST, Li FJ, Hsu TY, Liang SM, Yeh YC, Liao WY, et al. CLEC5A is a critical receptor in innate immunity against Listeria infection. *Nat Commun.* (2017) 8:299. doi: 10.1038/s41467-017-00356-3
32. Sprokholt J, Helgers LC, Geijtenbeek TB. Innate immune receptors drive dengue virus immune activation and disease. *Future Virol.* (2017) 13:287-305. doi: 10.2217/fvl-2017-0146
33. Fan HW, Ni Q, Fan YN, Ma ZX, Li YB. C-type lectin domain family 5, member A (CLEC5A, MDL-1) promotes brain glioblastoma tumorigenesis by regulating PI3K/Akt signalling. *Cell Prolif.* (2019) 52:e12584. doi: 10.1111/cpr.12584
34. Bouvet M, Dubois-Deruy E, Alayi TD, Mulder P, El Amranii M, Beseme O, et al. Increased level of phosphorylated desmin and its degradation products in heart failure. *Biochem Biophys Rep.* (2016) 6:54-62. doi: 10.1016/j.bbrep.2016.02.014
35. Brodehl A, Gaertner-Rommel A, Milting H. Molecular insights into cardiomyopathies associated with desmin (DES) mutations. *Biophys Rev.* (2018) 10:983-1006. doi: 10.1007/s12551-018-0429-0
36. Onder S, Ozogul E, Koksal D, Sarinc Ulasli S, Firat P, Emri S. Diagnostic value of BAP1, GLUT-1 and desmin expression in the discrimination between reactive mesothelial proliferation and malignant mesothelioma in tissues and effusions. *Cytopathology.* (2019). doi: 10.1111/cyt.12738. [Epub ahead of print].
37. Bao J, Wu Q, Song R, Jie Z, Zheng H, Xu C, et al. RANBP17 is localized to the XY body of spermatocytes and interacts with SPEM1 on the manchette of elongating spermatids. *Mol Cell Endocrinol.* (2011) 333:134-42. doi: 10.1016/j.mce.2010.12.021
38. Kutay U, Hartmann E, Treichel N, Calado A, Carmo-Fonseca M, Prehn S, et al. Identification of two novel RanGTP-binding proteins belonging to the importin beta superfamily. *J Biol Chem.* (2000) 275:40163-8. doi: 10.1074/jbc.M006242200
39. Molina-Navarro MM, Rosello-Lleti E, Tarazon E, Ortega A, Sanchez-Izquierdo D, Lago F, et al. Heart failure entails significant changes in human nucleocytoplasmic transport gene expression. *Int J Cardiol.* (2013) 168:2837-43. doi: 10.1016/j.ijcard.2013.03.192
40. Liu YJ, Zhu Y, Yuan HX, Zhang JP, Guo JM, Lin ZM. Overexpression of HOXC11 homeobox gene in clear cell renal cell carcinoma induces cellular proliferation and is associated with poor prognosis. *Tumour Biol.* (2015) 36:2821-9. doi: 10.1007/s13277-014-2909-6
41. Zhang X, Hamada J, Nishimoto A, Takahashi Y, Murai T, Tada M, et al. HOXC6 and HOXC11 increase transcription of S100beta gene in BrdU-induced *in vitro* differentiation of GOTO neuroblastoma cells into Schwannian cells. *J Cell Mol Med.* (2007) 11:299-306. doi: 10.1111/j.1582-4934.2007.00020.x
42. Sun B, Hua J, Cui H, Liu H, Zhang K, Zhou H. MicroRNA-1197 downregulation inhibits proliferation and migration in human non- small cell lung cancer cells by upregulating HOXC11. *Biomed Pharmacother.* (2019) 117:109041. doi: 10.1016/j.biopha.2019.109041
43. Benthani FA, Herrmann D, Tran PN, Pangon L, Lucas MC, Allam AH, et al. 'MCC' protein interacts with E-cadherin and beta-catenin strengthening cell-cell adhesion of HCT116 colon cancer cells. *Oncogene.* (2018) 37:663-672. doi: 10.1038/onc.2017.362
44. Giussani M, Triulzi T, Sozzi G, Tagliabue E. Tumor extracellular matrix remodeling: new perspectives as a circulating tool in the diagnosis and prognosis of solid tumors. *Cells.* (2019) 8:E81. doi: 10.3390/cells8020081
45. Dong D, Tang L, Li ZY, Fang MJ, Gao JB, Shan XH, et al. Development and validation of an individualized nomogram to identify occult peritoneal metastasis in patients with advanced gastric cancer. *Ann Oncol.* (2019) 30:431-8. doi: 10.1093/annonc/mdz001
46. Caulfield S, Menezes G, Marignol L, Poole C. Nomograms are key decision-making tools in prostate cancer radiation therapy. *Urol Oncol.* (2018) 36:283-292. doi: 10.1016/j.urolonc.2018.03.017
47. Hameed NUF, Qiu T, Zhuang D, Lu J, Yu Z, Wu S, et al. Transcortical insular glioma resection: clinical outcome and predictors. *J Neurosurg.* (2018) 1:1–11. doi: 10.3171/2018.4.Jns18424
48. Pei G, Chen L, Zhang W. WGCNA application to proteomic and metabolomic data analysis. *Methods Enzymol.* (2017) 585:135-158. doi: 10.1016/bs.mie.2016.09.016

3

Integrin Beta 5 is a Prognostic Biomarker and Potential Therapeutic Target in Glioblastoma

Lu-yang Zhang[1†], *Qing Guo*[1†], *Ge-fei Guan*[1], *Wen Cheng*[1], *Peng Cheng*[1*] and *An-hua Wu*[1,2*]

[1] *Department of Neurosurgery, The First Hospital of China Medical University, Shenyang, China,* [2] *College of Applied Technology, China Medical University, Shenyang, China*

***Correspondence:**
Peng Cheng
chengpengcmu@sina.com
An-hua Wu
wuanhua@yahoo.com

† These authors have contributed equally to this work

Background: Glioblastoma (GBM) is the most lethal cancer of the central nervous system. Integrin beta 5 (*ITGB5*) is thought to be involved in intercellular signal transduction and regulation of tumor initiation and progression. However, the function of *ITGB5* in GBM is not known.

Methods: To address this question, we evaluated the expression level of *ITGB5* in clinical specimens by immunohistochemistry and western blotting, as well as the association between *ITGB5* expression and GBM patient survival using data from Chinese Glioma Genome Atlas and The Cancer Genome Atlas. The biological function of *ITGB5* in GBM was investigated by Gene Ontology, gene set enrichment, and *in vitro* loss-of-function experiments using glioma cells.

Results: Among integrin family members, *ITGB5* showed the greatest difference in expression between low-grade glioma and GBM. Elevated ITGB5 expression was highly correlated with glioma progression and a mesenchymal subtype and poor survival in GBM patients. *ITGB5* was found to be associated with regulation of the immune response and angiogenesis in GBM, and was required for migration and invasion of glioma cells and tube formation by endothelial cells.

Conclusions: These data indicate that ITGB5 can serve as a predictive biomarker for GBM patient survival and is a potential therapeutic target in GBM treatment.

Keywords: integrin, ITGB5, Glioblastoma, prognosis, brain cancer

INTRODUCTION

Glioblastoma (GBM) is the most common primary malignant brain tumor in adults. Even when different treatment approaches such as surgical resection, chemotherapy, and radiotherapy are combined, tumor recurrence is inevitable and the prognosis of GBM patients is extremely poor, with a median survival of 12–15 months (1–3). Significant efforts are being made to identify GBM surface molecules and pathways that can be targeted by therapeutics (4).

Integrins are a group of integral transmembrane heterodimers with many functions including cell adhesion in the extracellular matrix and acting as receptors for various physiological ligands (5). Aberrant integrin expression profiles are often observed in aggressive tumors such as breast cancer; therefore, these proteins are potential drug targets (5). Integrins are the major determinant of the invasive phenotype of glioma (4, 6). Two integrin α subunits, ITGA6 and ITGA7, are key receptors in glioma stem-like cells (4, 7). Thus, antagonizing integrins may be a useful strategy for preventing

GBM progression, and characterizing the expression patterns of integrins and related signaling pathways in glioma—especially GBM—can provide insight into the molecular mechanisms of tumor recurrence and treatment resistance in malignant glioma.

Integrin β5 (ITGB5) encodes a subunit of integrin that can interact with several integrin α chains. ITGB5 mediates transforming growth factor (TGF)β-induced epithelial-mesenchymal transition (EMT) and contributes to the tumorigenic potential of breast cancer cells (8, 9). A recent study reported that ITGB5 promotes tumorigenesis in hepatocellular carcinoma by interacting with β-catenin (10). In addition, ITGB5 was enriched in liver metastatic pancreatic cancer exosomes (11). This indicated its potential role in intercellular communication during tumor progression and metastasis. In GBM, ITGB5 was shown to regulate GBM-infiltrating macrophages in the local microenvironment via modulation of osteopontin (12). However, the role of ITGB5 in the tumor microenvironment is not fully understood.

Characterizing ITGB5 expression and how this is related to patient prognosis may be useful for the development of more effective treatment strategies for GBM and for predicting the outcome of glioma patients. To this end, in the present study we examined the expression of ITGB5 in clinical glioma samples and its relationship with the outcome of glioma patients. We found that ITGB5 overexpression in GBM was associated with poor survival. Furthermore, ITGB5 not only promoted the migration and invasion of glioma cells but also regulated the function of endothelial cells. Conversely, ITGB5 silencing decreased the expression of EMT markers in glioma cells.

MATERIALS AND METHODS

Clinical Specimens and Ethics Approval

Clinical specimens were collected at the First Hospital of China Medical University from January 2011 to February 2018 (non-tumor, $n = 5$; grade II, $n = 7$; grade III, $n = 17$; and grade IV, $n = 61$). There were 53 grade IV (GBM) samples for which patient survival information was available that were used for immunohistochemical analysis. A total of 17 clinical specimens for western blotting were collected at the First Hospital of China Medical University from June 2017 to February 2018 (non-tumor, $n = 3$; grade II, $n = 4$; grade III, $n = 4$; and grade IV, $n = 6$). Histological diagnoses were confirmed by two neuropathologists according to the 2016 World Health Organization classification. The study protocol was approved by the Ethics Committee of the First Hospital of China Medical University.

Datasets for ITGB5 Expression and Survival Analyses

Gene expression profiles from Chinese Glioma Genome Atlas (CGGA) and The Cancer Genome Atlas (TCGA) were used for *ITGB5* expression and patient survival analyses. The CGGA RNA Sequencing (RNAseq) dataset and associated clinical information (http://www.cgga.org.cn) included 310 samples (grade II, $n = 105$; grade III, $n = 67$; and GBM, $n = 138$). The *ITGB5* expression and clinical data in TCGA and Ivy GAP were extracted from GlioVis (http://gliovis.bioinfo.cnio.es/) (13). TCGA RNAseq dataset included 625 samples (grade II, $n = 227$; grade III, $n = 243$; and GBM, $n = 155$); TCGA-4502A mRNA microarray dataset comprised 488 GBM samples. The Ivy GAP RNAseq dataset was used to analyze *ITGB5* expression in different GBM regions.

Cell Lines and Culture

LN229 cells were provided by Professor Tao Jiang (Department of Molecular Neuropathology, Beijing Neurosurgical Institute). Human umbilical vein endothelial cells (HUVECs) were provided by Professor Xin Meng (Department of Biochemistry, China Medical University). LN229 cells and HUVECs were maintained in Dulbecco's modified Eagle's medium (DMEM; Gibco, Grand Island, NY, USA) supplemented with 10% fetal bovine serum (FBS; Gibco) and 1% penicillin/streptomycin (Gibco) at 37°C with 5% CO_2. Patient-derived primary glioma cells (PGC1228) were cultured from fresh glioma samples according to a protocol approved by the Ethics Committee of the First Hospital of China Medical University. The cells were cultured in Roswell Park Memorial Institute (RPMI)-1640 medium (Gibco) containing 10% FBS and 1% penicillin/streptomycin (Gibco) at 37°C and 5% CO_2, and the established cell line was authenticated.

Immunohistochemistry and Western Blotting

Immunohistochemistry and immunoblotting were performed as described in our previous study (14). Antibody information is shown in **Table S1.**

RNA Isolation and Reverse Transcription Quantitative PCR (RT-qPCR)

After RNA isolation and first-strand cDNA synthesis, RT-qPCR was performed with SYBR Green Master Mix (Takara Bio, Otsu, Japan) according to the manufacturer's instructions. The forward and reverse primer sequences were as follows: *ITGB5*, GGA AGTTCGGAAACAGAGGGT and CTTTCGCCAGCCAAT CTTCTC; and *glyceraldehyde 3-phosphate dehydrogenase*, GGA GCGAGATCCCTCCAAAAT and GGCTGTTGTCATACTTCT CATGG).

Receiver Operator Characteristic (ROC) Curve

The ROC curve was plotted and the area under the ROC curve of each cutoff was determined as previously described (15, 16).

Gene Ontology (GO) Analysis

Genes whose expression was correlated with that of *ITGB5* were defined by a Pearson $r > 0.3$ and $P < 0.05$ in two GBM datasets (CGGA RNAseq and TCGA RNAseq). GO analysis was performed using DAVID 6.8 [https://david.ncifcrf.gov/tools.jsp (17)].

Gene Set Enrichment Analysis (GSEA) and Gene Set Variation Analysis (GSVA)

Patients were stratified into two groups according to the median *ITGB5* mRNA expression level. GSEA was performed

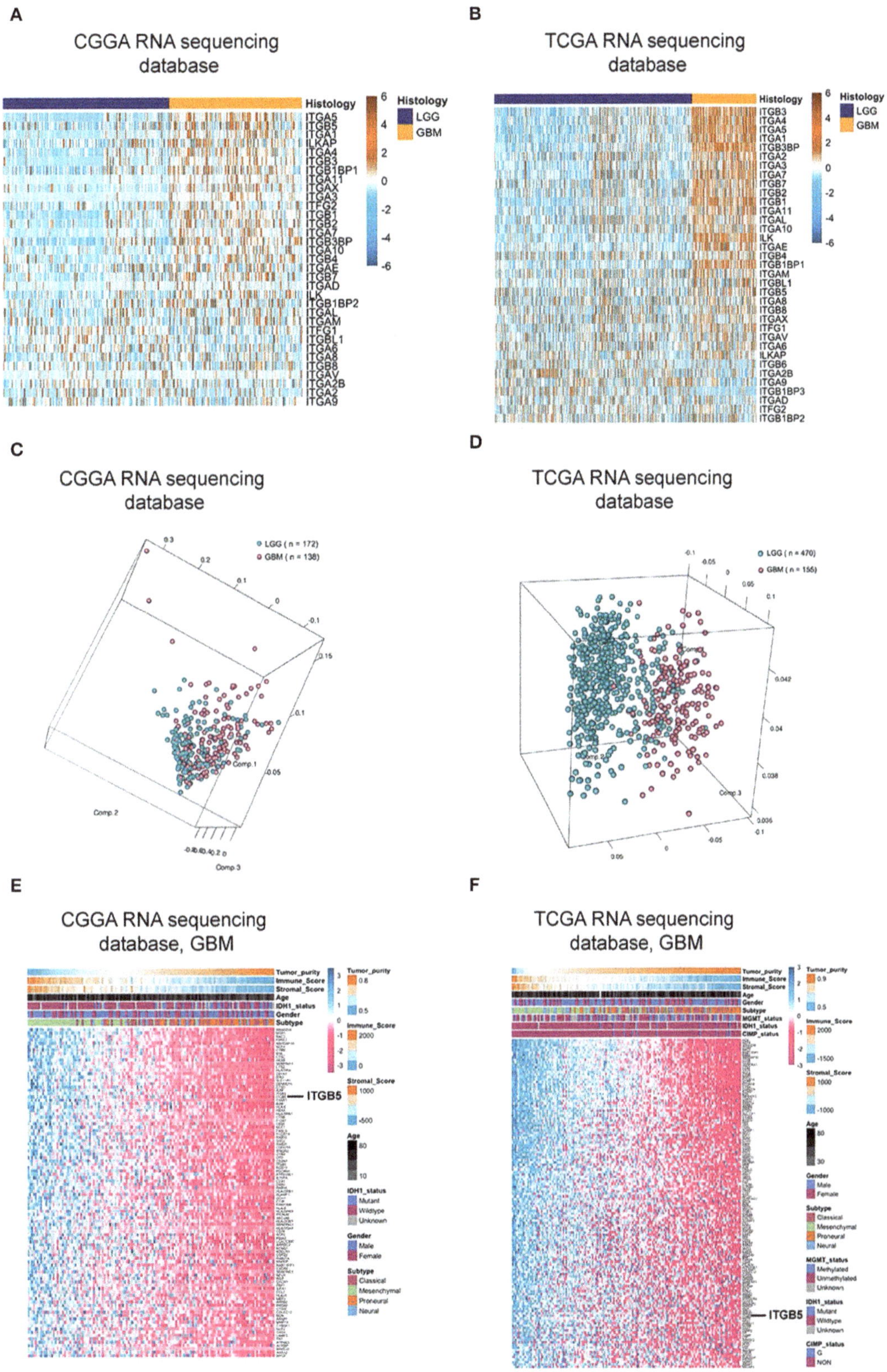

FIGURE 1 | *ITGB5* expression in glioma. **(A,B)** Heatmaps of expression patterns of integrin family genes in glioma based on CGGA **(A)** and TCGA RNAseq **(B)** data. **(C,D)** PCA based on vesicle-related genes in CGGA **(C)** and TCGA **(D)** stratifies LGG and GBM. **(E,F)** Heatmaps showing the positive correlation between vesicle-related genes and tumor purity and immune and stromal scores (**E**, CGGA; **F**, TCGA RNAseq). $r > 0.45$ or < -0.45 (Pearson's correlation analysis).

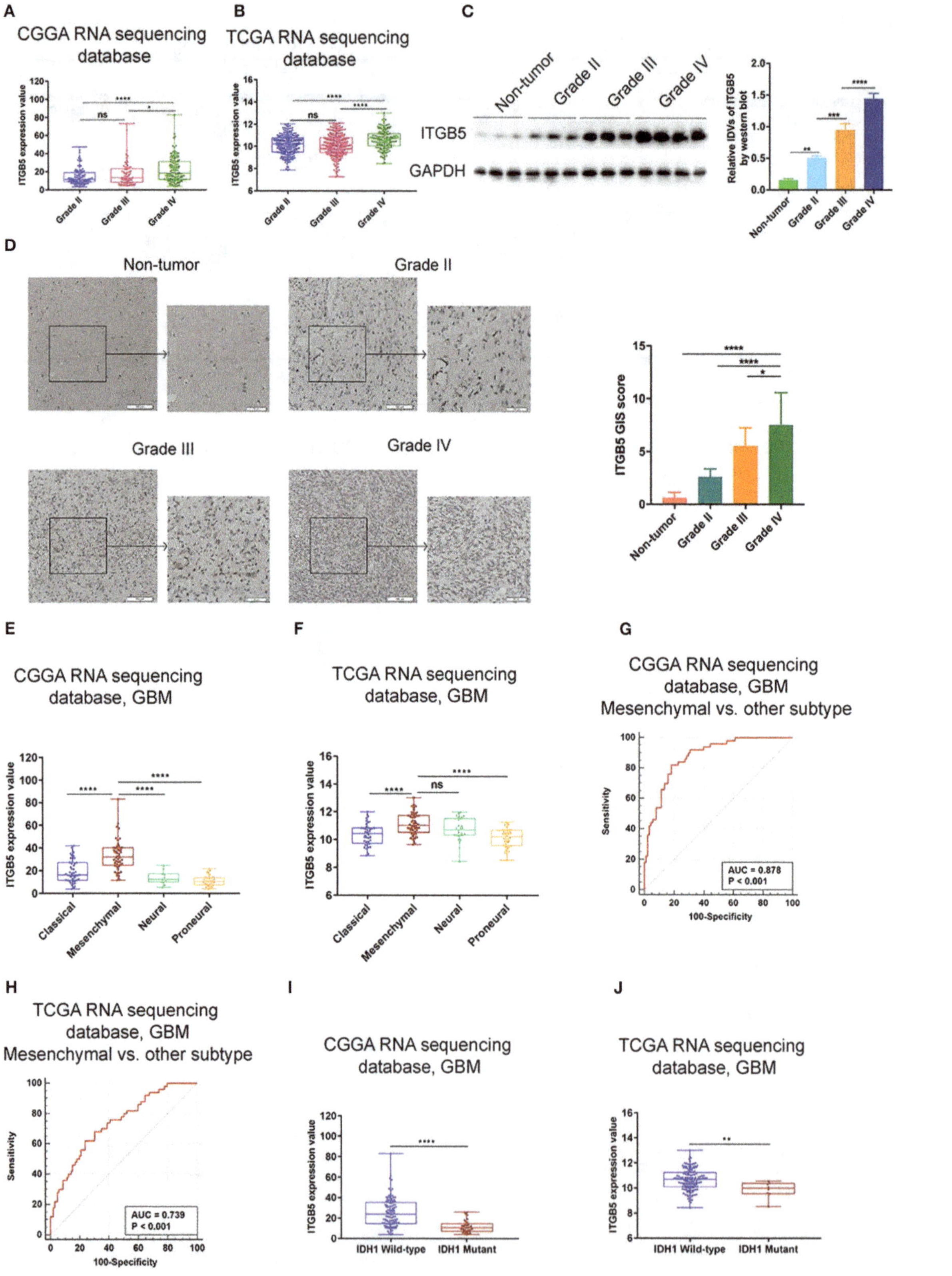

FIGURE 2 | Elevated *ITGB5* expression is associated with progressive malignancy and a mesenchymal subtype in glioma. **(A,B)** *ITGB5* expression according to glioma grade (**A**, CGGA RNA-seq; **B**, TCGA RNA-seq). ns, $P > 0.05$; *$P < 0.05$; **** $P < 0.0001$ (one-way analysis of variance [ANOVA]). **(C)** *ITGB5* expression is *(Continued)*

FIGURE 2 | elevated according to glioma grade, as determined by western blotting. $^{**}P < 0.01$; $^{***}P < 0.001$; $^{****}P < 0.0001$ (one-way ANOVA). **(D)** Representative images (left panel) of ITGB5 expression in clinical specimens and quantification of staining intensity (right panel). $^{*}P < 0.05$; $^{****}P < 0.0001$ (one-way ANOVA). **(E,F)** ITGB5 expression is highest in the mesenchymal subtype of GBM (**E**, CGGA RNA-seq; **F**, TCGA RNA-seq). ns, $P > 0.05$; $^{****}P < 0.0001$ (one-way ANOVA). **(G,H)** ROC curve for evaluating the sensitivity and specificity of ITGB5 as a diagnostic marker for the mesenchymal subtype of GBM vs. other subtypes (**G**, CGGA RNAseq, area under the ROC curve [AUC]: 0.878, $P < 0.001$; **H**, TCGA RNAseq, AUC: 0.739, $P < 0.001$). **(I,J)** ITGB5 expression is elevated in *IDH1*-wild-type as compared to *IDH1*-mutant GBM (**I**, CGGA RNAseq; **J**, TCGA RNAseq, $^{**}P < 0.01$; $^{****}P < 0.0001$ [*t*-test]).

to determine whether the identified sets of genes showed statistically significant differences between the two groups based on normalized enrichment score and false discovery rate (18). GSVA (http://www.bioconductor.org) was performed to further verify whether the genes were correlated with specific signaling pathways (19).

Tumor Purity, Immune and Stromal Scores, and Microenvironment Cell Populations-Counter (MCP-Counter)

Tumor purity and immune and stromal scores were calculated as previously described (20). Eight immune and two non-immune stromal cell populations [immune cells: T cells, cluster of differentiation (CD)8+ T cells, natural killer (NK) cells, cytotoxic T lymphocytes, B cells, monocytes, myeloid dendritic cells, and neutrophils) and stromal cell populations (endothelial cells and fibroblasts) were evaluated by the MCP-counter method (21).

Small Interfering (si)RNA and Cell Transfection

Specific siRNAs targeting *ITGB5* (siITGB5) and a negative control siRNA (siNC) were synthesized by Sangon Biotech (Shanghai, China). The *ITGB5* siRNA sense and antisense sequences were as follows: si*ITGB5*-368, GCUCGCAGGUCU CAACAUATT and UAUGUUGAGACCUGCGAGCTT; and si*ITGB5*-1218, GCCAACGAGUACACUGCAUTT and AUG CAGUGUACUCGUUGGCTT. The siRNAs were transfected using Lipofectamine 3000 reagent (Life Technologies, Carlsbad, CA, USA) according to the manufacturer's instructions.

In vitro Cell Proliferation Assays

Cell growth was evaluated with the MTS assay (Promega, Madison, WI, USA) according to the manufacturer's instructions.

Cell Migration and Invasion Assays

Transwell inserts with a pore size of 8 µm (Corning Inc., Corning, NY, USA; 3422) were used for *in vitro* cell migration and invasion assays. To assess cell migration, LN229 and PGC1228 cells transfected with siITGB5 or siNC were resuspended in DMEM containing 0.2% FBS and seeded into the upper chambers of the transwell insert at a density of 2×10^4/200 µl. A 600-µl volume of DMEM containing 20% FBS was added to the lower chamber and the number of cells that migrated into the lower chamber was counted. For the invasion assay, LN229 and PGC1228 cells transfected with siITGB5 or siNC were resuspended as described above and seeded into the upper chamber of the insert that was pre-coated with 500 ng/ml Matrigel solution (BD Biosciences, Franklin Lakes, NJ, USA) at a density of 4×10^4/200 µl. A 600-µl volume of DMEM containing 20% FBS was added to the lower chamber. After 24 h, cells on the upper side of the membrane were removed with a cotton swab; the membrane was fixed with methanol and stained with 1% crystal violet solution, and the number of cells on the lower side of the membrane in five random high-power fields per well was counted under a microscope.

Conditioned Medium

Conditioned medium was obtained by culturing equal numbers of treated glioma cells in DMEM or RPMI-1640 medium at 37°C and 5% CO_2 for 24 h. The media were passed thought a 0.2-µm pore filter prior to use in experiments (22).

Tube Formation Assay

The Matrigel assay was used to evaluate *in vitro* angiogenesis based on the quantification of tube formation (23). Briefly, each well of a 96-well culture plate was coated with 100 µl of Matrigel and the plate was incubated for 30 min at 37°C. HUVECs were resuspended in tumor-conditioned medium at a density of 2.0 $\times 10^5$ cells/ml. A 100-µl volume of the cell suspension was seeded in each Matrigel-coated well of the 96-well culture plate, followed by incubation at 37°C for 12 h. Images were acquired at 100× magnification using a fluorescence microscope (DP71; Olympus, Tokyo, Japan), and the total number of branched tubules was quantified (22).

Statistical Analysis

Data were analyzed with SPSS v.20 (SPSS Inc., Chicago, IL, USA) and Prism 7 software (GraphPad Inc., La Jolla, CA, USA) software. Heat maps were generated with R v.3.4.2 (https://www.r-project.org/). Statistical significance was defined as $P < 0.05$. Differences between and among groups were evaluated with the two-tailed *t*-test and by one-way analysis of variance followed by Turkey *post-hoc* test, respectively. Univariate and multivariate Cox regression analyses were performed with R v.3.4.2. A Kaplan-Meier survival analysis was used to estimate the survival distribution, followed by the log-rank test to evaluate differences among stratified groups using the median value as a cutoff. *ITGB5* copy number variation (CNV) frequency in glioma was evaluated with GISTIC2.0 (24); a locus with a GISTIC value ≥ 1 or $\leq$-1 was defined as an amplification or deletion, respectively.

RESULTS

ITGB5 Is Differentially Expressed Between Low-Grade Glioma (LGG) and GBM

Over 20 integrin proteins have been identified, including 18 α and eight β integrin subunits (5). The importance of integrins in cancer biology makes these proteins attractive therapeutic

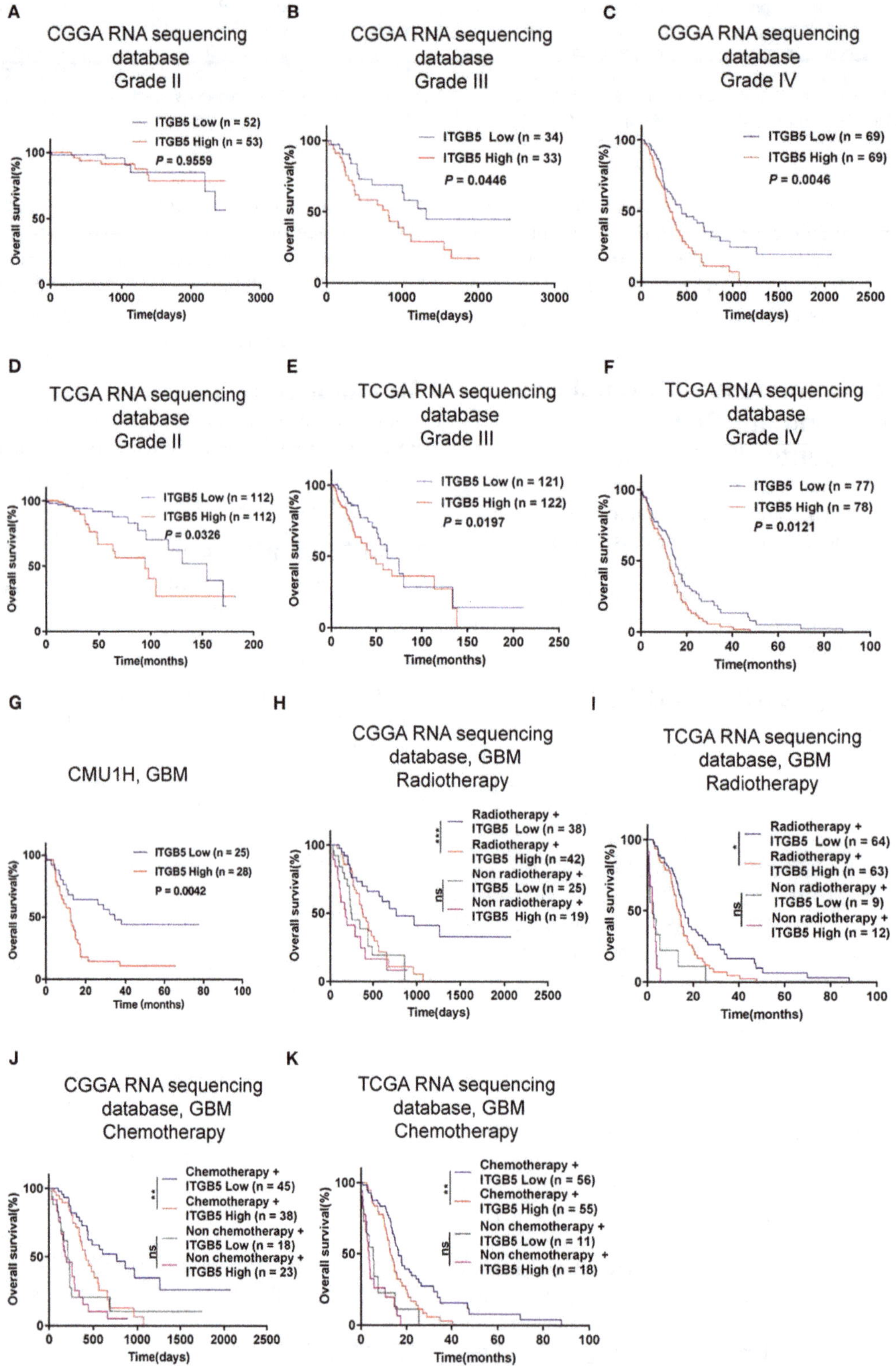

FIGURE 3 | *ITGB5* overexpression is a prognostic biomarker in GBM. **(A–F)**, Kaplan-Meier analysis of the association between *ITGB5* expression and patient survival according to glioma grade (**A**, CGGA grade II; **B**, CGGA grade III; **C**, CGGA grade IV; **D**, TCGA grade II; **E**, TCGA grade III; **F**, TCGA grade IV). **(G)** Kaplan-Meier analysis of the correlation between high ITGB5 expression and patient prognosis in GBM (ITGB5 high vs. low, $P = 0.0042$; log-rank test). **(H–K)** Results of the Kaplan-Meier analysis demonstrating that high ITGB5 expression is associated with poor survival in GBM patients receiving radiotherapy (**H**, CGGA RNAseq; **I**, TCGA RNAseq) or chemotherapy (**J**, CGGA RNAseq; **K**, TCGA RNAseq). ns, $P > 0.05$; $^{*}P < 0.05$; $^{**}P < 0.01$; $^{***}P < 0.001$ (log-rank test).

TABLE 1 | Univariate and multivariate Cox regression analyses of *ITGB5* in CGGA and TCGA RNAseq datasets and overall survival of GBM patients.

Variable	Univariate regression		Multivariate regression	
	HR	*P*-value	HR	*P*-value
CGGA RNAseq, GBM				
Age	1.0050	0.5665	0.96348	0.0029
IDH1	0.7071	0.2017	0.61566	0.1449
Radiotherapy	0.4119	0.0002	0.48658	0.0053
Chemotherapy	0.3359	0.0000	0.31579	0.0000
ITGB5	1.0189	0.0095	1.02759	0.0039
TCGA RNAseq, GBM				
Age	1.0267	0.0010	1.01027	0.2589
IDH1	0.2110	0.0081	0.30458	0.0023
Radiotherapy	0.2351	0.0000	0.86749	0.6752
Chemotherapy	0.4507	0.0001	0.35453	0.1654
ITGB5	1.3776	0.0027	1.32495	0.0132

targets (25, 26). In this study, we analyzed the expression of genes encoding integrin family members in glioma using CGGA and TCGA RNAseq datasets and found that *ITGB5* showed the greatest difference in expression between LGG and GBM (**Figures 1A,B**). We investigated the *ITGB5* copy number variation (CNV) frequency in glioma and observed the following: grade II: amplification, 0.89% and deletion, 5.80%; grade III: amplification, 2.88% and deletion, 7.82%; and GBM: amplification, 18.00% and deletion, 6.67%) (TCGA RNAseq dataset); and GBM: amplification, 12.61% and deletion, 10.04% (TCGA 4502A microarray dataset) (**Table S2**). These data indicate that no mutations are present in *ITGB5* in GBM.

ITGB5 Overexpression Is Associated With Tumor Purity and Immune and Stromal Scores

Extracellular vesicle (EV)-mediated cell-to-cell communication plays an important role in cancer (27, 28). We compiled a list of EV-related genes from intercellular and secretory vesicle gene sets (http://software.broadinstitute.org/gsea/) (**Table S3**), and a principal component analysis (PCA) revealed that these genes can distinguish GBM from LGG (**Figures 1C,D**). We examined the correlation between extracellular vesicle-related genes and tumor purity as well as immune and stromal scores in CGGA and TCGA datasets and determined that *ITGB5* is the only gene that is significantly correlated with all three factors along with unfavorable survival of GBM patients based on a univariate Cox regression analysis ($P < 0.01$; **Figures 1E,F; Figure S1; Table S4**).

Elevated ITGB5 Expression Is Associated With Progressive Malignancy and a Mesenchymal Subtype in Glioma

To further investigate the expression profile of *ITGB5* in glioma, we analyzed *ITGB5* expression in different glioma grades. ITGB5 levels increased with tumor grade (**Figures 2A,B**), and western blot and immunohistochemical analyses of clinical specimens showed that ITGB5 was overexpressed in GBM as compared to non-tumor and grades II and III glioma tissue (**Figures 2C,D**). We then analyzed ITGB5 expression in different GBM subtypes using CGGA and TCGA datasets and found that *ITGB5* was more closely associated with the mesenchymal phenotype (**Figures 2E,F; Figure S2A**), suggesting that it could serve as a diagnostic marker for this subtype (**Figures 2G,H; Figure S2B**). Moreover, according to data from the Ivy database, *ITGB5* was overexpressed in areas of microvascular proliferation relative to other regions of the tumor (**Figure S2C**) and in isocitrate dehydrogenase (*IDH*)*1*-wild-type as compared to *IDH1*-mutant GBM (**Figures 2I,J; Figure S2D**). However, there was no significant difference in *ITGB5* expression between GBM patients with and those without *O6-methylguanine DNA methyltransferase* promoter methylation (**Figures S2E,F**). Thus, elevated *ITGB5* expression is associated with progressive malignancy in glioma and is specific to the mesenchymal subtype.

High ITGB5 Levels Predict Poor Prognosis in GBM

Given the association between high ITGB5 expression and glioma grade, we speculated that ITGB5 could be a prognostic biomarker for glioma outcome. To test this hypothesis, we examined the correlation between ITGB5 expression and the survival of glioma patients. Elevated ITGB5 expression was associated with a favorable outcome for glioma patients (**Figures 3A–F; Figure S3A**). We also analyzed the relationship between ITGB5 expression and the survival of 53 GBM patients and determined that patients with higher ITGB5 levels had poorer outcomes compared to those with a lower ITGB5 expression level (**Figure 3G**). Furthermore, among GBM cases in CGGA and TCGA who underwent radio- and chemotherapy, those with higher ITGB5 expression had a significantly shorter survival time than those with lower expression (**Figures 3H–K; Figures S3B,C**). To assess the correlation between ITGB5 expression and the clinical characteristics in GBM, we performed univariate and multivariate Cox regression analyses with the clinical characteristics of age, *IDH1* mutation status, radiotherapy, and chemotherapy as variables. The results showed that ITGB5 is an independent prognostic factor for overall survival in GBM (**Table 1**). Taken together, these results suggest that ITGB5 is a useful biomarker for predicting survival in GBM patients.

ITGB5 May Be Involved in Immune Regulation and Angiogenesis in the GBM Microenvironment

To clarify the function of ITGB5 in GBM, we compiled a list of 1,043 genes whose expression is correlated with a high *ITGB5* expression level based on CGGA and TCGA GBM RNAseq datasets ($r > 0.3$, $P < 0.05$; **Table S5**). A GO analysis revealed an association between *ITGB5* expression and the GO terms vascular endothelial growth factor signaling pathway, migration, inflammatory response, immune response, cell adhesion, and angiogenesis (**Figure 4A**). As mentioned above, *ITGB5* was the only gene correlated with tumor purity and immune and

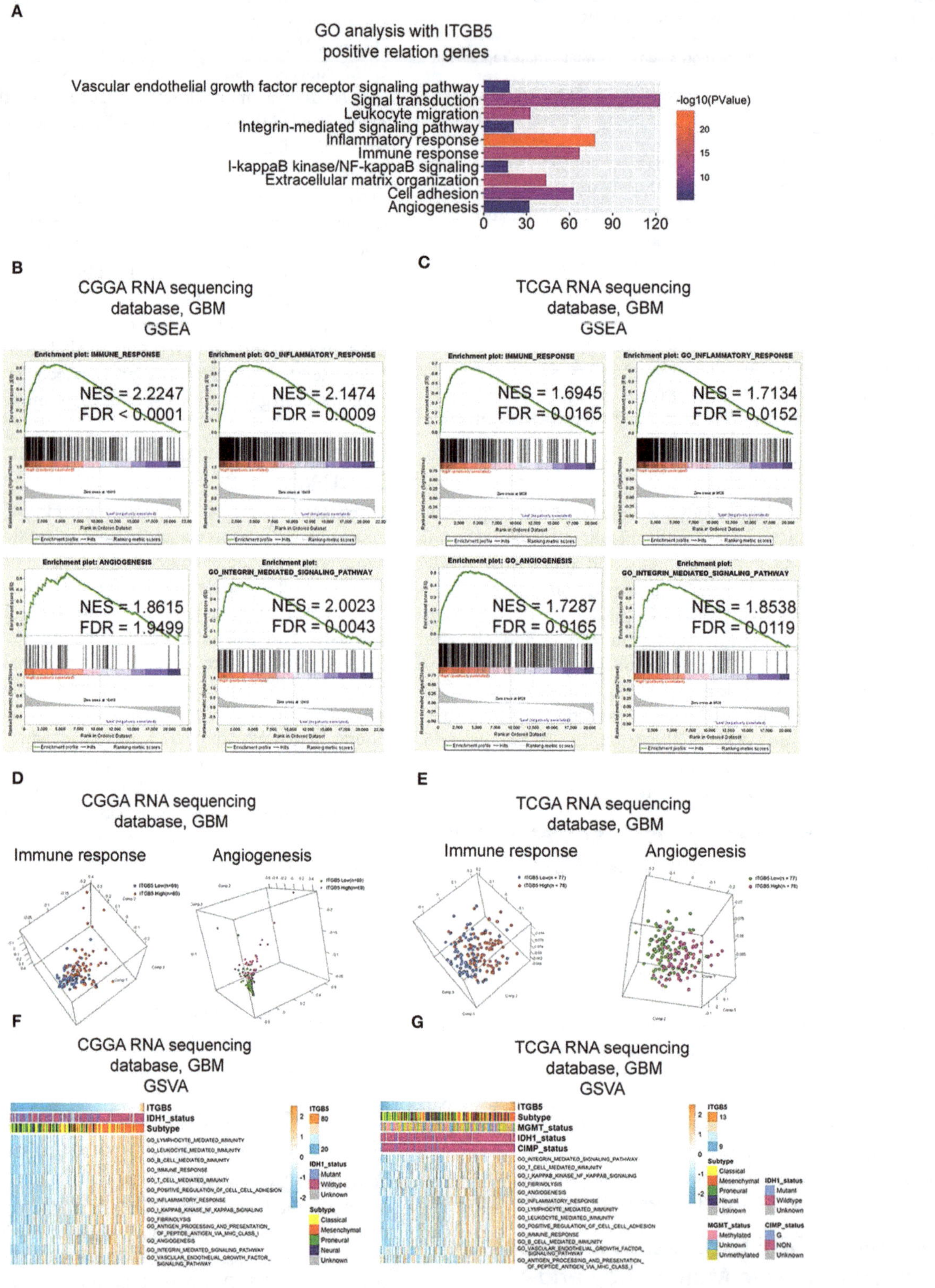

FIGURE 4 | Functional analysis of signaling pathways associated with high *ITGB5* expression level in GBM. **(A)** GO analysis of genes positively correlated with *ITGB5* based on CGGA and TCGA RNAseq datasets (Pearson's correlation analysis). **(B,C)** GSEA analyses of CGGA **(B)** and TCGA **(C)** GBM RNAseq datasets showing the enrichment of immune response, inflammatory response, angiogenesis, and integrin-mediated signaling pathways in patient samples with high *ITGB5* expression. **(D,E)** PCA analysis based on CGGA **(D)** and TCGA **(E)** GBM RNAseq datasets shows that high ITGB5 expression can stratify immune response and angiogenesis signaling. **(F,G)** GSVA showing the correlation between high *ITGB5* levels and immune response and angiogenesis-related signaling pathways.

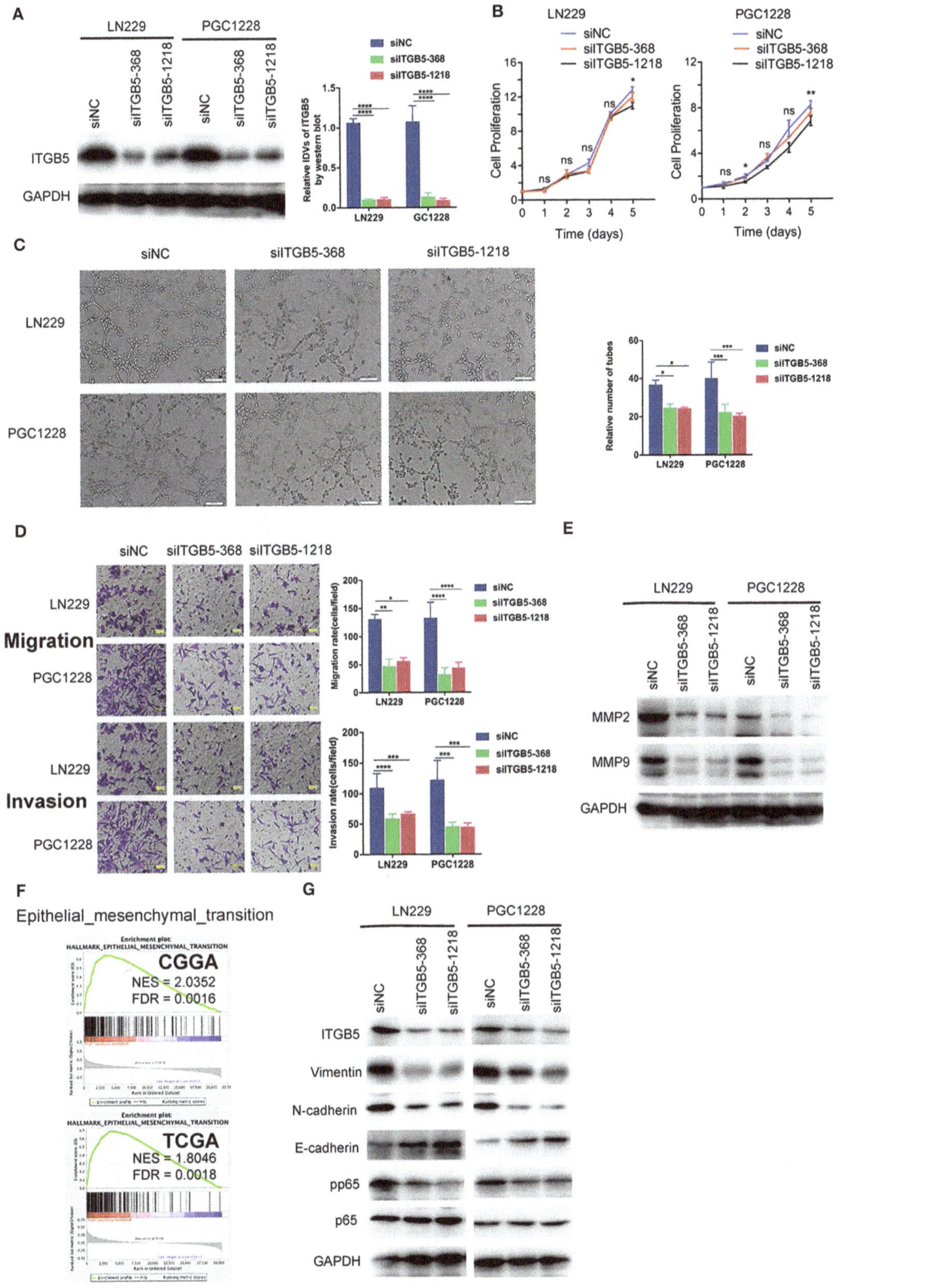

FIGURE 5 | *ITGB5* silencing attenuates the migration and angiogenesis of glioma cells and inhibits epithelial-mesenchymal transition marker expression. **(A)** Representative western blots (left panel) and analysis (right panel) of glioma cells transfected with indicated siRNAs targeting *ITGB5* (si*ITGB5*-368 and si*ITGB5*-1218)

(Continued)

FIGURE 5 | or siNC. **(B)** The effect of *ITGB5* silencing on the growth of LN229 and PGC1228 cells. **(C)** *ITGB5* knockdown suppresses tube formation by endothelial cells treated with conditioned medium from cultured glioma cells. **(D)** Glioma cell migration (upper panel) and invasion (lower panel) are inhibited by *ITGB5* knockdown. **(E)** Western blot analysis of glioma cells transfected with indicated siRNAs showing that *ITGB5* silencing attenuates MMP2 and MMP9 expression. **(F)** GSEA of CGGA and TCGA RNAseq datasets reveals the enrichment of epithelial–mesenchymal transition-related genes in specimens with high ITGB5 levels. **(G)** Western blot analysis of glioma cells transfected with indicated siRNAs targeting *ITGB5* (si*ITGB5*-368 and si*ITGB5*-1218) or siNC. *ITGB5* silencing suppressed EMT marker expression. ns, $P > 0.05$; $^*P < 0.05$; $^{**}P < 0.01$; $^{***}P < 0.001$; $^{****}P < 0.0001$ (one-way analysis of variance [ANOVA]).

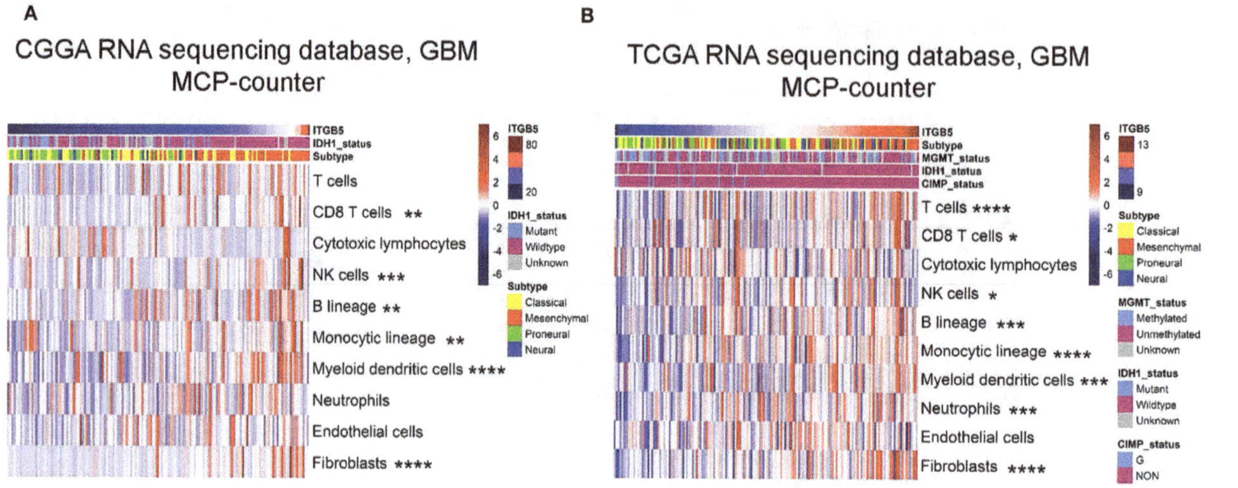

FIGURE 6 | Correlation between *ITGB5* expression and non-tumor immune and stromal cell populations in the GBM microenvironment. Cell populations were quantified with MCP-counter (**A**, CGGA GBM RNAseq; **B**, TCGA GBM RNAseq). $^*P < 0.05$; $^{**}P < 0.01$; $^{***}P < 0.001$; $^{****}P < 0.0001$ (Pearson's correlation analysis).

stromal scores in CGGA and TCGA datasets ($r > 0.45$ or <-0.45; **Table S4**). Based on this observation, we carried out GSEA to investigate the function of ITGB5 in GBM. The immune response, inflammatory response, angiogenesis, and integrin-mediated signaling were associated with elevated ITGB5 expression (**Figures 4B,C**). Additionally, PCA based on CGGA and TCGA GBM RNAseq datasets demonstrated that high *ITGB5* levels can stratify immune response and angiogenesis signaling (**Figures 4D,E**). Consistent with these results, GSVA revealed that ITGB5 contributes to the regulation of local immune response, cell adhesion, and vascular endothelial growth factor signaling (**Figures 4F,G**). Thus, ITGB5 is involved in the immune response and angiogenesis in the GBM microenvironment.

ITGB5 Is Required for Glioma Cell Migration and Invasion and for Tube Formation by Endothelial Cells

To examine the functions of ITGB5 in GBM in greater detail, we used two *ITGB5*-specific siRNAs to knock down *ITGB5* expression in a stable glioma cell line (LN229) and a primary glioma cell line derived from a clinical GBM specimen (PGC1228) (**Figure 5A**; **Figure S4**). ITGB5 silencing did not significantly affect the growth of LN229 at day 1, 2, 3, and 4 (**Figure 5B**, left panel). For PGC1228, there was significantly difference at day 2 and day 5, and there was no significant difference at dayl, 3, and 4 (**Figure 5B**, right panel); however, the tube formation capacity of endothelial cells induced with glioma cell-conditioned medium as well as glioma cell migration and invasion were inhibited (**Figures 5C,D**). The expression of matrix metalloproteinase (MMP)2 and MMP9—two proteins that regulate the migration and invasion of glioma cells—was also attenuated by ITGB5 knockdown (**Figure 5E**). In addition, GSEA revealed that EMT signaling was increased in association with high ITGB5 expression (**Figure 5F**). Consistent with this observation, western blot analysis of glioma cells transfected with siRNAs targeting *ITGB5* showed that the expression of several EMT markers including vimentin, N-cadherin, and phosphorylated p65 was downregulated by ITGB5 depletion (**Figure 5G**). These data indicate ITGB5 not only regulates the migration and invasion of glioma cells but also tube formation capacity in endothelial cells.

ITGB5 Expression Is Associated With Non-tumor Immune and Stromal Cell Populations in the Glioma Microenvironment

We evaluated the association between *ITGB5* and the immune and stromal cell populations in the GBM microenvironment with the MCP-counter method. The results showed that CD8+ T cell, NK cell, fibroblast, B cell, monocyte, and myeloid dendritic cell numbers were positively associated with ITGB5 expression (**Figures 6A,B**), providing further evidence for the regulatory role of ITGB5 in the local tumor microenvironment.

DISCUSSION

Despite the use of multimodal treatment strategies, the survival time of most GBM patients is <2 years (1). Reliable prognostic biomarkers for this disease are needed in order to improve patient outcome and monitor the response to standard radio-and chemotherapy. Moreover, the characterization of molecular changes has important clinical implications for predicting glioma outcome (29). Our analyses showed that ITGB5 was overexpressed in GBM, especially in the mesenchymal subtype. Another novel finding of this study was that high ITGB5 levels were independently correlated with shorter survival time in patients. These data highlight the value of ITGB5 as a predictive biomarker in GBM.

A typical feature of GBM is disruption of the local microenvironment (20). Our bioinformatic analyses revealed that high ITGB5 expression is correlated with integrin-related, immune, and angiogenesis signaling, suggesting that ITGB5 may play an important regulatory role in the GBM microenvironment. Tumor-associated macrophages have been implicated in brain tumor angiogenesis and resistance to anti-angiogenic therapies, in part due to their ability to modulate vessel integrity and function (30–32). We show that *ITGB5* expression is positively correlated with the number of monocyte lineage cells, which may reflect the mechanism by which ITGB5 regulates the tumor microenvironment. This result is consistent with a recent report, which indicated that the heterodimer of ITGB5 and ITGAV expressed by GBM-infiltrating macrophages constituted a major OPN receptor and mediated the recruitment of macrophages (12). In comparison with non-tumor tissue, glioma, especially GBM, have an elevated expression level of ITGB5 (**Figure 2C**). This may indicate the potential of ITGB5 as a therapeutic target in the treatment of GBM. Considering ITGB5 expressed in normal tissue and non-tumor cells, further study is needed to investigate whether systematic blockade of ITGB5 may lead to potential side effects, like immunosuppression.

To investigate the function of ITGB5 in GBM, we performed knockdown experiments using siRNAs and found that glioma cell growth was unaffected by *ITGB5* depletion, although their migration and invasion were reduced. Moreover, the decreased capacity for endothelial tube formation caused by ITGB5 knockdown indicates that ITGB5 is required for angiogenesis, which may be promoted by the release of factors via extracellular vesicles. However, further studies are needed to investigate this possibility.

In summary, our study shows that a high expression level of *ITGB5* is an indicator of progressive malignancy in glioma and predicts unfavorable outcome in GBM patients, even after radiotherapy. ITGB5 not only influences the migration and invasion of glioma cells, but is also involved in regulating the immune response and angiogenesis in the tumor microenvironment. Thus, ITGB5 is a useful prognostic biomarker and potential therapeutic target in GBM.

AUTHOR CONTRIBUTIONS

QG, PC, and AW conceived and designed the study. LZ, QG, and WC carried out the experiments and collected data and performed the bioinformatics analysis. PC, QG, GG, and AW drafted the manuscript. PC and AW obtained funding for the study. All authors read and approved the final manuscript.

FUNDING

This study was supported by the National Natural Science Foundation of China (nos. 81172409, 81472360, and 81872054 to AW and no. 81872057 to PC) and Liaoning Science and Technology Plan Projects (no. 2011225034 to AW).

ACKNOWLEDGMENTS

We thank all members of Dr. Wu Ah's laboratory for helpful discussions on this work.

SUPPLEMENTARY MATERIAL

Figure S1 | Heatmaps of correlations between intercellular vesicle-related gene expression and tumor purity and immune and stromal scores based on TCGA 4502A mRNA microarray data. $r > 0.45$ or < -0.45 (Pearson's correlation analysis).

Figure S2 | *ITGB5* expression in glioma. **(A)** *ITGB5* expression in different grades of glioma based on TCGA 4502A mRNA microarray data. ****$P < 0.0001$ (one-way ANOVA). **(C)** *ITGB5* expression in the Ivy GAP RNAseq dataset. **$P < 0.01$; ****$P < 0.0001$ (one-way ANOVA). **(B)** ROC curve for evaluating the sensitivity and specificity of *ITGB5* as a diagnostic marker for the mesenchymal subtype of GBM as compared to the other subtypes (TCGA 4502A mRNA microarray, area under the ROC curve [AUC]: 0.757; $P < 0.001$). **(D)** ITGB5 expression is elevated in *IDH1*-wild-type as compared to *IDH1*-mutant GBM (TCGA 4502A mRNA microarray; *t*-test). **(E,F)** ITGB5 expression in GBM patients with or without *O6-methylguanine DNA methyltransferase (MGMT)* promoter methylation. (**E**, TCGA RNAseq; **F**, TCGA 4502A microarray). ns, $P > 0.05$ (*t*-test).

Figure S3 | *ITGB5* is a prognostic biomarker in GBM. **(A)** *ITGB5* expression is associated with unfavorable prognosis in GBM (TCGA 4502A mRNA microarray). $P = 0.0008$ (log-rank test). **(B,C)** High *ITGB5* expression predicts the response of GBM patients to radiotherapy **(B)** and chemotherapy **(C)** (TCGA 4502A mRNA microarray) (*$P < 0.05$, **$P < 0.001$, log-rank test).

Figure S4 | *ITGB5* silencing has no effect on glioma cell growth. **(A)** Representative RT-qPCR analysis of glioma cells transfected with indicated siRNAs targeting *ITGB5* (siITGB5-368 and siITGB5-1218) or control siRNA (siNC). ****$P < 0.0001$ (one-way ANOVA).

Table S1 | Antibodies used in this study.

Table S2 | *ITGB5* copy number variation frequency in TCGA.

Table S3 | Intercellular vesicle-related genes.

Table S4 | Correlation analysis of intercellular vesicle-related genes with tumor purity and immune and stromal scores in CGGA and TCGA datasets (Pearson's correlation analysis).

Table S5 | Genes positively correlated with high *ITGB5* expression in CGGA and TCGA GBM RNAseq datasets.

REFERENCES

1. Stupp R, Hegi ME, Mason WP, van den Bent MJ, Taphoorn MJ, Janzer RC, et al. Effects of radiotherapy with concomitant and adjuvant temozolomide versus radiotherapy alone on survival in glioblastoma in a randomised phase III study: 5-year analysis of the EORTC-NCIC trial. *Lancet Oncol.* (2009) 10:459–66. doi: 10.1016/S1470-2045(09)70025-7
2. Chinot OL, Wick W, Mason W, Henriksson R, Saran F, Nishikawa R, et al. Bevacizumab plus radiotherapy-temozolomide for newly diagnosed glioblastoma. *N Engl J Med.* (2014) 370:709–22. doi: 10.1056/NEJMoa1308345
3. Wen PY, Kesari S. Malignant gliomas in adults. *N Engl J Med.* (2008) 359:492–507. doi: 10.1056/NEJMra0708126

4. Haas TL, Sciuto MR, Brunetto L, Valvo C, Signore M, Fiori ME, et al. Integrin alpha7 is a functional marker and potential therapeutic target in glioblastoma. *Cell Stem Cell.* (2017) 21:35–50.e9. doi: 10.1016/j.stem.2017.04.009
5. Hamidi H, Ivaska J. Every step of the way: integrins in cancer progression and metastasis. *Nat Rev Cancer.* (2018) 18:533–48. doi: 10.1038/s41568-018-0038-z
6. Ferrer VP, Moura Neto V, Mentlein R. Glioma infiltration and extracellular matrix: key players and modulators. *Glia.* 66:1542–65. (2018) doi: 10.1002/glia.23309
7. Lathia J, D., Gallagher J, Heddleston J, M., Wang J, Eyler C, E., Macswords J, et al. Integrin alpha 6 regulates glioblastoma stem cells. *Cell Stem Cell.* (2010) 6:421–32. doi: 10.1016/j.stem.2010.02.018
8. Bianchi A, Gervasi M, E., Bakin A. Role of beta5-integrin in epithelial-mesenchymal transition in response to TGF-beta. *Cell Cycle.* (2010) 9:1647–59. doi: 10.4161/cc.9.8.11517
9. Bianchi-Smiraglia A, Paesante S, Bakin AV. Integrin beta5 contributes to the tumorigenic potential of breast cancer cells through the Src-FAK and MEK-ERK signaling pathways. *Oncogene.* (2013) 32:3049–58. doi: 10.1038/onc.2012.320
10. Lin Z, He R, Luo H, Lu C, Ning Z, Wu Y, et al. Integrin-beta5, a miR-185-targeted gene, promotes hepatocellular carcinoma tumorigenesis by regulating beta-catenin stability. *J Exp Clin Cancer Res.* (2018) 37:17. doi: 10.1186/s13046-018-0691-9
11. Wortzel I, Dror S, Kenific CM, Lyden D. Exosome-mediated metastasis: communication from a distance. *Dev Cell.* (2019) 49:347–60. doi: 10.1016/j.devcel.2019.04.011
12. Wei J, Marisetty A, Schrand B, Gabrusiewicz K, Hashimoto Y, Ott M, et al. Osteopontin mediates glioblastoma-associated macrophage infiltration and is a potential therapeutic target. *J Clin Invest.* (2019) 129:137–49. doi: 10.1172/JCI121266
13. Bowman RL, Wang Q, Carro A, Verhaak RG, Squatrito M. GlioVis data portal for visualization and analysis of brain tumor expression datasets. *Neuro Oncol.* (2017) 19:139–41. doi: 10.1093/neuonc/now247
14. Wang J, Cheng P, Pavlyukov M, S., Yu H, Zhang Z, Kim SH, et al. Targeting NEK2 attenuates glioblastoma growth and radioresistance by destabilizing histone methyltransferase EZH2. *J Clin Invest.* (2017) 127:3075–89. doi: 10.1172/JCI89092
15. Yoshihara K, Shahmoradgoli M, Martinez E, Vegesna R, Kim H, Torres-Garcia W, et al. Inferring tumour purity and stromal and immune cell admixture from expression data. *Nat Commun.* (2013) 4:2612. doi: 10.1038/ncomms3612
16. Robin X, Turck N, Hainard A, Tiberti N, Lisacek F, Sanchez JC, et al. pROC: an open-source package for R and S+ to analyze and compare ROC curves. *BMC Bioinformatics.* (2011) 12:77. doi: 10.1186/1471-21 05-12-77
17. Huang da W, Sherman BT, Lempicki RA. Systematic and integrative analysis of large gene lists using DAVID bioinformatics resources. *Nat Protoc.* (2009) 4:44–57. doi: 10.1038/nprot.2008.211
18. Subramanian A, Tamayo P, Mootha V, K., Mukherjee S, Ebert BL, Gillette MA, et al. Gene set enrichment analysis: a knowledge-based approach for interpreting genome-wide expression profiles. *Proc Natl Acad Sci USA.* (2005) 102:15545–50. doi: 10.1073/pnas.0506580102
19. Hanzelmann S, Castelo R, Guinney J. GSVA: gene set variation analysis for microarray and RNA-seq data. *BMC Bioinformatics.* (2013) 14:7. doi: 10.1186/1471-2105-14-7
20. Zhang C, Cheng W, Ren X, Wang Z, Liu X, Li G, et al. Tumor purity as an underlying key factor in glioma. *Clin Cancer Res.* (2017) 23:6279–91. doi: 10.1158/1078-0432.CCR-16-2598
21. Becht E, Giraldo N, A., Lacroix L, Buttard B, Elarouci N, Petitprez F, et al. Estimating the population abundance of tissue-infiltrating immune and stromal cell populations using gene expression. *Genome Biol.* (2016) 17:218. doi: 10.1186/s13059-016-1070-5
22. Cai H, Liu X, Zheng J, Xue Y, Ma J, Li Z, et al. Long non-coding RNA taurine upregulated 1 enhances tumor-induced angiogenesis through inhibiting microRNA-299 in human glioblastoma. *Oncogene.* (2017) 36:318–31. doi: 10.1038/onc.2016.212
23. Wurdinger T, Tannous BA, Saydam O, Skog J, Grau S, Soutschek J, et al. miR-296 regulates growth factor receptor overexpression in angiogenic endothelial cells. *Cancer Cell.* (2008) 14:382–93. doi: 10.1016/j.ccr.2008.10.005
24. Mermel CH, Schumacher SE, Hill B, Meyerson ML, Beroukhim R, Getz G. GISTIC2.0 facilitates sensitive and confident localization of the targets of focal somatic copy-number alteration in human cancers. *Genome Biol.* (2011) 12:R41. doi: 10.1186/gb-2011-12-4-r41
25. Desgrosellier JS, Cheresh DA. Integrins in cancer: biological implications and therapeutic opportunities. *Nat Rev Cancer.* (2010) 10:9–22. doi: 10.1038/nrc2748
26. Paolillo M, Serra M, Schinelli S. Integrins in glioblastoma: still an attractive target? *Pharmacol Res.* (2016) 113(Pt A):55–61. doi: 10.1016/j.phrs.2016.08.004
27. Pavlyukov MS, Yu H, Bastola S, Minata M, Shender VO, Lee Y, et al. Apoptotic cell-derived extracellular vesicles promote malignancy of glioblastoma via intercellular transfer of splicing factors. *Cancer Cell.* (2018) 34:119–35.e10. doi: 10.1016/j.ccell.2018.05.012
28. Hoshino A, Costa-Silva B, Shen TL, Rodrigues G, Hashimoto A, Tesic Mark M, et al. Tumour exosome integrins determine organotropic metastasis. *Nature.* (2015) 527:329–35. doi: 10.1038/nature15756
29. Aquilanti E, Miller J, Santagata S, Cahill DP, Brastianos PK. Updates in prognostic markers for gliomas. *Neuro Oncol.* (2018) 20(suppl. 7):vii17–26. doi: 10.1093/neuonc/noy158
30. De Palma M, Venneri MA, Galli R, Sergi Sergi L, Politi LS, Sampaolesi M, et al. Tie2 identifies a hematopoietic lineage of proangiogenic monocytes required for tumor vessel formation and a mesenchymal population of pericyte progenitors. *Cancer Cell.* (2005) 8:211–26. doi: 10.1016/j.ccr.2005.08.002
31. Lu-Emerson C, Snuderl M, Kirkpatrick ND, Goveia J, Davidson C, Huang Y, et al. Increase in tumor-associated macrophages after antiangiogenic therapy is associated with poor survival among patients with recurrent glioblastoma. *Neuro Oncol.* (2013) 15:1079–87. doi: 10.1093/neuonc/not082
32. Piao Y, Liang J, Holmes L, Zurita A, J., Henry V, Heymach JV, et al. Glioblastoma resistance to anti-VEGF therapy is associated with myeloid cell infiltration, stem cell accumulation, and a mesenchymal phenotype. *Neuro Oncol.* (2012) 14:1379–92. doi: 10.1093/neuonc/nos158

4

Prognostic and Clinic Pathological Value of Cx43 Expression in Glioma

Chao Zhang[1,2]*, Cheng-fen Liu*[1]*, An-bin Chen*[1,2]*, Zhong Yao*[1,2]*, Wei-guo Li*[1,2]*, Shu-jun Xu*[1,2] *and Xiang-yu Ma*[1,2*]

[1] *Department of Neurosurgery, Qilu Hospital, Shandong University, Jinan, China,* [2] *Brain Science Research Institute, Shandong University, Jinan, China*

Correspondence:
Xiang-yu Ma
drmaxiangyu@hotmail.com

Gap junctional intercellular communication (GJIC) composed of connexin proteins is considered vital to cancer onset and progression since 50 years ago based on Lowenstein and Kano's works, however altered expression of connexins is still a lesser known "hallmark" of cancer. Although many studies support the hypothesis that connexins are tumor suppressors, recent evidence indicates that, in some tumor types including glioma, they may play contradictory role in some specific stages of tumor progression. We thus conduct a meta-analysis to evaluate the prognostic role of Cx43 in glioma for the unanswered questions that whether Cx43 is a beneficial or insalubrity factor for glioma. Eight studies with 1,706 patients were included for meta-analysis. The results showed that Cx43 expression was a clearly negative factor with tumor grades ($I^2 = 34\%$, $P < 0.001$) and beneficial for OS ($n = 3$, HR 2.62, 95%CI 1.47–4.68; $P = 0.001$). Subgroup analysis also found that Cx43 had different expression in Asian young patients vs. other groups. In conclusion, this article summarize the prognostic value of Cx43 and offer a clinical evidence for the notion that Cx43 is generally a tumor suppressor and beneficial for the patients' survival time.

Keywords: glioma, Cx43, gap junctional intercellular communication, glioma survival time, meta-analysis

INTRODUCTION

Brain tumors account for 1.9% of all new cancer cases and 2.3% of cancer related deaths globally. Among them, glioblastoma (GBM) is the most common primary malignant brain tumor (more than 45% of all malignant brain tumors) (1). However, the 5-year survival individuals with traditional treatment is still <5% since past decades, ranking it the 6th most lethal of all types among tumors (2). Standard procedure of care for newly diagnosed GBM includes maximum surgery resection, followed by ionizing radiation and chemotherapy with temozolomide (TMZ). Evidences showed that surgery resection is still the most effective way to cure GBM and excision extension is closely tied to patients' overall survival, so the importance of early-diagnosing GBM and exact-safe resection appeal to more and more focus (3). Therefore, it is necessary to identify molecular markers to help to distinguish surgical range and give a predicted clinical outcomes of high risk patients.

Cellular communication is vital in numerous processes critical for tumor biological homeostasis, for cell survival, proliferation, differentiation, and invasion. And in turn, it facilitated disease through a passive intercellular transmit of small molecules, second messengers, ions, microRNAs, and electrical signals (4). The structure of Connexins are tetra-span integral plasma membrane, consisting of two extracellular loops and one intracellular loop along with cytoplasmic amino (NH_2) and carboxyl-terminal (CT) tail domains. Up to now, numbers of Cx molecules have been explored in the CNS: Cx30, Cx32, Cx36, and Cx43 in neurons; Cx30, Cx40, Cx43, and Cx45 in astrocytes; Cx32, Cx36, and Cx43 in microglia; and Cx26, Cx32, Cx29, Cx36, and Cx47 in oligodendrocyte (5, 6).

Although the big family consisting of Connexins, Cx43 is one of the most important subtypes which highly expressed in GBM tissues in some patients and appeared to be a marker distinguishing glioma from other types of brain cancers such as oligodendrocytic (7, 8). Cx43 has also been reported to possess the tumor-suppressor-like activities, to cause cancer cell dedifferentiation (mesenchymal to epithelial transition), and to inhibit metastasis thus affecting the tumor progression (6). Recently, few cases reported that Cx43 expression was inversely correlated to tumor grade as a result Cx43 was considered to "normalize" the phenotype of rat and human glioma cells (4, 9, 10). However, these articles failed to find any association between Cx43 and OS in glioma in their study and no meta-analysis reported that. In order to give a convincing evidence for this issue, we thus gathered the most recent studies and performed a meta-analysis to pool the results from eligible studies to present a quantitative calculation.

METHODS

Literature Search Strategy

A systematic review and meta-analysis was conducted under the recommends of PRISMA guidelines. Data extraction was systematically performed in PubMed, Web of Science and EMBASE/Medlin, with different combinations of the following key words ["Glioma," "brain tumor" OR "glioblastoma"] AND ["Connexin43," "gap junction channels 43" OR "Cx43"] and no language restrictions. Terms ["Glioma," "brain tumor" OR "glioblastoma"] AND ["Connexin," "gap junction channels" OR "Cx"] were also searched and after eliminating papers focusing on other Cx proteins, the included results were same as the combination of glioma and Cx43. This search was finally renewed till May 1, 2019. References consists of studies, clinical cases and review articles were also included to find additional patients data.

Inclusion Criteria

Our purpose of this study was to identify whether Cx43 expression decreased the risk of glioma. Therefore, the criteria for enrolled study was as follows: (1) study should concerned the relationship between Cx43 and clinical outcomes among patients with gliomas. (2) Gliomas should be diagnosed by standard criteria, histopathologic analysis. (3) Cx43 expression was examined in glioma tissue obtained from glioma patients not experimental cells. (4) Cx43 expression was examined by immunohistochemistry (IHC) methods, PCR or tissue microarray. (5) The data should provide detailed information to calculate overall survival (OS) or disease free survival (DFS). Studies that could not meet any one of the above inclusion criteria were excluded. Studies which did not meet the above requirements were excluded and animal studies, letters were also precluded.

Data Extraction

Two authors independently evaluated all studies and selected eligible trials, and any discrepancies between the authors were resolved by discussion and consensus. Among the studies, data was extracted included following information: country of the population enrolled, first author's name, number of included patients, and year of publication, sample size, patients' age, histological grade, diagnosed technique, and positive standard, antibody used, overall survival rates and survival outcomes. Kaplan-Meier (K-M) curves of these studies were analyzed by Engauge Digitizer (http://sourceforge.net/projects/digitizer/) which was utilized to calculate the OR and DFS. When univariate analysis and multivariate analysis were all provided in studies, we prefer the former results to be analyzed in the study. If the extract information could not be retained directly from included studies, we would send an email to the correspond author to get the original relevant data, otherwise the item would be marked as "Not Documented (ND)."

Statistical Analysis

The Revman (version 5.3) was used to conduct all the calculations during the whole process of meta-analysis. Odds risks (OR) with 95% confidence intervals (CIs) were calculated and conducted to evaluate the correlation between Cx43 and clinical pathological outcomes in forest plots. I^2 test and Q test were used to estimate heterogeneity in these studies. If the I^2 test (>50%) or the Q test ($P < 0.05$) were abnormal, which indicated a significant heterogeneity between the selected studies, random-effect model would be introduced to assess the results, and otherwise the fixed-effect model would be used. Sub-group analyses based on research techniques (IHC or PCR), ethnicity and sample size were conducted. Sensitivity analysis was conducted to evaluate heterogeneity and stability of enrolled data. Potential publication

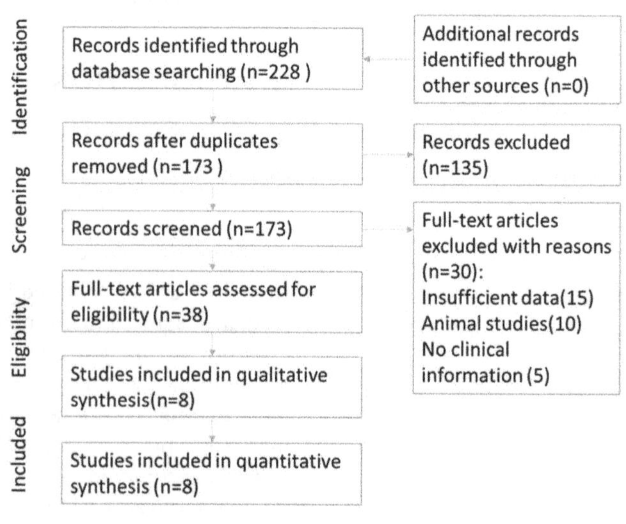

FIGURE 1 | Flow chart for selection of studies.

bias were assessed by the funnel plots and Egger's tests. Also the effect of Cx43 diagnostic sensitivity and specificity were also presented by forest plot and SROC curve.

RESULTS

Study Selection and Characteristics

The flow of study selection has been presented in **Figure 1**. Based on an extensive combination of keywords search and screened a total of 173 papers by article title as well as abstract, we picked up 8 (9, 11–17) published studies that fulfilled all inclusion criteria which required intact data, strict experiment design and minor publication bias in the present meta-analysis. The enrolled studies were well-controlled and accorded with selection criterions. Based on the expression level of Cx43, enrolled patients of all the studies were divided into different subgroups: the high Cx43 level patients confirming to every positive standard in papers were classified into the Cx43 High subgroup, and patients with low Cx43 levels were attributed into the Cx43 Low subgroup. Overall, 8 studies constituting 790 Cx43 High patients and 916 Cx43 Low patients were evaluated with tumor grades, ethnicity, research technique and overall survival (OS).

Study Characteristics and Quality Assessment

The enrolled studies and clinical characteristics of included articles are presented in **Table 1**. Eight studies were conducted

TABLE 1 | Characteristics of included studies into meta-analysis.

Author	Ethnicity	Year	Sample size	Age (yr)	Histology	Research techniques	Ab used	Positive standard
Peiyu Pu	China	2003	52	ND	Normal 8 Grade I 4 (pilocytic astrocytoma) Grade II 12 (protoplasmic and fibrillary astrocytoma) Grade III 14 (anaplastic astrocytoma) Grade IV 14 (glioblastoma multiforme)	IHC	Santa Cruz	No positive cells (0), positive cells <25% (1), between 25 and 50% (2), between 50 and 75% (3), >75% (4)
Rosario Caltabiano	Italy	2010	32	43.9 (2–80)	Grade I 7 Grade II 5 Grade III 7 Grade IV 13	IHC RT-PCR	Zymed	Negative (–) = absence of labeling, (+) = positivity <50% of the neoplastic glial cells, (++) = positivity from 50 to 100% of the neoplastic glial cells.
Paul R. Gielen	America	2013	208	45.5 (9–70)	Normal 8 Grade I 13 Grade II 42 Grade III 112 Grade IV 33	IHC RT-PCR	Sigma, C6219	No positive cells (0), positive cells <25% (1), between 25 and 50% (2), between 50 and 75% (3), >75% (4)
Joanna Reszeć	Poland	2014	131	65.9	Grade II 26 (diffuse astrocytoma anaplasic) Grade III 44 (astrocytomas) Grade IV 61 (glioblastoma)	IHC	Santa Cruz, C-20	≤10% positive cells (–), 11–50% (+), ≥51% (++)
Susan F. Murphy	America	2015	520	ND	Normal 62 Grade I 95 Grade II 214 Grade III 80 Grade IV 121	IHC RT-PCR	Sigma	≤10% positive cells (–), 11–50% (+), ≥51% (++)
WC Sin	Canada	2015	474	42.9 (2–72)	Normal 52 Grade I 86 Grade II 205 Grade III 71 Grade IV 112	IHC	Sigma,C6219	Negative (–) = absence of labeling, (+) = positivity <50% of the neoplastic glial cells, (++) = positivity from 50 to 100% of the neoplastic glial cells.
Xin-Yun Ye	China	2015	80	ND	Grade I 20 (pilocytic astrocytoma) Grade II 20 (protoplasmic and fibrillary astrocytoma) Grade III 20 (anaplastic astrocytoma) Grade IV 20 (glioblastoma multiforme)	IHC	Santa Cruz	No positive cells(0), positive cells <25% (1), between 25 and 50%(2), between 50 and 75% (3), >75% (4)
Sophie Crespin	France	2016	85	51.9 (16–78)	Grade II 19 Grade III 12 Grade IV 22	IHC	Transduction laboratories, USA	No positive cells (0), positive cells <25% (1), between 25 and 50% (2), between 50 and 75% (3), >75% (4)

ND, no details; IHC, immunohistochemistry; PCR, polymerase chain reaction.

TABLE 2 | Newcastle-Ottawa Quality Assessment Scale of included studies.

Study	Selection				Comparability	Outcome			
	Representativeness of exposed cohort 1	Selection of non-exposed group 2	Ascertartainment of expose 3	Outcome of interest 4	Comparability of cohorts 5	Assessment of outcome 6	Length of follow-up 7	Adequency of follow-up 8	Score
Peiyu Pu	1	1	1	1	1	1	0	0	6
Rosario Caltabiano	1	1	1	1	1	1	0	0	6
Paul R. Gielen	1	1	1	1	2	0	1	1	8
Joanna Reszeć	1	1	1	1	1	1	0	0	6
Susan F. Murphy	1	1	1	1	2	0	1	1	8
W. C. Sin	1	1	1	1	2	0	1	1	8
Xin-Yun Ye	1	1	1	1	1	1	0	0	6
Sophie crespin	1	1	1	1	1	1	0	0	6

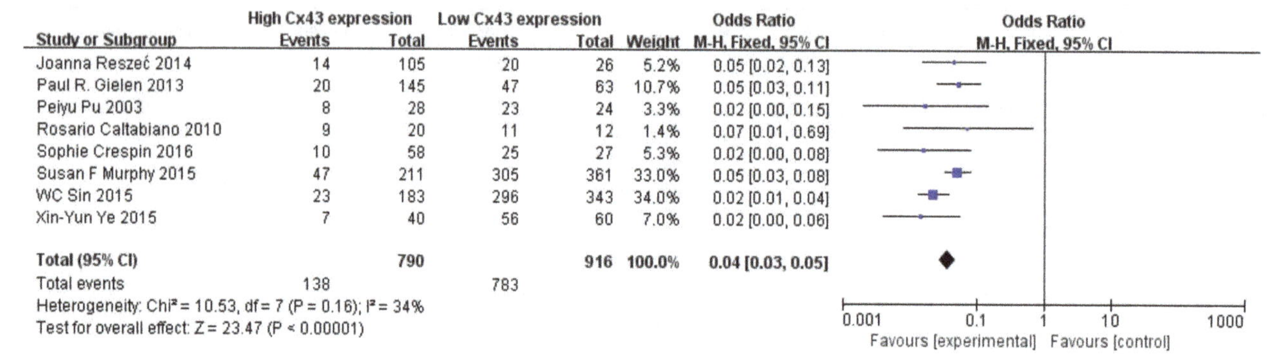

FIGURE 2 | Forest plot of studies evaluating the relationship between Cx43 expression and tumor grades.

within western countries, and two within Asia. Five studies including more than 100 patients while the other three studies had relatively smaller patient's numbers. Two studies examined Cx43 expression by RT-PCR and six studies used IHC methods. Three articles evaluated cancer survival and recurrence. The publication time of all papers ranged from 2003 to 2016. The number size of enrolled group ranged from 32 to 572, and the positive rates of Cx43 expression varied from 55.6 to 89.2%. To examine the quality of included studies, Newcastle-Ottawa Quality Assessment scores (NOS) were introduced and the data ranged from six to nine (detail listed in **Table 2**), which manifested that the quality of enrolled studies was high. Exacted clinical data could be browsed in **Tables 1, 2**.

Association Between Cx43 in Glioma and 3-Year Overall Survival

Methods described previously were introduced to evaluate the results, the association between Cx43 and tumor grades were estimated by forest plots. Cx43 showed clearly negative with tumor grades in glioma patients ($I^2 = 34\%$, $P < 0.001$) (**Figure 2**). Three studies enrolled 1,202 patients were examined for the relationship between Cx43 and 3-year OS. And data (**Figure 3A**) showed that less Cx43 level was related with poor prognosis of glioma patients (HR 2.62, 95%CI 1.47–4.68; $P = 0.001$). Otherwise, this meta-analysis indicated that Cx43 level was highly related with a higher OS rates. The P value and I^2 of this results showed they were eligible. There was no notable heterogeneities among these studies likely existed [Heterogeneity: $Chi^2 = 10.53$, $df = 7$ ($P = 0.16$); $I^2 = 34\%$] (**Figure 3B**), so the resulting was reliable and then random-effect model was introduced to assess the possible publication bias of clinic pathological features.

Association Between Cx43 and Clinic Pathological Features

To further confirm the potential value of Cx43 in clinical practice, the relationship between Cx43 and patients' clinic pathological characters including tumor grades, gender and average age were explored precisely. As seen in **Table 3** and **Figure 4**, forest plots of 8 eligible studies showed the downregulated Cx43 was associated with tumor grades ($P < 0.001$). No difference was found between Cx43 expression in gender group ($P = 0.86$) (**Figure 4A**), but in age group, it effected the positive rate of Cx43 ($P = 0.002$). The difference may come from the different morbidity in different age and also the criteria for young (<60) and old (>60) do have

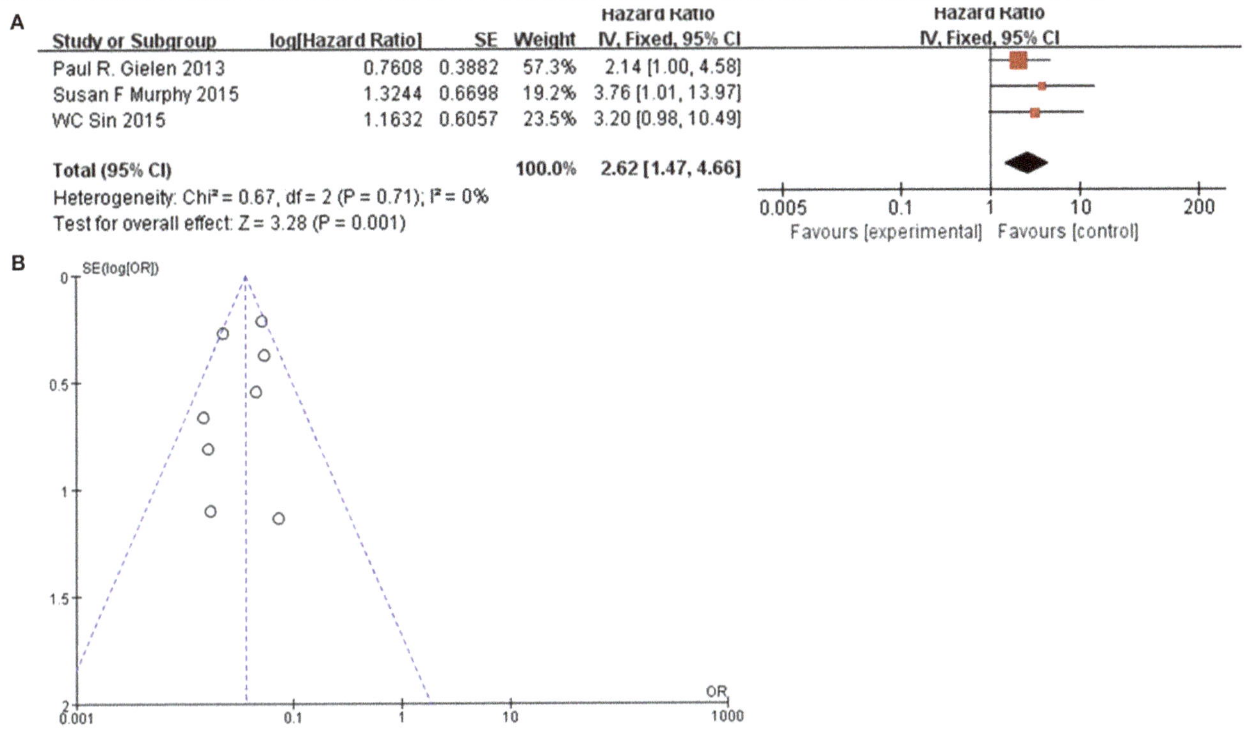

FIGURE 3 | (A) Forest plot of the association between Cx43 and OS in glioma patients. **(B)** Funnel plot for publication bias test of Cx43 related studies.

TABLE 3 | Data of subgroup for analyze of the gender and age effects.

	Male		Female		Old		Young	
	Positive	Total	Positive	Total	Positive	Total	Positive	Total
Reszec et al. (13)	38	66	29	65	25	30	42	101
Gielen et al. (12)	37	127	30	81	13	19	54	189
Pu et al. (11)	15	29	16	23	6	8	25	44
Caltabiano et al. (9)	9	15	11	17	5	8	15	24
Crespin et al. (17)	20	49	15	36	14	19	21	66
Murphy et al. (14)	178	282	174	290	57	79	275	493
Sin et al. (15)	154	301	165	325	106	194	213	432
Ye et al. (16)	27	44	36	56	11	18	52	82

influence on the bias (Heterogeneity: $Chi^2 = 22.49$, $P = 0.002$; $I^2 = 69\%$) (**Figure 4B**).

Sensitivity and Subgroup Analyses

Subgroup analysis was performed to explore the potential sources of heterogeneity, which were divided by research techniques, ethnicity and sample sizes. **Table 4** and **Figure 5** present the results of subgroup analyzed elucidate the correlations between Cx43 level and tumor grades. These results also indicated that low Cx43 expression was related to a significantly poorer results as compared to high expression. While sample size ($P = 0.21$) and research technique ($P = 0.20$) (IHC vs. PCR) did not obviously effect the prognosis rate of Cx43, but there might be a difference between Asian group and Western country group ($Chi^2 = 4.31$, $P = 0.04$, $I^2 = 76.8\%$) (**Figure 5B**).

Publication Bias

Potential publication bias was evaluated by using Begg's funnel plot and Egger's test. The results were presented in **Figure 5**. The results indicated that there was no significant publication bias for all studies, and no evidence of significant publication bias was found in this paper.

As seen in **Figure 6** and **Table 4**, group size didn't I effect the correlation between Cx43 level and tumor grades (*Test for subgroup differences:* $Chi^2 = 1.57, P = 0.21, I^2 = 36.5\%$). However, the heterogeneity of ethnicity existed in these subgroups (*Heterogeneity:* $Chi^2 = 29.29, P = 0.0001; I^2 = 76\%$). Additionally, research technique didn't influence the conclusion. And there

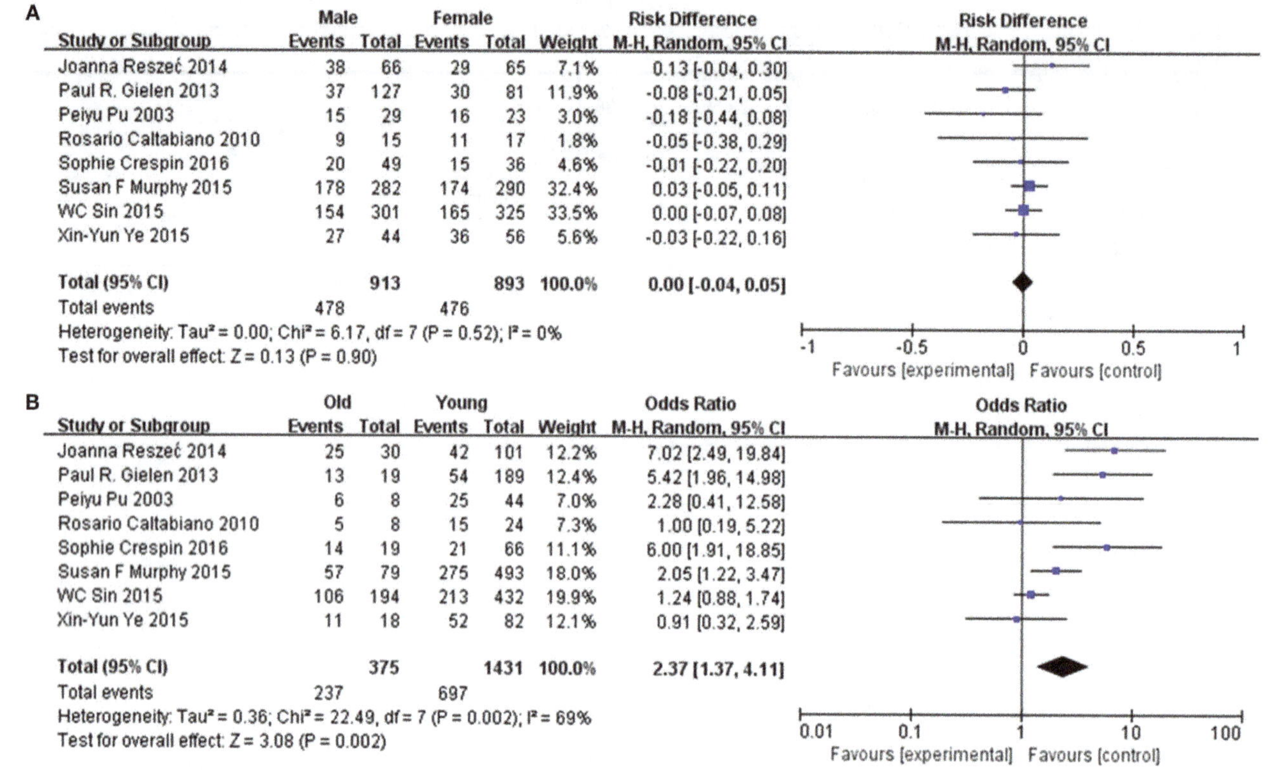

FIGURE 4 | Association between Cx43 and clinical pathological features in glioma patients. **(A)** Gender. **(B)** Age.

TABLE 4 | Subgroup analysis of region, sample size, and research technique.

Factors	Studies	Patients	Effect model	Test for subgroup differences:	Heterogeneity:
Region					
Asian countries	2	152	Odds Ratio (M-H, Randomed, 95% CI)	$Chi^2 = 4.31$, $df = 1$ ($P = 0.04$), $I^2 = 76.8\%$	$Chi^2 = 29.29$, $df = 7$ ($P = 0.0001$); $I^2 = 76\%$
Non-Asian countries	6	1,554	Odds Ratio (M-H, Randomed, 95% CI)		
Sample size					
>100	5	1,537	Odds Ratio (M-H, Randomed, 95% CI)	$Chi^2 = 1.57$, $df = 1$ ($P = 0.21$), $I^2 = 36.5\%$	$Chi^2 = 29.29$, $df = 7$ ($P = 0.0001$); $I^2 = 76\%$
<100	3	169	Odds Ratio (M-H, Randomed, 95% CI)		
Research technique					
IHC	6	1,367	Odds Ratio (M-H, Randomed, 95% CI)	Test for subgroup differences: $Chi^2 = 1.77$, $df = 1$ ($P = 0.18$), $I^2 = 43.5\%$	$Chi^2 = 10.53$, $df = 7$ ($P = 0.16$); $I^2 = 34\%$
RT-PCR	2	339	Odds Ratio (M-H, Randomed, 95% CI)		

were little heterogeneity among these subgroups (*IHC:* $I^2 = 45\%$, $P = 0.10$; *RT-PCR:* $I2 = 0\%$, $P = 0.80$). While in both subgroups divided by ethnicity, Cx43 expression was correlated to patients' ethnicity (*Test for subgroup differences:* $Chi^2 = 4.31$, $P = 0.04$, $I^2 = 76.8\%$). Heterogeneity in these subgroups was obvious, so further studies were still needed (*Heterogeneity:* $Chi^2 = 29.29$, $P = 0.0001$; $I^2 = 76\%$). With these results, the heterogeneity of tumor grades mainly resulted from the sample size and ethnicity.

Cx43 Diagnostic Sensitivity and Specificity

Sensitivity and specificity analyses were conducted to evaluate the diagnostic effect of Cx43 in glioma patients'. As seen in **Figure 7**,

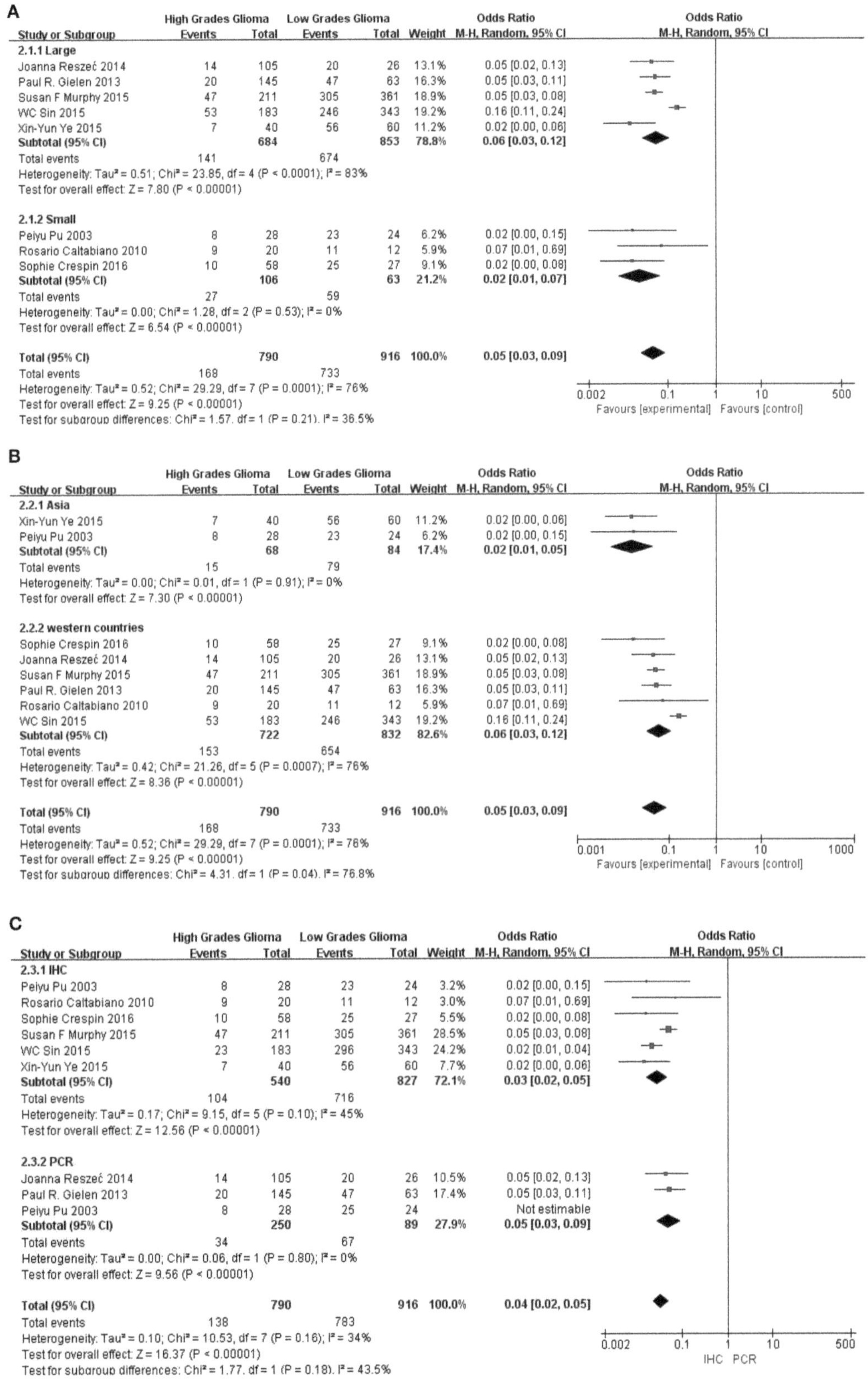

FIGURE 5 | Subgroup analysis of Cx43 with ethnicity, sample size and research technique: **(A)** sample size; **(B)** region; **(C)** research technique.

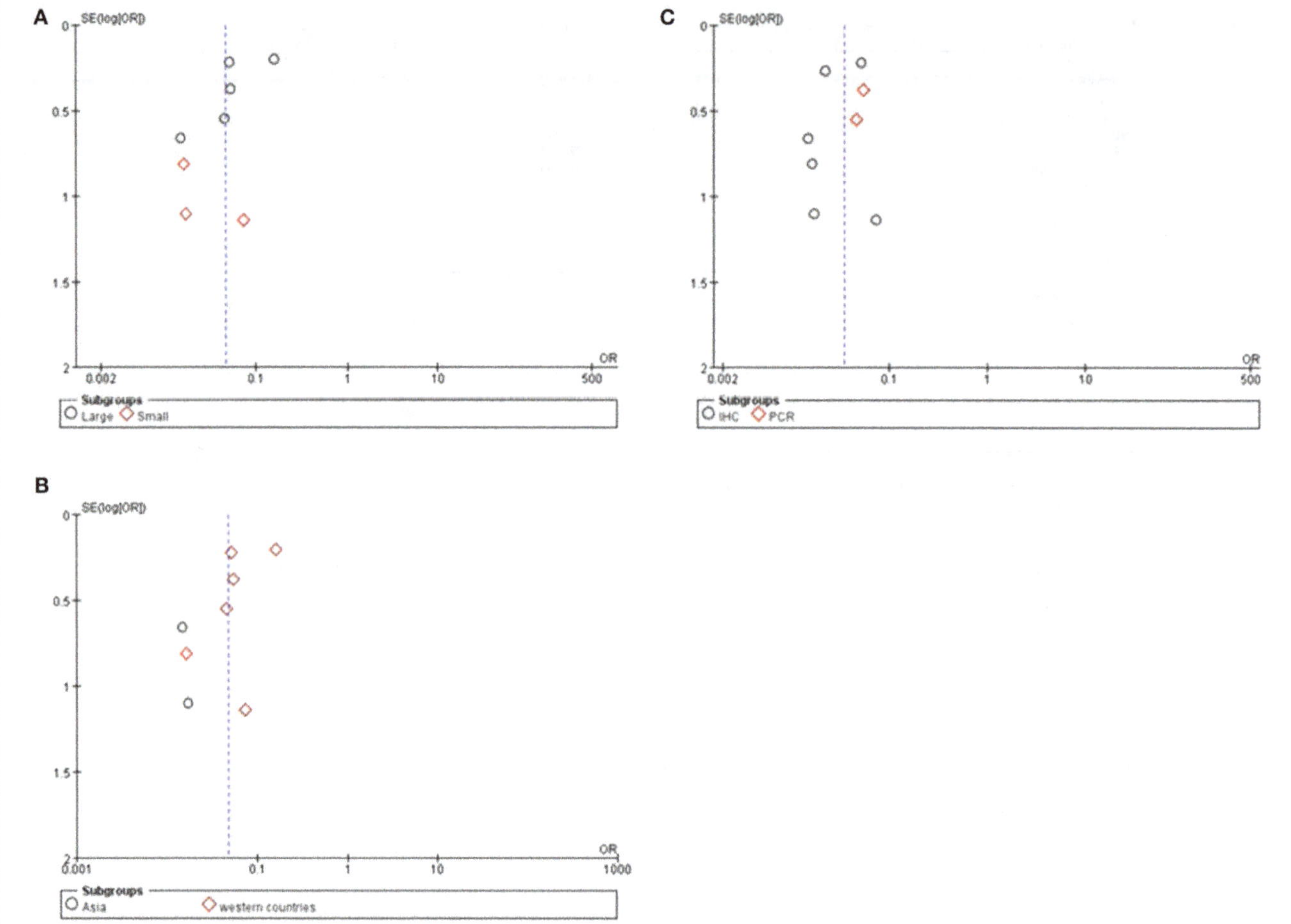

FIGURE 6 | Funnel plot for publication bias test of Cx43 related studies. **(A)** Sample size. **(B)** Region. **(C)** Research technique.

forest plot and SROC curve of 8 eligible studies showed the Cx43 is highly related to low grades glioma patients and shows good potential of sensitivity and specificity to define the tumor grades.

DISCUSSION

A huge number of studies have confirmed the relationship between cancer and connexins which was hypothesized more than 40 years ago (8, 18–20). However, the pivotal role of Cx43 in influencing tumor progression used to be overlooked because downregulation of Cx43-mediated intercellular communication is normally leading to increased malignancy in tumor cells (8, 19).As a result, Cx43 is usually considered as a tumor suppressor by its effect on reducing glioma proliferation (21, 22), anti-metastasis (23), and pro-apoptosis (24) and anti-inflammation (25). And our study is corresponded to these existing research that Cx43 expression is negatively associated with tumor grades.

In some studies, restoring Cx43 to glioma cells *in vitro* inhibits their tumorigenicity but this tumor suppressor effect could be glossed by its' promotion on invasion, adhesion and migration *in vivo* (1). Over-expression of Cx43 has been reported to enhance glioma migration in a channel-dependent manner, especially within the help of astrocytes (26, 27). Some experiments showed that Co-culture of glioma cells with astrocytes enhanced the invasiveness of the glioma cells and silencing Cx43 could extenuate this effect (25). Further study demonstrated this result and confirmed that junctions between glioma-glioma suppressed its invasiveness, while GJs of glioma–astrocyte and astrocyte–astrocyte promoted invasion (28). This seemed to be contrary to our findings that high Cx43 expression was beneficial to overall survive rate (OS). But it could be explained by the clinical experience that Cx43 usually highly expressed in low grades patients who could get gross-total resection (GTR) or even supra-total resection (SupTR) (29).

Due to nature of Cx43 that locates at the cell surface, Cx43 is associated with the brain endothelial barrier formation and the loss of Cx43 in glioma may lead to the infiltration of inflammation cells as well as more concentration of chemotherapy drugs (30). And further study of the correlationship between Cx43 and the popular glioma biomarkers is undergoing a proof study which would be published soon by our team. Besides Cx43 also the induction of inflammatory signaling, such as the treatment of anti-cancer agents and exposure to cytokines. One report demonstrated

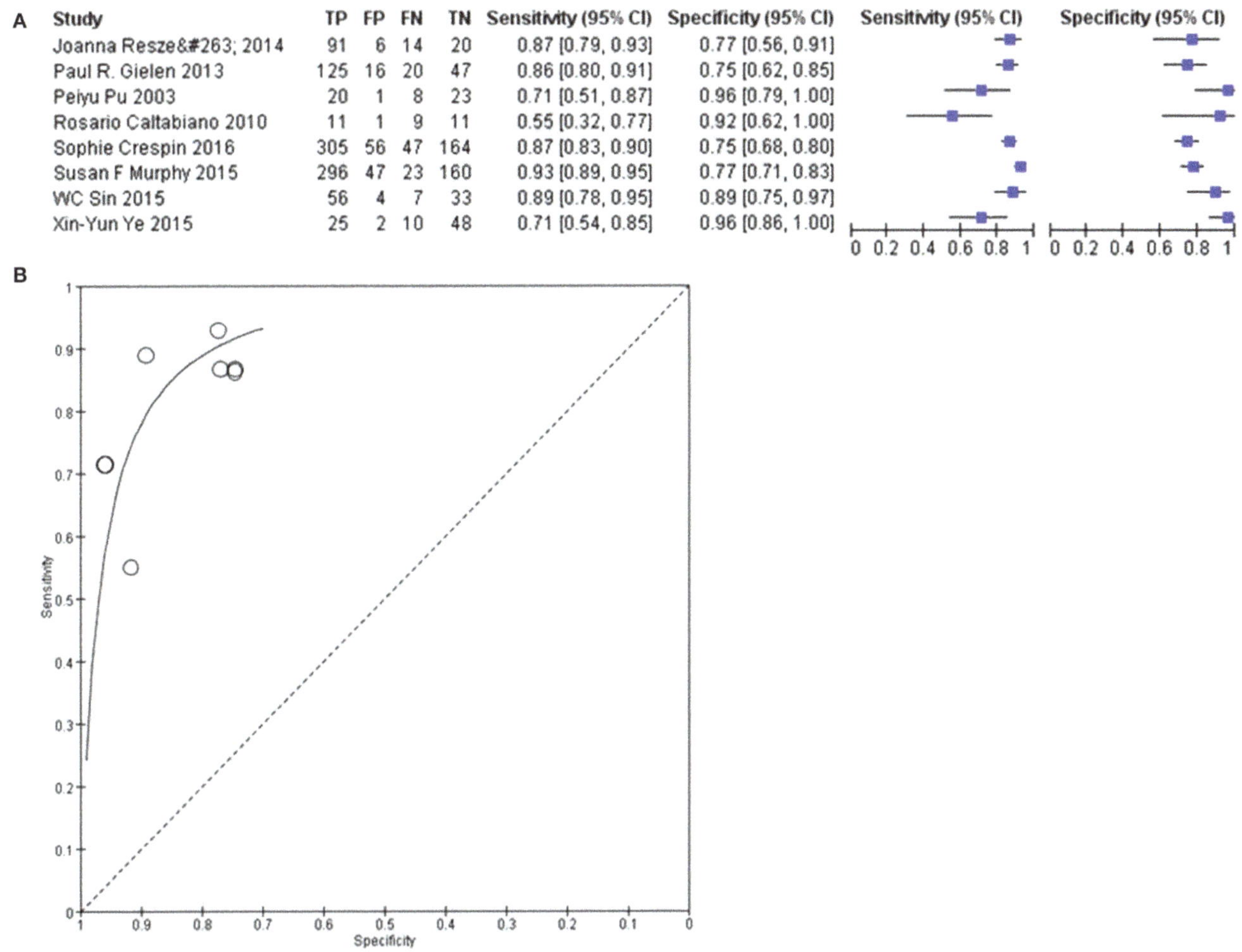

FIGURE 7 | Diagnosis effect of Cx43 in glioma patients. **(A)** The sensitivity and specificity of Cx43 in glioma patients. **(B)** The diagnostic curve of Cx43 among glioma patients.

that Cx43 promoted glioma cell resistance to temozolomide by a channel-dependent (31), and another study find that Cx43 interacted Bax signal pathway by modulating mitochondrial apoptosis (32). Therefore, it will be beneficial to examine Cx43 expression in glioma before physician apply temozolomide or develop a drug to target Cx43. Cx43 peptidomimetics provide a potential method to selectively modulate the activity of connexin GJs as well as the numerous factors that correlated with tumorigenesis, recently study shown that inhibiting Cx43 restored TMZ sensitivity in TMZ-resistant/Cx43-high GBM cells including GSCs (33).

Besides, Cx43 is the most abundant Cx isoform in adult astrocytes especially in reactive astrocytes (34, 35). It was also demonstrated that reactive astrocytes such as M2 cell (abbreviation of pro-tumorigenic macrophage) is vital for innate immune systems in brain tumor microenvironment (36) and might also be responsible for immune therapy results. As a result, a high Cx43 expression is often seen in low grade gliomas at the early stage (15).

Cx43 channels are well known for the direct passage of small ions and metabolites such as Ca2+, ATP, glutamate, glucose and peptides through (37). However, emerging evidence has shown that Cx43 is also permeable to oligonucleotides as long as 24 nucleotides in length. Other results also demonstrated that glioma–astrocyte GJs were capable to transfer miRNAs (28). These findings adding to recent studies confirmed that cancer cells might "reprogram" the normal stromal cells by miRNAs through Cx43 junctions and normal cell might be hijacked by tumor cells to form a favorable environment for tumor as a result.

One unique character of Cx43 is the relationship with metabolism. Under glucose uptake situation, GJs allow the transition of glucose and other metabolic substrates throughout the network (38). Recently, studies find the inhibition of gap junctional communication or the decreasing of Cx43 expression resulted in an increase in the rate of glucose uptake (39) and aerobic glycolysis, which may be an explanation of poor prognosis of OS and high negative relevance ratio of Cx43 in high grade gliomas.

The role of Cx43 in tumor hemostasis is actually a very complex relationship. The mechanisms underlying these effects suggest a complex balance of variety proteins in the whole process (18). Our meta-analysis directly indicated that lower Cx43 as associated with poorer patient prognosis and thus revealed the potential value of Cx43 in diagnosis and prognosis of gliomas, however need more studies are still needed to elaborate the exact mechanism of Cx43 to bring it into clinical practice.

AUTHOR CONTRIBUTIONS

CZ wrote the main part of the manuscript including introduction results, methods and materials, and abstract. CL collected the related papers. AC and ZY assessed the quality of included papers. WL, SX, and XM revised the paper. All authors reviewed the manuscript.

FUNDING

This paper was funded by Scientific and technological Innovation Plan for Clinical Medicine of Jinan City (201805037) and Natural Science Foundation of China (Grant 81702469).

ACKNOWLEDGMENTS

We appreciated to the clinical cases provided by CL, Dr. Yang, SX, and WL.

REFERENCES

1. Ferlay J, Shin HR, Bray F, Forman D, Mathers C, Parkin DM. Estimates of worldwide burden of cancer in 2008: GLOBOCAN 2008. *Int J Cancer.* (2010) 127:2893–917. doi: 10.1002/ijc.25516
2. Ameratunga M, Pavlakis N, Wheeler H, Grant R, Simes J, Khasraw M. Anti-angiogenic therapy for high-grade glioma. *Cochrane Database Syst Rev.* (2018) 11:Cd008218. doi: 10.1002/14651858.CD008218.pub4
3. Sanai N, Berger MS. Surgical oncology for gliomas: the state of the art. *Nat Rev Clin Oncol.* (2018) 15:112–25. doi: 10.1038/nrclinonc.2017.171
4. Grek CL, Rhett JM, Ghatnekar GS. Cardiac to cancer: connecting connexins to clinical opportunity. *FEBS Lett.* (2014) 588:1349–64. doi: 10.1016/j.febslet.2014.02.047
5. Nakase T, Naus CC. Gap junctions and neurological disorders of the central nervous system. *Biochim Biophys Acta.* (2004) 1662:149–58. doi: 10.1016/j.bbamem.2004.01.009
6. Giaume C, Leybaert L, Naus CC, Saez JC. Connexin and pannexin hemichannels in brain glial cells: properties, pharmacology, and roles. *Front Pharmacol.* (2013) 4:88. doi: 10.3389/fphar.2013.00088
7. Bai D. Structural analysis of key gap junction domains–Lessons from genome data and disease-linked mutants. *Semin Cell Dev Biol.* (2016) 50:74–82. doi: 10.1016/j.semcdb.2015.11.015
8. Naus CC, Laird DW. Implications and challenges of connexin connections to cancer. *Nat Rev Cancer.* (2010) 10:435–41. doi: 10.1038/nrc2841
9. Caltabiano R, Torrisi A, Condorelli D, Albanese V, Lanzafame S. High levels of connexin 43 mRNA in high grade astrocytomas. Study of 32 cases with *in situ* hybridization. *Acta Histochem.* (2010) 112:529–35. doi: 10.1016/j.acthis.2009.05.008
10. Huang R, Liu YG, Lin Y, Fan Y, Boynton A, Yang D, et al. Enhanced apoptosis under low serum conditions in human glioblastoma cells by connexin 43 (Cx43). *Mol Carcinog.* (2001) 32:128–38. doi: 10.1002/mc.1072
11. Pu P, Xia Z, Yu S, Huang Q. Altered expression of Cx43 in astrocytic tumors. *Clin Neurol Neurosurg.* (2004) 107:49–54. doi: 10.1016/j.clineuro.2004.03.006
12. Gielen PR, Aftab Q, Ma N, Chen VC, Hong X, Lozinsky S, et al. Connexin43 confers Temozolomide resistance in human glioma cells by modulating the mitochondrial apoptosis pathway. *Neuropharmacology.* (2013) 75:539–48. doi: 10.1016/j.neuropharm.2013.05.002
13. Reszec J, Szkudlarek M, Hermanowicz A, Bernaczyk PS, Mariak Z, Chyczewski L. N-cadherin, beta-catenin and connexin 43 expression in astrocytic tumours of various grades. *Histol Histopathol.* (2015) 30:361–71. doi: 10.14670/HH-30.361
14. Murphy SF, Varghese RT, Lamouille S, Guo S, Pridham KJ, Kanabur P, et al. Connexin 43 inhibition sensitizes chemoresistant glioblastoma cells to temozolomide. *Cancer Res.* (2016) 76:139–49. doi: 10.1158/0008-5472.CAN-15-1286
15. Sin WC, Aftab Q, Bechberger JF, Leung JH, Chen H, Naus CC. Astrocytes promote glioma invasion via the gap junction protein connexin43. *Oncogene.* (2016) 35:1504–16. doi: 10.1038/onc.2015.210
16. Ye XY, Jiang QH, Hong T, Zhang ZY, Yang RJ, Huang JQ, et al. Altered expression of connexin43 and phosphorylation connexin43 in glioma tumors. *Int J Clin Exp Pathol.* (2015) 8:4296–306.
17. Crespin S, Fromont G, Wager M, Levillain P, Cronier L, Monvoisin A, et al. Expression of a gap junction protein, connexin43, in a large panel of human gliomas: new insights. *Cancer Med.* (2016) 5:1742–52. doi: 10.1002/cam4.730
18. Tabernero A, Gangoso E, Jaraiz-Rodriguez M, Medina JM. The role of connexin43-Src interaction in astrocytomas: a molecular puzzle. *Neuroscience.* (2016) 323:183–94. doi: 10.1016/j.neuroscience.2015.02.029
19. Mesnil M, Crespin S, Avanzo JL, Zaidan-Dagli ML. Defective gap junctional intercellular communication in the carcinogenic process. *Biochim Biophys Acta.* (2005) 1719:125–45. doi: 10.1016/j.bbamem.2005.11.004
20. Aasen T, Mesnil M, Naus CC, Lampe PD, Laird DW. Gap junctions and cancer: communicating for 50 years. *Nat Rev Cancer.* (2017) 17:74. doi: 10.1038/nrc.2016.142
21. Saito T, Sato H, Virgona N, Hagiwara H, Kashiwagi K, Suzuki K, et al. Negative growth control of osteosarcoma cell by Bowman-Birk protease inhibitor from soybean; involvement of connexin 43. *Cancer Lett.* (2007) 253:249–57. doi: 10.1016/j.canlet.2007.01.021
22. Zhou JZ, Riquelme MA, Gu S, Kar R, Gao X, Sun L, et al. Osteocytic connexin hemichannels suppress breast cancer growth and bone metastasis. *Oncogene.* (2016) 35:5597–607. doi: 10.1038/onc.2016.101
23. Kou Y, Ji L, Wang H, Wang W, Zheng H, Zou J, et al. Connexin 43 upregulation by dioscin inhibits melanoma progression via suppressing malignancy and inducing M1 polarization. *Int J Cancer.* (2017) 141:1690–703. doi: 10.1002/ijc.30872
24. Uzu M, Sato H, Yamada R, Kashiba T, Shibata Y, Yamaura K, et al. Effect of enhanced expression of connexin 43 on sunitinib-induced cytotoxicity in mesothelioma cells. *J Pharmacol Sci.* (2015) 128:17–26. doi: 10.1016/j.jphs.2015.04.002
25. Uzu M, Sin WC, Shimizu A, Sato H. Conflicting roles of connexin43 in tumor invasion and growth in the central nervous system. *Int J Mol Sci.* (2018) 19:E1159. doi: 10.3390/ijms19041159
26. Oliveira R, Christov C, Guillamo JS, de Bouard S, Palfi S, Venance L, et al. Contribution of gap junctional communication between tumor cells and astroglia to the invasion of the brain parenchyma by human glioblastomas. *BMC Cell Biol.* (2005) 6:7. doi: 10.1186/1471-2121-6-7
27. Lin JH, Takano T, Cotrina ML, Arcuino G, Kang J, Liu S, et al. Connexin 43 enhances the adhesivity and mediates the invasion of malignant glioma cells. *J Neurosci.* (2002) 22:4302–11. doi: 10.1523/JNEUROSCI.22-11-04302.2002
28. Hong X, Sin WC, Harris AL, Naus CC. Gap junctions modulate glioma invasion by direct transfer of microRNA. *Oncotarget.* (2015) 6:15566–77. doi: 10.18632/oncotarget.3904
29. Roh TH, Kang SG, Moon JH, Sung KS, Park HH, Kim SH, et al. Survival benefit of lobectomy over gross-total resection without lobectomy in cases of glioblastoma in the noneloquent area: a retrospective study. *J Neurosurg.* (2019). doi: 10.3171/2018.12.JNS182558. [Epub ahead of print].

30. Kaneko Y, Tachikawa M, Akaogi R, Fujimoto K, Ishibashi M, Uchida Y, et al. Contribution of pannexin 1 and connexin 43 hemichannels to extracellular calcium-dependent transport dynamics in human blood-brain barrier endothelial cells. *J Pharmacol Exp Ther.* (2015) 353:192–200. doi: 10.1124/jpet.114.220210
31. Kim SW, Choi HJ, Lee HJ, He J, Wu Q, Langley RR, et al. Role of the endothelin axis in astrocyte- and endothelial cell-mediated chemoprotection of cancer cells. *Neuro Oncol.* (2014) 16:1585–98. doi: 10.1093/neuonc/nou128
32. Uzu M, Sato H, Shimizu A, Shibata Y, Ueno K, Hisaka A. Connexin 43 enhances Bax activation via JNK activation in sunitinib-induced apoptosis in mesothelioma cells. *J Pharmacol Sci.* (2017) 134:101–7. doi: 10.1016/j.jphs.2017.05.005
33. Rhett JM, Calder BW, Fann SA, Bainbridge H, Gourdie RG, Yost MJ. Mechanism of action of the anti-inflammatory connexin43 mimetic peptide JM2. *Am J Physiol Cell Physiol.* (2017) 313:C314–26. doi: 10.1152/ajpcell.00229.2016
34. Szilvasy-Szabo A, Varga E, Beliczai Z, Lechan RM, Fekete C. Localization of connexin 43 gap junctions and hemichannels in tanycytes of adult mice. *Brain Res.* (2017) 1673:64–71. doi: 10.1016/j.brainres.2017.08.010
35. Kozoriz MG, Bechberger JF, Bechberger GR, Suen MW, Moreno AP, Maass K, et al. The connexin43 C-terminal region mediates neuroprotection during stroke. *J Neuropathol Exp Neurol.* (2010) 69:196–206. doi: 10.1097/NEN.0b013e3181cd44df
36. Kolar K, Freitas-Andrade M, Bechberger JF, Krishnan H, Goldberg GS, Naus CC, et al. Podoplanin: a marker for reactive gliosis in gliomas and brain injury. *J Neuropathol Exp Neurol.* (2015) 74:64–74. doi: 10.1097/NEN.0000000000000150
37. Simon AM, Goodenough DA. Diverse functions of vertebrate gap junctions. *Trends Cell Biol.* (1998) 8:477–83. doi: 10.1016/S0962-8924(98)01372-5
38. Wolf A, Agnihotri S, Micallef J, Mukherjee J, Sabha N, Cairns R, et al. Hexokinase 2 is a key mediator of aerobic glycolysis and promotes tumor growth in human glioblastoma multiforme. *J Exp Med.* (2011) 208:313–26. doi: 10.1084/jem.20101470
39. Herrero-Gonzalez S, Valle-Casuso JC, Sanchez-Alvarez R, Giaume C, Medina JM, Tabernero A. Connexin43 is involved in the effect of endothelin-1 on astrocyte proliferation and glucose uptake. *Glia.* (2009) 57:222–33. doi: 10.1002/glia.20748

5

O^6-Methylguanine-DNA Methyltransferase (MGMT): Challenges and New Opportunities in Glioma Chemotherapy

Wei Yu [1,2], Lili Zhang [1,2], Qichun Wei [1,2] and Anwen Shao [3]**

[1] Department of Radiation Oncology, The Second Affiliated Hospital, Zhejiang University School of Medicine, Hangzhou, China, [2] Cancer Institute (Ministry of Education Key Laboratory of Cancer Prevention and Intervention), Zhejiang University Cancer Institute, Hangzhou, China, [3] Department of Neurosurgery, The Second Affiliated Hospital, Zhejiang University School of Medicine, Hangzhou, China

***Correspondence:**
Anwen Shao
2316040@zju.edu.cn;
anwenshao@sina.com
Qichun Wei
qichun_wei@zju.edu.cn

Chemoresistance has been a significant problem affecting the efficacy of drugs targeting tumors for decades. MGMT, known as O^6-methylguanine-DNA methyltransferase, is a DNA repair enzyme that plays an important role in chemoresistance to alkylating agents. Hence, MGMT is considered a promising target for tumor treatment. Several methods are employed to detect MGMT, each with its own advantages and disadvantages. Some of the detection methods are; immunohistochemistry, methylation-specific PCR (MSP), pyrophosphate sequencing, MGMT activity test, and real-time quantitative PCR. Methylation of MGMT promoter is a key predictor of whether alkylating agents can effectively control glioma cells. The prognostic value of MGMT in glioma is currently being explored. The expression of MGMT gene mainly depends on epigenetic modification–methylation of CpG island of MGMT promoter. CpG island covers a length of 762 bp, with 98 CpG sites located at the 5' end of the gene, ranging from 480 to 1,480 nucleotides. The methylation sites and frequencies of CpG islands vary in MGMT-deficient tumor cell lines, xenografts of glioblastoma and *in situ* glioblastoma. Methylation in some regions of promoter CpG islands is particularly associated with gene expression. The change in the methylation status of the MGMT promoter after chemotherapy, radiotherapy or both is not completely understood, and results from previous studies have been controversial. Several studies have revealed that chemotherapy may enhance MGMT expression in gliomas. This could be through gene induction or selection of high MGMT-expressing cells during chemotherapy. Selective survival of glioma cells with high MGMT expression during alkylating agent therapy may change MGMT status in case of recurrence. Several strategies have been pursued to improve the anti-tumor effects of temozolomide. These include the synthesis of analogs of O^6-meG such as O^6-benzylguanine (O^6-BG) and O^6-(4-bromothenyl) guanine (O^6-BTG), RNAi, and viral proteins. This review describes the regulation of MGMT expression and its role in chemotherapy, especially in glioma. Targeting MGMT seems to be a promising approach to overcome chemoresistance. Further studies exploring new agents targeting MGMT with better curative effect and less toxicity are advocated. We anticipate that these developments will improve the current poor prognosis of glioma patients.

Keywords: MGMT, methylation, alkylating agents, target therapy, chemotherapy

INTRODUCTION

O^6-methylguanine-DNA methyltransferase, known as MGMT, is a DNA "suicide" repair enzyme. It repairs damaged guanine nucleotides by transferring the methyl at O^6 site of guanine to its cysteine residues, thus avoiding gene mutation, cell death and tumorigenesis caused by alkylating agents. MGMT gene is located on chromosome 10q26.3 (**Figure 1A**), with a total length of 300,437 bp (3, 4). The expression of MGMT gene is mainly regulated by epigenetic modification. Many studies have shown that the loss of MGMT expression is not due to gene deletion, mutation, rearrangement or unstable RNA, but due to methylation of CpG island of MGMT promoter (5–9). In 1987, Gardiner and Frommer discovered that the human MGMT gene has a CpG island with a length of 762 bp, with 98 CpG sites located at the 5' end of the gene, ranging from 480 to 1,480 nucleotides (nt) (**Figure 1B**). The transcription initiation site of the gene is nt 956, and the CpG island spans about 500 bp (1) at the 5' and 3' ends of the transcription initiation site. The nt naming was initiated by Harris et al. beginning from the recognition site (2) of the restriction enzyme BamH1. In the non-methylated state, the transcriptional initiation sites of MGMT adhere to four precisely located nucleosome-like structures, which fine-tunes the transcription of the gene. Methylation of CpG islands leads to heterochromatinization, accompanied by rearrangement and random localization of nucleosomes, thus obscuring the transcription initiation sites and making transcription devices unable to bind (10, 11). Other studies have shown that methylation and chromatin status modulate the transcription of MGMT gene by determining whether Sp1 and other transcription factors access the MGMT promoter (12).

DETECTION METHODS FOR MGMT

Immunohistochemistry is a semi-quantitative method used to detect the expression of MGMT protein (13–15). It can distinguish between tumor cells and non-tumor cells, and thus the results are not confounded by the heterogeneity of tumors, but this method is greatly influenced by the subjectivity of the observer (16). In clinical research, many methods are used to detect the methylation status of MGMT promoter in glioma. The most frequently used method is methylation-specific PCR (MSP) (17, 18). This method was first established in 1996 for detection of promoter methylation (19). However, it can only detect the methylation of small fragments complementary to primers, and cannot determine the exact location of promoter methylation. Therefore, it is a semi-quantitative method (20). Whether conventional MSP primers (+120 toc +143, +173 to +196) bind to the key regions that regulate MGMT expression remains unclear. Pyrophosphate sequencing is a comprehensive sequencing method. In this method, methylation level of a single CpG site modified by sulfite can be quantitatively evaluated by efficient PCR amplification and sequencing. Therefore, Pyrophosphate sequencing is more reliable than MSP (21). However, the role of CpG island hypermethylation in gene silencing remains controversial (22–25). Many researchers hold the view that methylation of MGMT promoter directly inhibits gene transcription, thus detection of promoter methylation may serve as an indicator of susceptibility to alkylating agents. In fact, the most direct method used to detect the sensitivity of alkylating agents is MGMT activity test. The number of MGMT active molecules per unit protein or DNA detected by MGMT activity test can reflect the level of MGMT protein and RNA. However, because the test requires fresh or frozen tissues and *in situ* hybridization, it is not feasible for daily application. In contrast, quantitative detection of MGMT RNA expression by real-time quantitative PCR seems more suitable and highly sensitive, but few studies have applied it in MGMT RNA detection. Recently, Wang et al. found that a combination of immunohistochemistry and qMSP assays can provide high sensitivity and specificity for the prediction of MGMT status (26).

THE PREDICTION AND PROGNOSTIC VALUE OF MGMT PROMOTER STATUS IN GLIOMA

The MGMT gene encodes a DNA damage repair protein that removes alkylating agents resulting in resistance to chemotherapy. Because DNA methylation can inhibit transcription, methylation of MGMT promoter increases sensitivity to alkylating agents (27). Several studies have shown that methylation of MGMT promoter can predict whether alkylating agents can be of benefit in glioblastoma and low-grade gliomas (28–37). Two other clinical trials have revealed that methylation status of MGMT promoter can predict the prognosis of glioma patients. In these two studies, retrospective analysis of MGMT promoter methylation in elderly patients found that it could predict good prognosis in temozolomide (TMZ) group, but not in radiotherapy alone group (38, 39). The EORTC26951 clinical trial retrospectively analyzed the methylation status of MGMT promoter in anaplastic oligodendroglioma patients. It was found that methylation of MGMT promoter in anaplastic oligodendroglioma patients predicted better overall survival (OS) and PFS, whether in radiotherapy alone or in sequential radiotherapy and chemotherapy group [chemotherapy regimen: procarbacine, lomustine (CCNU), vincristine (PCV)]. But it had no prognostic value in glioblastoma patients. Elsewhere, it has been reported that methylation of MGMT promoter has no predictive value for chemosensitivity of anaplastic oligodendroglioma patients undergoing adjuvant PCV chemotherapy (40). Another phase III randomized clinical trial, NOA-04, drew a similar conclusion that methylation of MGMT promoter and IDH1 mutation reduces the risk of progression in anaplastic glioma patients, and patients with MGMT promoter methylation have a longer PFS (41) in both radiotherapy and chemotherapy groups (PVC). In addition,

Abbreviations: MGMT, O^6-methylguanine-DNA methyltransferase; MSP, methylation-specific PCR; IHC, immunohistochemistry; PCV, methylbenzylhydrazine, cyclohexanisolone and vincristine; OS, overall survival; PFS, progression-free survival; IDH1, isocitrate dehydrogenase; LMPCR, Linker-mediated PCR; TSS, transcription initiation site; BSP, Bisulfite Sequencing PCR; O^6-BG, O^6-benzylguanine; TMZ, temozolomide; CSF, cerebrospinal fluid; O^6-BTG, O^6-(4-bromothenyl) guanine; DSF, disulfiram.

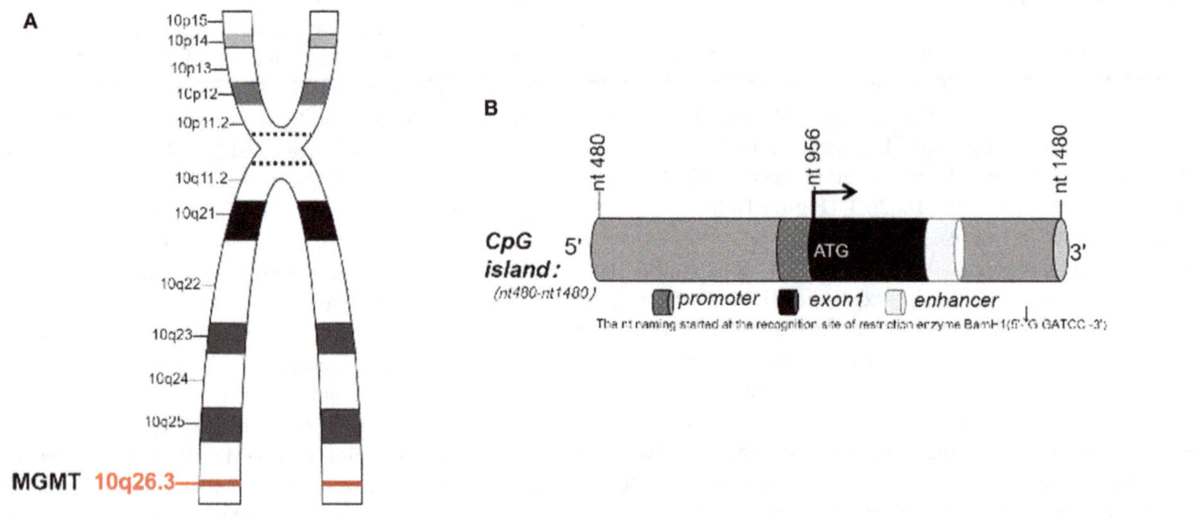

FIGURE 1 | (A) MGMT gene is located on chromosome 10, q26.3. **(B)** CpG island in MGMT. **(B)** In 1987, Gardiner-Garden and Frommer (1) identified the CpG island with 762 bp in MGMT gene. It has 98 CpG sites, located on about 480–1,480 nucleotide (nt) at the 5' end of this gene. The transcription start site (TSS) is located at nt956, CpG island covers a length of 500 bp at both 5' end and 3' end of TSS. The name of nt was first coined by Harris et al. (2), derived from the recognition site of restriction enzyme BamH1.

results from a phase III clinical trial prospectively indicate that MGMT promoter methylation status can be used as a biomarker to predict good prognosis of glioblastoma patients treated with TMZ (42) (**Table 1**).

EPIGENETIC REGULATION OF MGMT CPG ISLAND

The methylation sites and frequencies of CpG islands vary among MGMT-deficient tumor cell lines, xenografts of glioblastoma and *in situ* glioblastoma. Pieper et al. used Linker-mediated PCR (LMPCR) to detect the methylation status of MGMT promoter. It was found that the changes in methylation level of MGMT promoter mainly occurred at four CpG loci in cell lines expressing MGMT and those lacking MGMT, rather than being distributed uniformly throughout the CpG island. Two of them are located at about 130 nucleotides (+130) downstream of the transcription initiation site (TSS), including the sites recently studied using MPS. Two other nucleotides (−200) are located upstream of the transcription initiation site, and the transcription factor binding sites in both cell lines are not methylated. The transcription initiation site is defined as 0 (43). Watts et al. performed bisulfite sequencing PCR (BSP) on 108 CpG loci of 8226/s and 8226/v promoter CpG islands, respectively, and found that 8226/v has three methylation-rich regions which differs from those of 8226/s: −446 to −353, −265 to −162 and +112 to +212 (11). Costello et al. analyzed the methylation status of CpG loci in MGMT promoter −252 to −155 and −90 to +65 regions of glioma cell line by LM-PCR, and found that 21 of 25 loci were negatively correlated with MGMT gene expression (12). Because the authors detected the methylation level in high, low and non-expressing cell lines in these two regions, a quantitative relationship could not be established. Qian et al. used BSP method to detect the methylation level of CpG loci from −249 to +259 in MGMT CpG island region. It was found that HT29, a cell line expressing MGMT, was almost not methylated in this region, whereas BE, a cell line not expressing MGMT, was heavily methylated in each clone in this region. The most frequently methylated regions ranged from −249 to −103, +107 to +196 (44). Malley et al. used pyrophosphatic acid sequencing to detect the methylation of CpG islands in the entire MGMT promoter of glioblastoma cell lines, xenografts and normal brain tissues (41 samples). It was found that the +152 to +214 were the key regions promoting the transcription of MGMT (45). Subsequently, methylation of MGMT promoter was studied in human glioma samples. It was found that the methylation of CpG loci at −186 to −172 and +93 to +153 regions was most correlated with MGMT gene expression, but previous MSP loci were not found in this region, although the methylation level of MSP loci was similar to that reported previously (46). Bady et al. used human methylation 450 gene chip (HM-450K) to detect 14 CpG loci of MGMT promoter in 63 glioblastoma samples. It was found that the methylation of −193 and +173 CpG loci was negatively correlated with gene expression and had a good predictive accuracy for prognosis (47). Similarly, Mur et al. obtained genome-wide methylation profiles of 247 glioma samples from HM-450K platform, including 25 CpG loci in CpG island of MGMT promoter region. The methylation of + 173 CpG loci was significantly associated with overall survival (48). These researchers also found that MGMT promoter CpG islands are not suitable for methylation and this do not regulate expression or predict the prognosis of patients. Everhard et al. found that MGMT promoter regions −452 to −399 were highly methylated in both tumors and normal brain tissues. The region −90 to +69 is the first CpG region of small

TABLE 1 | Summary of the OS and PFS of patients receiving different treatments and characterized by non-methylated and methylated MGMT promoters in different studies.

References	Pathology	Treatment	OS (months)			PFS (months)		
			MGMTm	**MGMTu**	**All**	**MGMTm**	**MGMTu**	**ALL**
Criniere et al. (28)	GBM	RT+BCNU	17.1 (14.5–26.5)	13.1 (10.1–17.2)	NG	NG		
		RT	15.1 (9.8–n.r.)	10.2 (3.33–21.9)	NG			
		ALL☆	14.4 (13–16.1)	13.6 (11.4–15.7)	13.9 (12.5–15.3)	7.33 (5.8–8.43)	7.63 (6.47–8.63)	7.37 (6.5–8.43)
Hegi et al. (29)	GBM	RT+TMZ	21.7 (17.4–30.4)	12.7 (11.6–14.4)	NG	10.3 (6.5–14.0)	5.3 (5.0–7.6)	NG
		RT	15.3 (13.0–20.9)	11.8 (9.7–14.1)		5.9 (5.3–7.7)	4.4 (3.1–6.0)	
		ALL	18.2 (15.5–22.0)	12.2 (11.4–13.5)		NG	NG	
Reifenberger et al. (30)	GBM (age ≥ 70)	RT+TMZ	13.1 (11.0–15.3)	10.4 (8.4–12.4)	12.3(11.2–13.4)	7.3 (6.2–8.5)	7.2 (5.6–8.7)	7.2 (6.3–8.0)
		TMZ	7.2 (5.6–8.9)	2.6 (n.r.)	6.8(4.8–8.8)	6.8 (2.5–11.0)	0.5 (n.r.)	5.3 (0.1–10.5)
		RT	7.8 (3.4–12.2)	8.8 (7.5–10.1)	8.7(7.0–10.4)	4.5 (3.5–5.4)	5.2 (4.3–6.2)	5.0 (4.4–5.6)
		No treatment	2.3 (0.8–3.8)	2.0 (0.6–3.7)	2.3(0.9–3.7)	1.8 (1.1–2.4)	1.7 (0.4–3.1)	1.8 (1.0–2.5)
		ALL	8.4 (6.7–10.1)	6.4 (3.9–8.9)	7.7(6.3–9.0)	5.2 (4.3–6.1)	4.7 (3.8–5.5)	4.8 (4.3–5.3)
Esteller et al. (31)	AA/GBM	ALL (RT+BCNU)	MGMTu/MGMTm: HR = 9.5 (95% CI: 3.0–42.7, $p < 0.001$)			MGMTu/MGMTm: HR = 10.8 (95% CI: 4.4–30.8, $p < 0.001$)		
Hegi et al. (32)	GBM	ALL (RT+TMZ after surgery)	MGMTu/MGMTm: The risk of death within 18 months after surgery: 92% vs. 38%; $p = 0.002$			NG		
Everhard et al. (33)	LGG	ALL (TMZ)	NG			29.5 (21.5–n.r.)	6 (5–n.r.)	28 (20–n.r.)
Pandith et al. (37)	Gliomas	RT+TMZ	40.1 (29.8–50.3)	6.8 (3.8–9.6)	43.4 (32.5–54.1)	23.9 (20.0–27.7)	3.2 (0.6–5.8)	25.8 (21.9–29.6)
Malmstrom et al. (38)	GBM (age≥60)	TMZ	9.7 (8.0–11.4)	6.8 (5.9–7.7)	8.3 (7.1–9.5)	NG		
		Standard RT (60 Gy)	8.2 (6.6–9.9)※	7.0 (5.7–8.3)※	6.0 (5.1–6.8)			
		Hypofractioned RT (34 Gy)			7.5 (6.5–8.6)			
		ALL	9.0 (8.0–10.0)	6.9 (5.9–7.9)	NG			
Wick et al. (39)	AA/GBM (age ≥ 65)	TMZ	n.r. (10.1–n.r.)	7 (5.7–8.7)	8.6 (7.3–110.2)	8.4 (5.5–11.7)	3.3 (3.0–3.5)	3.3 (3.2–4.1)
		RT	9.6 (6.4–n.r.)	10.4 (8–11.6)	9.6 (8.2–10.8)	4.6 (4.2–5.0)	4.6 (3.7–6.3)	4.7 (4.2–5.2)
		ALL	11.9 (9.0–n.r.)	8.2 (7.0–10.0)	NG	5.7 (5.0–7.4)	3.5 (3.3–3.7)	NG
van den Bent et al. (40)	AOD/AOA (≥25% oligodendroglia elements)	RT RT+PVC	59.3 (30.0–66.2) n.r. (n.r.)	12.3 (11.5–28.5) 19.0 (12.3–34.5)	NG	17.9 (11.9–43.4) 49.0 (19.1–71.2)	7.8 (7.1–17.6) 10.5 (5.2–23.0)	NG
Wick et al. (41)	Anaplastic gliomas (WHO III)		NG			MGMTu/MGMTm:		
		RT			72.1 (n.r.)	HR = 2.0 (95% CI: 1.1–3.6, $p < 0.03$)		30.6 (16.3–42.8)
		TMZ/PCV			82.6 (n.r.)	HR = 2.7 (95% CI: 1.4–5.1, $p < 0.003$)		31.9 (21.1–37.3)
Gilbert et al. (42)	GBM	Standard dose TMZ	21.4 (17.6–29.0)	14.6 (13.2–16.5)	16.6 (14.9–18.0)	6.5 (4.1–9.6)	5.1 (4.3–5.7)	5.5 (4.7–6.1)
		Dense dose TMZ	20.2 (15.4–25.1)	13.3 (12.3–14.3)	14.9 (13.7–16.5)	10.1 (7.9–12.4)	6.0 (5.5–6.5)	6.7 (6.2–7.7)
		ALL	21.2 (17.9–24.8)	14.0 (12.9–14.7)	NG	8.7 (6.6–11.2)	5.7 (5.1–6.1)	NG

☆, included other treatments: BCNU alone or supportive care; ✱, standard RT and hypofractioned RT is grouped together; GBM, glioblastoma; LGG, low-grade gliomas; AA, anaplastic astrocytoma; AOD, anaplastic oligodendroglia tumors; AOA, anaplastic oligoastrocytoma; RT, radiotherapy; TMZ, temozolomide; BCNU, carmustine; PCV, procarbazine, lomustine, and vincristine; OS, median overall survival; PFS, median progression-free survival; MGMTm, MGMT promoter methylated status; MGMTu, MGMT promoter unmethylated status; NG, not given; n.r., not reached; HR, hazard ratio; 95%CI, 95 percent confidence interval.

promoter, TSS and non-coding exon, which is equivalent to the methylation-free region (46) in both normal brain tissue and tumors. Thus, transcriptional silencing does not require methylation of the entire CpG island, but only methylation of several gene-specific core CpG sites. Therefore, methylation at some regions of promoter CpG islands is particularly associated with gene expression.

THE INFLUENCE OF CHEMOTHERAPY AND RADIOTHERAPY ON THE METHYLATION STATUS, ACTIVITY AND PROTEIN EXPRESSION OF MGMT

Methylation of the promoter region of the MGMT gene is known to predict the response to alkylating agent's treatment in glioma patients. However, knowledge about the change in the methylation status of the MGMT promoter after chemotherapy, radiotherapy or both is still incomplete. Wiewrodt et al. analyzed MGMT activity in 40 paired primary and recurrent glioblastomas, 16 patients after RT only, 24 patients with RT combined with chemotherapy (TMZ and/or CCNU or ACNU). In both recurrent groups, the MGMT activity was higher than in primary tumors. In contrast, for patients who received RT only, there was no significant difference between primary glioblastomas and recurrences. The MGMT activity was significant, however, in patients with primary glioblastomas and recurrences that received RT plus alkylating agent therapy (49). Brandes et al. analyzed MGMT promoter methylation status of 38 paired primary and recurrent glioblastomas treated with adjuvant radiotherapy and chemotherapy. They found that MGMT methylation status was changed in 14 patients (37%) who had recurrent tumors and more frequently in those with methylated MGMT than in unmethylated patients (50). Christmann et al. compared MGMT activity and MGMT promoter methylation in 46 primary glioblastoma samples and 19 recurrent glioblastoma samples. They found that MGMT activity increased after treatment, and methylation of MGMT promoter was detected in 39% primary tumors, while only 5.3% recurrent glioblastomas displayed MGMT promoter methylation (17). Elsewhere, Felsberg et al. analyzed the methylation status of MGMT promoter in 80 paired primary and recurrent glioblastomas, of which 16 patients received radiotherapy alone and 64 patients received radiotherapy and TMZ chemotherapy. They found the MGMT methylation status of 89% patients was not altered (51). It is worth noting, besides, that the response of the human MGMT promoter to genotoxic stress may be weak. Although Fritz et al. and Chan et al. had reported MGMT mRNA transcription can be induced by DNA-damaging treatments, both of their experiments were limited in rat H4IIE hepatoma cells (52, 53). As for human MGMT promoter, Grombacher et al. found that it could be induced by dexamethasone when transfected into rat H4IIE and human HeLa S3 (Mex+) cells, but methylating agents and ionizing radiation only worked in H4IIE cells (54). Boldogh et al. analyzed the mechanism of human MGMT expression induction, they found that protein kinase C-mediated signaling played an important role, involving activation of AP-1 sites on MGMT promoter by TPA (55). Aasland et al. further identified that human MGMT promoter can be induced by glucocorticoids, but not by genotoxic stress, in human malignant glioblastoma cells (56). They put forward that a cluster of SP1 sites in human MGMT promoter prevented transcriptional up-graduation and overshadowed activation signals from other weaker transcriptional factors. The transcription factor SP1 was sequestrated by p53, which was induced following radiochemotherapy (57). Coincidentally, an earlier retrospective clinical data from Pitter at al. showed longer survival of no glucocorticoid usage GBM patient cohorts, alongside corresponding data in animal models (58). Thus, radiation and chemotherapy may have minor influence on transient transcriptional activation of human MGMT. The finding of a protection of tumor cells by dexamethasone and other steroids suggests that a controlled use of glucocoricoids in GBM therapy is desirable. In conclusion, these studies revealed that chemotherapy may provoke an up-regulation of MGMT expression in gliomas through selection of high MGMT expressing cells during chemotherapy. Selective survival of glioma cells with high MGMT expression during alkylating agent therapy may change MGMT status when recurrence.

MGMT IN GLIOBLASTOMA STEM CELLS

Cancer stem cells have been implicated in the progression and recurrence of GBMs. It has been recognized that even after effective treatment of tumors, minimal residual stem cells may be activated to enter a new stage of differentiation and proliferation. In this way, cancer stem cells promote the recurrence of tumors. Thus, we postulate that glioblastoma stem cells may cause resistance to TMZ, which enables them survive during chemotherapy. Liu et al. and Pistollato et al. revealed that glioblastoma (GBM) stem cells, identified with the stem cell marker CD133, express high level of MGMT and displayed strong tumor resistance to TMZ (59, 60). Beier et al. reported that there are distinct stem cell populations that, despite having similar MGMT promoter methylation status, differ in MGMT protein expression. And they also found that TMZ preferentially kills cancer stem cells in glioblastoma in MGMT-negative cell lines (61, 62). Mantwill et al. stated that MGMT is not expressed in all stem cell lines, which indicates that these cells have different grades of TMZ resistance (63). Happold et al. observed that differentiation of glioma stem cells resulted in a gradual loss of MGMT expression and increased TMZ sensitivity (64, 65). Although MGMT is highly expressed in stem cells, it is not clear why the alkylating agents are not effective in recurrent GBMs. Do the differentiated cells retain the TMZ resistance features of stem cells? These challenges necessitate the search for the mechanisms that regulate the expression of MGMT in different cell stages.

TARGETING MGMT PROTEIN

O^6-benzylguanine (O^6-BG) is the analog of O^6-meG which is a low molecular weight pseudosubstrate for MGMT. It inactivates MGMT through alkyl group transfer (**Figure 2**). It can pass the

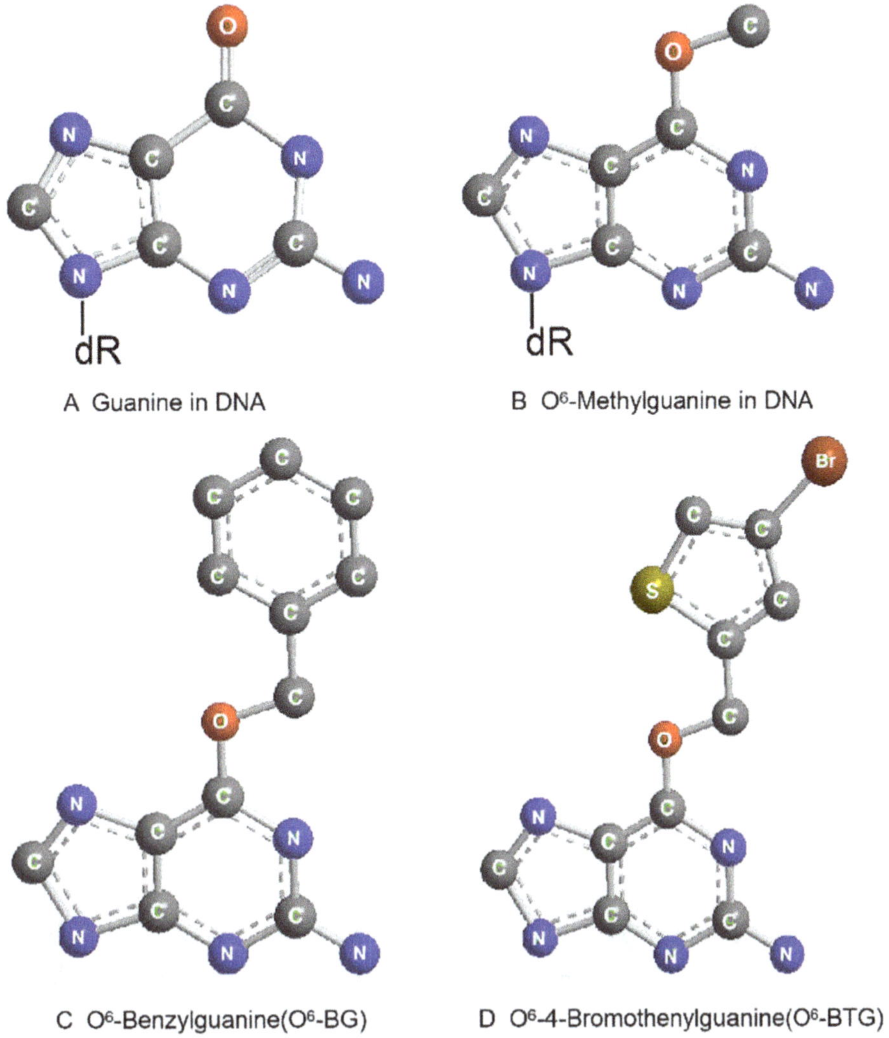

FIGURE 2 | Molecular structure of guanine in DNA **(A)**, O^6-Methylguanine in DNA **(B)**, O^6-Benzylguanine **(C)**, and O^6-4-Bromothenylguanine **(D)**.

blood brain barrier and has, therefore, the potential to be a treatment for gliomas. It has been widely used as an MGMT inhibitor and as a sensitizer of glioma cells to alkylating agent TMZ (66, 67). Koch et al. found that local intracranial interaction of O^6-BG with TMZ after intraoperative removal of brain tumors might delay tumor recurrence without any side effect (68). Phase I, II and III clinical trials of O^6-BG combined with TMZ have revealed that this combination successfully aberrates other tumors, such as brain tumor, melanoma, lymphoma and colon cancer (69–72). A later phase II clinical research by Quinn et al. found that 06-BG combined with gliadel wafer prolonged the survival time of patients. However, it also increased the risk of hydrocephalus, cerebrospinal fluid (CSF) leak, and CSF/brain infection (73).

Another pseudosubstrate, O^6-(4-bromothenyl) guanine (O^6-BTG), has 10-fold higher potency than O^6-BG in inactivating MGMT protein and is orally bioavailable without inherently toxic (**Figure 2**). It has been reported that O^6-BTG efficiently and rapidly inactivates MGMT in various tumors *in vivo* and *in* v *vitro* and significantly increases tumor sensitivity to TMZ (74–77). A phase I trial of O^6-BTG in combination with TMZ in advanced solid tumors established an oral ATase-depleting dose of lomeguatrib (Trade name for O6-BTG) and developed a combination regimen with TMZ that was 75% of the maximum tolerable dose of the single agent. The dose-limiting toxicity of O^6-BTG was myelosuppression (78). Papachristodoulou et al. reported that a liposomal O^6BTG can efficiently target MGMT, thereby sensitizing murine and human glioma cells to TMZ *in vitro* and magnetic resonance image-guided microbubble-enhanced low-intensity pulsed focused ultrasound mediates the delivery of the stable liposomal MGMT inactivator into the tumor region resulting in complete MGMT depletion *in vivo* (79).

Although the developed MGMT inhibitors, O^6-BG and O^6-BTG, are effective, their systemic toxicity due to non-specific targeting to normal cells cannot be ignored. Going forward, the high glucose consumption hallmark of tumor cells presents a new avenue that can be exploited for development of selective inhibitors by conjugating agents to glucose. It has been reported that both O^{6}BG-Glu and O^{6}BTG-Glu are highly effective at inhibiting MGMT in several cancer cell lines, including T98G glioblastoma. These agents also enhance the cell-killing effect of temozolomide (80–82). Besides, Tomaszowski et al. found that glucose conjugates are subject of transport out of the cell by the ATP-binding cassette (ABC) transporter mediated efflux, which impacts the efficiency of MGMT inhibition. In this study, the importance of proper linker selection for a successful ligand-based drug delivery strategy was underscored (83). Similarly, conjugating pseudosubstrates to folate esters is another promising strategy to target tumor cells (84). So far, few studies have investigated the cellular effects of glucose or folate esters conjugated inhibitors. Further detailed studies should unravel the mechanisms of these inhibitors to provide better treatment agents.

Watson et al. conducted phase II clinical trials to evaluate the efficacy of lomeguatrib in patients with melanoma. They found that lomeguatrib plus TMZ had a greater MGMT inactivation than did TMZ treatment alone (85). Another study by the same group also reported that lomeguatrib can be applied in prostate, primary CNS, and colorectal cancers to inactivate MGMT (86). However, lomeguatrib increases myelosuppression, and other studies revealed that it did not improve the response rate to TMZ (69, 70, 74, 87–89).

RNA interference is another promising therapy targeting MGMT. Kato et al. reported that when combined with TMZ, the MGMT-siRNA/liposome complex exerted a strong synergistic antitumor effect (90). Zhang et al. found that miR-181d downregulated MGMT by directly interacting with MGMT 3'UTR, and this potentiated the TMZ sensitizer as an MGMT targeting therapy (91). Nie et al. found that miR-198 directly targeted MGMT by binding to the 3′-UTR of MGMT, thereby inhibiting the MGMT mRNA translation in GBM cells. MiR-198 restored the tumor sensitivity to TMZ in glioblastomas overexpressing MGMT (92).

Oncolytic viruses which inactivate or leverage the cellular DNA-repair machinery to achieve productive replication have also been exploited to design agents targeting MGMT. Adenoviruses express proteins which can downregulate MGMT expression. It has been reported that overexpression of adenovirus E1A, which binds p300, efficiently inhibits both basal and TSA inducible promoter activity of MGMT and may thus reduce chemoresistance (93, 94). CBP/p300 is a transcriptional coactivator which interacts with multiple transcription factors including those involved in MGMT gene. It plays an important

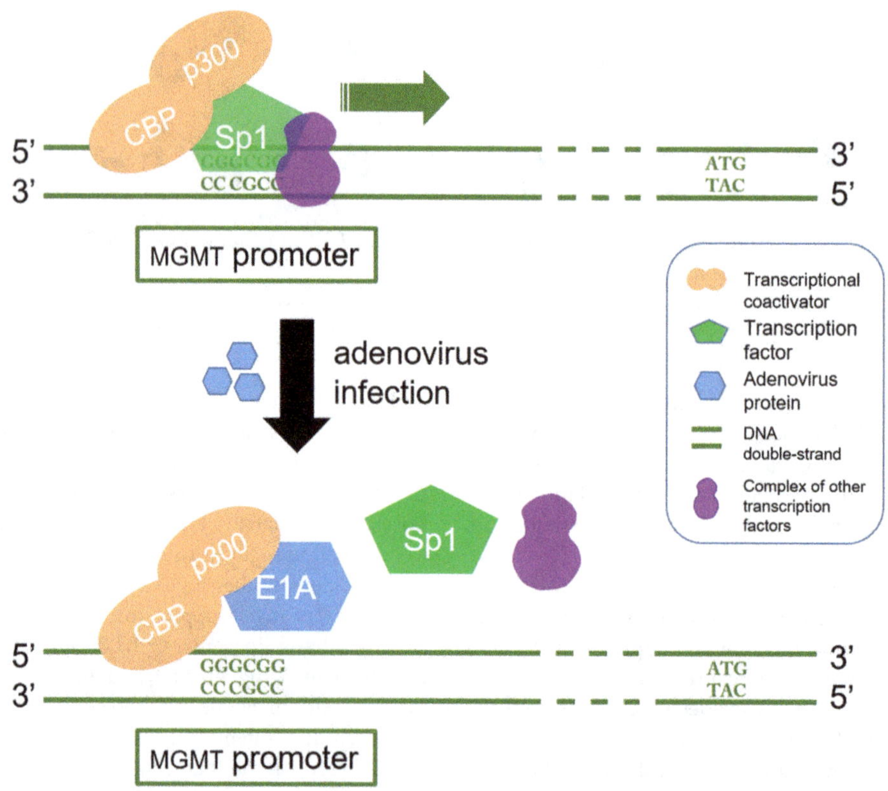

FIGURE 3 | E1A interferes with CBP/p300 in which regulate the transcription process of MGMT gene. CBP/p300 is a transcription coactivator and Sp1 is a transcription factor. CBP/p300 recruits Sp1 protein to recognize and bind to the GC region (5'-GGGCGG-3') in the MGMT promoter, which in turn acts as a transcriptional activator. On the other hand, E1A is a product of oncolytic adenovirus. It stops the Sp1 from being recruited by binding to p300. This blocks the MGMT gene transcription signal.

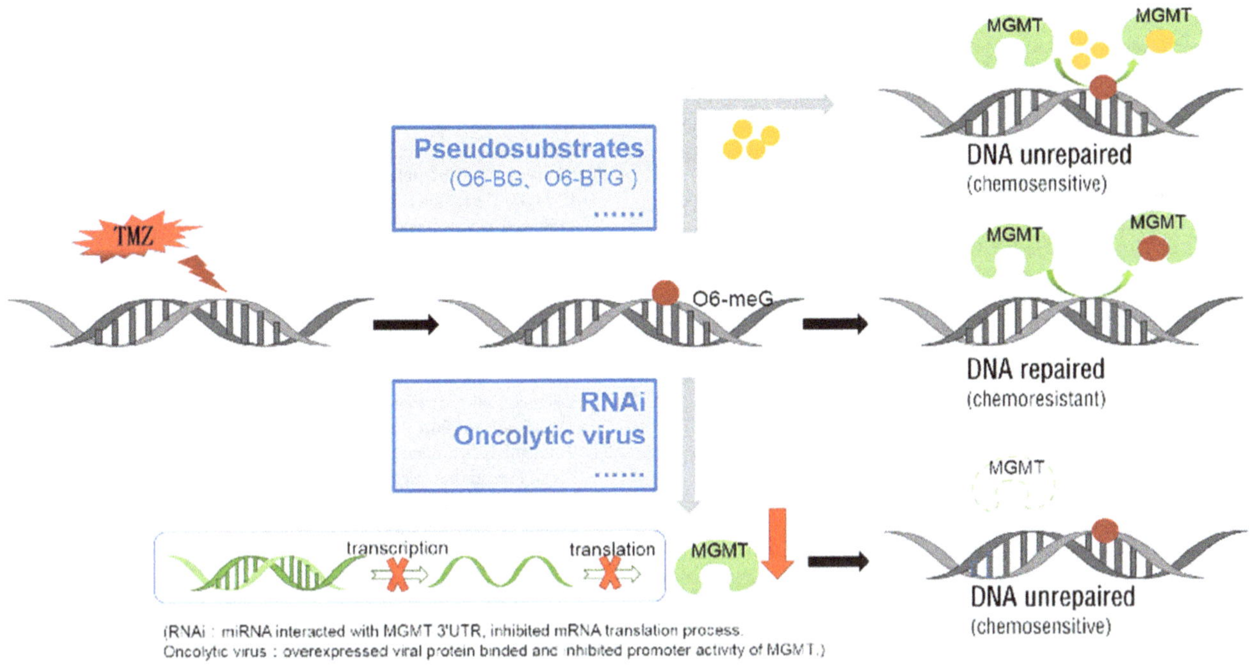

FIGURE 4 | Two main approaches to block methylated DNA repair by targeting the MGMT protein. TMZ can add methyl to the guanine on the DNA molecule (form as 06-meG), which then induce DNA cross-linking. MGMT protein can repair DNA damage by binding and transferring the methyl on it. Low molecular weight O^6-meG analogs, like O^6-BG and O^6-BTG, are used as pseudosubstrates to bind MGMT protein and reduce the methyl transfer activity. Specific miRNA/ liposome complexes which interact with MGMT 3'UTR then inhibit the MGMT mRNA translation process (RNAi). The proliferated oncolytic virus in a host can inhibit the host's MGMT promoter's activation, by means of the E1A binding to the p300.

role in many cellular processes, and the structural and functional versatility of CBP/p300 are yet to be fully elucidated. For this reason, the utilization of adenovirus targeting MGMT is far from being clinically implemented (95) (**Figure 3**).

Jiang et al. reported that a combination of TMZ and viral therapy may overcome the chemoresistance of gliomas to TMZ (96). Further, it has been shown that oncolytic virus-mediated manipulation of DNA damage responses can also be applied to kill GSCs (97). The discovery of this oncolytic viral therapy opens a new era in cancer therapy. However, there are safety concerns regarding the use of virus-based therapy.

Other drugs that target MGMT protein such as disulfiram (DSF) have also been studied. For instance, Paranjpe reported that DSF directly suppressed MGMT protein expression through sole site Cys145 (98).

CONCLUSION AND PERSPECTIVES

MGMT is a DNA methyltransferase which repairs damaged DNA thus avoiding cell death caused by alkylating agents. The expression of MGMT gene is mainly regulated by epigenetic modification. Several methods have been developed for MGMT detection including immunohistochemistry, methylation-specific PCR, pyrophosphate sequencing, MGMT activity test, real-time quantitative PCR among others. Methylation of MGMT promoter can predict whether alkylating agents are effective for glioblastoma and low-grade gliomas. The prognostic value of MGMT methylation is still controversial and calls for further clarification. Epigenetic regulation of specific sites of MGMT CpG island influences MGMT transcription. Chemotherapy and radiotherapy may modulate MGMT methylation status, activity and protein expression. TMZ is a promising chemotherapeutic agent for glioma, but the rapid development of drug resistance poses a huge challenge. Overexpression of MGMT is an important mechanism of TMZ resistance. Several strategies have been pursued to improve the anti-tumor effects of TMZ. These include development of pseudosubstrates, RNAi, viral proteins and many others agents (**Figure 4**). Given on-going research advancements in this field, the current poor prognosis of glioma patients is expected to improve.

AUTHOR CONTRIBUTIONS

AS designed the study and determined the final version. QW revised the manuscript and polished the language. WY drafted the manuscript. LZ made the figures and tables. All authors read and approved the final manuscript.

FUNDING

This work was supported by the National Natural Science Foundation of China (81701144) and China Postdoctoral Science Foundation (2017M612010).

REFERENCES

1. Gardiner-Garden M, Frommer M. CpG islands in vertebrate genomes. *J Mol Biol.* (1987) 196:261–82. doi: 10.1016/0022-2836(87)90689-9
2. Harris LC, Potter PM, Tano K, Shiota S, Mitra S, Brent TP. Characterization of the promoter region of the human O6-methylguanine-DNA methyltransferase gene. *Nucleic Acids Res.* (1991) 19:6163–7. doi: 10.1093/nar/19.22.6163
3. Kent WJ. BLAT–the BLAST-like alignment tool. *Genome Res.* (2002) 12:656–64. doi: 10.1101/gr.229202
4. Pruitt KD, Tatusova T, Maglott DR. NCBI Reference Sequence (RefSeq): a curated non-redundant sequence database of genomes, transcripts and proteins. *Nucleic Acids Res.* (2005) 33:D501–4. doi: 10.1093/nar/gki025
5. Day RS III, Ziolkowski CH, Scudiero DA, Meyer SA, Lubiniecki AS, Girardi AJ, et al. Defective repair of alkylated DNA by human tumour and SV40-transformed human cell strains. *Nature.* (1980) 288:724–7. doi: 10.1038/288724a0
6. Fornace AJ Jr, Papathanasiou MA, Hollander MC, Yarosh DB. Expression of the O6-methylguanine-DNA methyltransferase gene MGMT in MER+ and MER- human tumor cells. *Cancer Res.* (1990) 50:7908–11.
7. Pieper RO, Futscher BW, Dong Q, Ellis TM, Erickson LC. Comparison of O-6-methylguanine DNA methyltransferase (MGMT) mRNA levels in Mer+ and Mer- human tumor cell lines containing the MGMT gene by the polymerase chain reaction technique. *Cancer Commun.* (1990) 2:13–20. doi: 10.3727/095535490820874812
8. Kroes RA, Erickson LC. The role of mRNA stability and transcription in O6-methylguanine DNA methyltransferase (MGMT) expression in Mer+ human tumor cells. *Carcinogenesis.* (1995) 16:2255–7. doi: 10.1093/carcin/16.9.2255
9. Bouras E, Karakioulaki M, Bougioukas KI, Aivaliotis M, Tzimagiorgis G, Chourdakis M. Gene promoter methylation and cancer: an umbrella review. *Gene.* (2019) 710:333–40. doi: 10.1016/j.gene.2019.06.023
10. Costello JF, Futscher BW, Tano K, Graunke DM, Pieper RO. Graded methylation in the promoter and body of the O6-methylguanine DNA methyltransferase (MGMT) gene correlates with MGMT expression in human glioma cells. *J Biol Chem.* (1994) 269:17228–37.
11. Watts GS, Pieper RO, Costello JF, Peng YM, Dalton WS, Futscher BW. Methylation of discrete regions of the O6-methylguanine DNA methyltransferase (MGMT) CpG island is associated with heterochromatinization of the MGMT transcription start site and silencing of the gene. *Mol Cell Biol.* (1997) 17:5612–9. doi: 10.1128/MCB.17.9.5612
12. Costello JF, Futscher BW, Kroes RA, Pieper RO. Methylation-related chromatin structure is associated with exclusion of transcription factors from and suppressed expression of the O-6-methylguanine DNA methyltransferase gene in human glioma cell lines. *Mol Cell Biol.* (1994) 14:6515–21. doi: 10.1128/MCB.14.10.6515
13. Micko ASG, Hoftberger R, Wohrer A, Millesi M, Knosp E, Wolfsberger S. MGMT assessment in pituitary adenomas: comparison of different immunohistochemistry fixation chemicals. *Pituitary.* (2018) 21:266–73. doi: 10.1007/s11102-018-0862-x
14. Jiang X, Reardon DA, Desjardins A, Vredenburgh JJ, Quinn JA, Austin AD, et al. O6-methylguanine-DNA methyltransferase (MGMT) immunohistochemistry as a predictor of resistance to temozolomide in primary CNS lymphoma. *J Neurooncol.* (2013) 114:135–40. doi: 10.1007/s11060-013-1162-y
15. Mason S, McDonald K. MGMT testing for glioma in clinical laboratories: discordance with methylation analyses prevents the implementation of routine immunohistochemistry. *J Cancer Res Clin Oncol.* (2012) 138:1789–97. doi: 10.1007/s00432-012-1312-1
16. Preusser M, Charles Janzer R, Felsberg J, Reifenberger G, Hamou MF, Diserens AC, et al. Anti-O6-methylguanine-methyltransferase (MGMT) immunohistochemistry in glioblastoma multiforme: observer variability and lack of association with patient survival impede its use as clinical biomarker. *Brain Pathol.* (2008) 18:520–32. doi: 10.1111/j.1750-3639.2008.00153.x
17. Christmann M, Nagel G, Horn S, Krahn U, Wiewrodt D, Sommer C, et al. MGMT activity, promoter methylation and immunohistochemistry of pretreatment and recurrent malignant gliomas: a comparative study on astrocytoma and glioblastoma. *Int J Cancer.* (2010) 127:2106–18. doi: 10.1002/ijc.25229
18. Yachi K, Watanabe T, Ohta T, Fukushima T, Yoshino A, Ogino A, et al. Relevance of MSP assay for the detection of MGMT promoter hypermethylation in glioblastomas. *Int J Oncol.* (2008) 33:469–75. doi: 10.3892/ijo_00000029
19. Herman JG, Graff JR, Myohanen S, Nelkin BD, Baylin SB. Methylation-specific PCR: a novel PCR assay for methylation status of CpG islands. *Proc Natl Acad Sci USA.* (1996) 93:9821–6. doi: 10.1073/pnas.93.18.9821
20. Switzeny OJ, Christmann M, Renovanz M, Giese A, Sommer C, Kaina B. MGMT promoter methylation determined by HRM in comparison to MSP and pyrosequencing for predicting high-grade glioma response. *Clin Epigenetics.* (2016) 8:49. doi: 10.1186/s13148-016-0204-7
21. Tost J, El abdalaoui H, Gut IG. Serial pyrosequencing for quantitative DNA methylation analysis. *Biotechniques.* (2006) 40:721–2. doi: 10.2144/000112190
22. Schnell O, Albrecht V, Pfirrmann D, Eigenbrod S, Krebs B, Romagna A, et al. MGMT promoter methylation is not correlated with integrin expression in malignant gliomas: clarifying recent clinical trial results. *Med Oncol.* (2018) 35:103. doi: 10.1007/s12032-018-1162-z
23. Toffolatti L, Scquizzato E, Cavallin S, Canal F, Scarpa M, Stefani PM, et al. MGMT promoter methylation and correlation with protein expression in primary central nervous system lymphoma. *Virchows Arch.* (2014) 465:579–86. doi: 10.1007/s00428-014-1622-6
24. Melguizo C, Prados J, Gonzalez B, Ortiz R, Concha A, Alvarez PJ, et al. MGMT promoter methylation status and MGMT and CD133 immunohistochemical expression as prognostic markers in glioblastoma patients treated with temozolomide plus radiotherapy. *J Transl Med.* (2012) 10:250. doi: 10.1186/1479-5876-10-250
25. Uno M, Oba-Shinjo SM, Camargo AA, Moura RP, Aguiar PH, Cabrera HN, et al. Correlation of MGMT promoter methylation status with gene and protein expression levels in glioblastoma. *Clinics.* (2011) 66:1747–55. doi: 10.1590/S1807-59322011001000013
26. Wang L, Li Z, Liu C, Chen L, Liu L, Hu Z, et al. Comparative assessment of three methods to analyze MGMT methylation status in a series of 350 gliomas and gangliogliomas. *Pathol Res Pract.* (2017) 213:1489–93. doi: 10.1016/j.prp.2017.10.007
27. Kaina B, Christmann M. DNA repair in personalized brain cancer therapy with temozolomide and nitrosoureas. *DNA Repair.* (2019) 78:128–41. doi: 10.1016/j.dnarep.2019.04.007
28. Criniere E, Kaloshi G, Laigle-Donadey F, Lejeune J, Auger N, Benouaich-Amiel A, et al. MGMT prognostic impact on glioblastoma is dependent on therapeutic modalities. *J Neurooncol.* (2007) 83:173–9. doi: 10.1007/s11060-006-9320-0
29. Hegi ME, Diserens AC, Gorlia T, Hamou MF, de Tribolet N, Weller M, et al. MGMT gene silencing and benefit from temozolomide in glioblastoma. *N Engl J Med.* (2005) 352:997–1003. doi: 10.1056/NEJMoa043331
30. Reifenberger G, Hentschel B, Felsberg J, Schackert G, Simon M, Schnell O, et al. Predictive impact of MGMT promoter methylation in glioblastoma of the elderly. *Int J Cancer.* (2012) 131:1342–50. doi: 10.1002/ijc.27385
31. Esteller M, Garcia-Foncillas J, Andion E, Goodman SN, Hidalgo OF, Vanaclocha V, et al. Inactivation of the DNA-repair gene MGMT and the clinical response of gliomas to alkylating agents. *N Engl J Med.* (2000) 343:1350–4. doi: 10.1056/NEJM200011093431901
32. Hegi ME, Diserens AC, Godard S, Dietrich PY, Regli L, Ostermann S, et al. Clinical trial substantiates the predictive value of O-6-methylguanine-DNA methyltransferase promoter methylation in glioblastoma patients treated with temozolomide. *Clin Cancer Res.* (2004) 10:1871–4. doi: 10.1158/1078-0432.CCR-03-0384
33. Everhard S, Kaloshi G, Criniere E, Benouaich-Amiel A, Lejeune J, Marie Y, et al. MGMT methylation: a marker of response to temozolomide in low-grade gliomas. *Ann Neurol.* (2006) 60:740–3. doi: 10.1002/ana.21044
34. Aoki K, Natsume A. Overview of DNA methylation in adult diffuse gliomas. *Brain Tumor Pathol.* (2019) 36:84–91. doi: 10.1007/s10014-019-00339-w
35. Qi F, Yin Z, Wang G, Zeng S. Clinical and prognostic significance of O(6)-methylguanine-DNA methyltransferase promoter methylation in patients with melanoma: a systematic meta-analysis. *Ann Dermatol.* (2018) 30:129–35. doi: 10.5021/ad.2018.30.2.129
36. Dahlrot RH, Larsen P, Boldt HB, Kreutzfeldt MS, Hansen S, Hjelmborg JB, et al. Posttreatment effect of MGMT methylation level on

glioblastoma survival. *J Neuropathol Exp Neurol.* (2019) 78:633–40. doi: 10.1093/jnen/nlz032

37. Pandith AA, Qasim I, Zahoor W, Shah P, Bhat AR, Sanadhya D, et al. Concordant association validates MGMT methylation and protein expression as favorable prognostic factors in glioma patients on alkylating chemotherapy (Temozolomide). *Sci Rep.* (2018) 8:6704. doi: 10.1038/s41598-018-25169-2
38. Malmstrom A, Gronberg BH, Marosi C, Stupp R, Frappaz D, Schultz H, et al. Temozolomide versus standard 6-week radiotherapy versus hypofractionated radiotherapy in patients older than 60 years with glioblastoma: the Nordic randomised, phase 3 trial. *Lancet Oncol.* (2012) 13:916–26. doi: 10.1016/S1470-2045(12)70265-6
39. Wick W, Platten M, Meisner C, Felsberg J, Tabatabai G, Simon M, et al. Temozolomide chemotherapy alone versus radiotherapy alone for malignant astrocytoma in the elderly: the NOA-08 randomised, phase 3 trial. *Lancet Oncol.* (2012) 13:707–15. doi: 10.1016/S1470-2045(12)70164-X
40. van den Bent MJ, Dubbink HJ, Sanson M, van der Lee-Haarloo CR, Hegi M, Jeuken JW, et al. MGMT promoter methylation is prognostic but not predictive for outcome to adjuvant PCV chemotherapy in anaplastic oligodendroglial tumors: a report from EORTC Brain Tumor Group Study 26951. *J Clin Oncol.* (2009) 27:5881–6. doi: 10.1200/JCO.2009.24.1034
41. Wick W, Hartmann C, Engel C, Stoffels M, Felsberg J, Stockhammer F, et al. NOA-04 randomized phase III trial of sequential radiochemotherapy of anaplastic glioma with procarbazine, lomustine, and vincristine or temozolomide. *J Clin Oncol.* (2009) 27:5874–80. doi: 10.1200/JCO.2009.23.6497
42. Gilbert MR, Wang M, Aldape KD, Stupp R, Hegi M, Jaeckle KA, et al. RTOG 0525: a randomized phase III trial comparing standard adjuvant temozolomide (TMZ) with a dose-dense (dd) schedule in newly diagnosed glioblastoma (GBM). *J Clin Oncol.* (2011) 29:2006. doi: 10.1200/jco.2011.29.15_suppl.2006
43. Pieper RO, Patel S, Ting SA, Futscher BW, Costello JF. Methylation of CpG island transcription factor binding sites is unnecessary for aberrant silencing of the human MGMT gene. *J Biol Chem.* (1996) 271:13916–24. doi: 10.1074/jbc.271.23.13916
44. Qian XC, Brent TP. Methylation hot spots in the 5' flanking region denote silencing of the O6-methylguanine-DNA methyltransferase gene. *Cancer Res.* (1997) 57:3672–7.
45. Malley DS, Hamoudi RA, Kocialkowski S, Pearson DM, Collins VP, Ichimura K. A distinct region of the MGMT CpG island critical for transcriptional regulation is preferentially methylated in glioblastoma cells and xenografts. *Acta Neuropathol.* (2011) 121:651–61. doi: 10.1007/s00401-011-0803-5
46. Everhard S, Tost J, El Abdalaoui H, Criniere E, Busato F, Marie Y, et al. Identification of regions correlating MGMT promoter methylation and gene expression in glioblastomas. *Neuro Oncol.* (2009) 11:348–56. doi: 10.1215/15228517-2009-001
47. Bady P, Sciuscio D, Diserens AC, Bloch J, van den Bent MJ, Marosi C, et al. MGMT methylation analysis of glioblastoma on the Infinium methylation BeadChip identifies two distinct CpG regions associated with gene silencing and outcome, yielding a prediction model for comparisons across datasets, tumor grades, and CIMP-status. *Acta Neuropathol.* (2012) 124:547–60. doi: 10.1007/s00401-012-1016-2
48. Mur P, Rodriguez de Lope A, Diaz-Crespo FJ, Hernandez-Iglesias T, Ribalta T, Fiano C, et al. Impact on prognosis of the regional distribution of MGMT methylation with respect to the CpG island methylator phenotype and age in glioma patients. *J Neurooncol.* (2015) 122:441–50. doi: 10.1007/s11060-015-1738-9
49. Wiewrodt D, Nagel G, Dreimuller N, Hundsberger T, Perneczky A, Kaina B. MGMT in primary and recurrent human glioblastomas after radiation and chemotherapy and comparison with p53 status and clinical outcome. *Int J Cancer.* (2008) 122:1391–9. doi: 10.1002/ijc.23219
50. Brandes AA, Franceschi E, Tosoni A, Bartolini S, Bacci A, Agati R, et al. O(6)-methylguanine DNA-methyltransferase methylation status can change between first surgery for newly diagnosed glioblastoma and second surgery for recurrence: clinical implications. *Neuro Oncol.* (2010) 12:283–8. doi: 10.1093/neuonc/nop050
51. Felsberg J, Thon N, Eigenbrod S, Hentschel B, Sabel MC, Westphal M, et al. Promoter methylation and expression of MGMT and the DNA mismatch repair genes MLH1, MSH2, MSH6 and PMS2 in paired primary and recurrent glioblastomas. *Int J Cancer.* (2011) 129:659–70. doi: 10.1002/ijc.26083
52. Fritz G, Tano K, Mitra S, Kaina B. Inducibility of the DNA repair gene encoding O6-methylguanine-DNA methyltransferase in mammalian cells by DNA-damaging treatments. *Mol Cell Biol.* (1991) 11:4660–8. doi: 10.1128/MCB.11.9.4660
53. Chan CL, Wu Z, Eastman A, Bresnick E. Irradiation-induced expression of O6-methylguanine-DNA methyltransferase in mammalian cells. *Cancer Res.* (1992) 52:1804–9.
54. Grombacher T, Mitra S, Kaina B. Induction of the alkyltransferase (MGMT) gene by DNA damaging agents and the glucocorticoid dexamethasone and comparison with the response of base excision repair genes. *Carcinogenesis.* (1996) 17:2329–36. doi: 10.1093/carcin/17.11.2329
55. Boldogh I, Ramana CV, Chen Z, Biswas T, Hazra TK, Grosch S, et al. Regulation of expression of the DNA repair gene O6-methylguanine-DNA methyltransferase via protein kinase C-mediated signaling. *Cancer Res.* (1998) 58:3950–6.
56. Aasland D, Reich TR, Tomicic MT, Switzeny OJ, Kaina B, Christmann M. Repair gene O(6) -methylguanine-DNA methyltransferase is controlled by SP1 and up-regulated by glucocorticoids, but not by temozolomide and radiation. *J Neurochem.* (2018) 144:139–51. doi: 10.1111/jnc.14262
57. Tomicic MT, Meise R, Aasland D, Berte N, Kitzinger R, Kramer OH, et al. Apoptosis induced by temozolomide and nimustine in glioblastoma cells is supported by JNK/c-Jun-mediated induction of the BH3-only protein BIM. *Oncotarget.* (2015) 6:33755–68. doi: 10.18632/oncotarget.5274
58. Pitter KL, Tamagno I, Alikhanyan K, Hosni-Ahmed A, Pattwell SS, Donnola S, et al. Corticosteroids compromise survival in glioblastoma. *Brain.* (2016) 139(Pt 5):1458–71. doi: 10.1093/brain/aww046
59. Pistollato F, Abbadi S, Rampazzo E, Persano L, Della Puppa A, Frasson C, et al. Intratumoral hypoxic gradient drives stem cells distribution and MGMT expression in glioblastoma. *Stem Cells.* (2010) 28:851–62. doi: 10.1002/stem.415
60. Liu G, Yuan X, Zeng Z, Tunici P, Ng H, Abdulkadir IR, et al. Analysis of gene expression and chemoresistance of CD133+ cancer stem cells in glioblastoma. *Mol Cancer.* (2006) 5:67. doi: 10.1186/1476-4598-5-67
61. Beier D, Hau P, Proescholdt M, Lohmeier A, Wischhusen J, Oefner PJ, et al. CD133(+) and CD133(-) glioblastoma-derived cancer stem cells show differential growth characteristics and molecular profiles. *Cancer Res.* (2007) 67:4010–5. doi: 10.1158/0008-5472.CAN-06-4180
62. Beier D, Rohrl S, Pillai DR, Schwarz S, Kunz-Schughart LA, Leukel P, et al. Temozolomide preferentially depletes cancer stem cells in glioblastoma. *Cancer Res.* (2008) 68:5706–15. doi: 10.1158/0008-5472.CAN-07-6878
63. Mantwill K, Naumann U, Seznec J, Girbinger V, Lage H, Surowiak P, et al. YB-1 dependent oncolytic adenovirus efficiently inhibits tumor growth of glioma cancer stem like cells. *J Transl Med.* (2013) 11:216. doi: 10.1186/1479-5876-11-216
64. Happold C, Stojcheva N, Silginer M, Weiss T, Roth P, Reifenberger G, et al. Transcriptional control of O(6) -methylguanine DNA methyltransferase expression and temozolomide resistance in glioblastoma. *J Neurochem.* (2018) 144:780–90. doi: 10.1111/jnc.14326
65. Chumakova A, Lathia JD. Outlining involvement of stem cell program in regulation of O6-methylguanine DNA methyltransferase and development of temozolomide resistance in glioblastoma: an editorial highlight for 'Transcriptional control of O(6) -methylguanine DNA methyltransferase expression and temozolomide resistance in glioblastoma' on page 780. *J Neurochem.* (2018) 144:688–90. doi: 10.1111/jnc.14280
66. Middleton MR, Margison GP. Improvement of chemotherapy efficacy by inactivation of a DNA-repair pathway. *Lancet Oncol.* (2003) 4:37–44. doi: 10.1016/S1470-2045(03)00959-8
67. Bobola MS, Silber JR, Ellenbogen RG, Geyer JR, Blank A, Goff RD. O6-methylguanine-DNA methyltransferase, O^6-benzylguanine, and resistance to clinical alkylators in pediatric primary brain tumor cell lines. *Clin Cancer Res.* (2005) 11:2747–55. doi: 10.1158/1078-0432.CCR-04-2045
68. Koch D, Hundsberger T, Boor S, Kaina B. Local intracerebral administration of O(6)-benzylguanine combined with systemic chemotherapy with temozolomide of a patient suffering from a recurrent glioblastoma. *J Neurooncol.* (2007) 82:85–9. doi: 10.1007/s11060-006-9244-8

69. Quinn JA, Desjardins A, Weingart J, Brem H, Dolan ME, Delaney SM, et al. Phase I trial of temozolomide plus O^6-benzylguanine for patients with recurrent or progressive malignant glioma. *J Clin Oncol.* (2005) 23:7178–87. doi: 10.1200/JCO.2005.06.502
70. Quinn JA, Jiang SX, Reardon DA, Desjardins A, Vredenburgh JJ, Rich JN, et al. Phase I trial of temozolomide plus O^6-benzylguanine 5-day regimen with recurrent malignant glioma. *Neuro Oncol.* (2009) 11:556–61. doi: 10.1215/15228517-2009-007
71. Verbeek B, Southgate TD, Gilham DE, Margison GP. O6-methylguanine-DNA methyltransferase inactivation and chemotherapy. *Br Med Bull.* (2008) 85:17–33. doi: 10.1093/bmb/ldm036
72. Broniscer A, Gururangan S, MacDonald TJ, Goldman S, Packer RJ, Stewart CF, et al. Phase I trial of single-dose temozolomide and continuous administration of O^6-benzylguanine in children with brain tumors: a pediatric brain tumor consortium report. *Clin Cancer Res.* (2007) 13(22 Pt 1):6712–8. doi: 10.1158/1078-0432.CCR-07-1016
73. Quinn JA, Jiang SX, Carter J, Reardon DA, Desjardins A, Vredenburgh JJ, et al. Phase II trial of gliadel plus O^6-benzylguanine in adults with recurrent glioblastoma multiforme. *Clin Cancer Res.* (2009) 15:1064–8. doi: 10.1158/1078-0432.CCR-08-2130
74. Barvaux VA, Lorigan P, Ranson M, Gillum AM, McElhinney RS, McMurry TB, et al. Sensitization of a human ovarian cancer cell line to temozolomide by simultaneous attenuation of the Bcl-2 antiapoptotic protein and DNA repair by O6-alkylguanine-DNA alkyltransferase. *Mol Cancer Ther.* (2004) 3:1215–20.
75. Turriziani M, Caporaso P, Bonmassar L, Buccisano F, Amadori S, Venditti A, et al. O6-(4-bromothenyl)guanine (PaTrin-2), a novel inhibitor of O6-alkylguanine DNA alkyl-transferase, increases the inhibitory activity of temozolomide against human acute leukaemia cells *in vitro*. *Pharmacol Res.* (2006) 53:317–23. doi: 10.1016/j.phrs.2005.12.001
76. Middleton MR, Kelly J, Thatcher N, Donnelly DJ, McElhinney RS, McMurry TB, et al. O(6)-(4-bromothenyl)guanine improves the therapeutic index of temozolomide against A375M melanoma xenografts. *Int J Cancer.* (2000) 85:248–52. doi: 10.1002/(SICI)1097-0215(20000115)85:2%3C248::AID-IJC16%3E3.0.CO;2-V
77. Clemons M, Kelly J, Watson AJ, Howell A, McElhinney RS, McMurry TB, et al. O6-(4-bromothenyl)guanine reverses temozolomide resistance in human breast tumour MCF-7 cells and xenografts. *Br J Cancer.* (2005) 93:1152–6. doi: 10.1038/sj.bjc.6602833
78. Ranson M, Middleton MR, Bridgewater J, Lee SM, Dawson M, Jowle D, et al. Lomeguatrib, a potent inhibitor of O6-alkylguanine-DNA-alkyltransferase: phase I safety, pharmacodynamic, and pharmacokinetic trial and evaluation in combination with temozolomide in patients with advanced solid tumors. *Clin Cancer Res.* (2006) 12:1577–84. doi: 10.1158/1078-0432.CCR-05-2198
79. Papachristodoulou A, Signorell RD, Werner B, Brambilla D, Luciani P, Cavusoglu M, et al. Chemotherapy sensitization of glioblastoma by focused ultrasound-mediated delivery of therapeutic liposomes. *J Control Release.* (2019) 295:130–9. doi: 10.1016/j.jconrel.2018.12.009
80. Reinhard J, Eichhorn U, Wiessler M, Kaina B. Inactivation of O(6)-methylguanine-DNA methyltransferase by glucose-conjugated inhibitors. *Int J Cancer.* (2001) 93:373–9. doi: 10.1002/ijc.1336
81. Kaina B, Muhlhausen U, Piee-Staffa A, Christmann M, Garcia Boy R, Rosch F, et al. Inhibition of O6-methylguanine-DNA methyltransferase by glucose-conjugated inhibitors: comparison with nonconjugated inhibitors and effect on fotemustine and temozolomide-induced cell death. *J Pharmacol Exp Ther.* (2004) 311:585–93. doi: 10.1124/jpet.104.071316
82. Tomaszowski KH, Schirrmacher R, Kaina B. Multidrug efflux pumps attenuate the effect of MGMT inhibitors. *Mol Pharm.* (2015) 12:3924–34. doi: 10.1021/acs.molpharmaceut.5b00341
83. Tomaszowski KH, Hellmann N, Ponath V, Takatsu H, Shin HW, Kaina B. Uptake of glucose-conjugated MGMT inhibitors in cancer cells: role of flippases and type IV P-type ATPases. *Sci Rep.* (2017) 7:13925. doi: 10.1038/s41598-017-14129-x
84. Javanmard S, Loktionova NA, Fang Q, Pauly GT, Pegg AE, Moschel RC. Inactivation of O(6)-alkylguanine-DNA alkyltransferase by folate esters of O(6)-benzyl-2'-deoxyguanosine and of O(6)-[4-(hydroxymethyl)benzyl]guanine. *J Med Chem.* (2007) 50:5193–201. doi: 10.1021/jm0705859
85. Watson AJ, Middleton MR, McGown G, Thorncroft M, Ranson M, Hersey P, et al. O(6)-methylguanine-DNA methyltransferase depletion and DNA damage in patients with melanoma treated with temozolomide alone or with lomeguatrib. *Br J Cancer.* (2009) 100:1250–6. doi: 10.1038/sj.bjc.6605015
86. Watson AJ, Sabharwal A, Thorncroft M, McGown G, Kerr R, Bojanic S, et al. Tumor O(6)-methylguanine-DNA methyltransferase inactivation by oral lomeguatrib. *Clin Cancer Res.* (2010) 16:743–9. doi: 10.1158/1078-0432.CCR-09-1389
87. Quinn JA, Jiang SX, Reardon DA, Desjardins A, Vredenburgh JJ, Rich JN, et al. Phase II trial of temozolomide plus O^6-benzylguanine in adults with recurrent, temozolomide-resistant malignant glioma. *J Clin Oncol.* (2009) 27:1262–7. doi: 10.1200/JCO.2008.18.8417
88. Tawbi HA, Villaruz L, Tarhini A, Moschos S, Sulecki M, Viverette F, et al. Inhibition of DNA repair with MGMT pseudosubstrates: phase I study of lomeguatrib in combination with dacarbazine in patients with advanced melanoma and other solid tumours. *Br J Cancer.* (2011) 105:773–7. doi: 10.1038/bjc.2011.285
89. Romani M, Pistillo MP, Banelli B. Epigenetic targeting of glioblastoma. *Front Oncol.* (2018) 8:448. doi: 10.3389/fonc.2018.00448
90. Kato T, Natsume A, Toda H, Iwamizu H, Sugita T, Hachisu R, et al. Efficient delivery of liposome-mediated MGMT-siRNA reinforces the cytotoxity of temozolomide in GBM-initiating cells. *Gene Ther.* (2010) 17:1363–71. doi: 10.1038/gt.2010.88
91. Zhang W, Zhang J, Hoadley K, Kushwaha D, Ramakrishnan V, Li S, et al. miR-181d: a predictive glioblastoma biomarker that downregulates MGMT expression. *Neuro Oncol.* (2012) 14:712–9. doi: 10.1093/neuonc/nos089
92. Nie E, Jin X, Wu W, Yu T, Zhou X, Shi Z, et al. MiR-198 enhances temozolomide sensitivity in glioblastoma by targeting MGMT. *J Neurooncol.* (2017) 133:59–68. doi: 10.1007/s11060-017-2425-9
93. Bhakat KK, Mitra S. Regulation of the human O(6)-methylguanine-DNA methyltransferase gene by transcriptional coactivators cAMP response element-binding protein-binding protein and p300. *J Biol Chem.* (2000) 275:34197–204. doi: 10.1074/jbc.M005447200
94. Alonso MM, Gomez-Manzano C, Bekele BN, Yung WK, Fueyo J. Adenovirus-based strategies overcome temozolomide resistance by silencing the O6-methylguanine-DNA methyltransferase promoter. *Cancer Res.* (2007) 67:11499–504. doi: 10.1158/0008-5472.CAN-07-5312
95. Wang F, Marshall CB, Ikura M. Transcriptional/epigenetic regulator CBP/p300 in tumorigenesis: structural and functional versatility in target recognition. *Cell Mol Life Sci.* (2013) 70:3989–4008. doi: 10.1007/s00018-012-1254-4
96. Jiang H, Alonso MM, Gomez-Manzano C, Piao Y, Fueyo J. Oncolytic viruses and DNA-repair machinery: overcoming chemoresistance of gliomas. *Expert Rev Anticancer Ther.* (2006) 6:1585–92. doi: 10.1586/14737140.6.11.1585
97. Kanai R, Rabkin SD, Yip S, Sgubin D, Zaupa CM, Hirose Y, et al. Oncolytic virus-mediated manipulation of DNA damage responses: synergy with chemotherapy in killing glioblastoma stem cells. *JNCI J Natl Cancer Inst.* (2012) 104:42–55. doi: 10.1093/jnci/djr509
98. Paranjpe A, Zhang R, Ali-Osman F, Bobustuc GC, Srivenugopal KS. Disulfiram is a direct and potent inhibitor of human O6-methylguanine-DNA methyltransferase (MGMT) in brain tumor cells and mouse brain and markedly increases the alkylating DNA damage. *Carcinogenesis.* (2014) 35:692–702. doi: 10.1093/carcin/bgt366

6

Spatial Distance Correlates with Genetic Distance in Diffuse Glioma

Evan D. H. Gates[1,2†], Jie Yang[2,3†], Kazutaka Fukumura[4†], Jonathan S. Lin[1,5,6], Jeffrey S. Weinberg[7], Sujit S. Prabhu[7], Lihong Long[8], David Fuentes[1], Erik P. Sulman[3], Jason T. Huse[4,9] and Dawid Schellingerhout[10*]*

[1] Department of Imaging Physics, The University of Texas MD Anderson Cancer Center, Houston, TX, United States, [2] Graduate School of Biomedical Sciences, The University of Texas MD Anderson Cancer Center UTHealth, Houston, TX, United States, [3] Department of Radiation Oncology, NYU Langone School of Medicine, New York, NY, United States, [4] Department of Translational Molecular Pathology, The University of Texas MD Anderson Cancer Center, Houston, TX, United States, [5] Medical Scientist Training Program, Baylor College of Medicine, Houston, TX, United States, [6] Department of Bioengineering, Rice University, Houston, TX, United States, [7] Department of Neurosurgery, The University of Texas MD Anderson Cancer Center, Houston, TX, United States, [8] Department of Radiation Oncology, The University of Texas MD Anderson Cancer Center, Houston, TX, United States, [9] Department of Pathology, The University of Texas MD Anderson Cancer Center, Houston, TX, United States, [10] Departments of Neuroradiology and Cancer Systems Imaging, University of Texas MD Anderson Cancer Center, Houston, TX, United States

***Correspondence:**
Dawid Schellingerhout
dawid.schellingerhout@mdanderson.org
Jason T. Huse
jhuse@mdanderson.org

† These authors have contributed equally to this work

Background: Treatment effectiveness and overall prognosis for glioma patients depend heavily on the genetic and epigenetic factors in each individual tumor. However, intra-tumoral genetic heterogeneity is known to exist and needs to be managed. Currently, evidence for genetic changes varying spatially within the tumor is qualitative, and quantitative data is lacking. We hypothesized that a greater genetic diversity or "genetic distance" would be observed for distinct tumor samples taken with larger physical distances between them.

Methods: Stereotactic biopsies were obtained from untreated primary glioma patients as part of a clinical trial between 2011 and 2016, with at least one biopsy pair collected in each case. The physical (Euclidean) distance between biopsy sites was determined using coordinates from imaging studies. The tissue samples underwent whole exome DNA sequencing and epigenetic methylation profiling and genomic distances were defined in three separate ways derived from differences in number of genes, copy number variations (CNV), and methylation profiles.

Results: Of the 31 patients recruited to the trial, 23 were included in DNA methylation analysis, for a total of 71 tissue samples (14 female, 9 male patients, age range 21–80). Samples from an 8 patient subset of the 23 evaluated patients were further included in whole exome and copy number variation analysis. Physical and genomic distances were found to be independently and positively correlated for each of the three genomic distance measures. The correlation coefficients were 0.63, 0.65, and 0.35, respectively for (a) gene level mutations, (b) copy number variation, and (c) methylation status. We also derived quantitative linear relationships between physical and genomic distances.

Conclusion: Primary brain tumors are genetically heterogeneous, and the physical distance within a given glioma correlates to genomic distance using multiple orthogonal genomic assessments. These data should be helpful in the clinical diagnostic and therapeutic management of glioma, for example by: managing sampling error, and estimating genetic heterogeneity using simple imaging inputs.

Keywords: glioma, genomics, epigenetics, stereotactic biopsy, medical image analysis, radiomics, imaging genomics, radiologic-pathologic correlation

INTRODUCTION

Gliomas are thought to be genetically heterogeneous within a single specimen, as manifested by spatial morphological diversity observed on imaging. Genetic analyses are increasingly important in the delineation of glioma subgroups with distinct clinical behavior, as evidenced by the strong influence of genomic classifiers in the WHO 2016 grading system (1). Previous work has shown that biopsies taken from non-representative regions of tumor can produce errors in histopathological grading (2), and while modern image guidance may improve histopathological accuracy (3, 4), there are strong suggestions from the literature that genetic heterogeneity may also be underrepresented by standard surgical sampling (5, 6). Additionally, we know from work in other tumors that genomic signatures can vary depending on regional sampling (7).

If, therefore, molecular heterogeneity varies as a function of location in space, then it is reasonable to *hypothesize* that such variability might correlate with physical (Euclidean) distance between biopsy sites. A formal relationship between Euclidean and molecular distance *per se* has not (to our knowledge) been described for glioma. In this study, we seek to address this *gap in knowledge*, both qualitatively and with a quantitative statistical assessment.

To do so, we obtained multiple sets of stereotactic biopsies in previously untreated glioma patients, carefully noted the physical coordinates of each sample, and calculated the Euclidean distances between each pair of samples within a single tumor. Multidimensional genomic analysis was then performed on each sample, and distinct measures of genomic distance were derived from: (1) mutation number, (2) copy number variation, and (3) the extent of CpG island methylation. We found that in each case, meaningful and positive correlations were present between Euclidean and genetic distance.

METHODS

Biopsy Collection

Our study retrospectively analyzed glioma tissue samples collected as part of an IRB approved, HIPAA-compliant clinical trial protocol (NCT03458676). All subjects gave written informed consent in accordance with the Declaration of Helsinki. Biopsies were collected from previously untreated adult (>18 years old) patients with primary glioma immediately prior to tumor resection. Each patient underwent pre-surgical MRI within 3 days prior to craniotomy. During surgery, two or more image-guided biopsies were collected from each patient. The biopsy locations were chosen based on one or more findings in pre-operative MRI including contrast enhancement, reduced diffusivity, or increased cerebral blood flow. This approach mimics clinical workflow and targets areas likely to harbor malignant tumor tissue. Samples were collected using either a side-cutting, Nashold-type, image-guided biopsy needle (0.9 mm width and 10 mm side port) or by image-registered surgical biopsy forceps based on surgeon preference and patient anatomy. Samples were collected before tumor resection in order to minimize brain shift and we estimate the variance in the distance measurements based on the recorded image coordinates to be <2 mm. Tissue samples were immediately placed on ice for transport to a pathology lab where the tissue was frozen in OCT until analysis.

Biopsy Euclidean Distance

At the time of the biopsy collection, we recorded the image coordinates of the instruments using the surgical navigation software. The distance between separate biopsy sites i and j is calculated by the Euclidean distance of the captured 3D coordinates (x, y, z): $d_{ij} = \sqrt{(x_i - x_j)^2 + (y_i - y_j)^2 + (z_i - z_j)^2}$ (**Figure 2**). When possible for needle biopsies, the "shallow" and "deep" ends of the cylindrical specimens were divided. These specimens were analyzed separately with a distance of 5 mm assigned to the two parts of the divide sample, based on the needle geometry. The exact geometry is illustrated in **Supplementary Figure S2**.

DNA Extraction

Using light microscopy, each sample was microscopically confirmed to be comprised of tumor before DNA extraction. Percent wise quantification was not attempted due to the small amount of tissue in each sample. DNA was extracted from frozen biopsies and matched normal white blood cells (WBCs) using QIAamp DNA Mini Kit (Qiagen), and DNA concentrations were measured with Qubit fluorometer (Thermo Fisher Scientific).

Whole-Exome Sequencing

Between 200 and 1,000 ng of DNA were used for enrichment of all exonic fragments with SureSelect Human All Exon V6 (Agilent Technologies), followed by massively parallel sequencing on HiSeq4000 platform (Illumina) using 75-bp paired-end option. For the validation of somatic mutations identified by the HiSeq platform, custom PCR primer panels corresponding to the mutations were made with Ion AmpliSeq Designer. The libraries were prepared with Ion AmpliSeq Library Kit Plus (Thermo Fisher Scientific) according to the manufacture's protocol, and then subjected to Ion Proton sequencing (Thermo Fisher Scientific). Where available, we estimated tumor cellularity and ploidy using the whole-exome data and the sequenza (8). This confirmed the tumor content identified microscopically.

Mutation Count Genetic Distance

With the whole-exome sequencing (WES) fastq files, we used the BWA-MEM (9) software for read mapping. With the bam files, we used MuTect2 (10) software to call genetic variations between tumor samples and blood control samples and used ANNOVAR (11) to annotate the specific mutations (pseudocode provided on Github).[1] We then filtered the resulting mutations based on the five following criteria: (1) mutations must be located in exonic regions; (2) mutation function must be frameshift deletion, frameshift insertion, non-synonymous SNV, stopgain or stoploss; (3) reference read count, the read having same base call as reference, must be $\geq$10; (4) alterative read count, the reads detected as mutations, must be $\geq$8; and (5) the alternative read frequency must be $\geq$0.1. These filters ensure the mutations are real, not statistical artifacts, and that they likely lead to molecular tumor changes such as reduced expression levels, truncated proteins, or errors in DNA transcription and translation. The mutation count genetic difference between samples from the same tumor in one patient was measured using the Jaccard distance (12).

$$d_{Jaccard} = \frac{\sum (P_i - Q_i)^2}{\sum P_i^2 + \sum Q_i^2 - \sum (P_i * Q_i)}$$

Where P_i and Q_i are the alternative allele frequency for the ith mutation. The mutation count genetic distance between samples is small when the gene mutations are present in both samples and maximum when the sets of mutations are disjoint. Pearson correlation coefficients were calculated between the number of genes/mutation genetic distance and the Euclidean distance for all available biopsy pairs.

Copy Number Variation Genetic Distance

Copy number variations (CNV) for paired biopsies were obtained using WES data with CNVKit (13), which has high CNV calling accuracy (14) and can infer information in uncovered intron regions. With the segmentation information for each biopsy, we combined all break points available from all biopsies, created a list of CNV events, and assigned the corresponding log2 ratio value to each event and each biopsy. The CNV distance was calculated using the Canberra distance

$$d_{Canberra} = \sum \frac{|P_i - Q_i|}{P_i + Q_i}$$

Where P_i and Q_i are the log ratio values of the first and second samples at event i (12) between paired biopsies from the same patients. The Canberra distance is effectively the L_1 distance but scaled at each value by the average signal of the samples. This normalizes the differences so that samples with larger relative absolute difference will be a greater distance apart under this metric. So, CNV distance is a measure of the total amount of DNA variation between samples. Also note that the distance between a sample and itself is zero. Pearson correlation coefficients were calculated between the CNV distance and the Euclidean distance for each biopsy pair.

[1]https://github.com/JieYang031/WGS-analysis

Methylation Distance

DNA was subjected to bisulfite conversion with EZ DNA Methylation-Gold Kit (Zymo Research), and analyzed for methylation profiling using Infinium Methylation EPIC Beadchip and iScan (Illumina). We evaluated differences in DNA methylation as a way to quantify the epigenetic distance between samples and investigate correlation with physical distance. Raw DNA methylation data were processed with default pre-processing steps in UniD (15) as implemented in R. Samples with more than 10% of values missing and probes with more than 3 missing values were excluded. The isocitrate dehydrogenase (*IDH*) mutation status for each sample was predicted using UniD predictive models (15). The methylation level was represented as a β value [methylated signal divided by the sum of methylated and unmethylated signal (16)]. We first applied unsupervised clustering and t-distributed stochastic neighbor embedding (t-SNE) (17) analysis with the top 200 and 500 probes with the highest median absolute deviation (MAD) values across all samples. Then, using only the most variant probes, we removed probes that are likely uninformative and only reduce statistical power (18). In order to calculate the methylation distance between biopsies pairs from the same patients, we used the top 500 probes with highest variance within each patient to calculate the L_1 distance:

$$d_{L1} = \sum_i |P_i - Q_i|$$

Where P_i is the ith beta value of the first sample in the pair and Q_i is the beta value of the second sample in the pair (12). The L_1 distance metric measures the total variation in methylation values and identical profiles have zero distance. Since the beta values are already normalized as the sum of methylated and unmethylated signal, we used the standard L_1 distance metric rather than the Canberra distance used for CNV genetic distance. The correlation between the methylation distance and Euclidean distance was measured with the Pearson correlation coefficient.

RESULTS

In total, 31 patients were recruited between 2013 and 2016. Patients with no tissue harvest due to surgical complexity, cardiac issues, or technical difficulties or patients with insufficient tissue for downstream molecular analysis were excluded from our study cohort ($n = 8$) (**Figure 1A**) leaving 23 patients with 71 biopsies.

After exclusions (4 samples) for ambiguous imaging coordinates, 67 samples from 23 patients were subjected to global methylation array-based profiling (**Figure 1C**). Seventeen of these samples from 8 patients were processed for WES

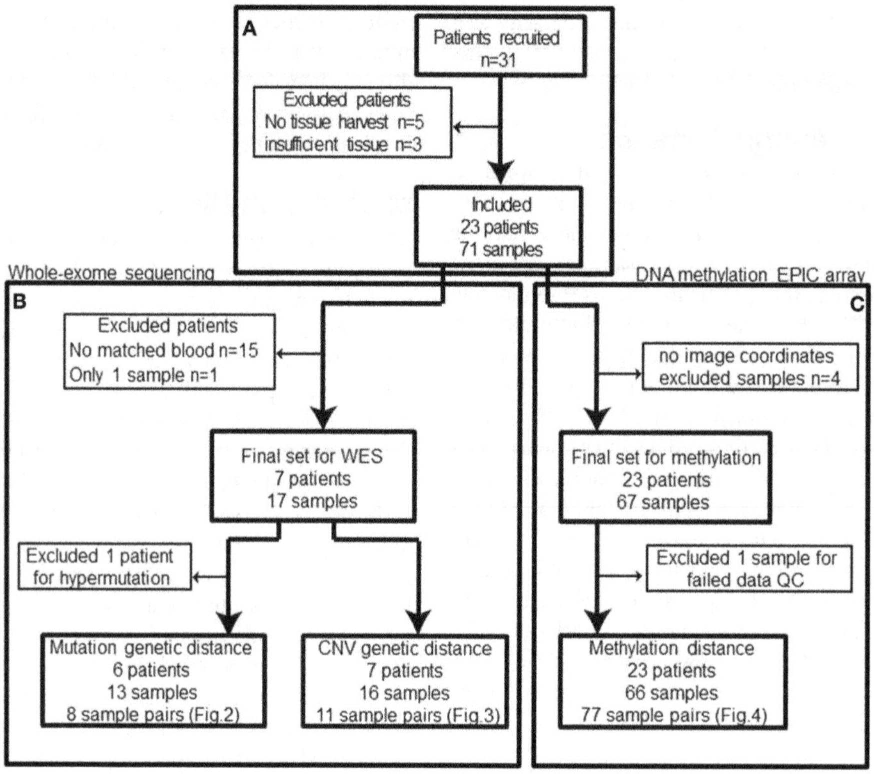

FIGURE 1 | Patient and samples cohort processing flowchart. **(A)** 31 patients were recruited between 2013 and 2016. Five patients had no tissue harvest due to surgical complexity ($n = 3$), cardiac issues, or technical difficulties and three patients had no sufficient tissue. In total, eight patients were excluded from the cohort. **(B)** Among the remaining patients, only eight patients had normal blood samples available for whole-exome sequencing and one of those patients only had a single sample sequenced. Based on the mutation calls, one patient was excluded due to abnormally high mutation burden (TMB). The remaining 13 biopsies from 6 patients constitute 8 biopsy pairs for mutation genetic distance. **(C)** After excluding samples without image coordinates, we have 67 samples from 23 patients for methylation profiling. One sample was excluded from methylation analysis due to poor data quality: 12.85% of available probes returned missing values. In summary, 66 samples from 42 unique image guided biopsy sites in 23 patients were available for methylation data analysis, comprising 77 unique biopsy pairs. The specific patients included in each analysis is available in **Table 1**.

(**Figure 1B**). These patients were selected because patient-matched blood samples were retrospectively available for somatic DNA assessment thanks to an institutional tumor banking initiative. A summary of the patient demographic information is given in **Table 1**. Of the 67 total samples in the final analysis, 46 samples were shallow/deep pairs from needle biopsy, 4 were single samples from needle biopsy, 15 were single samples from forceps biopsy, and 2 were a shallow/deep pair collected from the same spatial location using forceps.

Genomic and physical distances were only calculated on an intra-tumor basis, meaning samples were not compared between patients, but only to other samples in the same patient/tumor.

Mutation Count Genetic Distance

WES was performed to identify gene mutations in the biopsy tissue samples. The mean coverage was 117 and 103 for tumor tissues and WBCs, respectively. We used the MuTect2 (10) and ANNOVAR (11) for somatic mutation calling and annotation. After filtering mutations, we identified a total of 257 single nucleotide variants (SNVs) and 19 insertions/deletions (indels) in our final 14 tissue samples analyzed.

In further examining the profiles of three biopsies (P12S1, P12S2, and P12S3) from one patient (patient 12), we found significantly higher mutation calls than in the other patients. Even after applying mutation filters, we found patient 12 had on average 2438 mutations per biopsy while all other patients/samples averaged 22 mutations per biopsy. In published literature (19), the median mutation rate per million base (Mb) is <1 for lower grade gliomas. So, the median mutation number for the whole exome (about 30 Mb) is <30. Therefore, we believe these three biopsies show hypermutation. We eliminated the possibility of a mismatched blood sample by comparing the non-conserved long insertion sequence between the blood and tumor samples, which were found to be consistent. Further review of this case revealed a prominent history of cancer in the patient's family, suggesting a fundamentally distinct mechanism of tumor evolution from those utilized in the remaining cohort. For these reasons, we excluded these samples from mutation count genetic distance analysis (**Figure 1B**), leaving 14 biopsies in 7 patients for analysis.

A total of 74 somatic mutations identified in our initial WES were then validated by focused Ion Proton

TABLE 1 | Patient demographic information.

Patient information				Clinical information							Test applied	
Pt #	# biopsy samples	# blood samples	# sample pairs	Age	Sex	Primary diagnosis	WHO	1p/19q status	IDH1	EPIC	WES
1	3	1	3	36	F	OA	II	Codel	WT	Yes	Yes
2	2	0	1	25	F	Anaplastic Diffuse Glioma	III	Codel	Mut	Yes	No
3	2	0	1	21	F	Anaplastic Diffuse Mixed OA	III	Codel	Mut	Yes	No
4	6	0	10	26	F	GB	IV	Neg	Mut	Yes	No
5	4	0	6	75	F	Diffuse Astrocytoma	II	Neg	WT	Yes	No
6	2	0	1	56	F	Diffuse Glioma	II	Neg	Mut	Yes	No
7	4	0	6	54	F	GB	IV	Neg	WT	Yes	No
8	4	0	6	45	M	Anaplastic Astrocytoma	III	Neg	WT	Yes	No
9	4	0	6	28	M	OD	II	Codel	Mut	Yes	No
10	3	0	3	30	F	Anaplastic Astrocytoma	III	Neg	Mut	Yes	No
11	2	0	1	62	M	GB	IV	Neg	WT	Yes	No
12	3	1	3	80	M	GB	IV	Neg	WT	Yes	Yes
13	2	0	1	44	M	Anaplastic Astrocytoma	III	Neg	Mut	Yes	No
14	6	0	15	55	F	OD	II	Codel	Mut	Yes	No
15	2	1	1*	67	M	GB	IV	Neg	WT	Yes	Yes*
16	2	1	1	32	M	OD	III	Codel	Mut	Yes	Yes
17	2	1	1	66	M	Diffuse Astrocytoma, GB	IV	Neg	Mut	Yes	Yes
18	2	0	1	41	F	Anaplastic OD	III	Codel	Mut	Yes	No
19	2	0	1	58	F	Diffuse Astrocytoma, GB	IV	Neg	WT	Yes	No
20	2	1	1	35	F	OD	II	Codel	Mut	Yes	Yes
21	2	1	1	49	F	GB	IV	Neg	WT	Yes	Yes
22	2	1	1	32	M	Anaplastic Astrocytoma	III	Neg	Mut	Yes	Yes
23	4	0	6	39	F	Diffuse Astrocytoma	II	Neg	Mut	Yes	No

*List of each patient included in the final analysis. EPIC indicates DNA methylation EPIC array was performed on that patient's samples (for methylation genetic distance) and WES indicated whole-exome sequencing (for mutation and copy number variation genetic distance). Sample pairs refers to the number of biopsy sample pairs that were available to calculate spatial and genetic distance. Patient age, sex, primary diagnosis, WHO grade, 1p/19q, and IDH mutation status are listed for reference. GB, Glioblastoma; OD, oligodendroglioma; OA, oligoastrocytoma. *WES only applied to one of two samples due to insufficient tumor content in one sample. EPIC methylation assay was performed on both samples.*

sequencing, yielding a concordance rate of 100% (74/74 mutations, **Supplementary Table S1** with primer sequences in **Supplementary Table S2**). Confident in the quality of our sequencing data, we proceeded to determine the genetic distance as measured by mutation count between patient-matched samples for our remaining pairs as a function of number of distinct mutations. Similar approaches have been applied in recent work (20). We then correlated mutation count genetic distance to Euclidean distance and found a strong correlation (Pearson correlation coefficient $= 0.63$, $p = 0.091$) (**Figure 2**), supporting the notion that as the physical distance between biopsy samples increases, so too does the number of mutated genes. Indeed, some of the most closely clustered samples (Patient 1) by Euclidean distance (5 mm) exhibited only one distinct mutation whereas two samples biopsied 21 mm apart (Patient 22) had 36 distinct mutations between them. On average a one unit increase in mutation count genetic distance unit was equivalent to an increased Euclidean distance of 0.6 mm, and 10 mm of additional Euclidean distance was equivalent to 17 additional mutation counts. The equation of the best fit regression line was: Genetic count distance $= -11.6 + 1.7\cdot$ Euclidean distance in mm.

Using the three samples from patient 1 as unique samples for further exploration, the hierarchical structure between biopsies was investigated (**Figure 2**). By comparing mutation calls among biopsies, we found that all three samples shared 10 common mutations, while P1S1 or P1S3 each had one additional distinct mutation (**Figure 2**). Finally, the allele frequency of mutation calls (**Figure 2**) were generally higher for the shared mutations between the three samples than for the private mutations, suggestive of sub-clonality within independently evolving tumor clones.

Copy Number Variation Genetic Distance

Copy number variation (CNV) for each biopsy was derived from WES data using CNVkit and visualized with Integrative Genomics Viewer (IGV, version 2.4.8) (21, 22) (**Figure 3A**). We obtained 255 CNV events after combining all break points available. WES data also estimated cellularity to be >50% for a majority of samples used in CNV analysis (**Supplementary Table S3**). Reassuringly, we found that our data recapitulated well-known glioma-associated patterns such as 1p/19q co-deletion and co-incident 7-gain/10-loss,

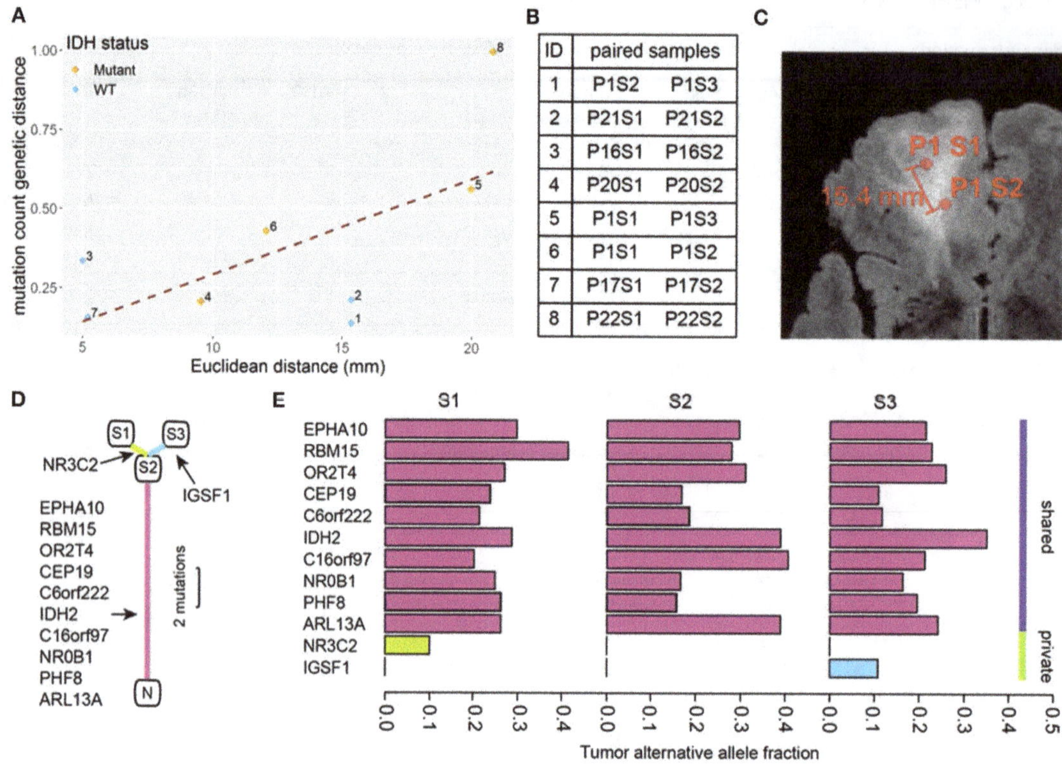

FIGURE 2 | Mutation count genetic distance. **(A)** Scatter plot shows a high correlation between Euclidean distance and the Jaccard distance between biopsy pairs (Pearson $r = 0.63$). **(B)** The pairs of biopsy points whose distances are graphed in **(A)**. The samples are listed by patient number (P) and sample number (S) so for example pair 1 consists of sample 2 from patient 1 (P1S2) and sample 3 from patient 1 (P1S3). **(C)** Physical distance illustration. On this magnetic resonance image, a biopsy pair in patient 1 (samples P1S1, P1S2) are indicated by circles. The Euclidean distance between the sample sites is shown. **(D)** The phylogenetic tree of three biopsies from the same patient (P1). N represents normal brain (no mutations), and S1-3 are the three biopsy sites sampled. The detected mutations events are shown in the annotations, the segment length is proportional to the number of mutations. **(E)** The tumor alternative allele fraction for all mutation events were compared between biopsies shown in **(D)**. The shared mutations between all samples generally show a higher alternative allele frequency.

characteristic of IDH-mutant oligodendroglioma and IDH-wild type glioblastoma, respectively (**Table 1**).

Using the log2 ratio value as input, CNV distance was calculated between each biopsy pair. Since the algorithm inferring CNV using WES data relies on the read counts instead of mutation calls, we included the hypermutated case of patient 12 in our CNV analysis (**Figure 3C**). We compared CNV distance with Euclidean distance for each paired set of biopsy specimens and once again obtained a strong correlation (Pearson correlation coefficient = 0.65, $p = 0.04$, **Figure 3B**). Moreover, linear regression between CNV distance and Euclidean distance (slope constant was approximately 6.8 log2 CNV per mm) showed the same trend as was seen between mutation count genetic distance and Euclidean distance. IDH mutant and wild-type samples both demonstrated the same general relationship between CNV distance and Euclidean distance. On average 10 mm additional distance increased the CNV distance by 68.4 units. Each unit of CNV distance corresponded to about 0.15 mm Euclidean distance. The equation of the best fit regression line is: CNV distance = − 93.8 + 6.9· Euclidean distance in mm.

Methylation Genetic Distance

After data pre-processing with the UniD algorithm (see materials and methods), one sample was excluded due to high probe fail percentage (>10%) (**Figure 1**). Unsupervised hierarchical clustering of the remaining 500 probes and 66 samples delineated two subgroups within the cohort as evidenced by a heatmap (**Figure 4**, **Supplementary Figure S1**). The strong separation of the two clusters was further illustrated by t-SNE analysis and visualization (**Figure 4**). The composition of the two clusters showed a well-established concordance to *IDH* mutational status (23) (**Supplementary Table S4**).

Methylation distance was then independently calculated between all possible biopsy pairs from each patient using the L_1 distance between the values of the top 500 most variant methylation probes. Comparing these findings with Euclidean distance once again revealed a significant correlation (Pearson correlation coefficient 0.35, $p = 0.002$) (**Figure 4**). The abundance of sample pairs at a Euclidean distance of 5 mm is due to the shallow and deep portions of the same biopsy specimen, separated from each other by 5 mm, being analyzed separately (**Supplementary Figure S2**). The methylation distance between

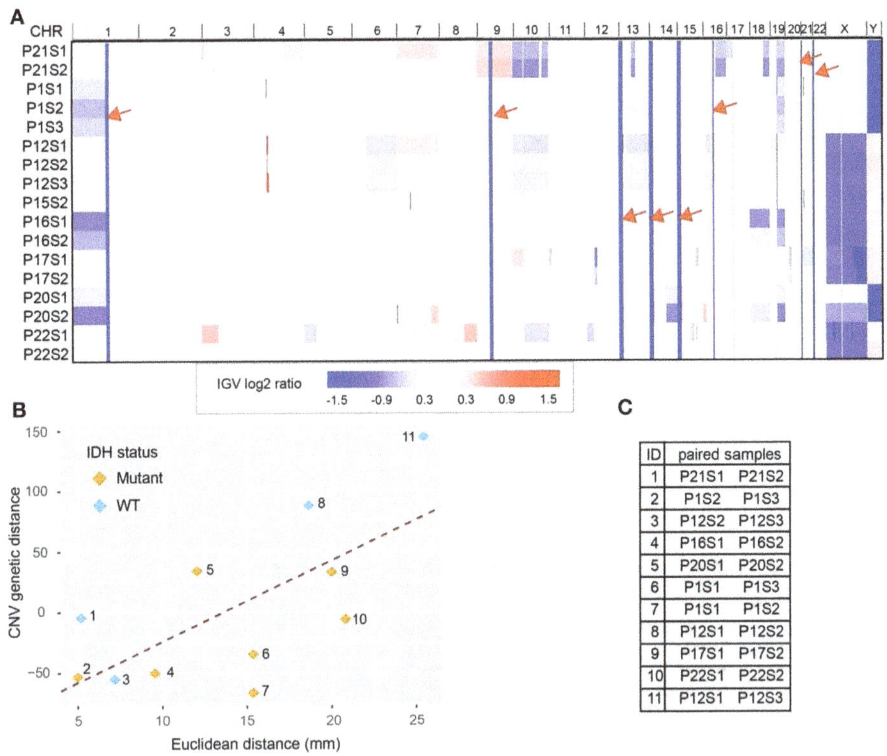

ID	paired samples	
1	P21S1	P21S2
2	P1S2	P1S3
3	P12S2	P12S3
4	P16S1	P16S2
5	P20S1	P20S2
6	P1S1	P1S3
7	P1S1	P1S2
8	P12S1	P12S2
9	P17S1	P17S2
10	P22S1	P22S2
11	P12S1	P12S3

FIGURE 3 | Whole Exome Sequencing (WES) derived copy number variations (CNV) distance. **(A)** CNV shown in Integrative Genomics Viewer (IGV). Chromosomes are labeled at the top of the panel and sorted in order from chromosome 1 to chromosome Y. Each row represents one sample identified by patient number (P) and sample number (S). The color blocks show the CNV log2 ratio value: blue indicated loss of copies while red indicated amplification. For regions with the same CNV across samples (solid column of blue marked with red arrows) there is no information across all samples. **(B)** CNV distance showed high correlation with the Euclidean distance between biopsy pairs from the same patient (Pearson $r = 0.65$). Pairs were drawn with color indicating IDH mutation status. **(C)** The paired sample details based on the label in **(B)**. Each sample is labeled by patient number (P) and sample number (S).

these shallow/deep pairs spanned the entire dynamic range, a finding not seen for other measures of molecular distance (see above). This discrepancy may be due to greater fluctuation in the DNA methylation profile between samples compared to mutational or copy number variation or may be due to the increased number of samples available for methylation analysis. Regardless, there is a significant correlation (correlation coefficient = 0.35, $p = 0.002$) between methylation distance and Euclidean distance and the minimum methylation distance between samples increased substantially with a Euclidean distance above about 2 cm. Based on the best-fit regression line we estimate an increase in the methylation distance of about 1.8 per 10 mm Euclidean distance, with each unit of methylation genetic distance corresponding to about 5.6 mm of Euclidean distance. The best-fit regression line equation was: Methylation genetic distance = 5.27 + 0.18. Euclidean distance in mm. The relation between methylation genetic distance and Euclidean distance is fairly consistent between samples from IDH wild-type and IDH mutant tumors as seen visually in **Figure 4**. The correlation remains statistically significant even when only samples with similar IDH mutation or 1p/19q co-deletion status are considered. See the **Supplementary Figures S3, S4** for details.

DISCUSSION

Many recent studies have documented the heterogeneity characterizing malignant glioma (24–26). Delineating the molecular mechanisms driving this heterogeneity remains an active area of investigation, as does the optimization of techniques for its non-invasive assessment. In this study, we aimed to establish informative and quantitative links between heterogeneity and spatial distance in a small glioma patient cohort. Among the most basic measures of spatial variability is simple Euclidean distance, and we found strong correlations between this metric and multiple assessments of molecular distance for distinct genomic/epigenomic variables. Two of these "molecular distances" were based on some form of total variation, or L_1 distance, an additional similarity, and the third (mutation count genetic distance) used a sum-of-squared distances. Future work may incorporate image data to develop a more complex measure of "radiographic distance" to complement physical distance. Our findings confirm prior work showing that gliomas exhibit spatial variability in their genomic signatures dependent on precise biopsy site location (5, 6, 24, 27). Moreover, they establish, for our limited patient population, a set of correlation constants for the various measures of molecular distance and

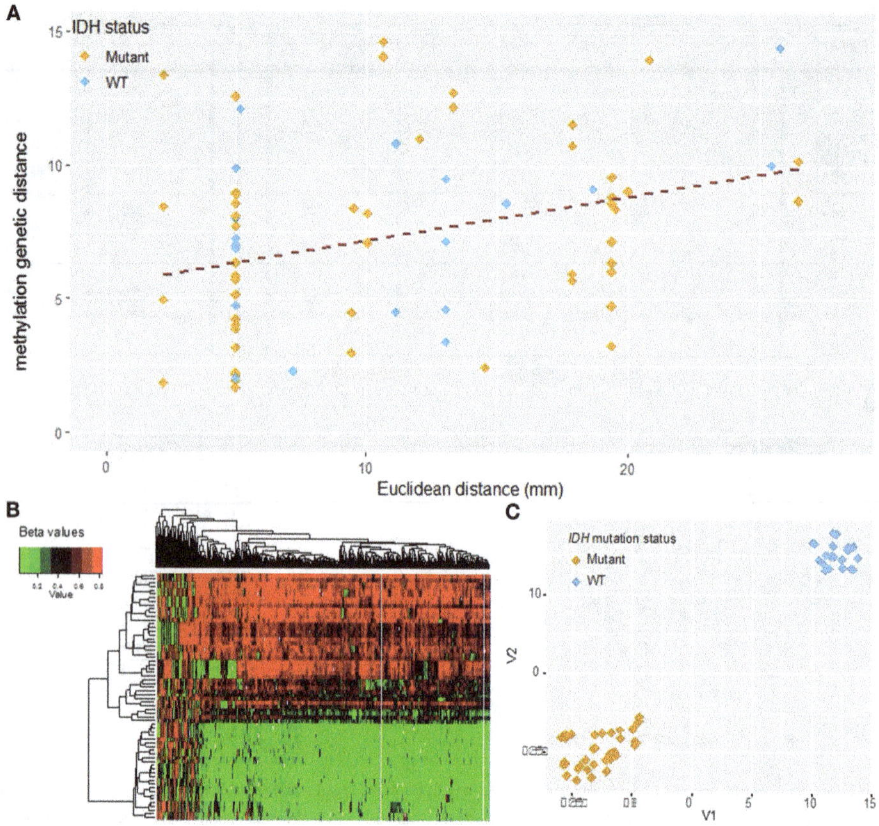

FIGURE 4 | DNA methylation L_1 distance vs. Euclidean distance. **(A)** The L_1 distance measures total variability in the methylation profile. This measure shows moderate correlation with Euclidean distance (Pearson $r = 0.35$, $p = 0.002$). Shallow/deep pairs from the same biopsy sample are assumed to be 5 mm distant. **(B)** Heatmap of hierarchical clustering with the top 500 probes with highest median absolute deviation (MAD) values. Each row represents one sample and each column one probe. **(C)** t-SNE plot of the top 500 probes with highest MAD values (probes with missing values were removed). The marker color indicates IDH mutation status. A natural clustering into IDH mutated and wild type tumors is evident in both the heatmap and t-SNE plot.

position in Euclidean space. The fact that three distinct molecular features, (1) somatic mutations, (2) CNVs, and (3) global methylation profiles, tracked similarly with Euclidean distance is notable.

Similar work includes a study conducted recently by Lee et al. (5), where the authors calculated Nei's genetic distance in multisector samples of glioblastomas and found that this metric was greater for samples that were farther apart in space (i.e., distant vs. local recurrence). Note: the Nei's distance analyzes genetic variability within populations which is not applicable to our sample size, hence why we used other distance measures in our analysis. Additional work by Sottoriva et al. analyzed copy number and gene expression data from multiple samplings of glioblastomas to illustrate how tumor phylogeny can be related to the approximate spatial position (24). Our study is consistent with these earlier reports. In addition, we measure the actual physical distance between samples and demonstrate a significant linear relationship between spatial and molecular distance in glioma. This correlation suggests that the processes of molecular and spatial evolution in tumor cells may be fundamentally linked.

A proposed mechanism for tumor heterogeneity is that distinct molecular characteristics become apparent in cancer cell clones as they distribute themselves across a given tumor mass over time (28, 29). While our present study does not investigate this mechanism directly, it is one potential explanation for the correlation between spatial and genetic distance. Whether acquired molecular alterations actively drive cellular motility as a rule, however, remains less certain. Recent literature suggests that branching mutational profiles of multiple tumor samples are due in part to differences in selective pressures (6, 7, 29), from environmental factors such as hypoxia (30). Such constraints could fundamentally drive molecular evolution as a means to escape suboptimal microenvironments. However, simple expansion of a tumor mass would also be expected to passively drive clones apart that, over time, would acquire increasing molecular distinctiveness.

This proposed mechanism does not account for hypermutated cases such as the patient we discussed previously. Given that the patients in our study were previously untreated, we can exclude the possibility of these mutations being caused by alkylating chemotherapeutic agents. In the absence of prior treatment the hypermutation status suggests an underlying germ line mutation, although our analysis precludes certainty. This is further supported by the patient's strong family history of cancer (31, 32).

Although our results show substantial differences in the number of mutations between samples from the same patient (**Supplementary Table S5**), we found that some root-level carcinogenic mutations like IDH1 were consistently present or absent in all samples from a given patient (**Supplementary Table S4**). Genomic findings thus support a branched evolution pattern, where some genetic events, in particular IDH1 mutations, are fundamental, required for tumorigenesis and are thus present in all samples. Accordingly, these alterations are truncal, with more unusual mutations relegated to sub-clonal events in selected populations (5, 6). These early, required mutations, tend to be diagnostically important, as reflected by the inclusion of IDH1 in the WHO grading criteria (1). These findings also reflect multiple published reports on clonal evolution within malignant glioma (5, 27).

As the classification and prognosis of gliomas is substantially influenced by genomic features, we suspect that the specific relationship between spatial and molecular distance might depend on the grade and type of the glioma. Within our sample set, additional subgroupings could be made based on established and prognostically relevant molecular stratifiers such as IDH mutation status and MGMT promotor methylation. However, our patient population is not large enough to examine distinctions within these smaller subgroups with sufficient statistical power. Nevertheless, our results using a combined glioma population across grades and subtypes suggests the positive and linear relationship between spatial and genetic distance is a characteristic of gliomas in general.

The concept of genetic heterogeneity is not novel, but our work is the first attempt (to our knowledge) to formally quantitate the relationship between spatial and genetic distances. We chose to use the simplest measure of correlation between spatial and genetic distance (i.e., linear) as the initial avenue of investigation. More complex methods of quantitating this relationship in the future may provide better correlation or interpretability. We also look to future investigations to elucidate the undoubtedly complex relationships between glioma subtypes, grades, and diverse genomic selectors, and the spatial distribution of genomic heterogeneity.

We propose that the further exploration of such genomic-spatial relationships in clinical trials similar to the current study, is justified. Establishing first the fundamental, and later on, more sophisticated imaging-genomic correlates, will put the field of imaging genomics on a firm scientific footing, and develop it into something that could be made useful for patient care.

CONCLUSION

The genetic heterogeneity of gliomas is correlated to physical distance within individual tumors, as confirmed by quantitative relationships using multiple independent methods. These findings likely support a diverging clonal evolutionary model of glioma expansion.

AUTHOR CONTRIBUTIONS

EG, JY, KF, JL, JW, SP, DF, ES, JH, and DS: study design. EG, JY, KF, JW, SP, LL, DF, JH, and DS: data collection, analysis, and interpretation. EG, JY, KF, JL, DF, ES, JH, and DS: manuscript writing. EG, JY, JH, and DS: figures.

FUNDING

UT MD Anderson Institutional Research Grant (DS). UT MD Anderson Clinical Research Trial Support (DS). UT MD Anderson Diagnostic Imaging Clinical Research Committee Imaging costs support (DS). UT MD Anderson Sequencing and Microarray Facility Core grant CA016672(SMF) provided support for exome sequencing. EG is supported by a fellowship from the Gulf Coast Consortia on the NLM Training Program in Biomedical Science and Data Science T15LM007093.

REFERENCES

1. Louis DN, Perry A, Reifenberger G, von Deimling A, Figarella-Branger D, Cavenee WK, et al. The 2016 World Health Organization classification of tumors of the central nervous system: a summary. *Acta Neuropathol.* (2016) 131:803–20. doi: 10.1007/s00401-016-1545-1
2. Jackson RJ, Fuller GN, Abi-Said D, Lang FF, Gokaslan ZL, Shi WM, et al. Limitations of stereotactic biopsy in the initial management of gliomas. *Neuro Oncol.* (2001) 3:193–200. doi: 10.1215/S1522851701000011
3. McGirt MJ, Villavicencio AT, Bulsara KR, Friedman AH. MRI-guided stereotactic biopsy in the diagnosis of glioma: comparison of biopsy and surgical resection specimen. *Surg Neurol.* (2003) 59:279–83. doi: 10.1016/S0090-3019(03)00048-X
4. Gates ED, Lin JS, Weinberg JS, Hamilton J, Prabhu SS, Hazle JD, et al. Guiding the first biopsy in glioma patients using estimated Ki-67 maps derived from MRI: conventional versus advanced imaging. *Neuro Oncol.* (2019) 21:527–36. doi: 10.1093/neuonc/noz004
5. Lee JK, Wang J, Sa JK, Ladewig E, Lee HO, Lee IH, et al. Spatiotemporal genomic architecture informs precision oncology in glioblastoma. *Nat Genet.* (2017) 49:594–9. doi: 10.1038/ng.3806
6. Suzuki H, Aoki K, Chiba K, Sato Y, Shiozawa Y, Shiraishi Y, et al. Mutational landscape and clonal architecture in grade II and III gliomas. *Nat Genet.* (2015) 47:458–68. doi: 10.1038/ng.3273
7. Gerlinger M, Rowan AJ, Horswell S, Larkin J, Endesfelder D, Gronroos E, et al. Intratumor heterogeneity and branched evolution revealed by multiregion sequencing. *N Engl J Med.* (2012) 366:883–92. doi: 10.1056/NEJMoa1113205
8. Eklund AC, Marquard AM, Favero F, Krzystanek M, Birkbak NJ, Li Q, et al. Sequenza: allele-specific copy number and mutation profiles from tumor sequencing data. *Ann Oncol.* (2014) 26:64–70. doi: 10.1093/annonc/mdu479
9. Li H, Durbin R. Fast and accurate short read alignment with Burrows-Wheeler transform. *Bioinformatics.* (2009) 25:1754–60. doi: 10.1093/bioinformatics/btp324

10. Cibulskis K, Lawrence MS, Carter SL, Sivachenko A, Jaffe D, Sougnez C, et al. Sensitive detection of somatic point mutations in impure and heterogeneous cancer samples. *Nat Biotechnol.* (2013) 31:213–9. doi: 10.1038/nbt.2514
11. Wang K, Li M, Hakonarson H. ANNOVAR: functional annotation of genetic variants from high-throughput sequencing data. *Nucleic Acids Res.* (2010) 38:e164–e. doi: 10.1093/nar/gkq603
12. Cha SH. Comprehensive survey on distance/similarity measures between probability density functions. *Int J Math Models Methods Appl Sci.* (2007) 1:300–7. Available online at: http://www.naun.org/main/NAUN/ijmmas/2007.htm
13. Talevich E, Shain AH, Botton T, Bastian BC. CNVkit: genome-wide copy number detection and visualization from targeted DNA sequencing. *PLoS Comput Biol.* (2016) 12:e1004873. doi: 10.1371/journal.pcbi.1004873
14. Seed G, Yuan W, Mateo J, Carreira S, Bertan C, Lambros M, et al. Gene copy number estimation from targeted next-generation sequencing of prostate cancer biopsies: analytic validation and clinical qualification. *Clin Cancer Res.* (2017) 23:6070–7. doi: 10.1158/1078-0432.CCR-17-0972
15. Yang J, Wang Q, Long L, Ezhilarasan R, Sulman E. UniD: unified and integrated diagnostic pipeline for malignant gliomas based on DNA methylation data. *Cancer Res.* (2017) 77(13 Suppl.):3348. doi: 10.1158/1538-7445.AM2017-3348
16. Bock C. Analysing and interpreting DNA methylation data. *Nat Rev Genet.* (2012) 13:705–19. doi: 10.1038/nrg3273
17. van der Maaten LJP, Hinton GE. Visualizing high-dimensional data using t-SNE. *J Mach Learn Res.* (2008) 9:2579–605. Available online at: http://www.jmlr.org/papers/volume9/vandermaaten08a/vandermaaten08a.pdf
18. Brocks D, Assenov Y, Minner S, Bogatyrova O, Simon R, Koop C, et al. Intratumor DNA methylation heterogeneity reflects clonal evolution in aggressive prostate cancer. *Cell Rep.* (2014) 8:798–806. doi: 10.1016/j.celrep.2014.06.053
19. Alexandrov LB, Nik-Zainal S, Wedge DC, Aparicio SA, Behjati S, Biankin AV, et al. Signatures of mutational processes in human cancer. *Nature.* (2013) 500:415–21. doi: 10.1038/nature12477
20. Gerlinger M, Horswell S, Larkin J, Rowan AJ, Salm MP, Varela I, et al. Genomic architecture and evolution of clear cell renal cell carcinomas defined by multiregion sequencing. *Nat Genetics.* (2014) 46:225. doi: 10.1038/ng.2891
21. Robinson JT, Thorvaldsdottir H, Winckler W, Guttman M, Lander ES, Getz G, et al. Integrative genomics viewer. *Nat Biotechnol.* (2011) 29:24–6. doi: 10.1038/nbt.1754
22. Thorvaldsdottir H, Robinson JT, Mesirov JP. Integrative genomics viewer (IGV): high-performance genomics data visualization and exploration. *Brief Bioinform.* (2013) 14:178–92. doi: 10.1093/bib/bbs017
23. Turcan S, Rohle D, Goenka A, Walsh LA, Fang F, Yilmaz E, et al. IDH1 mutation is sufficient to establish the glioma hypermethylator phenotype. *Nature.* (2012) 483:479. doi: 10.1038/nature10866
24. Sottoriva A, Spiteri I, Piccirillo SG, Touloumis A, Collins VP, Marioni JC, et al. Intratumor heterogeneity in human glioblastoma reflects cancer evolutionary dynamics. *Proc Natl Acad Sci USA.* (2013) 110:4009–14. doi: 10.1073/pnas.1219747110
25. Cancer Genome Atlas Research Network. Comprehensive genomic characterization defines human glioblastoma genes and core pathways. *Nature.* (2008) 455:1061. doi: 10.1038/nature07385
26. Patel AP, Tirosh I, Trombetta JJ, Shalek AK, Gillespie SM, Wakimoto H, et al. Single-cell RNA-seq highlights intratumoral heterogeneity in primary glioblastoma. *Science.* (2014) 344:1396. doi: 10.1126/science.1254257
27. Johnson BE, Mazor T, Hong C, Barnes M, Aihara K, McLean CY, et al. Mutational analysis reveals the origin and therapy-driven evolution of recurrent glioma. *Science.* (2014) 343:189. doi: 10.1126/science.1239947
28. Swanton C. Intratumor heterogeneity: evolution through space and time. *Cancer Res.* (2012) 72:4875. doi: 10.1158/0008-5472.CAN-12-2217
29. Greaves M, Maley CC. Clonal evolution in cancer. *Nature.* (2012) 481:306. doi: 10.1038/nature10762
30. Zagzag D, Zhong H, Scalzitti Joanne M, Laughner E, Simons Jonathan W, Semenza Gregg L. Expression of hypoxia-inducible factor 1α in brain tumors. *Cancer.* (2000) 88:2606–18. doi: 10.1002/1097-0142(20000601)88:11<2606::AID-CNCR25>3.3.CO;2-N
31. van Thuijl HF, Mazor T, Johnson BE, Fouse SD, Aihara K, Hong C, et al. Evolution of DNA repair defects during malignant progression of low-grade gliomas after temozolomide treatment. *Acta Neuropathol.* (2015) 129:597–607. doi: 10.1007/s00401-015-1403-6
32. Campbell BB, Light N, Fabrizio D, Zatzman M, Fuligni F, de Borja R, et al. Comprehensive analysis of hypermutation in human cancer. *Cell.* (2017) 171:1042–56.e10. doi: 10.1016/j.cell.2017.09.048

7

Lcn2-Derived Circular RNA (hsa_circ_0088732) Inhibits Cell Apoptosis and Promotes EMT in Glioma via the miR-661/RAB3D Axis

Tao Jin[1,2], Mingfa Liu[2], Yan Liu[2], Yuanzhi Li[3], Zhennan Xu[2], Haoqi He[1], Jie Liu[1], Yuxuan Zhang[1] and Yiquan Ke[1,4]**

[1] The National Key Clinical Specialty, Guangdong Provincial Key Laboratory on Brain Function Repair and Regeneration, Department of Neurosurgery, The Engineering Technology Research Center of Education Ministry of China, Zhujiang Hospital, Southern Medical University, Guangzhou, China, [2] Department of Neurosurgery, Shantou Central Hospital, Affiliated Shantou Hospital of Sun Yat-sen University, Shantou, China, [3] Department of Neurosurgery, Affiliated Hengyang Hospital of Southern Medical University (Hengyang Central Hospital), Hengyang, China, [4] Key Laboratory of Mental Health of the Ministry of Education, Guangdong-Hong Kong-Macao Greater Bay Area Center for Brain Science and Brain-Inspired Intelligence, Southern Medical University, Guangzhou, China

***Correspondence:**
Tao Jin
doctor_jin@qq.com
Yiquan Ke
kyquan@smu.edu.cn

Background: Glioma is the most common malignant tumor of the central nervous system, and often displays invasive growth. Recently, circular RNA (circRNA), which is a novel non-coding type of RNA, has been shown to play a vital role in glioma tumorigenesis. However, the functions and mechanism of lipocalin-2 (Lcn2)-derived circular RNA (hsa_circ_0088732) in glioma progression remain unclear.

Methods: We evaluated hsa_circ_0088732 expression by fluorescence *in situ* hybridization (FISH), Sanger sequencing, and PCR assays. Cell apoptosis was evaluated by flow cytometry and Hoechst 33258 staining. Transwell migration and invasion assays were performed to measure cell metastasis and viability. In addition, the target miRNA of hsa_circ_0088732 and the target gene of miR-661 were predicted by a bioinformatics analysis, and the interactions were verified by dual-luciferase reporter assays. RAB3D expression was analyzed by an immunochemistry assay, and E-cadherin, N-cadherin, and vimentin protein expression were examined by western blot assays. A mouse xenograft model was developed and used to analyze the effects of hsa_circ_0088732 on glioma growth *in vivo*.

Results: We verified that hsa_circ_0088732 is circular and highly expressed in glioma tissues. Knockdown of hsa_circ_0088732 induced glioma cell apoptosis and inhibited glioma cell migration, invasion, and epithelial-mesenchymal transition (EMT). We found that hsa_circ_0088732 negatively regulated miR-661 by targeting miR-661, and *RAB3D* was a target gene of miR-661. In addition, inhibition of miR-661 promoted glioma cell metastasis and suppressed cell apoptosis. Knockdown of *RAB3D* induced cell apoptosis and suppressed cell metastasis. Moreover, hsa_circ_0088732 accelerated glioma progression through its effects on the miR-661/RAB3D axis. Finally, results from a mouse xenograft model confirmed that knockdown of hsa_circ_0088732 induced miR-661 expression, resulting in suppression of RAB3D expression and inhibition of tumor growth *in vivo*.

Conclusion: We demonstrated that hsa_circ_0088732 facilitated glioma progression by sponging miR-661 to increase RAB3D expression. This study provides a theoretical basis for understanding the development and occurrence of glioma, as well as for the development of targeted drugs.

Keywords: glioma, EMT, hsa_circ_0088732, miR-661, RAB3D

INTRODUCTION

Glioma is caused by the cancerous transformation of glial cells in the brain and spinal cord (1, 2). When compared with other types of tumors, glioma has a poor prognosis, and the median patient survival time is ≤2 years (3). Furthermore, the incidence of glioma has been continuously increasing (4). Although surgery is the main method for treating glioma, the tumor tissue cannot be completely removed (5, 6). While radiotherapy and chemotherapy provide certain curative effects on glioma, various side effects associated with those treatments limit their therapeutic effect (7, 8). At present, glioblastoma is associated with a short survival time and a uniformly fatal outcome, irrespective of the treatment provided (9). Therefore, it is of great importance to study the mechanism for the occurrence and development of glioma, and identify new therapeutic targets and treatment strategies.

The development of glioma is a complex biological process that involves multiple mechanisms and factors (10, 11). Numerous tumor suppressor genes, oncogenes, and growth factors have been confirmed to be involved in glioma progression (12–14). Recent studies have proven that other types of biomolecules, such as circular RNAs (circRNAs), also play essential roles in this process (15, 16). CircRNAs are a class of single-stranded covalently closed circular non-coding RNAs (ncRNAs) with neither a 5′-terminal nor 3′-terminal poly A tail (17). CircRNAs cannot be degraded by RNAase enzymes due to their uniquely stable structure, and are thus highly conserved (18). Numerous studies have suggested circRNAs as potential biomarkers for use in tumor diagnosis and therapy, based on their stability and specificity of expression (19). In recent years, studies have suggested that circRNAs are closely associated with the occurrence and development of tumors (20, 21), such as oral cancers (22), bladder cancer (23), non-small cell lung cancer (24), and hepatocellular carcinoma (25). However, the expression and function of circRNAs in glioma have rarely been studied.

The recently discovered tumor biomarker lipocalin-2 (Lcn2) was initially found to be associated with iron absorption, antimicrobial activity, and epithelial cell differentiation (26, 27). Several studies have demonstrated that Lcn2 expression is increased in the presence of acute or chronic inflammation, as well as in cancer (28, 29). In addition, Lcn2 is capable of interacting with matrix metalloproteinases via the formation of complexes, and then participating in the cancer cell invasion process (30). Our previous studies showed that NGAL, coded by *Lcn2*, is associated with the clinical prognosis of glioma (31, 32). It is known that circRNA is formed by the variable splicing of mRNA (33). Currently, the underlying functions and mechanisms of Lcn2-derived circRNAs, and especially hsa_circ_0088732 in glioma, remain largely undetermined.

Recently, growing numbers of studies have reported that circRNAs can function as "miRNA sponges" and negatively regulate miRNAs (34, 35). Current studies have also confirmed that circRNAs can inhibit miRNA activity, and thus block the inhibitory effects of miRNAs on their target genes (36–38). MicroRNAs (miRNAs) are a type of highly conserved endogenous non-coding small RNA molecules consisting of 19–25 nucleotides, and directly regulate the levels of more plentiful mRNAs involved in different biological functions (39, 40). Increasing evidence suggests that miRNAs are abnormally expressed in glioma cells and involved in cell proliferation, differentiation, metabolism, apoptosis, and metastasis (41–43). However, the role played by hsa_circ_0088732 as an "miRNA sponge" in glioma has not been fully elucidated.

Rab GTPases are highly conserved intracellular transporter molecules, and basic components and major regulators of exocytic and endocytic membrane transport signaling pathways (44). RAB3D is one of the most important members of the Rab GTPase family, and an essential regulator of protein secretion. Within cancer cells, RAB3D activates intracellular AKT/GSK3β signaling to induce cell growth and metastasis (45). In the present study, we examined the expression levels of a novel circRNA (hsa_circ_0088732) in glioma tissues and cells, and also examined the function and mechanism of hsa_circ_0088732 in LN229 and U87-MG cells. In addition, we observed and analyzed the effects of hsa_circ_0088732 on miR-661, and proved that RAB3D is a direct target of miR-661. Taken together, our data indicate that hsa_circ_0088732 regulates RAB3D expression by targeting miR-661. Therefore, we for the first time suggest that the hsa_circ_0088732/miR-661/RAB3D axis may be a signaling pathway that can be of assistance in diagnosing and treating glioma.

MATERIALS AND METHODS

Clinical Samples

Twenty pairs of glioma and adjacent non-tumor tissues [Normal, and located 2 cm from the contrast enhancement in a T1-weighted image's so-called clinical target volume (46)] were obtained from glioma patients who were treated at the Affiliated Shantou Hospital of Sun Yat-sen University (Shantou, Guangdong, P.R. China) between March 2017 and January 2018. All patients provided their written informed consent for sample collection prior to the operation. The protocol for this study was reviewed and approved by the Ethics Committee of the Affiliated Shantou Hospital of Sun Yat-sen University. The tissue biopsies were immediately stored at the −80°C. None of the patients enrolled in this study had received chemotherapy or radiotherapy prior to surgery. The patients were diagnosed and re-evaluated according to World Health Organization (WHO) criteria by two pathologists, and any differences of opinion were resolved by careful discussion.

Fluorescence *in situ* Hybridization (FISH) Assay

The glioma tissues were fixed with 4% paraformaldehyde (Servicebio, China, G1113) for 6 h; after which, they were dehydrated in a graded ethanol series and embedded with paraffin (Sakura, Japan). After being sliced into sections (4 μm thick), the embedded tissues were incubated at 62°C for 2 h. Next, the sections were sequentially treated with dimethylbenzene xylene for 15 min, dimethylbenzene xylene for 15 min, anhydrous ethanol for 5 min, 85% alcohol for 5 min, and 75% alcohol for 5 min. The slide-mounted tissue sections were then treated with 3% H_2O_2 and proteinase K (2 μg/mL, Servicebio, G3016-1) at 37°C for 30 min, washed, pre-hybridized at 37°C for 1 h, and finally hybridized overnight at 46°C with 1 μL of hybrid solution that contained hsa_circ_0088732 probes (GenePharma, Shanghai, China). After washing, the slides were treated with 4′6-diamidino-2-phenylindole (DAPI, cat. no. 28718-90-3) solution for 8 min, and then visualized with a fluorescence microscope.

Cell Culture

Normal HEB glial cells, 293T cells, and glioma cell lines LN229, U87-MG, U251, and A172 were obtained from the Type Culture Collection of the Chinese Academy of Sciences (Shanghai, China). The 293T, HEB, LN229, U87-M, and A172 cells were cultured in Dulbecco's Modified Eagle's Medium (DMEM, cat # 11965-118), and the U251 cells were cultured in RPMI 1640 medium (ATCC, cat #: 30-2001). All culture media were supplemented with 10% fetal bovine serum (FBS, cat # SH30071.03), 1% penicillin/streptomycin, and 2 mM glutamine. All the cells were grown at 37°C in a humidified atmosphere containing 5% CO_2.

RNA Interference and miRNA Transfection

The small interfering RNAs (siRNAs) mixture targeting hsa_circ_0088732 and *RAB3D*, as well as a negative control (NC), miR-661 mimics, and miR-661 inhibitors were purchased from GenePharma Co., Ltd. (Shanghai, China). LN229 and U87-MG cells were seeded into 6-well plates (1×10^5/cells per well) and transfected with 10 nM NC, 10 nM hsa_circ_0088732 siRNAs and 10 nM RAB3D siRNAs or 10 nM miR-661 mimics, 10 nM miR-661 inhibitors and 10 nM control by using Lipofectamine® 2000 (Invitrogen) according to the manufacturer's protocol.

Plasmid Construction and Transfection

hsa_circ_0088732 and *RAB3D* were amplified by using 2 × Phanta Max Buffer, dNTP Mix (10 mM each), and Phanta Max Super-Fidelity DNA Polymerase. The PCR products were recycled with a Gel Extraction kit (Omega Bio-tek, Norcross, GA, USA), and then inserted into a psiCHECK-2 vector (Promega, Madison, WI, USA Cat Number C8021).

TABLE 1 | The sequences of primers used in real-time PCR.

Gene	Sequence(5′- 3′)
GAPDH F	TGTTCGTCATGGGTGTGAAC
GAPDH R	ATGGCATGGACTGTGGTCAT
hsa_circ_0088732 F	ATAAACATGTGCCCTCAGGC
hsa_circ_0088732 R	TTGGGACAGGGAAGACGATG
U6 F	CTCGCTTCGGCAGCACA
U6 R	AACGCTTCACGAATTTGCGT
All R	CTCAACTGGTGTCGTGGA
Hsa-miR-661	TGCCTGGGTCTCTGGCCTGCGCGT
Hsa-miR-661 RT	CTCAACTGGTGTCGTGGAGTCGGCAATTCAGTTGAGAC GCGCA
Hsa-miR-661 F	ACACTCCAGCTGGGTGCCTGGGTCTCTGGCCTGC
Hsa-miR-7	TGGAAGACTAGTGATTTTGTTGTT
Hsa-miR-7 RT	CTCAACTGGTGTCGTGGAGTCGGCAATTCAGTTGAGAA CAACA
Hsa-miR-7 F	ACACTCCAGCTGGGTGGAAGACTAGTGATTTTGT

F, forward primer; R, reversed primer; RT, reverse transcription primer.

The primers for hsa_circ_0088732 consisted of a forward primer containing an XhoI site: 5′-CCGCTCGAGGGAGAACCAAGGAGCTGACTTCG-3′, and a reverse primer containing a NotI site: 5′-ATTTGCGGCCGCGGCCTGAGGGCACATGTTTATTTAG-3′. The primers for RAB3D consisted of a forward primer containing a Kpn site: 5′-CCGCTCGAGTGGAACTATGGACCACATTAGACTG-3′, and a reverse primer containing an XhoI site: 5′-ATTTGCGGCCGCGACAAGGATTGGGAAATGGACA-3′. LN229 and U87-MG cells were seeded into 6-well plates (1×10^5 cells/well) and transfected with the hsa_circ_0088732-expression vector. The RAB3D-expression vector and control (pcDNA3.0) were transfected into cells by using Lipofectamine 3000 (Cat. No. L3000015) according to the manufacturer's protocol.

RNA Extraction and Quantitative Real-Time PCR (RT-PCR)

Total RNA was extracted from glioma cells and tissues by using TRIzol reagent (Invitrogen, Carlsbad, CA, USA). A NanoDrop2000c system (Thermo Fisher Scientific, Waltham, USA) was used to evaluate the concentrations of various RNAs, and a First Strand cDNA Synthesis Kit (Thermo Fisher) was used to produce cDNA by reverse transcription. PCR assays were performed by using SYBR GREEN PCR Master Mix (Takala) on an ABI7500 Real-time PCR system (Applied Biosystems, Foster City, CA, USA). The sequences of the primers used are shown in **Table 1**. The relative levels of mRNA or miRNA were measured by the $2^{-\Delta\Delta Ct}$ method, and normalized to those for GAPDH or U6, respectively.

Polymerase Chain Reaction (PCR) Assay

The cDNA template (5 ng) was mixed with Ex Taq DNA Polymerase (1.25 U), the upstream primer (0.2 μM), the downstream primer (0.2 μM), dNTPs (4 μL, 1 mM each), and 10 × Ex Taq buffer (5 μL) according to the manufacturer's instructions. The reaction conditions were 30 cycles of 94°C for 4 min, followed by 94°C for 40 s, 65°C for 30 s, and 72°C for 1 min, and then by 72°C for 5 min. The PCR products were assessed by electrophoresis with a 1.0% agarose gel.

Sanger Sequencing

The amplification product of the hsa_circ_0088732 sequence, including the splice sites, was verified by Sangon Biotech (Shanghai, China).

Western Blot Assays

RIPA lysis buffer was used to extract the total proteins from treated glioma cells, and the protein concentration in each extract was quantified using a BCA protein assay kit (Amresco, Fountain Parkway Solon, OH, USA, FA016-50G). An aliquot of total protein from each treatment group was separated by 10% SDS-PAGE, and the protein bands were transferred onto polyvinylidene fluoride (PVDF) membranes (Millipore, Burlington, MA, USA, IPVH00010). The membranes were subsequently blocked with non-fat milk and then incubated with primary antibodies against RAB3D (1:10,000, Abcam, Cambridge, UK, ab128997), E-cadherin (1:1,000; Abcam, ab76055), N-cadherin (1:500; Abcam, ab18203), vimentin (1:500; Abcam, ab137321) or GAPDH (1:2,000; Abcam, ab8245) for 1 h at room temperature. After washing, the membranes were incubated with an HRP-conjugated secondary antibody (1:20,000; BOSTER, Pleasanton, CA, USA, BA1054) for 40 min. The immunostained proteins were visualized by using ECL reagent (Applygen Technologies, Beijing, China) and X-ray film (SUPER RX-N-C; Fuji, Japan).

Transwell Assays

Transfected LN229 and U87-MG cells were harvested and counted. Next, 200 μL of cells (1×10^5 cells/mL) were seeded into the upper chamber of a Transwell plate (8 μm pore size, Costor, Cat. No. 3422), and 500 μL of culture medium containing 15% FBS was added to the lower chamber. After incubation for 24 h at 37°C, the migrated cells were fixed with 4% paraformaldehyde for 20 min and then stained with 0.5% crystal violet (Beyotime Institute of Biotechnology, China) for 5 min. After washing, the cells in the upper chamber were removed, and the migrated cells were observed under a microscope (OLYMPUS CX41). Transwell plates used for invasion assays had their upper chambers coated with Matrigel 30 min prior to being used for assays.

Cell Apoptosis Detection

Flow Cytometry Detection

The treated cells were harvested and counted, and then centrifuged at 1,000 g for 5 min; after which, they were washed and then stained for 15 min with reagents contained in an Annexin V-FITC Apoptosis Detection Kit (A211-01). Finally, the results for apoptosis were obtained by flow cytometry (FACSCalibur, BD, Franklin Lakes, NJ, USA).

Hoechst 33258 Staining

The treated cells were stained using Hoechst 33258 (Sigma-Aldrich, St. Louis, MO, USA) as recommended by the manufacturer. The morphology of the cell nucleus was observed using a fluorescence microscope (Olympus Corporation, Japan).

Immunohistochemistry Assays

Paraffin embedded tissue sections (5 μm thick) were dewaxed with pure xylene and then rehydrated in a series of ethanol solutions. The sections were then blocked with serum and incubated with anti-RAB3D antibody (Abcam, ab3337) at 4°C overnight; after which, they were incubated with goat anti-rabbit serum for 20 min. Following incubation, the sections were treated with diaminobenzidine (DAB, Sigma Aldrich, Cat# 5637), and then counterstained with hematoxylin. Images of the stained tissues were analyzed by microscopy, and results are expressed as a staining intensity and positive rate.

Dual-Luciferase Reporter Assays

The wild type (WT) and mutant (Mut) fragments of hsa_circ_0088732 and the 3′untranslated region (3′UTR) of RAB3D were amplified by PCR and inserted into the psiCHECK2 vector (Promega). The primer used for WT-hsa_circ_0088732 consisted of a forward primer containing an XhoI site: 5′-CCGCTCGAGGGAGAACCAAGGAGCTGA CTTCG-3′, and a reverse primer containing a NotI site: 5′-ATT TGCGGCCGCGGCCTGAGGGCACATGTTTATTTAG-3′. The primers used for MUT-hsa_circ_0088732 were 5′-CCCATGCAG CTGCTCTGATTAGCACCCCGCTGATGGA-3′ (forward) and 5′-TCCATCAGCGGGGTGCTAATCAGAGCAGCTGCA TGGG-3′ (reverse). The primers used for 3′UTR-RAB3D-WT consisted of a forward primer containing an XhoI site: 5′-CCG CTCGAGTGAAACTGACATCTTCTCAAATCTT-3′, and a reverse primer containing a NotI site: 5′-ATTTGCGGCCGC TATAGCCCTACACTGGAGGTCAA-3′. The primers used for 3′UTR-RAB3D-MUT were 5′-GTCCCCCTGCAGGTC TAACTCAAGCAGACAATTCCAC-3′ (forward) and 5′-GTG GAATTGTCTGCTTGAGTTAGACCTGCAGGGGGAC-3′ (reverse). The 293T cells were seeded into 96-well plates (1×10^4 cells/well) and incubated at 37°C. The next day, the cells were co-transfected with miR-661 mimics plus WT-hsa_circ_0088732 or MUT-hsa_circ_0088732 or 3′UTR-RAB3D-WT or 3′UTR-RAB3D-MUT. The transfection rates determined by flow cytometry were >90%. Next, luciferase activity was assessed by using the Dual-Luciferase Assay System (Promega) according to manufacturer's instructions. Firefly luciferase activity was normalized to that of Renilla luciferase activity.

The Xenograft Model

Male BALB/c Nude mice ($n = 24$; age = 5 weeks) were purchased from Charles River (Beijing, China). Treated LN229 cells in log phase growth were digested with trypsin and collected. After adjusting the cell density to 1×10^7 cells/mL, 0.1 mL of digested cells ($\sim 1 \times 10^6$ cells) was subcutaneously injected into the right axilla of each nude mouse. Tumor formation was examined every 3 days after injection. The mice were euthanized on day 21, and the tumor volumes were calculated by using the following modified ellipsoid formula: $(L \times W \times W)/2$, L: length, W: width. Tumor growth curves were drawn at the end of the experiment.

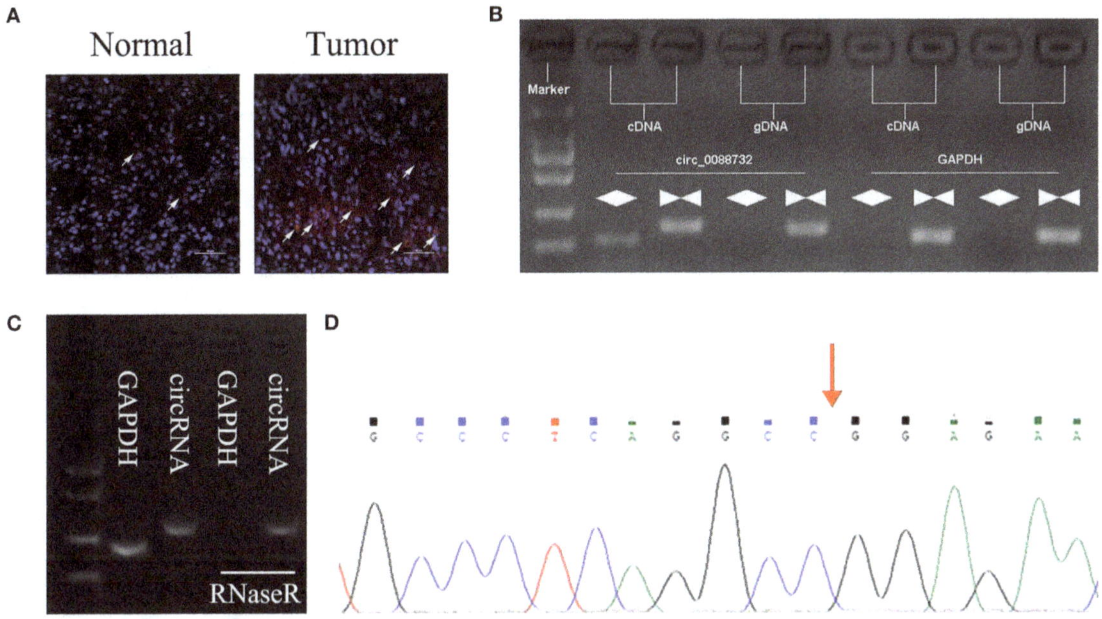

FIGURE 1 | Identification of hsa_circ_0088732. **(A)** Fluorescence *in situ* hybridization (FISH) was performed to show the levels and locations of Lcn2-derived circRNA (hsa_circ_0088732) expression. Red indicates circRNA and blue indicates nuclei (DAPI). The white arrow indicates hsa_circ_0088732. Magnification, ×200; Scale bar = 100 μm. **(B)** The linear and circular Lcn2 in cDNA and gDNA were amplified by using convergent and divergent primers, respectively. **(C)** qRT-PCR was used to analyze the expression of GAPDH and hsa_circ_0088732 RNA after treatment with RNaseR. **(D)** Sanger sequencing was used to verify the circular structure of hsa_circ_0088732; red arrow shows the site of the backsplice junction.

Hematoxylin-Eosin (H&E) Staining

The heterotransplanted tumors were fixed in 4% paraformaldehyde solution and embedded in paraffin; after which, 4 μm sections were cut and stained with hematoxylin and eosin (H&E). The sections were examined under a light microscope at ×200 magnification.

Immunohistochemistry (IHC)

Tissues were fixed in 4% paraformaldehyde solution and embedded in paraffin; after which, 4 μm sections were cut and immunostained. The slide-mounted sections were first incubated with Ki-67 primary antibody (1:100, Abcam, ab15580) for 1 h at 37°C, and then incubated with an HRP-conjugated secondary antibody for 60 min at room temperature. The sections were then counterstained with hematoxylin for 5 min, and images were collected under a microscope (Olympus, Tokyo, Japan) at ×200 magnification.

Terminal Deoxynucleotidyl Transferase-Mediated dUTP Nick End-Labeling (TUNEL) Assay

TUNEL assays were performed to assess cell death. The assays were conducting using an *in situ* cell death detection kit (Roche Applied Science, Indianapolis, IN, USA) according to the manufacturer's instructions.

Statistical Analysis

Each experiment was repeated three times, and results were expressed as the mean ± SD. All data were analyzed using Graphpad Prism software, Ver. 7 (GraphPad Prism Software, La Jolla, CA, USA). One-way analysis of variance was used to assess the significance of differences between different groups; the correlation between hsa_circ_0088732 and miR-661 was analyzed by Pearson's correlation coefficient. A P-value < 0.05 was considered to be statistically significant.

RESULTS

Identification of Lcn2-derived circRNAs

According to the circbase and circNet databases, Lcn2 can form hsa_circ_0088732 by cyclization. To explore the role of Lcn2-derived circRNA (hsa_circ_0088732) in glioma, a FISH probe was designed and used to examine the levels and locations of hsa_circ_0088732 expression in glioma tissues. The results showed that hsa_circ_0088732 was highly expressed in glioma tissues, and mainly located in the cytoplasm (**Figure 1A**; the white arrow indicates hsa_circ_0088732 expression). To verify the formation of hsa_circ_0088732, we designed convergent primers and divergent primers that could amplify the reference gene (GAPDH) and circLcn2 (hsa_circ_0088732) by using cDNA and gDNA as templates. The results revealed that

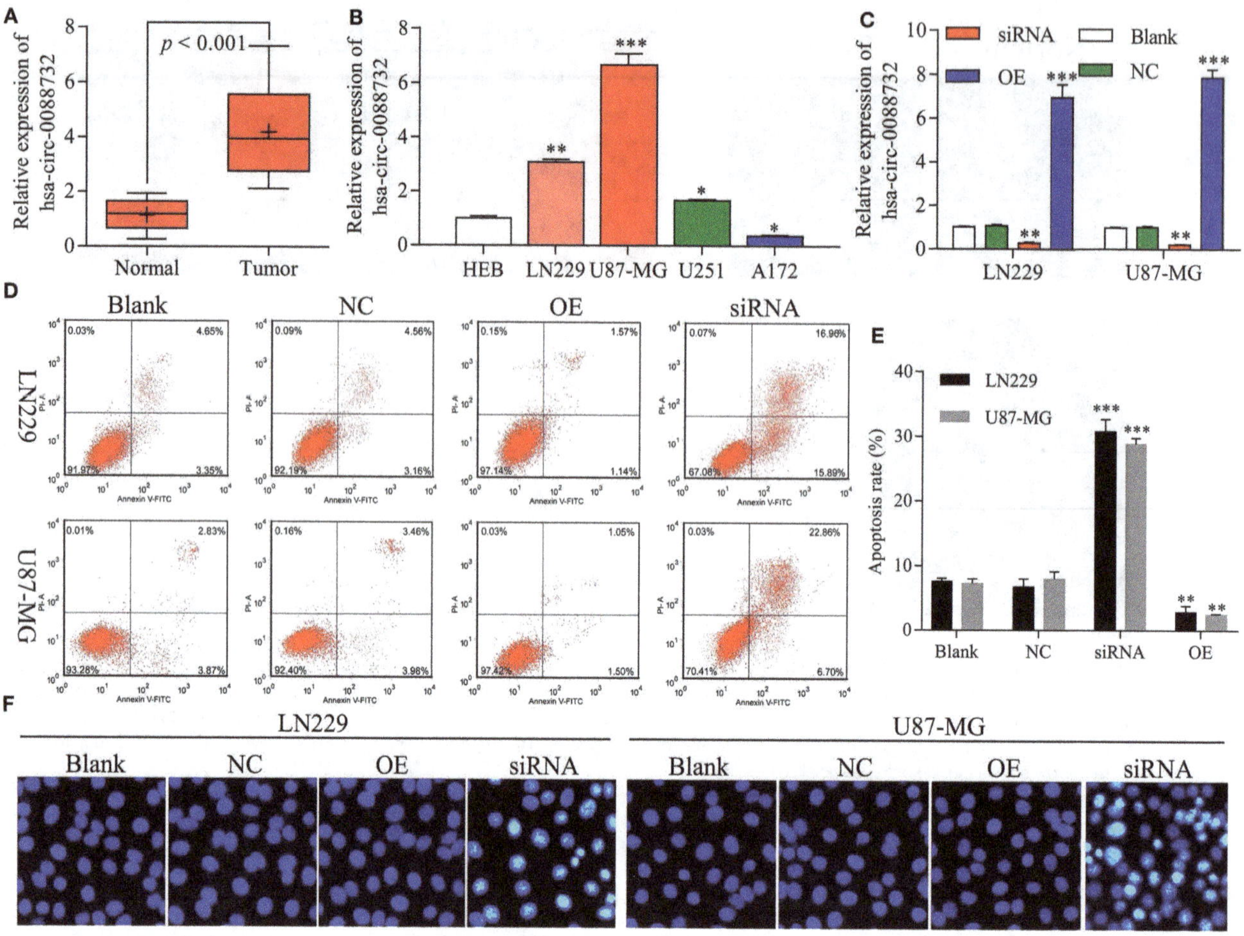

FIGURE 2 | hsa_circ_0088732 regulated glioma cell apoptosis. **(A)** qRT-PCR assays were performed to detect the expression of hsa_circ_0088732 in 20 pairs of glioma and adjacent non-tumor tissues ($P < 0.001$). **(B)** qRT-PCR assays were performed to assess the expression of hsa_circ_0088732 in HEB and glioma cells, including LN229, U87-MG, U251, and A172 cells (*$P < 0.05$, **$P < 0.01$, ***$P < 0.001$). **(C)** Knockdown or overexpression of hsa_circ_0088732 in LN229 and U87-MG cells was determined by qRT-PCR assays (**$P < 0.01$). **(D–F)** PI/Annexin V FITC and Hoechst 33258 staining were used to evaluate cell apoptosis (**$P < 0.01$). NC: negative control, siRNA: hsa_circ_0088732 siRNAs, OE: hsa_circ_0088732 overexpression plasmids.

hsa_circ_0088732 could be amplified by divergent cDNA primers, and no products were observed in the gDNA groups, suggesting that hsa_circ_0088732 could be formatted (**Figure 1B**). Furthermore, we found that the PCR products of GAPDH were not observed in cDNA after treatment with RNaseR, but hsa_circ_0088732 could be amplified (**Figure 1C**). In addition, we used Sanger sequencing to verify the circular structure, and found that the sequence was in accordance with hsa_circ_0088732 (**Figure 1D**; red arrow shows the site of the backsplice junction).

hsa_circ_0088732 Regulated Glioma Cell Apoptosis

Our results revealed that hsa_circ_0088732 was significantly upregulated in samples of glioma tissue when compared to samples of adjacent non-tumor tissue ($P < 0.001$, **Figure 2A**). We also found that hsa_circ_0088732 expression was significantly increased in glioma cells (LN229, U87-MG, and U251) when compared with HEB cells ($P < 0.05$, $P < 0.01$, $P < 0.001$, **Figure 2B**). Because hsa_circ_0088732 was highly expressed in glioma, the LN229 and U87-MG cell lines were used for further studies. To further investigate the biological functions and molecular mechanisms of hsa_circ_0088732 in glioma, hsa_circ_0088732 siRNA and overexpression plasmids were used to transfect LN229 and U87-MG cells. The qRT-PCR assay was used to determine the efficiency of hsa_circ_0088732 knockdown, and the results indicated that hsa_circ_0088732 expression was significantly decreased in the siRNA group relative to the control group, suggesting that hsa_circ_0088732 expression had been effectively blocked. Furthermore, hsa_circ_0088732 expression was significantly increased in the overexpression (OE) groups ($P < 0.01$, **Figure 2C**). Flow cytometry and Hoechst 33258 staining results showed that cell apoptosis was markedly increased in the siRNA group when compared with the blank group, and significantly decreased in the OE group when compared with the blank group. Therefore, these results demonstrated that knockdown of hsa_circ_0088732 could

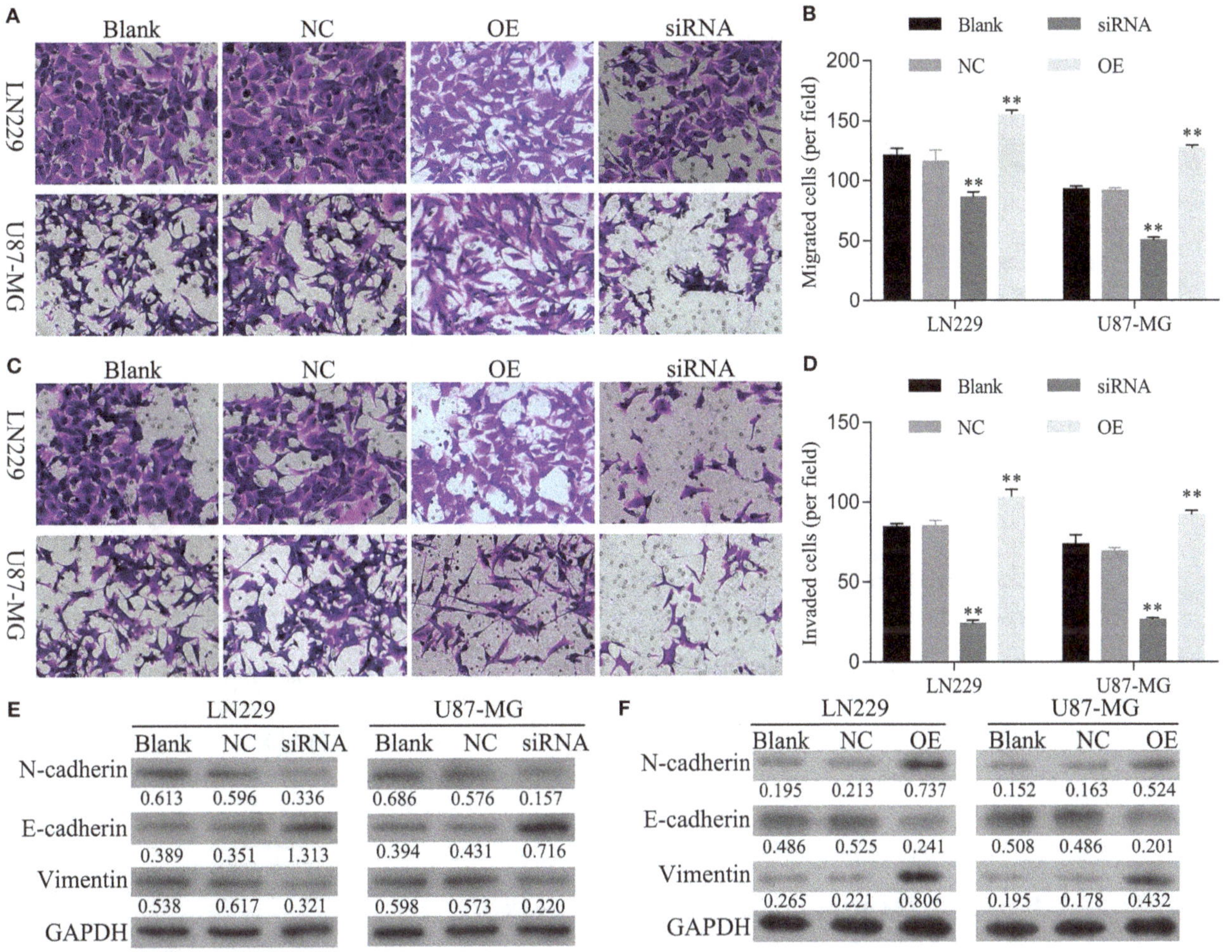

FIGURE 3 | hsa_circ_0088732 regulated glioma cell migration, invasion, and epithelial-mesenchymal transition (EMT). **(A–D)** The effect of hsa_circ_0088732 knockdown or overexpression on cell migration and invasion was evaluated by Transwell assays. **(E,F)** The expression of EMT-related proteins (E-cadherin, N-cadherin, and vimentin) was examined by western blotting. NC: negative control, siRNA: hsa_circ_0088732 siRNAs, OE: hsa_circ_0088732 overexpression plasmids.

promote cell apoptosis, and overexpression of hsa_circ_0088732 could inhibit apoptosis in glioma cell lines ($P < 0.01$, **Figures 2D–F**).

hsa_circ_0088732 Regulated Glioma Cell Migration, Invasion, and Epithelial-Mesenchymal Transition (EMT)

Next, the effects of hsa_circ_0088732 on glioma cell migration and invasion were assessed by Transwell assays. First, we analyzed the migration and invasion abilities of different glioma cell lines, and found that both abilities were positively correlated with levels of hsa_circ_0088732 expression (**Figure S1**). We also found that overexpression of hsa_circ_0088732 promoted HEB and A172 cell migration and invasion (**Figure S2**). Our results revealed that the numbers of migrated and invaded cells were significantly reduced in the siRNA group and markedly increased in OE group when compared with the blank group ($P < 0.05$, **Figures 3A–D**). In addition, the western blot results showed that knockdown of hsa_circ_0088732 downregulated N-cadherin and vimentin expression and upregulated E-cadherin expression, while overexpression of hsa_circ_0088732 induced N-cadherin and vimentin expression and reduced E-cadherin expression, suggesting that knockdown or overexpression of hsa_circ_0088732 inhibited or promoted glioma cell EMT, separately (**Figures 3E,F**).

hsa_circ_0088732 Sponged miR-661 and Negatively Regulated miR-661 Expression

To explore the underlying molecular mechanisms of hsa_circ_0088732 in glioma, a bioinformatics analysis was performed using the public database CircInteractome (https://circinteractome.nia.nih.gov/) to identify the target miRNAs of hsa_circ_0088732. We found that current publications had reported that miR-661 was clinically associated with glioma. Next, we performed qRT-PCR assays to identify the levels of miR-7 and miR-661 in glioma tissues, and found a

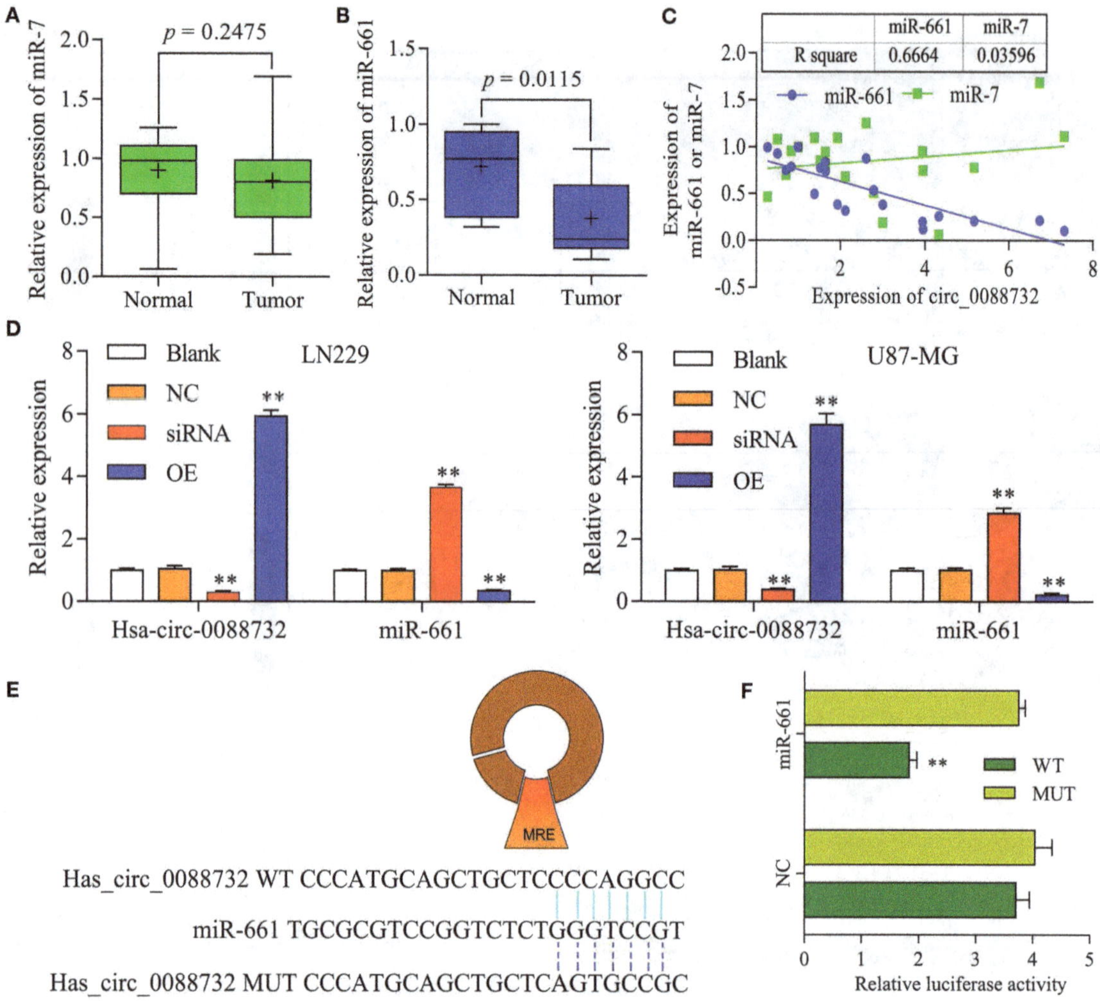

FIGURE 4 | hsa_circ_0088732 sponged miR-661 and negatively regulated miR-661 expression. **(A,B)** The levels of miR-7 and miR-661 expression in 20 pairs of glioma and adjacent non-tumor tissues were analyzed by qRT-PCR. **(C)** Person's correlation coefficient was used to analyze the correlation between hsa_circ_0088732 and miR-7 ($R^2 = 0.03596$) and miR-661 ($R^2 = 0.6664$). **(D)** LN229 and U87-MG cells were transfected with hsa_circ_0088732 siRNAs or overexpression plasmids, respectively. hsa_circ_0088732 and miR-661 expression were analyzed by qRT-PCR assays (**$P < 0.01$). **(E)** The potential targets of hsa_circ_0088732 were analyzed by a bioinformatics analysis, and a binding site between hsa_circ_0088732 and miR-661 was identified. **(F)** 293T cells were co-transfected with WT-hsa_circ_0088732 or MUT-hsa_circ_0088732, and with miR-661 or the NC, and the relative levels of luciferase activity were analyzed (**$P < 0.01$). NC: negative control, siRNA: hsa_circ_0088732 siRNAs, OE: hsa_circ_0088732 overexpression plasmids.

decrease in miR-661 levels ($P = 0.0115$) but no change in miR-7 levels ($P = 0.2475$) in glioma tissues when compared with adjacent non-tumor tissues (**Figures 4A,B**). In addition, we analyzed the correlation of hsa_circ_0088732 with miR-7 and miR-661. The results showed that hsa_circ_0088732 displayed a significant negative correlation with miR-661, but not with miR-7 (**Figure 4C**). To further explore the regulatory effect of hsa_circ_0088732 on miR-661, LN229 and U87-MG cells were transfected with hsa_circ_0088732 siRNA or overexpression plasmids. Results from qRT-PCR assays revealed that knockdown of hsa_circ_0088732 promoted miR-661 expression, and overexpression of hsa_circ_0088732 inhibited the expression of miR-661 ($P < 0.01$, **Figure 4D**). In addition, a bioinformatics analysis performed to predict and screen miRNAs that might be targeted by hsa_circ_0088732 showed that a hsa_circ_0088732 binding site existed for miR-661 (**Figure 4E**). The results also showed that there was a decreased luciferase intensity between the WT-hsa_circ_0088732 and miR-661, while there was no difference between the luciferase intensities of MUT-hsa_circ_0088732 and miR-661 ($P < 0.01$, **Figure 4F**). Our results confirmed that hsa_circ_0088732 could serve as a sponge to directly regulate miR-661 expression.

The Restoration of miR-661 Inhibition Led to Inhibition of Apoptosis and Promoted Glioma Cell Migration, Invasion, and EMT Mediated by hsa_circ_0088732 Knockdown

To confirm that knockdown of miR-661 could restore the inhibition of apoptosis and promotion of glioma cell migration,

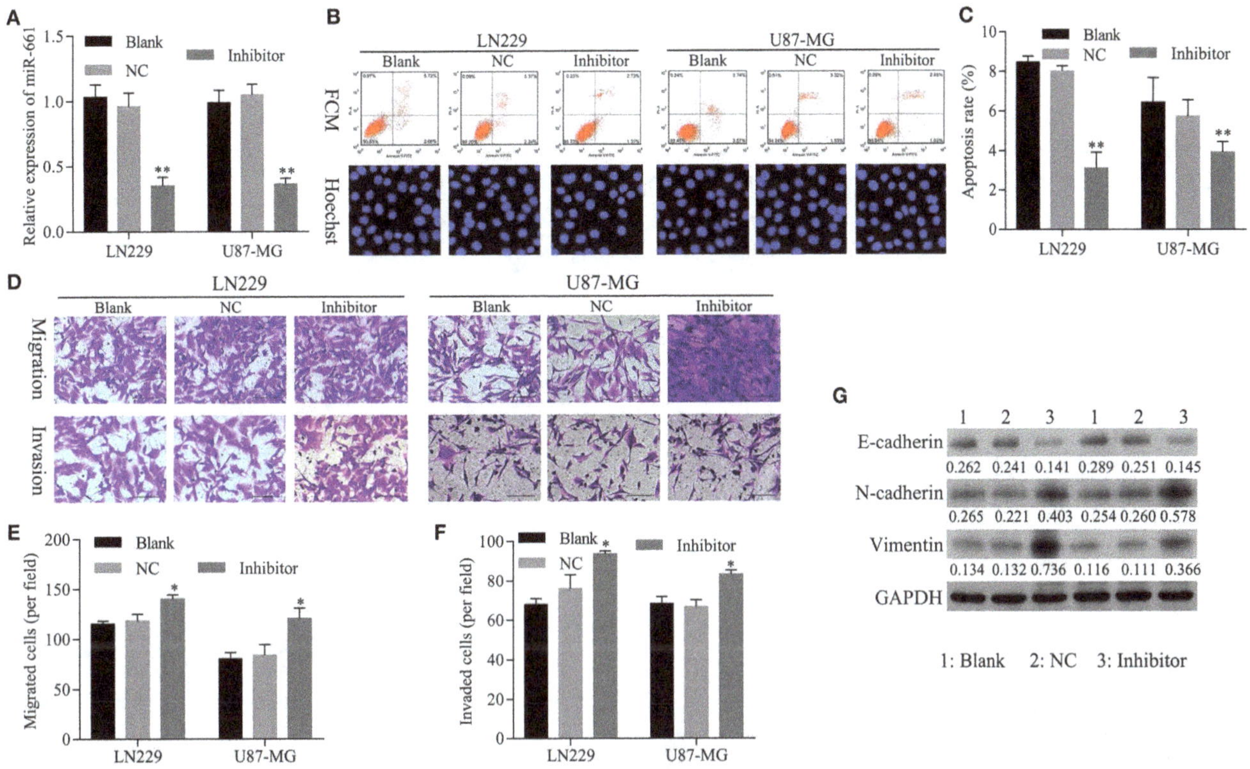

FIGURE 5 | Transfection with an miR-661 inhibitor suppressed glioma cell apoptosis and induced cell migration and invasion. **(A)** qRT-PCR assays were performed to detect miR-661 expression. **(B,C)** Flow cytometry and Hoechst 33258 staining were used to detect cell apoptosis. **(D–F)** The effect of miR-661 knockdown on cell migration and invasion was evaluated by Transwell assays. **(G)** The expression of EMT-related proteins (E-cadherin, N-cadherin, and vimentin) was examined by western blot assays (*$P < 0.05$, **$P < 0.01$). NC: negative control, Inhibitor: miR-661 inhibitor.

invasion, and EMT mediated by hsa_circ_0088732 knockdown, we first verified that transfection of an miR-661 inhibitor could inhibit LN229 and U87-MG cell apoptosis and promote the migration and invasion capabilities of LN229 and U87-MG cells by regulating N-cadherin, vimentin, and E-cadherin expression (**Figure 5**). Furthermore, we investigated the effects of hsa_circ_0088732 knockdown on glioma cell migration and invasion by suppressing miR-661. LN229 and U87-MG cells were transfected with hsa_circ_0088732 siRNA and/or an miR-661 inhibitor, respectively. Our data showed that the miR-661 inhibitor could attenuate the increase in glioma cell apoptosis induced by hsa_circ_0088732 knockdown ($P < 0.05$, $P < 0.01$, **Figures 6A,B**). Results from Transwell assays showed that cellular migration and invasion capabilities were significantly enhanced in the hsa_circ_0088732 siRNA+miR-661 inhibitor group when compared with the hsa_circ_0088732 siRNA group, indicating that an miR-661 inhibitor could reverse the inhibitory effect of hsa_circ_0088732 knockdown on glioma cell migration and invasion ($P < 0.05$, **Figures 6C–E**). Our results also revealed that N-cadherin and vimentin expression levels were increased and E-cadherin expression was decreased in the hsa_circ_0088732 siRNA+miR-661 inhibitor group relative to the hsa_circ_0088732 siRNA group (**Figure 6F**). These results suggested that knockdown of miR-661 could restore the inhibition of apoptosis and promotion of glioma cell migration, invasion, and EMT process mediated by hsa_circ_0088732 knockdown.

RAB3D Served as a Target of miR-661

Our qRT-PCR results showed that RAB3D expression was significantly upregulated in samples of glioma tissue when compared with samples of adjacent non-tumor tissue (**Figure 7A**), and that levels of RAB3D expression were negatively correlated with those of miR-661 expression (**Figure 7B**). Meanwhile, results of immunochemistry assays obtained from the public database The Human Protein Atlas (https://www.proteinatlas.org/) showed that RAB3D was expressed at much higher levels in glioma tissues than in adjacent non-tumor tissues ($P < 0.05$, **Figure 7H**). qRT-PCR and western blot results showed that overexpression miR-661 significantly suppressed the expression of RAB3D (**Figures 7C,D**). In addition, we used TargetScan, miRDB, and microorna.org to identify a binding site for miR-661 on RAB3D mRNA (**Figure 7E**), and the results of dual-luciferase reporter assays indicated that miR-661 significantly decreased the luciferase intensity of WT-RAB3D, while miR-661 had no effect on the MUT-RAB3D ($P < 0.05$, **Figure 7F**). Moreover, a search of information in Gene Expression Profiling Interactive Analysis (GEPIA, http://gepia.cancer-pku.cn/index.html) revealed that glioma patients with tumors that displayed high levels of RAB3D expression had

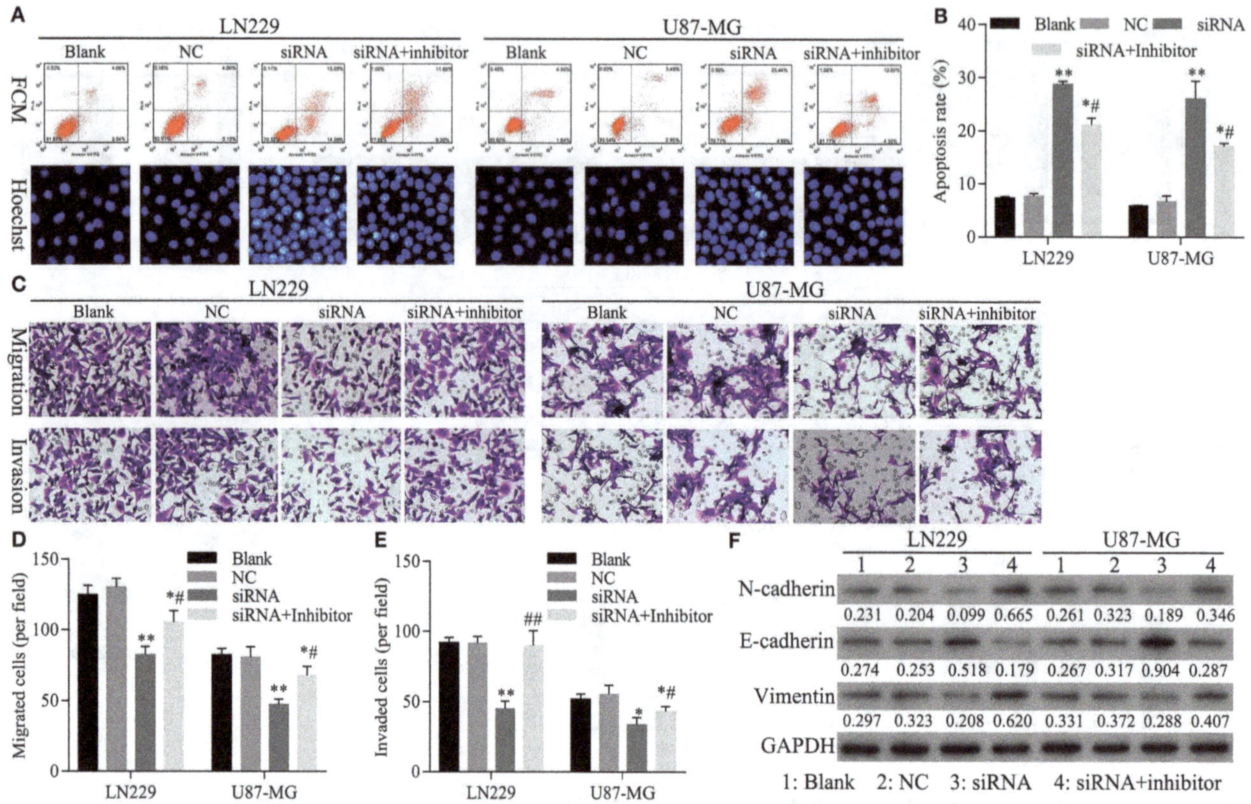

FIGURE 6 | The restoration of miR-661 inhibition led to inhibition of apoptosis, and promoted glioma cell migration, invasion, and EMT mediated by hsa_circ_0088732 knockdown. LN229 and U87-MG cells were transfected with hsa_circ_0088732 siRNAs and/or an miR-661 inhibitor, respectively. **(A,B)** Cell apoptosis was detected by PI/Annexin V FITC and Hoechst 33258 staining (*P < 0.05, **P < 0.01 vs. NC group; #P < 0.05 vs. siRNA group). **(C–E)** Cell migration and invasion capabilities were evaluated by Transwell assays. **(F)** The levels of E-cadherin, N-cadherin, and vimentin expression were determined by western blotting. NC: negative control, siRNA: hsa_circ_0088732 siRNAs, Inhibitor: miR-661 inhibitor.

shorter survival times (P = 0.0001), suggesting the relevance of RAB3D to the survival of glioma patients (**Figure 7G**). Taken together, our results suggest that *RAB3D* is a target gene of miR-661.

Knockdown of RAB3D Facilitated Glioma Cell Apoptosis and Inhibited Glioma Cell Migration, Invasion, and EMT

Next, we further investigated the effects of RAB3D on glioma progression. To assess the biological functions of RAB3D, specific siRNAs against RAB3D were synthesized and used to downregulate RAB3D expression in LN229 and U87-MG cells. The results showed that the RAB3D siRNAs could effectively knock down RAB3D expression (P < 0.01, **Figure 8A**). Flow cytometry and Hoechst 33258 staining results showed a significant promotion of cell apoptosis among RAB3D-silenced LN229 and U87-MG cells (P < 0.01, **Figures 8B,C**). Transwell assays showed that the migration and invasion capabilities of LN229 and U87-MG glioma cells transfected with RAB3D siRNA were significantly reduced when compared to those capabilities for control cells (P < 0.05, **Figures 8D–G**). Moreover, we demonstrated that after RAB3D knockdown, E-cadherin expression was upregulated, while N-cadherin and vimentin expression were downregulated (**Figure 8H**). These data indicated that knockdown of *RAB3D* could promote glioma cell apoptosis, and inhibit glioma cell migration and invasion by regulating the EMT process.

hsa_circ_0088732 Inhibited Apoptosis and Accelerated the Migration, Invasion, and EMT of Glioma Cells via miR-661 and RAB3D

Rescue experiments were performed to verify that hsa_circ_0088732 could regulate apoptosis, migration, and invasion through its effects on miR-661 and RAB3D in LN229 and U87-MG cells co-transfected with miR-661 mimics, RAB3D or hsa_circ_0088732. Results of flow cytometry and Hoechst 33258 staining studies showed that miR-661 promoted glioma cell apoptosis, while transfection of RAB3D partially rescued the apoptosis mediated by miR-661 mimics; furthermore, hsa_circ_0088732 further inhibited the glioma cell apoptosis mediated by miR-661 mimics and RAB3D (P < 0.05, P < 0.01, **Figures 9A,B**). Results of Transwell assays showed that miR-661 suppressed glioma cell migration and invasion,

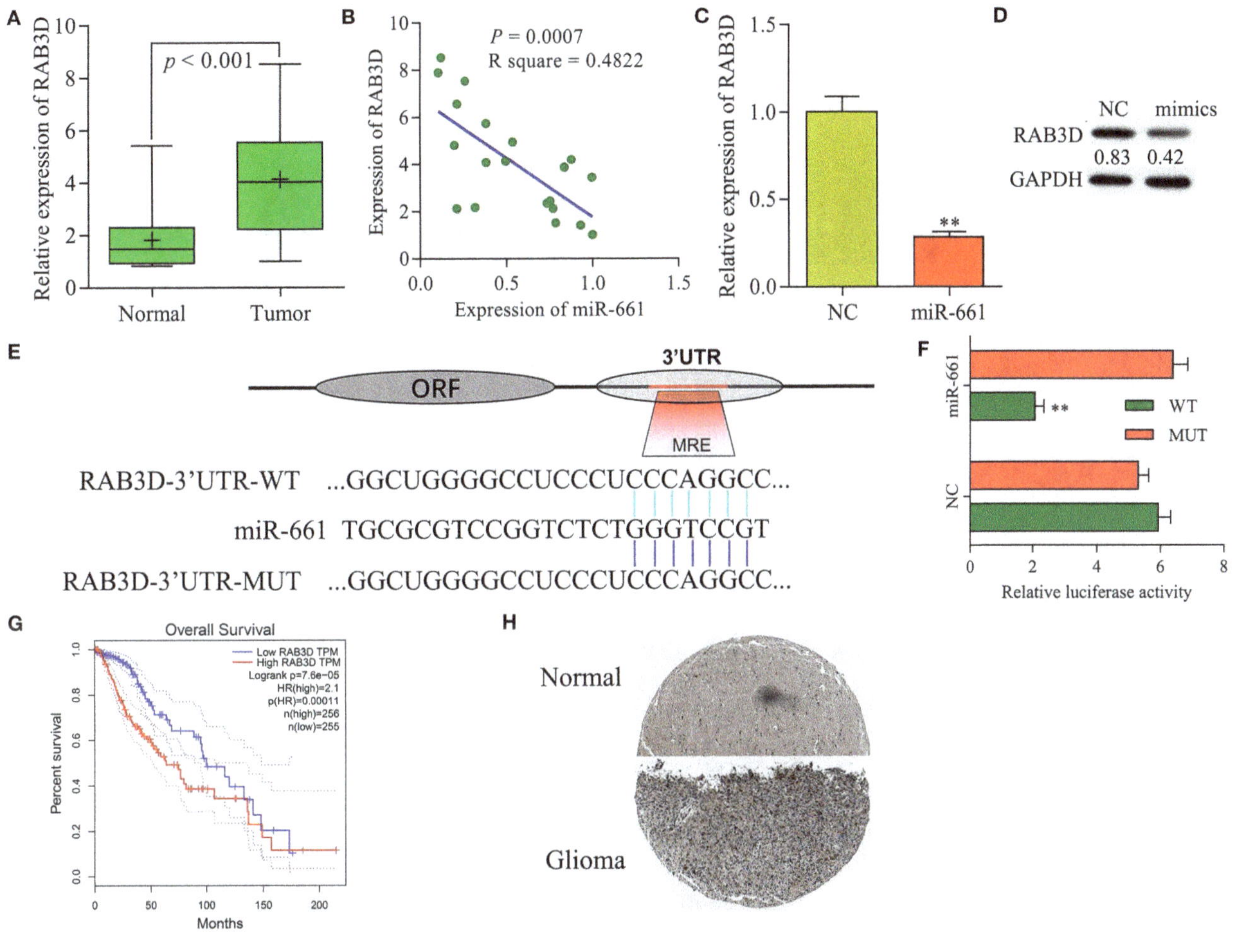

FIGURE 7 | RAB3D served as a target of miR-661. **(A)** RAB3D mRNA expression in samples of normal and tumor tissues was examined by qRT-PCR. **(B)** Person's correlation coefficient was used to analyze the correlation between RAB3D and miR-661. **(C,D)** RAB3D expression was measured by qRT-PCR and western blot assays after transfection with miR-661 mimics ($^{**}P < 0.01$). **(E)** The binding site between RAB3D and miR-661 was identified. **(F)** 293T cells were co-transfected with WT-RAB3D or MUT-RAB3D and miR-661 or NC; dual luciferase reporter assays were used to analyze relative luciferase activity. **(G)** GEPIA showing the overall survival of glioma patients. **(H)** RAB3D expression in glioma and adjacent non-tumor tissues was assessed by immunochemistry (online database: The human protein atlas).

while transfection of RAB3D partially rescued the migration and invasion mediated by miR-661 mimics. Additionally, hsa_circ_0088732 further accelerated the glioma cell migration and invasion mediated by miR-661 mimics and RAB3D, suggesting that the combined effects of hsa_circ_0088732 and RAB3D could rescue the migration and invasion mediated by miR-661 mimics ($P < 0.05$, $P < 0.01$, **Figures 9C–E**). Therefore, we demonstrated that the effects of hsa_circ_0088732 on glioma cell apoptosis, migration, and invasion were partially due to miR-661 and RAB3D. Our results also proved that miR-661 mimics could inhibit N-cadherin and vimentin expression and promote E-cadherin expression, while transfection of RAB3D rescued the N-cadherin, vimentin, and E-cadherin expression-mediated by miR-661 mimics. Finally, hsa_circ_0088732 further increased N-cadherin and vimentin expression, and decreased the E-cadherin expression mediated by miR-661 mimics and RAB3D (**Figure 9F**).

Knockdown of hsa_circ_0088732 Suppressed Glioma Growth *in vivo*

To further confirm all the above *in vitro* results showing that knockdown of hsa_circ_0088732 suppressed glioma cell proliferation and metastasis by regulating the miR-661/RAB3D axis, we generated four groups of LN229 cells transfected with (1) transfection reagent (Blank), (2) NC, (3) hsa_circ_0088732 siRNA or (4) hsa_circ_0088732 overexpression plasmids. We then inoculated the cells (1×10^6) into the right axilla of each nude mouse. After 21 days, we found that the mice inoculated with hsa_circ_0088732 siRNA-transfected LN229 cells had smaller tumor sizes than mice in the blank group, and the mice inoculated with LN229 cells transfected with hsa_circ_0088732 overexpression plasmids had larger tumor sizes than mice in the blank group (**Figures 10A,B**). qPCR results showed that hsa_circ_0088732 levels were decreased and miR-661 levels were increased in the hsa_circ_0088732 siRNA

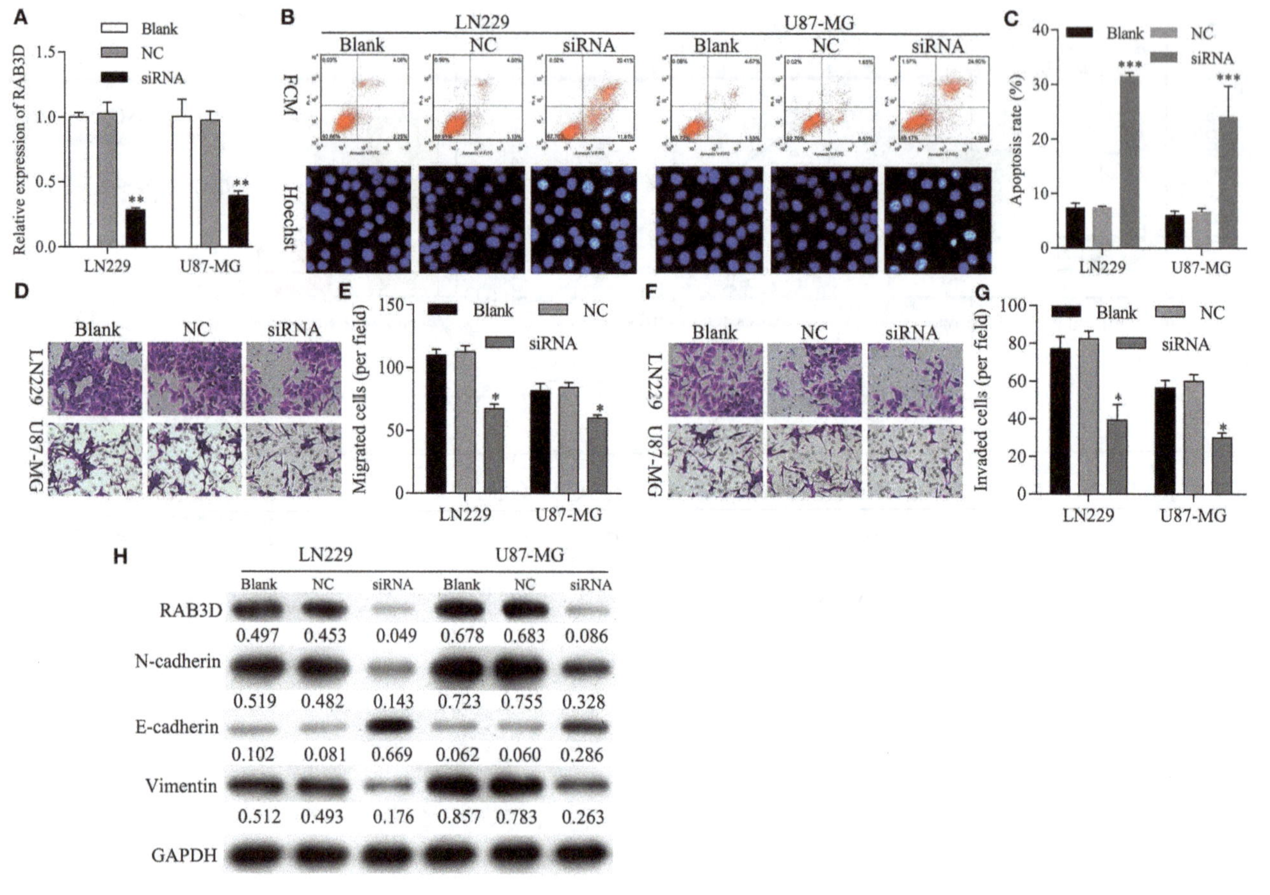

FIGURE 8 | Knockdown of RAB3D facilitated glioma cell apoptosis and inhibited glioma cell migration, invasion, and EMT. **(A)** RAB3D expression in LN229 and U87-MG cells was inhibited by transfection with RAB3D siRNA, and the efficiency of RAB3D knockdown was evaluated by qRT-PCR assays (*$P < 0.05$, **$P < 0.01$, ***$P < 0.001$). **(B,C)** Cell apoptosis in RAB3D-silenced LN229 and U87-MG cells was examined by flow cytometry and Hoechst 33258 staining. **(D–G)** The migration and invasion capabilities of LN229 and U87-MG cells with RAB3D knockdown were assessed by Transwell assays. **(H)** The levels of E-cadherin, N-cadherin, and vimentin were examined by western blotting. NC: negative control, siRNA: RAB3D siRNA.

group, while hsa_circ_0088732 expression was increased and miR-661 expression was decreased in the hsa_circ_0088732 overexpression group (**Figure 10C**). In addition, Ki-67 staining and Tunel assay results showed that knockdown of hsa_circ_0088732 suppressed tumor growth and induced apoptosis, while overexpression of hsa_circ_0088732 promoted tumor growth and inhibited cell apoptosis (**Figure 10D**). Moreover, western blot results showed that RAB3D expression was significantly decreased in the hsa_circ_0088732 siRNA group and increased in the hsa_circ_0088732 overexpression group (**Figure 10E**). When taken together, these results confirmed that knockdown of hsa_circ_0088732 suppressed glioma growth *in vivo*. Overall, our study suggested that hsa_circ_0088732 was formed by the *Lcn2* gene by cyclization, hsa_circ_0088732 negatively regulated miR-661, and *RAB3D* was a target gene of miR-661 (**Figure 11**).

DISCUSSION

Numerous studies have reported the abnormal expression of various ncRNAs, and particularly miRNAs and lncRNAs found in a variety of cancers. Most of those studies concentrated on the epigenetic regulation of cancer progression (47, 48). Recent studies have suggested that most miRNAs and circRNAs might play regulatory roles in the development and occurrence of glioma (49, 50). However, whether circRNAs have momentous effects on glioma development is far from clear. *hsa_circ_0088732* is located on chr9:130914461-130915734 with a 1273bp genomic length, and is formed by the *Lcn2* gene with the best transcript (NM_005564). Our study is the first report concerning the function and mechanism of hsa_circ_0088732 in glioma. Our results revealed that hsa_circ_0088732 is highly expressed in glioma, and that knockdown of hsa_circ_0088732 can facilitate glioma cell apoptosis *in vitro* and *in vivo*, and also inhibit glioma cell migration and invasion. In addition, we verified that knockdown of hsa_circ_0088732 reduced N-cadherin and vimentin expression, and induced E-cadherin expression. According to previous studies, the EMT is associated with a decreased expression of epithelial markers (E-cadherin), and an increased expression of mesenchymal markers (vimentin and N-cadherin) (51, 52). The EMT is a major biological process by which various malignant tumor cells migrate and invade, and

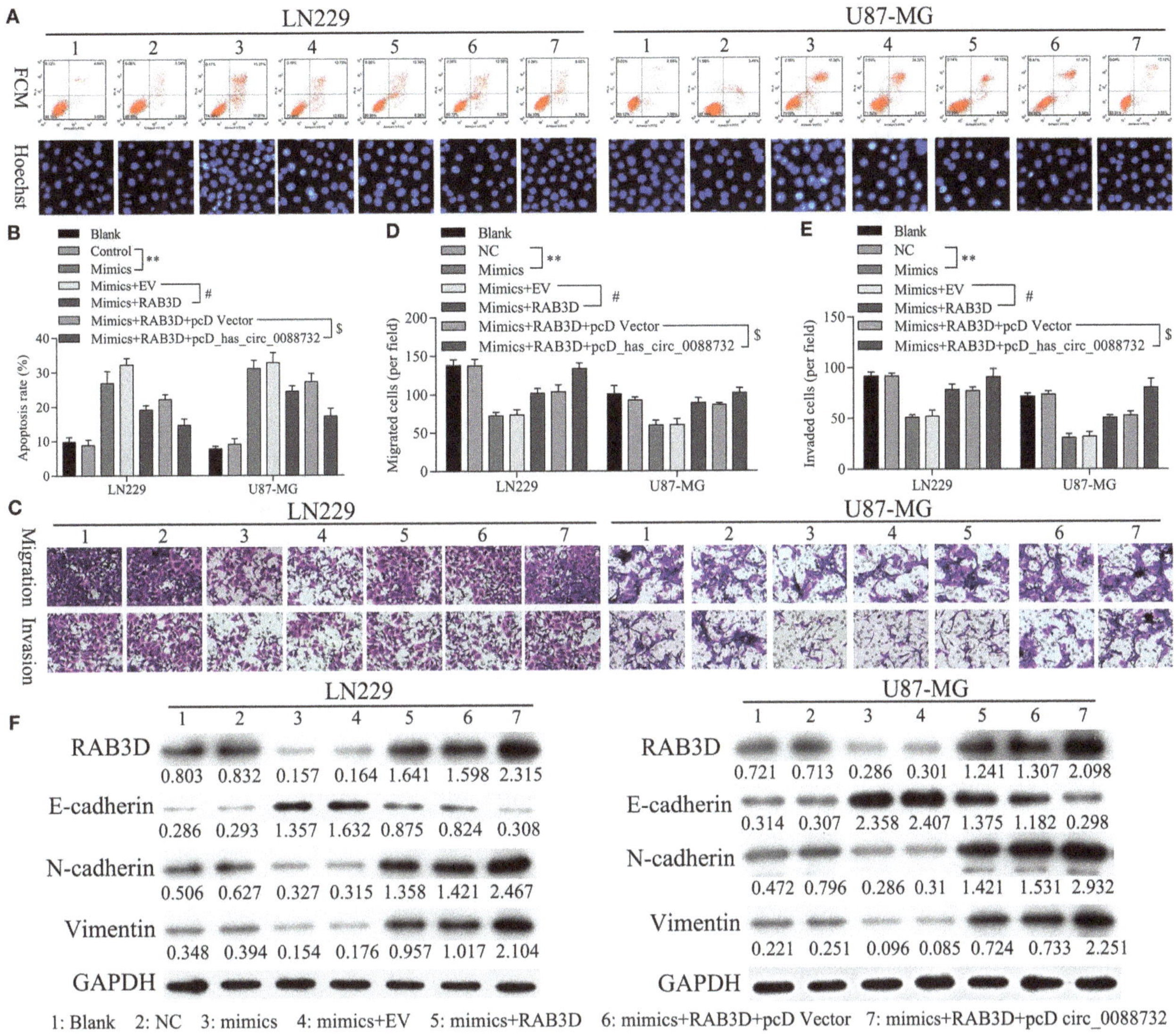

FIGURE 9 | hsa_circ_0088732 inhibited apoptosis and accelerated the migration, invasion, and EMT of glioma cells via miR-661 and RAB3D. LN229 and U87-MG cells were transfected with miR-661 mimics, RAB3D, and hsa_circ_0088732, respectively. The cell apoptosis rates **(A,B)** and numbers of migrated **(C,D)** and invaded **(C,E)** cells were assessed (**$P < 0.01$ vs. control group; $^{\#}P < 0.05$ vs. mimics + EV group; $^{\$}P < 0.05$ vs. mimics + RAB3D + pcDNA vector group). EV, overexpression vector; pcD, pcDNA3.1 plasmid; circ, hsa_circ_0088732. Western blot assays were performed to determine the levels of E-cadherin, N-cadherin, and vimentin expression in the transfected LN229 and U87-MG cells **(F)**.

also a key step in the invasion and metastasis of tumor cells (53). Our study is also the first to confirm that knockdown of hsa_circ_0088732 suppresses the EMT process in glioma cells.

In recent years, studies have revealed that circRNAs play a crucial role in regulating gene expression by serving as competing endogenous RNAs (ceRNAs). In addition, with the decreased polymorphism of miRNA response elements (MREs), exonic circRNAs become more effective as miRNA sponges. For example, the circular RNA ciRS-7 (Cdr1as) contains 74 binding sites for miR-7, which has been extensively isolated from CDR1, and makes it an effective "miR-7 sponge" (34); another circRNA designated as sex-determining region Y (Sry) was also verified to act as a sponge for miR-138 (35). In our study, we confirmed that hsa_circ_0088732 serves as a sponge for miR-661. In addition, we demonstrated that miR-661 was expressed at low levels in glioma, and negatively correlated with hsa_circ_0088732 expression. With regard to function, our results verified that knockdown of miR-661 suppressed cell apoptosis and promoted glioma cell migration, invasion, and the EMT. We also showed that a miR-661 inhibitor could attenuate the increase in glioma cell apoptosis induced by hsa_circ_0088732 knockdown, suggesting that hsa_circ_0088732 contributes to glioma progression by targeting miR-661. Previous studies have also shown that numerous miRNAs can regulate the EMT process, including members of the miRNA-200 family, miRNA-141, and miRNA-429 (54–58). Furthermore, miRNAs were shown to play vital roles in the development and occurrence of glioma by regulating the EMT (59, 60).

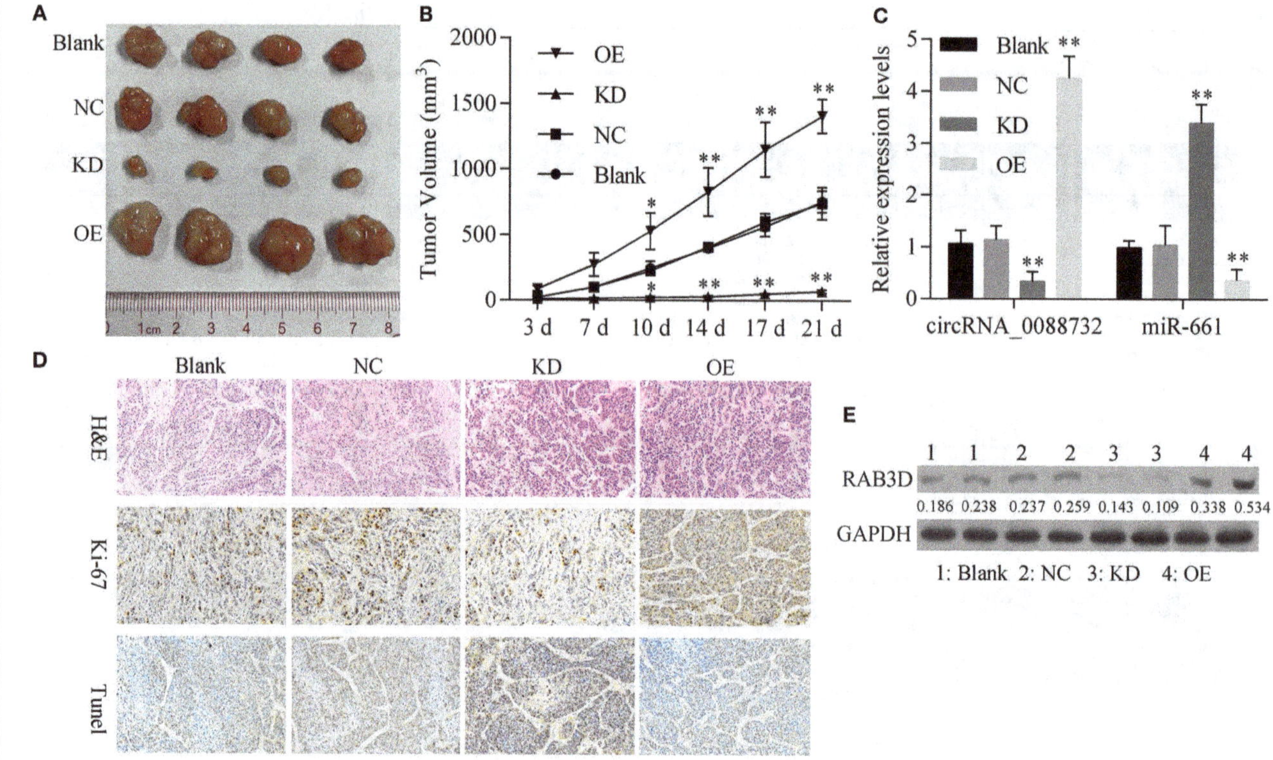

FIGURE 10 | Knockdown of hsa_circ_0088732 suppressed glioma growth *in vivo*. **(A,B)** Gross glioma tumor samples were taken from nude mice at 21 days after injection of LN229 cells (*$P < 0.05$, **$P < 0.01$). **(C)** qRT-PCR was used to analyze hsa_circ_0088732 and miR-661 expression (**$P < 0.01$). **(D)** Representative images of H&E, Ki-67, and Tunel staining assays. **(E)** Western blot analysis of RAB3D expression. NC: negative control, KD: hsa_circ_0088732 siRNAs, OE: hsa_circ_0088732 overexpression plasmids.

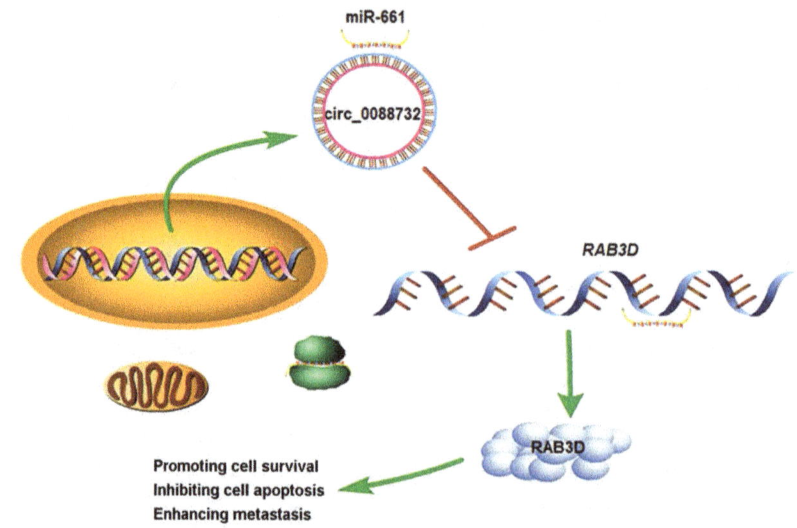

FIGURE 11 | A schematic diagram of the hsa_circ_0088732/miR-661/RAB3D axis in glioma. hsa_circ_0088732 was formed by the *Lcn2* gene by cyclization, hsa_circ_0088732 negatively regulated miR-661, and *RAB3D* was a target gene of miR-661.

We also proved the effect of miR-661 on the EMT process in glioma.

Scientific studies have proven that stable mRNA transcripts contain several RNA-binding sites or MREs, which might also serve as miRNA sponges. This might allow miRNA to regulate gene expression at the post-transcription level by binding to the 3′-untranslated regions (3′-UTRs) (61). In our study, we found that RAB3D was significantly upregulated in glioma, and negatively correlated with miR-661 expression. Additionally, a bioinformatics analysis showed there was a binding site for miR-661 in the 3′UTR of RAB3D mRNA, and luciferase reporter assays confirmed that *RAB3D* was a target gene of miR-661. *RAB3D* is a member of the RAS gene family of proto-oncogenes, and the RAB3D protein is a guanosine triphosphate (GTP) binding protein (62). RAB3D involvement has been implicated in multiple regulatory processes, such as vesicle transport, protein secretion, and signal transduction (63, 64). It was reported that RAB3D is highly expressed in tumor tissues and cells, and promotes the migration and invasion of tumor cells (65, 66). In our study, we found that RAB3D can act as an oncogene in glioma, and hsa_circ_0088732 can regulate RAB3D expression by sponging miR-661.

CONCLUSIONS

We suggest that hsa_circ_0088732 suppresses apoptosis and promotes the migration and invasion of glioma cells via the miR-661/RAB3D axis, whose function may involve molecular targets useful for diagnosing and treating glioma. This study highlights the diagnostic and therapeutic potential of the hsa_circ_0088732/miR-661/RAB3D axis in glioma, and provides a theoretical mechanism for the development and occurrence of glioma.

AUTHOR CONTRIBUTIONS

YK conceived the method and the experiments, and supervised the project. TJ, YLiu, ZX, and YZ performed experiments. TJ, ML, YLi, HH, and JL analyzed the results. TJ, ML, YLiu, and YZ wrote the first draft. YK revised the manuscript.

FUNDING

This study was supported by grants from the National Natural Science Foundation of China (Nos. 81772651, 81772652, and 81802481), and Natural Science Foundation of Guangdong Province (Nos. 2018A030310423 and 2018A030313597), and the Program for Changjiang Scholars and Innovative Research Team in University (IRT_16R37).

REFERENCES

1. Engwer C, Knappitsch M, Surulescu C. A multiscale model for glioma spread including cell-tissue interactions and proliferation. *Math Biosci.* (2015) 13:443–60. doi: 10.3934/mbe.2015011
2. Li X, Xue L, Peng Q. Tunicamycin inhibits progression of glioma cells through downregulation of the MEG-3-regulated wnt/β-catenin signaling pathway. *Oncol Lett.* (2018) 15:8470–6. doi: 10.3892/ol.2018.8416
3. Sørensen MD, Dahlrot RH, Boldt HB, Hansen S, Kristensen BW. Tumor-associated microglia/macrophages predict poor prognosis in high-grade gliomas and correlate with an aggressive tumor subtype. *Neuropathol Appl Neurobiol.* (2017) 44:185–206. doi: 10.1111/nan.12428
4. Ostrom QT, Cote DJ, Ascha M, Kruchko C, Barnholtz-Sloan JS. Adult glioma incidence and survival by race or ethnicity in the united states from 2000 to 2014. *JAMA Oncol.* (2018) 4:1254–62. doi: 10.1001/jamaoncol. 2018.1789
5. Senders JT, Muskens IS, Schnoor R, Karhade AV, Cote DJ, Smith TR, et al. Agents for fluorescence-guided glioma surgery: a systematic review of preclinical and clinical results. *Acta Neurochir.* (2017) 159:151–67. doi: 10.1007/s00701-016-3028-5
6. Weil S, Osswald M, Solecki G, Grosch J, Jung E, Lemke D, et al. Tumor microtubes convey resistance to surgical lesions and chemotherapy in gliomas. *Neuro Oncol.* (2017) 19:1316–26. doi: 10.1093/neuonc/nox070
7. Elazab A, Bai H, Zhang X, Hu Q. Low grade glioma growth modeling considering chemotherapy and radiotherapy effects from magnetic resonance images. In: *International Conference of the IEEE Engineering in Medicine & Biology Society.* Seogwipo (2017). p. 3077–80.
8. Wu J, Neale N, Huang Y, Bai HX, Li X, Zhang Z, et al. Comparison of adjuvant radiation therapy alone and chemotherapy alone in surgically resected low-grade gliomas: survival analyses of 2253 cases from the National Cancer Data Base. *World Neurosurg.* (2018) 112:e812–22. doi: 10.1016/j.wneu.2018. 01.163
9. Behin A, Hoang-Xuan K, Carpentier AF, Delattre JY. Primary brain tumours in adults. *Lancet.* (2003) 361:323–31. doi: 10.1016/S0140-6736(03)12328-8
10. Dong H, Zhou XW, Wang X, Yang Y, Luo JW, Liu YH, et al. Complex role of connexin 43 in astrocytic tumors and possible promotion of glioma-associated epileptic discharge (Review). *Mol Med Rep.* (2017) 16:7890–900. doi: 10.3892/mmr.2017.7618
11. Gritsenko PG, Friedl P. Adaptive adhesion systems mediate glioma cell invasion in complex environments. *J Cell Sci.* (2018) 131:jcs.216382. doi: 10.1242/jcs.216382
12. Beyer S, Fleming J, Meng W, Singh R, Haque SJ, Chakravarti A. The role of miRNAs in angiogenesis, invasion and metabolism and their therapeutic implications in gliomas. *Cancers.* (2017) 9:E85. doi: 10.3390/cancers9070085
13. Kondo T. Molecular mechanisms involved in gliomagenesis. *Brain Tumor Pathol.* (2017) 34:1–7. doi: 10.1007/s10014-017-0278-8
14. Szczepny A, Wagstaff KM, Dias M, Gajewska K, Wang C, Davies RG, et al. Overlapping binding sites for importin β1 and suppressor of fused (SuFu) on glioma-associated oncogene homologue 1 (Gli1) regulate its nuclear localization. *Biochem J.* (2014) 461:469–76. doi: 10.1042/BJ20130709
15. Li G, Yang H, Han K, Zhu D, Lun P, Zhao Y. A novel circular RNA, hsa_circ_0046701, promotes carcinogenesis by increasing the expression of miR-142-3p target ITGB8 in glioma. *Biochem Biophys Res Commun.* (2018) 498:254–61. doi: 10.1016/j.bbrc.2018.01.076
16. Yang Y, Gao X, Zhang M, Yan S, Sun C, Xiao F, et al. Novel role of FBXW7 circular RNA in repressing glioma tumorigenesis. *J Natl Cancer Inst.* (2018) 110:304–15. doi: 10.1093/jnci/djx166
17. Meng S, Zhou H, Feng Z, Xu Z, Tang Y, Li P, et al. CircRNA: functions and properties of a novel potential biomarker for cancer. *Mol Cancer.* (2017) 16:1–8. doi: 10.1186/s12943-017-0663-2
18. Zhou FY, Yang QZ, Zhu XC, Lan XY, Cheng H. Molecular feature, action mechanism and biology function of circular RNA. *J Agric Biotechnol.* (2017) 25:485–501.
19. Liu L, Wang J, Khanabdali R, Kalionis B, Tai X, Xia S. Circular RNAs: isolation, characterization and their potential role in diseases. *RNA Biol.* (2017) 14:1715–21. doi: 10.1080/15476286.2017.1367886
20. He J, Xie Q, Xu H, Li J, Li Y. Circular RNAs and cancer. *Cancer Lett.* (2017) 396:138–44. doi: 10.1016/j.canlet.2017.03.027
21. Zhang P, Zuo Z, Shang W, Wu A, Bi R, Wu J, et al. Identification of differentially expressed circular RNAs in human colorectal cancer. *Tumour Biol.* (2017) 39:101042831769454. doi: 10.1177/1010428317694546
22. Chen L, Zhang S, Wu J, Cui J, Zhong L, Zeng L, et al. circRNA_100290 plays a role in oral cancer by functioning as a sponge of the miR-29 family. *Oncogene.* (2017) 36:4551–61. doi: 10.1038/onc.2017.89
23. Li B, Xie F, Zheng FX, Jiang GS, Zeng FQ, Xiao XY. Overexpression of CircRNA BCRC4 regulates cell apoptosis and MicroRNA-101/EZH2 signaling in bladder cancer. *J Huazhong Univ Sci.* (2017) 37:886–90. doi: 10.1007/s11596-017-1822-9

24. Yao JT, Zhao SH, Liu QP, Lv MQ, Zhou DX, Liao ZJ, et al. Over-expression of CircRNA_100876 in non-small cell lung cancer and its prognostic value. *Pathol Res Pract.* (2017) 213:453–6. doi: 10.1016/j.prp.2017.02.011
25. Wang BG, Li JS, Liu YF, Xu Q. MicroRNA-200b suppresses the invasion and migration of hepatocellular carcinoma by downregulating RhoA and circRNA_000839. *Tumour Biol.* (2017) 39:1–10. doi: 10.1177/1010428317719577
26. Moschen AR, Adolph TE, Gerner RR, Wieser V, Tilg H. Lipocalin-2: a master mediator of intestinal and metabolic inflammation. *Trends Endocrinol Metab.* (2017) 28:388–97. doi: 10.1016/j.tem.2017.01.003
27. Xiao X, Yeoh BS, Vijay-Kumar M. Lipocalin 2: an emerging player in iron homeostasis and inflammation. *Annu Rev Nutr.* (2017) 37:103–30. doi: 10.1146/annurev-nutr-071816-064559
28. Asimakopoulou A, Weiskirchen S, Weiskirchen R. Lipocalin 2 (LCN2) expression in hepatic malfunction and therapy. *Front Physiol.* (2016) 7:430. doi: 10.3389/fphys.2016.00430
29. Li C, Chan YR. Lipocalin 2 regulation and its complex role in inflammation and cancer. *Cytokine.* (2011) 56:435–41. doi: 10.1016/j.cyto.2011.07.021
30. Srdelić Mihalj S, Kuzmić-Prusac I, Zekić-Tomaš S, Šamija-Projić I, Capkun V. Lipocalin-2 and matrix metalloproteinase-9 expression in high-grade endometrial cancer and their prognostic value. *Histopathology.* (2015) 67:206–15. doi: 10.1111/his.12633
31. Liu MF, Hu YY, Jin T, Xu K, Wang SH, Du GZ, et al. Matrix metalloproteinase-9/neutrophil gelatinase-associated lipocalin complex activity in human glioma samples predicts tumor presence and clinical prognosis. *Dis Markers.* (2015) 2015:138974. doi: 10.1155/2015/138974
32. Liu MF, Jin T, Shen JH, Shen ZY, Zheng ZC, Zhang ZL, et al. NGAL and NGALR are frequently overexpressed in human gliomas and are associated with clinical prognosis. *J Neurooncol.* (2011) 104:119–27. doi: 10.1007/s11060-010-0486-0
33. Ashwal-Fluss R, Meyer M, Pamudurti NR, Ivanov A, Bartok O, Hanan M, et al. circRNA biogenesis competes with pre-mRNA splicing. *Mol Cell.* (2014) 56:55–66. doi: 10.1016/j.molcel.2014.08.019
34. Memczak S, Jens M, Elefsinioti A, Torti F, Krueger J, Rybak A, et al. Circular RNAs are a large class of animal RNAs with regulatory potency. *Nature.* (2013) 495:333–8. doi: 10.1038/nature11928
35. Hansen TB, Jensen TI, Clausen BH, Bramsen JB, Finsen B, Damgaard CK, et al. Natural RNA circles function as efficient microRNA sponges. *Nature.* (2013) 495:384–8. doi: 10.1038/nature11993
36. Caiment F, Gaj S, Claessen S, Kleinjans J. High-throughput data integration of RNA–miRNA–circRNA reveals novel insights into mechanisms of benzo[a]pyrene-induced carcinogenicity. *Nucleic Acids Res.* (2015) 43:2525–34. doi: 10.1093/nar/gkv115
37. Liu YC, Hong HC, Yang CD, Lee WH, Huang HT, Huang HD. Ouroboros resembling competitive endogenous loop (ORCEL) in circular RNAs revealed through transcriptome sequencing dataset analysis. *BMC Genomics.* (2018) 19:171. doi: 10.1186/s12864-018-4456-9
38. Zhang J, Jiang J, Huang R, Wang Y, Nie X, Gui R. Circular RNA expression profiles are significantly altered in mice bone marrow stromal cells after total body irradiation. *Leuk Res.* (2018) 70:67–73. doi: 10.1016/j.leukres.2018.05.010
39. Dejima H, Iinuma H, Kanaoka R, Matsutani N, Kawamura M. Exosomal microRNA in plasma as a non-invasive biomarker for the recurrence of non-small cell lung cancer. *Oncol Lett.* (2017) 13:1256–63. doi: 10.3892/ol.2017.5569
40. Rupaimoole R, Slack FJ. MicroRNA therapeutics: towards a new era for the management of cancer and other diseases. *Nat Rev Drug Discov.* (2017) 16:203–22. doi: 10.1038/nrd.2016.246
41. Santangelo A, Imbrucè P, Gardenghi B, Belli L, Agushi R, Tamanini A. A microRNA signature from serum exosomes of patients with glioma as complementary diagnostic biomarker. *J Neuro Oncol.* (2018) 136:51–62. doi: 10.1007/s11060-017-2639-x
42. Zhi T, Jiang K, Xu X, Yu T, Wu W, Nie E. MicroRNA-520d-5p inhibits human glioma cell proliferation and induces cell cycle arrest by directly targeting PTTG1. *Am J Transl Res.* (2017) 9:4872–87.
43. Zhu Y, Zhao H, Rao M, Xu S. MicroRNA-365 inhibits proliferation, migration and invasion of glioma by targeting PIK3R3. *Oncol Rep.* (2017) 37:2185–92. doi: 10.3892/or.2017.5458
44. Pylypenko O, Hammich H, Yu IM, Houdusse A. Rab GTPases and their interacting protein partners: structural insights into Rab functional diversity. *Small GTPases.* (2018) 9:22–48. doi: 10.1080/21541248.2017.1336191
45. Yang J, Liu W, Lu X, Fu Y, Li L, Luo Y. High expression of small GTPase Rab3D promotes cancer progression and metastasis. *Oncotarget.* (2015) 6:11125–38. doi: 10.18632/oncotarget.3575
46. Niyazi M, Brada M, Chalmers AJ, Combs SE, Erridge SC, Fiorentino A. ESTRO-ACROP guideline "target delineation of glioblastomas". *Radiother Oncol.* (2016) 118:35–42. doi: 10.1016/j.radonc.2015.12.003
47. Kentwell J, Gundara JS, Sidhu SB. Noncoding RNAs in endocrine malignancy. *Oncologist.* (2014) 19:483–91. doi: 10.1634/theoncologist.2013-0458
48. Redis RS, Berindan-Neagoe I, Pop VI, Calin GA. Non-coding RNAs as theranostics in human cancers. *J Cell Biochem.* (2012) 113:1451–9. doi: 10.1002/jcb.24038
49. Xie G. Circular RNA hsa-circ-0012129 promotes cell proliferation and invasion in 30 cases of human glioma and human glioma cell lines U373, A172, and SHG44, by targeting microRNA-661 (miR-661). *Med Sci Monit.* (2018) 24:2497–507. doi: 10.12659/MSM.909229
50. Yuan Y, Jiaoming L, Xiang W, Yanhui L, Shu J, Maling G, et al. Analyzing the interactions of mRNAs, miRNAs, lncRNAs and circRNAs to predict competing endogenous RNA networks in glioblastoma. *J Neuro Oncol.* (2018) 137:1–10. doi: 10.1007/s11060-018-2757-0
51. Theys J, Jutten B, Habets R, Paesmans K, Groot AJ, Lambin P, et al. E-Cadherin loss associated with EMT promotes radioresistance in human tumor cells. *Radiotherapy.* (2011) 99:392–7. doi: 10.1016/j.radonc.2011.05.044
52. Yao X, Wang X, Wang Z, Dai L, Zhang G, Yan Q, et al. Clinicopathological and prognostic significance of epithelial mesenchymal transition-related protein expression in intrahepatic cholangiocarcinoma. *Oncotargets Ther.* (2012) 2012:255–61. doi: 10.2147/OTT.S36213
53. Ding Y, Li X, Hong D, Jiang L, He Y, Fang H. Silence of MACC1 decreases cell migration and invasion in human malignant melanoma through inhibiting the EMT. *Biosci Trends.* (2016) 10:258–64. doi: 10.5582/bst.2016.01091
54. Wang L, Mezencev R, Švajdler M, Benigno BB, McDonald JF. Ectopic over-expression of miR-429 induces mesenchymal-to-epithelial transition (MET) and increased drug sensitivity in metastasizing ovarian cancer cells. *Gynecol Oncol.* (2014) 134:96–103. doi: 10.1016/j.ygyno.2014.04.055
55. Al-Khalaf HH, Aboussekhra A. p16(INK4A) induces senescence and inhibits EMT through microRNA-141/microRNA-146b-5p-dependent repression of AUF1. *Mol Carcinogen.* (2016) 56:985–99. doi: 10.1002/mc.22564
56. Arunkumar G, Deva Magendhra Rao AK, Manikandan M, Prasanna Srinivasa Rao H, Subbiah S, Ilangovan R, et al. Dysregulation of miR-200 family microRNAs and epithelial-mesenchymal transition markers in oral squamous cell carcinoma. *Oncol Lett.* (2018) 15:649–57. doi: 10.3892/ol.2017.7296
57. Bhardwaj M, Sen S, Chosdol K, Sharma A, Pushker N, Kashyap S, et al. miRNA-200c and miRNA-141 as potential prognostic biomarkers and regulators of epithelial-mesenchymal transition in eyelid sebaceous gland carcinoma. *Br J Ophthalmol.* (2017) 101:536–42. doi: 10.1136/bjophthalmol-2016-309460
58. Choi PW, Ng SW. The functions of MicroRNA-200 family in ovarian cancer: beyond epithelial-mesenchymal transition. *Int J Mol Sci.* (2017) 18:E1207. doi: 10.3390/ijms18061207
59. Wang Y, Lin G. TP53INP1 3'-UTR functions as a ceRNA in repressing the metastasis of glioma cells by regulating miRNA activity. *Biotechnol Lett.* (2016) 38:1699–707. doi: 10.1007/s10529-016-2159-3
60. Yan Y, Wang Q, Yan XL, Zhang Y, Li W, Tang F, et al. miR-10a controls glioma migration and invasion through regulating epithelial-mesenchymal transition via EphA8. *FEBS Lett.* (2016) 589:756–65. doi: 10.1016/j.febslet.2015.02.005
61. Mohr AM, Mott JL. Overview of microRNA biology. *Semin Liver Dis.* (2015) 35:3–11. doi: 10.1055/s-0034-1397344
62. Larkin JM, Woo B, Balan V, Marks DL, Oswald BJ, LaRusso NF, et al. Rab3D, a small GTP-binding protein implicated in regulated secretion, is associated with the transcytotic pathway in rat hepatocytes. *Hepatology.* (2000) 32:348–56. doi: 10.1053/jhep.2000.9110
63. Millar AL, Pavios NJ, Xu J, Zheng MH. Rab3D: a regulator of exocytosis in non-neuronal cells. *Histol Histopathol.* (2002) 17:929–36. doi: 10.14670/HH-17.929

64. Evans E, Zhang W, Jerdeva G, Chen CY, Chen X, Hamm-Alvarez SF, et al. Direct interaction between Rab3D and the polymeric immunoglobulin receptor and trafficking through regulated secretory vesicles in lacrimal gland acinar cells. *Am J Physiol Cell Physiol.* (2008) 294:C662–72. doi: 10.1152/ajpcell.00623.2006
65. Wang JS, Chuang A, Zhang ZJ, Wang GB, Li B, He M. MicroRNA-506–3p inhibits osteosarcoma cell proliferation and metastasis by suppressing RAB3D expression. *Aging.* (2018) 10:1294–305. doi: 10.18632/aging.101468
66. Zhang J, Kong R, Sun L. Silencing of Rab3D suppresses the proliferation and invasion of esophageal squamous cell carcinoma cells. *Biomed Pharmacother.* (2017) 91:402–7. doi: 10.1016/j.biopha.2017.04.010

8

Tissues Harvested Using an Automated Surgical Approach Confirm Molecular Heterogeneity of Glioblastoma and Enhance Specimen's Translational Research Value

*Edie Zusman[1], Maxim Sidorov[2], Alexandria Ayala[3], Jimmin Chang[3], Eric Singer[2], Michelle Chen[2], Pierre-Yves Desprez[2], Sean McAllister[2], Nathan Salomonis[4], Kashish Chetal[4], Gautam Prasad[3], Tyler Kang[3], Joseph Mark[5], Lawrence Dickinson[3] and Liliana Soroceanu[2]**

[1] NorthBay Medical Center, Fairfield, CA, United States, [2] California Pacific Medical Center (CPMC) Research Institute, San Francisco, CA, United States, [3] Pacific Brain and Spine Medical Group, Eden Medical Center-Sutter Research, Castro Valley, CA, United States, [4] Cincinnati Children's Hospital Medical Center (CCHMC) Biomedical Informatics, Cincinnati, OH, United States, [5] NICO Corporation, Indianapolis, IN, United States

***Correspondence:**
Liliana Soroceanu
sorocel@cpmcri.org;
liliana.soroceanu@gmail.com

Glioblastoma (GBM) is the most aggressive primary brain tumor in adults. Designing effective individualized therapies for GBM requires quality fresh tissue specimens, and a comprehensive molecular profile of this highly heterogenous neoplasm. Novel neuro-surgical approaches, such as the automated resection NICO Myriad^{TM} system, are increasingly used by neurosurgeons to better reach the invasive front of tumors. However, no information exists on how harvesting GBM tissue using this approach may impact the translational research value of the sample. Here, we set out to characterize matched specimens from 15 patients, where one tissue sample was obtained using traditional tumor de-bulking (herein referred to as "en bloc" sample), and the other sample was obtained using the Myriad^{TM} System (herein referred to as "Myriad" sample). We investigated the fidelity of patient derived xenografts (PDXs) for each sample type to the corresponding human tissues and evaluated the added value of sequencing both samples for each patient. Matched en bloc and Myriad samples processed in parallel, were subjected to the following assays: cell viability, self-renewal, *in vivo* tumorigenicity using an orthotopic model of glioma, genomic sequencing, and pharmacological testing using PI3K-MTOR pathway inhibitors. Our results demonstrate that primary GBM cultures derived from matched specimens grew at similar rates (correlation coefficient $R = 0.72$), generated equivalent number of neurospheres, and had equivalent tumorigenic potential *in vivo* (mouse survival correlation coefficient $R = 0.93$). DNA Sequencing using the Illumina tumor panel amplicons revealed over 70% concordance in non-synonymous mutations between matched human GBM specimens. PDX genomic profiles were also highly concordant with the corresponding patient tissues (>70%). RNA sequencing of paired GBM samples revealed unique genomic variants and differential gene expression between the en bloc and Myriad specimens, with the former molecularly resembling the "tumor core" and the latter resembling the "invasive tumor front" signature. Functionally, we show that primary-derived GBM cells—obtained after fresh specimen's dissociation—are more effectively growth-inhibited by co-targeting non-overlapping mutations enriched in each sample type, suggesting that profiling both specimens more adequately capture the molecular heterogeneity of GBM and may enhance the design accuracy and efficacy of individualized therapies.

Keywords: glioblastoma, PDX, tumor heterogeneity, Myriad, RNA seq

INTRODUCTION

Glioblastoma (GBM), a grade IV glioma, according to World Health Organization (WHO) classification, is the most lethal primary glioma in adults. GBM has a prevalence of 26,000 cases, with a mortality rate of 15,000 cases yearly in the US, and an incidence of two to three per 100,000 adults per year (1). Currently approved therapies for GBM include surgery, radiation and Temozolomide (2). Surgical removal of the tumor via gross total resection is a critical determinant of patient outcome. Gross total resection of GBM increases the median survival rate by 200%, when compared to survival rates for patients subjected to a subtotal resection (3–5). While preserving as much uninvolved brain tissue as possible, the surgeons aim to harvest sufficient tissue for molecular and pathological diagnosis, and for translational research (6). As such, patient derived cancer models, including patient derived xenografts (PDXs) and related cultures (PDX-C) have unique value in integrating the genomic data with drug sensitivity toward designing personalized care for GBM patients (7). Successful generation of PDX from freshly harvested GBM samples is an important measure of the specimen's translational value (6, 8).

The traditional GBM collection technique has been to remove a contiguous portion of the neoplasm from the surgical field with forceps and transport this *en bloc* specimen for processing. This method is less effective for collecting deep-seated, smaller lesions, and those located in eloquent brain regions, or for removing the "leading edge" of the neoplasm while preserving the adjacent normal white matter anatomy. The NICO Myriad^{TM} System (NICO Corporation, Indianapolis, IN) is a multi-functional, non-ablative, tissue resection device that uses a guillotine-like cutting aperture and variable suction to grasp and cut small targeted blocks of architecturally intact tissue (several cubic millimeters are harvested each minute). As the use of automated resection devices is showing improved outcome (especially for deep lesions), an important question arises regarding the translational research value of tissues harvested in this manner and how it compares molecularly with samples harvested en bloc. In this study, we set out to compare matched en bloc and Myriad-derived GBM samples obtained during tumor removal in 15 patients diagnosed with glioblastoma. For each pair, we generated primary cultures to assess cell viability, primary GBM neurosphere growth, as well as "mouse avatars" (patient derived xenografts, PDXs) to compare *in vivo* tumorigenicity and histopathological characteristics of matched xenografts. Next generation sequencing was used to interrogate mutations in genomic DNA using the Illumina tumor amplicon panel, both in matched patient samples and corresponding PDXs. Furthermore, RNA sequencing was used to identify genomic variants and analyze gene expression patterns in matched patients' samples.

Ethics Statement

All patients included in the study were enrolled and consented for the study using an IRB approved non-treatment protocol (Sutter IRB# 25.125-2). All animal studies were pursued in accordance with CPMC approved IACUC protocols (protocol #15.08.03 and # 18.08.03).

METHODS

Patient Selection and Preoperative Assessment

All patients participating in this study provided informed consent to have their tumor tissue collected for research purposes. All patients underwent magnetic resonance imaging (MRI) that was also used for intra-operative navigation to direct and assist with tumor resection.

Operative Techniques and Tissue Collection Method

All tissues collected for the study were in excess of the sample required for pathological diagnosis (to guide patient treatment), per our IRB approved research protocol. Two methods of surgical access and tissue collection were used in this series including:

- Standard Craniotomy and en bloc collection followed by collection with the Myriad System.
- Minimally Invasive Parafascicular Surgery (MIPS) with en bloc collection followed by collection with the Myriad System.

For large, more superficial tumors, a standard craniotomy was performed, general practice guidelines were used to access the tumor through a large margin dural opening. Upon gaining access, an en bloc removal technique with tumor forceps was used to collect tissue in a traditional manner. At this time, sample for intra-operative pathological diagnosis was obtained. After GBM diagnosis confirmation by the pathologist, the collected specimen above mentioned is set-aside for tissue banking and transport in Hypothermosol solution (4°C). In each of these cases, a full time technician was present in the operating room during the full procedure dedicated to collecting and transporting the sample. Following en bloc resection of the tumor "core," the NICO Myriad System was then utilized to remove additional tumor tissue bordering the uninvolved normal brain parenchyma; this sample was immediately refrigerated and placed in Hypothermosol solution and transported to the research lab together with the en bloc specimen, within 1.5 h.

For some deep-seated tumors, minimally-invasive parafascicular surgery (MIPS) was employed. This involved a small cranial flap and dural opening, and introduction of a 13.5 mm diameter, navigable, trans-sulcal tubular retractor (BrainPath®) at the base of a sulcus, staying parallel to DTI defined fiber tracts. Tumor was collected using a conventional en bloc technique with tumor forceps first. Then the adjacent tissue was removed with the Myriad System. Care was taken to assure that both specimens had identical MRI signal characteristics, suggesting that they shared morphologic and physiologic attributes. In both types of cases, substantial volume of tumor could be collected for both en bloc and Myriad-derived samples.

The Myriad System

The NICO Myriad™ System (NICO Corporation, Indianapolis, IN) is a multi-functional, non-ablative, targetable tissue resection tool used for tumor removal (9). It is used in conjunction with NICO's automated tissue preservation system (TPS) designed to standardize and automate the process of tissue collection, increase the volume of tissue collected for research, and potentially improve biological preservation through an intraoperative, automated process of refrigeration, and buffering of the collected tissue. The system also allows for regional targeting, resection, and annotation. **Supplementary Figure 1** shows a diagram of the Myriad System as used in this study.

Primary GBM Cultures

Primary GBM cultures were generated as previously described (10). Cell viability was measured using automated cell counting (Countess II system) and performed in accordance with manufacturer instructions (ThermoFisher).

Next Generation Sequencing of Genomic DNA

Isolation of genomic DNA was performed using Qiagen kits after tissue disruption using ruptor disposable probes; DNA was quantified using PicoGreen (Thermo Fisher Scientific). A sequencing library targeting 212 amplicons in 48 genes was generated using the Illumina TruSeq Amplicon—Cancer Panel. Concordance between the original sample and its derivative was calculated as follows: Concordance: $C = 100\% * (x/y)$, where x = number of variants confirmed in both the en bloc and Myriad tissue and y = number of similar variants confirmed in en bloc tumor tissue or the Myriad tissue (11).

RNA Sequencing and Bioinformatics Data Analysis

RNA extraction from flash-frozen tissue samples was performed as previously described (12–14). Total RNA Extraction. RNA was processed from frozen tumor biopsies, following resuspension with Trizol (ThermoFisher Scientific). The total RNA was extracted by Direct-zol RNA Kit (Zymo Research) and the concentration was measured by Qubit RNA HS Assay Kit (ThermoFisher Scientific). RNA-Seq was performed from ~500 ng of total RNA processed using TruSeq polyA selection, at a target depth of 40 million paired-end, stranded reads on an Illumina 2500. Normalized gene expression data is available as **Supplementary Table 2** in connection with this manuscript.

Gene Expression Analyses

For RNA-Seq analysis, gene expression values were obtained using the Kallisto algorithm in AltAnalyze version 2.1.1 from all FASTQ files, to obtain transcript per million (TPM) estimates. Differential gene expression was performed using an empirical Bayes moderated *t*-test, following FDR correction ($p < 0.05$). Additional gene set enrichment, hierarchical clustering and data visualizations were generated using AltAnalyze.

Identification of Cancer Genomic Variants

Genome variants were detected from the RNA-Seq data using the GATK RNA-Seq analysis workflow and annotated using the COSMIC database and Ensembl Variant Effect Predictor. Oncofusions were detected with the FusionCatcher pipeline. Additional variant and clinical annotations were obtained from the TCGA and TARGET consortiums. Variants were evaluated for statistical enrichment on biological Pathways (WikiPathways) using the GO-Elite algorithm in AltAnalyze and subsequently visualized through this software. Variant and oncofusion enrichment analyses were performed using a Chi-squared test ($p < 0.05$) aggregating variants at the gene level. Disease free and overall survival analyses were performed in R using the multivariate cox proportional hazard (coxph) tests for each splicing subtype. The R packages glmnet and coxph were used to test for other clinical covariates such as subtype/grade, cytogenetic abnormalities, relapse, induction failure, or secondary site of metastasis, while accounting for potential confounding variables such as age, gender, ethnicity, smoking, drug therapy, or subtype/grade. Enrichment analyses were assessed using Fisher's Exact Test *p*-values following FDR correction.

Taqman Validation of Gene Expression

Taqman Validation of Gene Expression for *REST* and *SEMA6B* was performed using primers and probes from Applied Biosystems according to the manufacturer's protocol as previously described by our group (15). Normal human brain RNA (Invitrogen, Cat# AM7962) was used as a positive control.

Pharmacological Studies and Cell Viability

Drugs were obtained from Selleckchem and master stocks were primarily made at half maximum solubility with DMSO. After drug treatment, cells were incubated for 72 h. CellTiter-Glo (Promega) was used to quantify cell viability/proliferation. Data from luminescence reads were used to calculate cell viability.

Glioma Neurosphere (Tumorsphere) Assays

Glioma Neurosphere (Tumorsphere) Assays were used to measure self-renewal potential of the glioma neurospheres, as previously described (10).

Immunofluorescence and Immunohistochemistry

Primary cultures were fixed using methanol (10 min, RT) and immunostained using the following primary antibodies

TABLE 1 | Clinical annotation of GBM specimens included in this study.

Case ID	Diagnosis	Age/Sex	MGMT methylation	IDH1/IDH2
GBM 172	GBM	71 M	Not detected	N/D
GBM 177	GBM	66 F	Not detected	N/D
GBM 179	GBM	69 M	Not detected	N/D
GBM 180	GBM	54 F	Not detected	N/D
GBM 181	GBM	60 M	Not detected	N/D
GBM 183	Astrocytoma III	60 F	Not detected	R132H
GBM 190	GBM	77 F	Not detected	wild type
GBM 192	GBM	65 F	3.8%	Wild type
GBM 193	GBM	56 F	Not detected	Wild type
GBM 197	GBM	44 M	Not detected	Wild type
GBM 199	GBM	66 M	77%	Wild Type
GBM 203	GBM	65 M	70%	Wild type
GBM 208	GBM	82 M	Not detected	Wild type
GBM 213	GBM	49 F	Not detected	Wild type
GBM 215	GBM	72 M	Not detected	Wild type
GBM 216	GBM	68 M	Not detected	Wild type

(overnight incubation, 4C). Sox2 (1/1000, Epitomics), Tuj1 (Beta III Tubulin; 1/1000, Abcam). Nuclei were stained with DAPI or Propidium Iodide containing mounting medium from Vector Labs.

Intracranial Xenografts of Human GBMs

Intracranial Xenografts of Human GBMs were generated as previously published by our group (10, 12). Brains of euthanized mice were collected, fixed in formalin, paraffin embedded, and sectioned. Slides were stained with Hematoxlyin and Eosin, and then scanned using the Mirax MIDI whole slide high resolution scanning system.

RESULTS

Patient Cohort

Fifteen patients who underwent surgical resection for glioblastoma standard of treatment were enrolled in the study. **Table 1** lists patients' clinical information, including MGMT gene promoter methylation and IDH1 mutational status. Samples collected for this study were obtained using two different surgical approaches, as detailed below.

GBM Specimen Collection: Surgical Approaches

Standard Craniotomy

Standard craniotomy with the option of using the Myriad System for tissue collection is the preferred approach whenever the tumor can be easily accessed. **Figure 1** shows a representative case of one of the patients in our cohort undergoing a standard "open" craniotomy for resection of the tumor. **Figure 1A** shows the intraoperative navigation defining the area of tumor to be collected for the study. **Figure 1B** shows the tumor cavity after *en bloc* resection with biopsy forceps has been completed and the collection with the Myriad System (NICO Myriad™ and Automated Preservation System) initiated. Note the grayish blue color of the tumor, relative to the non-neoplastic edematous white matter appreciated after resection in **Figure 1C**.

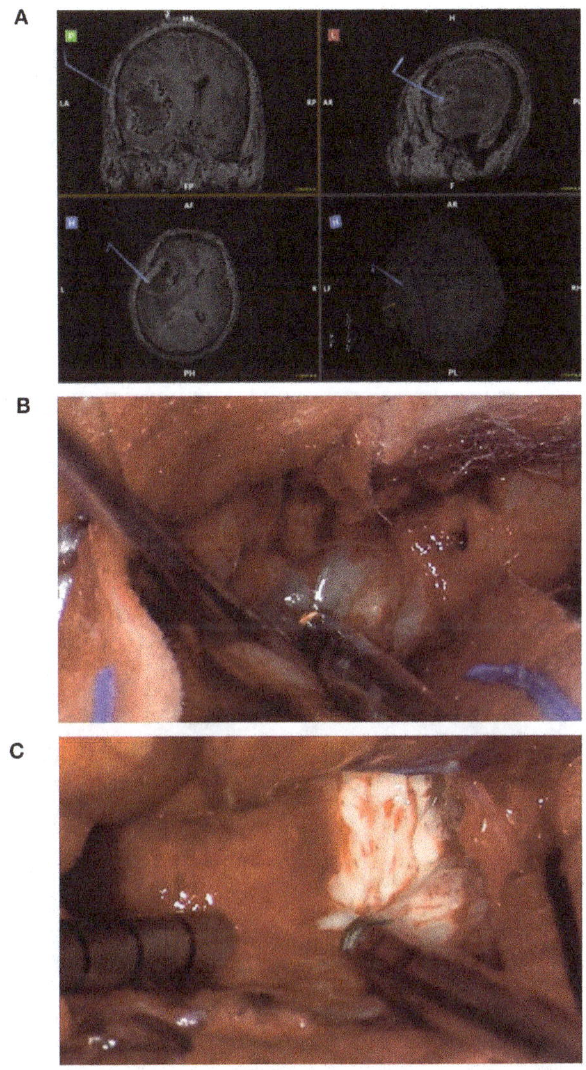

FIGURE 1 | Standard craniotomy and the use of Myriad tool for surgical GBM removal. **(A)** Intraoperative navigation defining the area of tumor to be collected for the study. **(B)** Tumor cavity after *en bloc* resection with biopsy forceps has been completed and the collection with the Myriad System initiated. **(C)** Note the grayish blue color of the tumor, relative to the non-neoplastic edematous white matter.

Minimally Invasive Parafascicular Surgery (MIPS) With BrainPath

Minimally Invasive Parafascicular Surgery (MIPS) with BrainPath was used to remove deep-seated tumors. This approach is also compatible with the use of the NICO Myriad System. **Figure 2** is a representative case of a patient enrolled in our study who underwent MIPS for tumor resection. **Figure 2A** shows the use of Synaptive BrightMatter® software to define a parafascicular trans-sulcal approach to the deep white matter neoplasm. The size of the craniotomy necessary

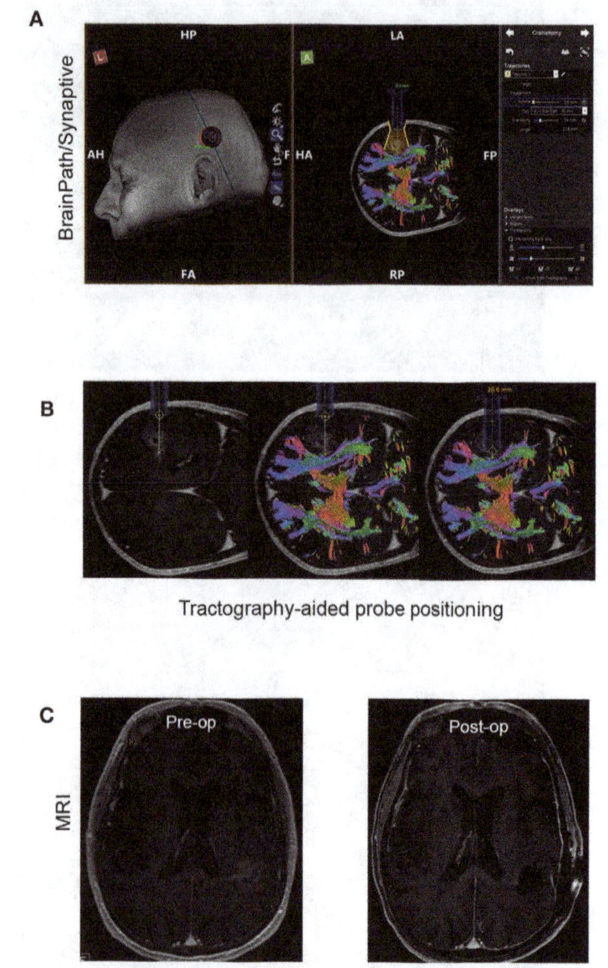

FIGURE 2 | Representative case of a patient that had MIPS resection of the tumor. **(A)** Use of the planning software (Synaptive BrightMatter) to define a parafascicular trans-sulcal approach to the deep white matter neoplasm. **(B)** Intraoperative navigation with the target positioned at the deepest enhancing portion of the tumor (left panel). Tractography (shown in the middle panel) suggests that this area disease is within the corticospinal tract and this portion should not be resected. **(C)** Pre- and post op post gadolinium T1 MRI images with the small "tail" of residual enhancement in the corticospinal tract purposefully left behind.

to access the full dimension of the tumor through the 13.5 mm tubular retractor (NICO BrainPath®) is also shown on the planning image. **Figure 2B** shows the intraoperative navigation with the target positioned at the deepest enhancing portion of the tumor (left panel). However, it is evident on the tractography (middle panel) that this area of disease is within the corticospinal tract and this portion should not be resected, as it would cause right hemiparesis. The right panel in **Figure 2B** shows the operating channel in position for resection of the deepest portion of tumor collection that could be performed safely. **Figure 2C** shows the pre- and post op post gadolinium T1 MRI images with the small "tail" of residual enhancement in the corticospinal tract purposefully left behind. This patient had no neurologic deficit following the procedure.

After collection, both en bloc and Myriad specimens, were maintained according to this institution's protocol, in Hyothermosol solution (4°C) and transported within 1.5 h from surgery to the research lab for processing.

In vitro Growth and Characterization of Primary-Derived GBM Neurospheres From Matched En Bloc and Myriad-Derived GBM Samples

Matched en bloc and Myriad-derived samples were processed in parallel to generate a single cell culture. Primary GBM cultures were established as previously described by our group (10). Initial cell viability and long term growth of neurosphere cultures from matched specimens were compared. Cell counts were obtained for 15 matched specimens following enzymatic and mechanical dissociation of fresh tissues, using the Countess II automated cell counter system. This approach is ideal for distinguishing between live and dead cells and also can accurately estimate cell viability of "clumpy" cultures which may result following GBM tissue dissociation. Median tumor cell viability was 56% for the en bloc specimen and 53% for the Myriad-derived specimen, with a correlation factor $R = 0.72$ between matched specimens (**Figure 3A**). GBM cultures were maintained as neurospheres for implantation and additional assays. Representative GBM-derived neurospheres obtained from matched patients' samples are shown in **Figure 3B**. Four day viability assays in three matched GBM samples demonstrate that similar growth rates characterize both the en bloc and Myriad-derived cultures, as shown in **Figure 3C** ($p > 0.5$ in all comparisons, Student *t*-Test). Neurosphere formation assays (a surrogate readout for tumor initiation potential) showed no difference between the en bloc and Myriad-derived samples. **Figure 3D** shows two examples of this assay performed using GBM 179 and GBM 193 samples ($p = 0.8$, Student *t*-Test). Next, we stained matched samples of primary patient GBM tumorspheres for markers associated with neural and glioma cancer stem cells which have previously shown to be enriched in primary glioblastoma samples (10, 15–17). Examples are shown in **Figures 3E,F** which display immunofluorescence-based detection of two neural stem markers—Sox2 and tubulin III (Tuj1) in matched specimens.

In vivo Tumorigenicity and Histological Evaluation of Matched Patient and PDX Samples

For *in vivo* tumorigenicity assessment, 300,000 cells were intracranially injected in two mice/specimen (four mice per patient) to generate PDXs. Mice bearing intracranial tumors were euthanized at the onset of neurological symptoms and animal survival was recorded for all samples. Intracranial xenografts are considered the best approach to test the ability of primary GBM cells to recapitulate the disease *in vivo*, and are characterized by high molecular and histological fidelity to patient's tumor (6). To validate the origin of tumors developed intracranially in nude mice, we performed hematoxylin and

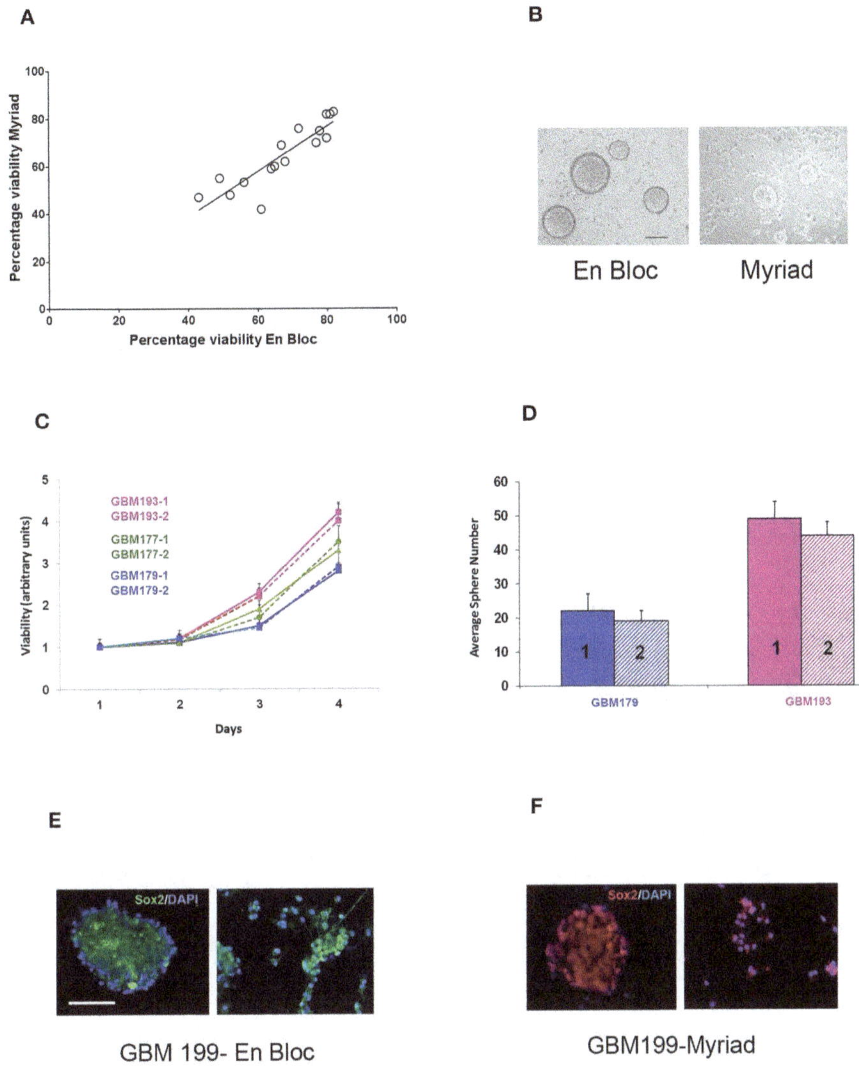

FIGURE 3 | *In vitro* assessment of matched en-bloc and Myriad GBM samples. **(A)** Tumor cell viability was calculated based on counting 3 fields/sample. Initial cell viability values compared across 15 samples are shown. Correlation coefficient $R = 0.72$. **(B)** Representative photomicrographs of GBM tumor neurospheres from matched en bloc and Myriad–derived cultures. Bar= 200 μm. **(C)** Matched GBM primary cells from three patients (GBM 193, GBM177, GBM179) were cultured in complete growth media (96 well microplates, 5,000/well). Luminescence based viability readouts were obtained on days 2, 3, 4. Comparisons within each patient for matched cultures, $p > 0.5$ (student *t*-Test). Samples were run in triplicates; data is representative of two assays. **(D)** Tumorspheres growth in 24 well plates was quantified 7 days post initial culturing. 20,000 cells/well from matched GBM179 and GBM193 samples were allowed to form spheres in complete growth medium. Six replicates/condition were used and data is representative of 3 repeat assays; $p = 0.4$ Student *t*-Test. **(E,F)** Immunofluorescence analysis of primary GBM199 neurospheres. Sox2 and Tuj1 (right panels) are detected in both en bloc and Myriad-derived neurosphere cultures. *GBM 199-1* (en bloc): FITC- conjugated secondary antibodies and DAPI nuclear stain were used in **(E)**. *GBM 199-2* (Myriad) Cy3-conjugated secondary antibodies and PI nuclear stain were used in **(F)**. Bar: 150 μm.

eosin (H&E) staining and evaluation of PDX tissue samples. **Figure 4A** shows an example of tissue sections from the *patient* (GBM 193, **Figure 4A**) and the corresponding *mouse PDX* (i.e., GBM193X, **Figure 4B**) stained using hematoxylin and eosin (H&E). GBM hallmarks, including high cellularity and areas of microvascular proliferation are noted. In another example, histological evaluation of GBM199-derived PDX tumor, is shown in **Figure 4C**. The H&E staining shows overall similar histological features between the matched xenografts, including areas of pseudo-palisading, another hallmark feature of GBM (18).

In vivo tumor take for all 15 paired samples (60 mice) was 100%. The time required for intracranial development of tumors (measured from time of implantation until neurological symptoms were present) was proportional to the tumor grade, as previously described (19). *In vivo* tumorigenicity correlation between matched en bloc and Myriad-derived samples was *high*, $R = 0.93$ (**Figure 4D**). Survival of mice implanted with either

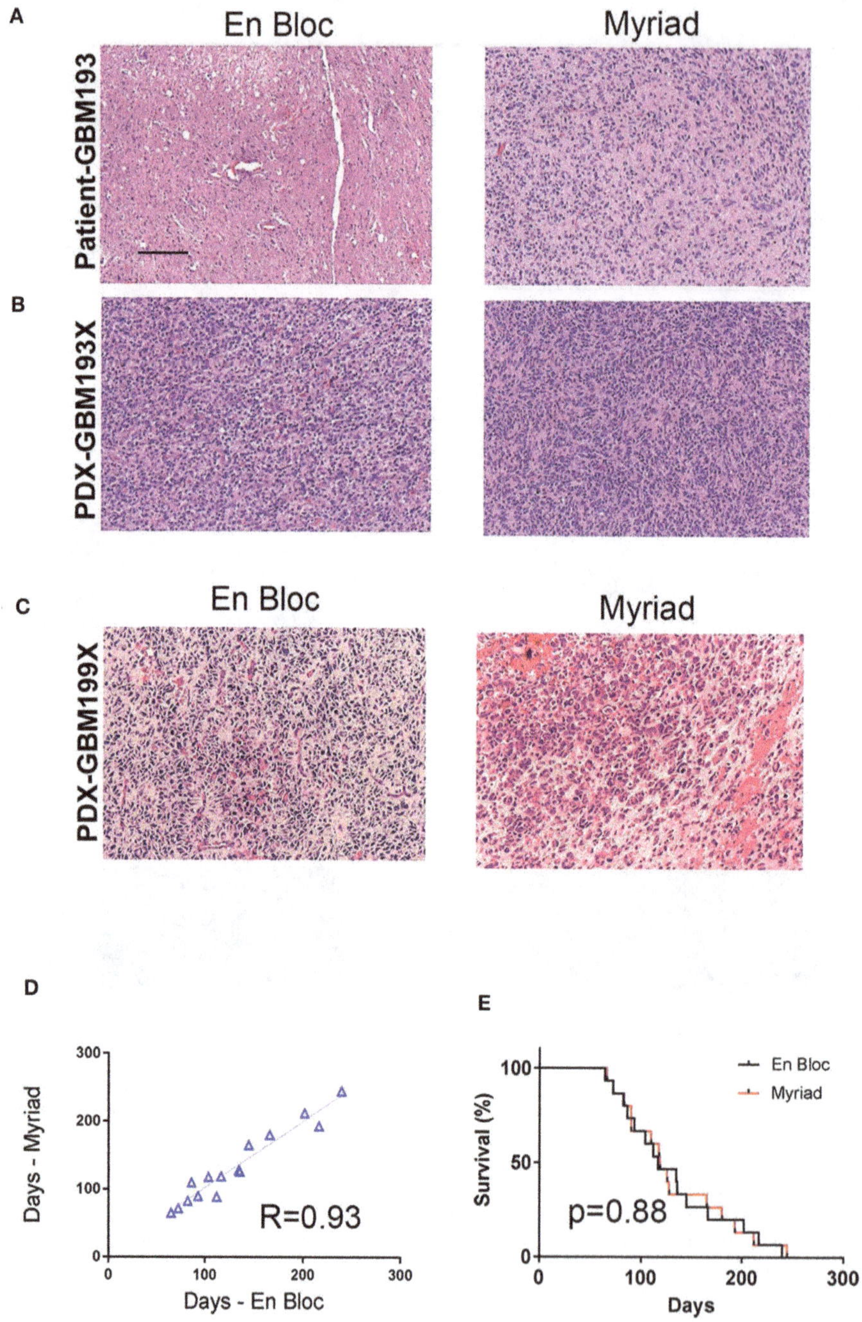

FIGURE 4 | *In vivo* tumorigenicity assessment of matched en-bloc and Myriad GBM samples. **(A)** H&E staining of matched patient (GBM 193) samples are shown. **(B)** H&E for corresponding PDX–derived from GBM193. **(C)** H&E staining of PDX- derived from GBM199 en bloc (left panel) and Myriad (right panel) specimens; bar = 50 μm. **(D)** Survival correlation for mice intra-cranially implanted with 15 matched GBM samples (3,000,000 cells/mouse). Each sample was implanted in 2 mice (4 mice/patient). **(E)** Kaplan Meyer survival curves comparing survival between mice implanted with either en bloc or Myriad-derived tumor cells, for 15 patients. No significant difference in survival between the 2 cohorts is noted.

en bloc or Myriad-derived GBM cells (300,000/mouse, intracranially) is shown in **Figure 4E** for all 15 patients. Kaplan Mayer survival analysis shows no significant difference in survival between the two cohorts (Log-rank Mantel-Cox test, $p = 0.88$).

Genomic Characterization of Matched GBM DNA Samples

Next generation sequencing using MiSeq tumor panel was performed on genomic DNA extracted from 13 matched

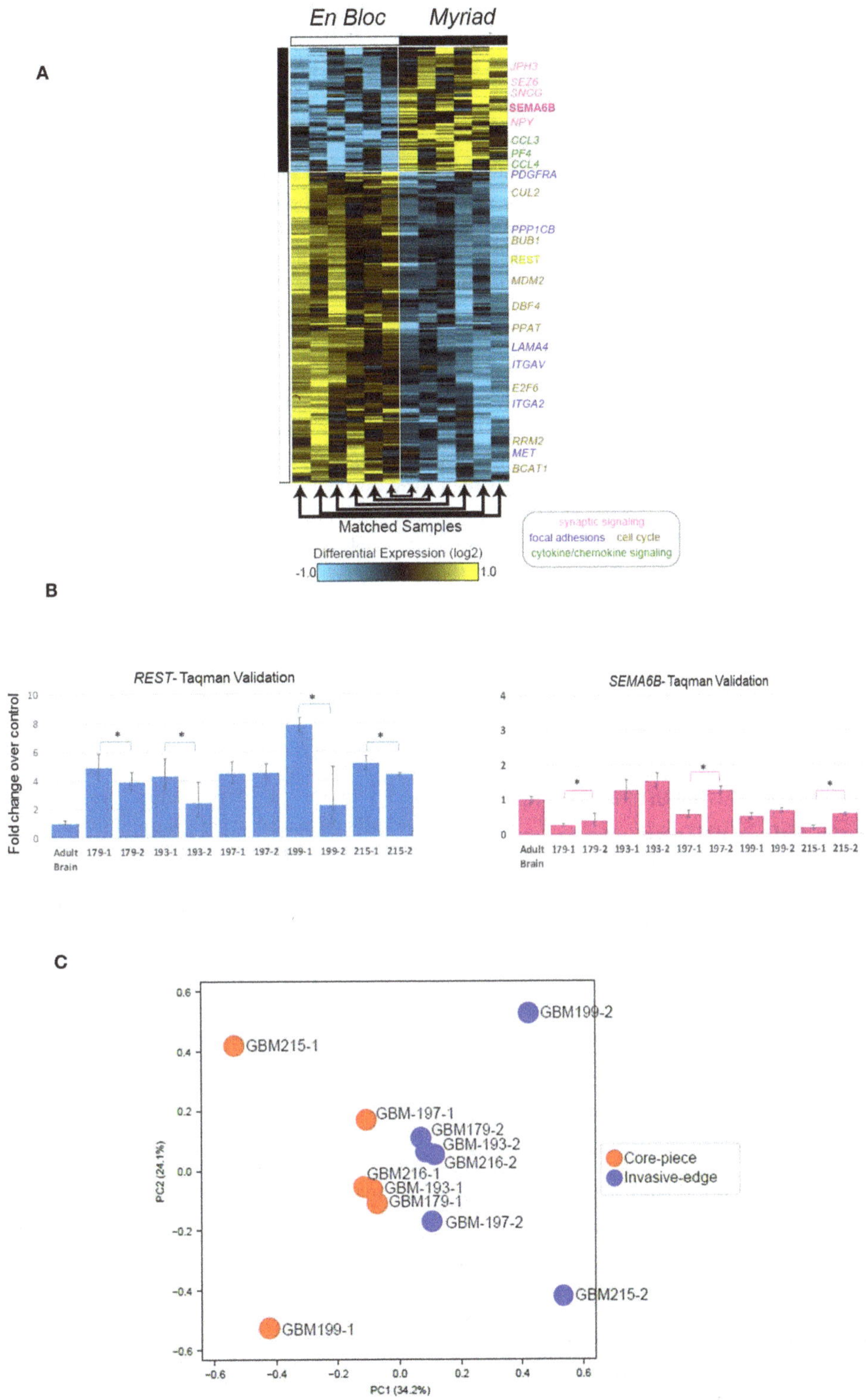

FIGURE 5 | Differentially expressed genes in paired GBM specimens. **(A)** Heatmap displaying genes differentially expressed in the en bloc and Myriad specimens across 12 GBM specimens. Genes with a fold change > 1.5 and FDR adjusted, e Bayes moderated *t*-test $p < 0.05$. Yellow indicates up-regulation and blue, down-regulation, relative to the median expression across all samples. Highlighted genes are indicated to the right of the heatmap, colored according to their indicated biological process (i.e., synaptic signaling, cell cycle, etc). **(B)** Taqman validation in 5 matched GBM samples for REST (left panel) and SEMA3B (right panel). $^*p < 0.02$ Student *T*-test. **(C)** Principal component analysis of all expressed genes (TPM > 1), followed intra-patient normalization.

patient samples. Additionally, five distinct PDX samples were sequenced to interrogate fidelity of the PDX model. Genomic DNA sequencing was performed using the AmpliSeq for Illumina Cancer Hotspot Panel v2. This is a targeted assay for identification of somatic mutations across the hotspot regions of 50 genes with known associations to cancer, as identified in the Catalog of Somatic Mutations in Cancer (COSMIC) database. **Supplementary Table 1** shows allele frequency information for the non-synonymus mutations identified in 7 genes previously shown to be involved in GBM pathogenesis (20, 21).The numbers shown in each cell represent variant allele frequencies (VAF). VAF in this case refers to the fraction of sequencing reads overlapping a genomic coordinate that support the mutant allele. The values shown correspond to the most deleterious variant identified within each gene. We calculated the percentage concordance between en bloc and Myriad samples from the same patient. Our data shows between 71 and 100% concordance in VAF between matched GBM samples from the same patient. This high degree of concordance is not surprising, given that the Illumina tumor amplicon panel used here includes a subset of genomic alterations frequently reported in GBM. Concordance between each PDX and its corresponding patient tumor was calculated to be 70% or higher.

Taken together, the data so far supports the notion that the use of the Myriad tool for GBM resection results in highly viable and tumorigenic tissue samples, similar to those obtained using the traditional, en bloc approach.

RNA Sequencing and Differential Gene Expression in Paired Samples

We used RNA Seq to interrogate gene expression in matched GBM specimens, in order to test the hypothesis that tissue samples from different anatomical regions of the tumor exhibit distinct molecular profiles, corresponding to multiple cancer driving signaling pathways (21). **Figure 5A** illustrates hierarchical clustering of differentially expressed genes in 12 specimens (6 matched en bloc and Myriad samples). Highlighted genes are shown to the right of the heatmap, colored according to their indicated biological process (e.g., cell cycle in yellow font, cytokine signaling in green font, synaptic signaling in purple font). Note that genes involved in cell cycle and focal adhesion regulation were enriched in the en bloc specimen, while genes regulating chemokine and synaptic signaling were upregulated in the Myriad sample, respectively. Next, we performed Taqman validation measuring expression levels for the cell cycle related gene *REST*, and a gene associated with synaptic signaling - *SEMA6B*, in 10 matched en bloc and myriad RNA samples. Significant differences in expression levels for each of these genes are noted in individual sample pairs (**Figure 5B**).

GBM Regional Heterogeneity Is Revealed by Analysis of Both En Bloc and Myriad Samples

Principal component analysis followed by intra-patient normalization, of all expressed genes demonstrates that the en bloc samples from all six patients cluster *together* (red full circles) and *away* from the matched Myriad samples for the same patients (blue full circles; **Figure 5C**). This suggests distinct biological pathways are enriched in each sample type, across all analyzed patients; these pathways may play complementary roles in GBM progression. GBM regional heterogeneity has been extensively documented (22). In a recent study, single cell RNA Seq of neoplastic cells, showed differential gene expression between cells retrieved from the tumor core and those collected from the invasive/migrating tumor edge (23). This study identified differentially expressed genes in these two tumor regions, associated with distinct signaling pathways. As such, the tumor-core enriched gene ontology (GO) pathways were cell proliferation, hypoxia-induced pathways, and cancer stem cells-related pathways, while GO pathways associated with the tumor edge and immune cell infiltrates included chemokine and chemokine receptors, cytokines, nervous system development, and cell migration related pathways (21). Using the open source software and data base available in conjunction with this publication (http://www.gbmseq.org) we analyzed RNA Seq data from the 6 matched GBM tissues (total 12 samples) and identified several genes overexpressed in the *en bloc* samples corresponding to the *tumor core* (as defined by single cell RNA expression profiling), while a number of genes overexpressed in the *Myriad samples* were enriched in the *invasive edge* of the tumor as defined by single cell RNA expression profiling. Relative abundance levels and corresponding tumor region for six genes are shown in **Supplementary Figure 2**. Statistically enriched Gene Ontology terms associated with up- or downregulated genes in the en bloc (tumor core) vs. Myriad (tumor edge) samples are shown in **Supplementary Figure 3**. Enrichment Fisher Exact was $p < 0.001$ for all pathways (GO-Elite). Taken together, these data suggest that molecular sequencing of both samples provides a comprehensive molecular tumor fingerprint in GBM, which is also actionable information for guiding individualized therapy.

Genomic Variants and Wiki-Pathway Analyses in Paired Samples

The 12 matched samples analyzed by RNA Seq were further interrogated to identify specific genomic variants for each patient. These data were analyzed using the AltAnalyze and WikiPathways platforms to identify signaling pathways specifically activated within each sample, based on predicted activating mutations. Examples of WikiPathway analyses for three matched GBM samples are shown in **Supplementary Figures 4–6**, where mutated genes are shown in red. Overall consistency in pathway activation is noted between matched samples. However, a subset of genomic alterations are identified in one specimen, but not the other (blue open circles). For example, an *ATM* mutation is only present in GBM 179-1 (en bloc sample), but not in GBM179-2 (Myriad; **Supplementary Figure 4**). *EGFR/ERBB2* alterations were identified only in the GBM199-2 (Myriad) but not in the GBM 199-1 (en bloc) sample (**Supplementary Figure 5**), while a *CDK4* mutation is uniquely present in the GBM216-1 (en bloc) but not in GBM216-2 (Myriad; **Supplementary Figure 6**).

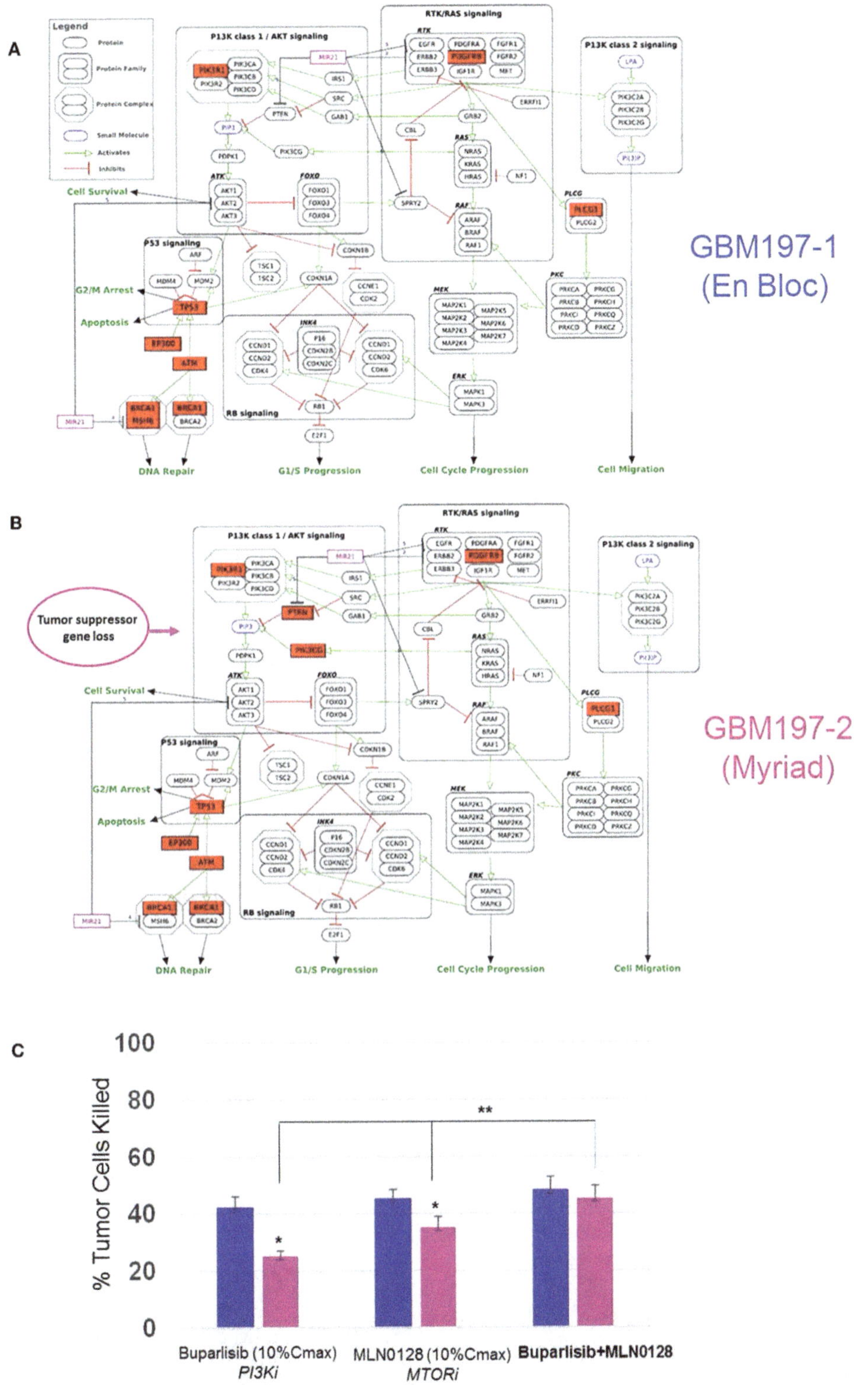

FIGURE 6 | Genomic and drug sensitivity testing in matched en bloc and Myriad GBM samples. **(A,B)** Wikipathways analysis for en bloc (GBM197-1, **A**) and Myriad (GBM197-2, **B**) samples. Arrow indicates the presence of a PTEN alteration in the Myriad specimen only (7B). **(C)** Cell viability data for GBM197-1 (blue bars) and GBM197-2 (pink bars) treated with a PI3K inhibitor (Buparlisib, 0.2 μM) and an MTOR inhibitor (MLN0128, 0.1 μM) 72h. Dug concentrations used in this assay represent 10% Cmax measured in the plasma from patients. $^{*}p = 0.04$, comparing single drug treatment and $^{**}p = 0.01$ comparing combination drug treatment with single drug treatment in the Myriad -derived specimen. Student *t*-Test.

While mechanistic studies are required to fully investigate the significance of these sample-specific genomic alterations, it is clear that gathering sequencing information from both specimens results in a more accurate and complete molecular characterization of the tumor.

To test the functional significance of these genomic findings, we generated primary cultures from matched GBM197-1 (en bloc) and GBM197-2 (Myriad) samples and subjected the cells to pharmacological testing. Pathway analyses for GBM197-1 (en bloc) and GBM 197-2 (Myriad) are shown in **Figures 6A,B**. Note that a critical tumor suppressor gene (*PTEN)* is altered in GBM197-2 only. Drug sensitivity testing was performed using Buparlisib which inhibits the PI3K pathway and MLN0128, an investigational MTOR inhibitor. As shown in **Figure 6C**, the 197-2 derived cells appear more resistant to treatment with either inhibitor compared to 197-1 cells, which is consistent with enhanced activation of the PI3K pathway driven by alterations in *PTEN* uniquely present in this sample. Combining both drugs was significantly more efficacious in inhibiting the growth of GBM197-2 cells.

Taken together, these data suggest that capturing the genomic heterogeneity of GBM by closely analyzing both en bloc and the Myriad-derived specimens may be required for designing effective personalized targeted or immunotherapy approaches, including neoantigen-based vaccine therapy for GBM patients (24).

DISCUSSION

Clinical trials for GBM are investigating efficacy of individualized targeted therapy based on genomic profiling as well immunotherapy options. The availability of high quality, viable tumor tissue is critical for the aforementioned efforts. In this study, we demonstrate that an automatic tissue collection and preservation strategy used to harvest GBM specimens proved equal to the traditional "en bloc" tumor resection in terms of providing viable samples for translational research. Our data attest to the viability and tumorigenicity of both Myriad (NICO Myriad^{TM}) and en bloc-derived specimens as shown by cell viability and tumor sphere growth assays in culture. In addition we document expression of molecular markers associated with self-renewal in primary GBM cultures derived from both types of specimens. The ability of tumor cells to recapitulate the disease in an immunocompromised mouse constitutes critical evidence of tissue viability. Our data shows that primary GBM cells from 15 matched specimens uniformly generated intracranial tumors in nude mice. Histo-pathologically, PDXs derived from each specimen recapitulated hallmark features of glioblastoma (7). Genomic sequencing confirmed the presence of "hot spots" in both specimens, with a high degree of concordance. Interestingly, RNA sequencing and bioinformatics analyses revealed salient gene expression differences between the two specimens and identified sample-specific genomic variants. In terms of gene expression, all en bloc samples clustered together and away from the Myriad-samples, as demonstrated by the principal component analysis. Furthermore, the gene expression signature enriched in the en bloc specimen was characteristic of the "tumor core," while the gene expression profile of the Myriad specimens corresponded to the "invasive tumor front" (23). In a recent study by Sottoriva et al., intra-tumor heterogeneity was assessed using surgical multisampling from same patient (similar to our approach) and various glioblastoma subtypes were identified within the same tumor (25). Similarly, our study demonstrates the presence of distinct tumor-promoting signaling pathways in the two matched GBM specimens, driven by non-overlapping genomic variants. These results are in agreement with previous studies who documented GBM gene expression heterogeneity at the single cell level. The study by Patel et al. (26) demonstrated the presence of diverse transcriptional programs related to oncogenic signaling, proliferation, and immune response in glioblastoma and their implication for disease progression. Regional molecular heterogeneity may have important consequences for designing combinatorial therapies for GBM. The PTEN-PI3K-MTOR pathway is altered in over 70% of GBMs (27, 28). Preliminary results from clinical trials in a subset of GBMs suggested that inhibition of any of the pathway's nodes alone was not efficacious, because of paradoxical pathway activation (29, 30). Concordantly, our data show that combined inhibition of PI3K and MTOR was significantly more efficacious in inhibiting GBM197 growth than either drug alone. Together, these results suggest that identification of molecular "fingerprints" in GBM samples by sequencing both the en bloc and the Myriad specimens, provides more comprehensive information about disease-driving pathways. The ability to annotate anatomical features with distinct genomic makers can be used for drug target validation and thus aid in designing of combinatorial therapies for patients with GBM (31).

In summary, this novel method of GBM collection and preservation was at least equivalent to or an improvement on traditional tissue harvesting, and permitted more controlled tissue removal at the tumor edges. We also found that en bloc tissues, usually obtained from the tumor "core" cluster *together* and display distinctly different RNA signatures than the Myriad derived tissues, usually obtained from the tumor edge. These data highlight the important issue of GBM heterogeneity as it relates to distinct regions within the tumor, harvested using specific surgical approaches (suitable for each location). Our results further support the need to harvest and sequence multiple specimens for each GBM, in order to capture the genomic diversity within each patient's tumor and improve the design of molecularly-directed therapeutics.

AUTHOR CONTRIBUTIONS

LS, EZ, LD, and JM conceived and designed the study. MS, AA, JC, ES, MC, P-YD, SM, and LS collected samples and performed experiments. EZ, LD, GP, and TK contributed patient samples and annotation. NS and KC performed bioinformatics analyses. EZ, LS, LD, and JM analyzed the data. LS, LD, and JM wrote the manuscript.

FUNDING

This study was funded by California Pacific Medical Center

Foundation (CPMCF) through the Cancer Avatar Program. Additional funds were provided by Nico Corporation.

SUPPLEMENTARY MATERIAL

Supplementary Figure 1 | (A) Minimally Invasive Parafascicular Surgery (MIPS) Access Device, the BrainPath® (NICO Corporation, Indianapolis, IN) of various lengths and diameters. **(B,C)** The NICO Myriad^{TM} System Components: **(B)** Side mouth aperture, filter element and specimen collector of the Myriad System are indicated. **(C)** Tissue Preservation System (TPS) components are shown, including the Tissue Filter Assembly, as well as Specimen Preserver and Chiller.

Supplementary Figure 2 | Genes enriched in the en bloc samples are enriched in the tumor core and genes overexpressed in Myriad samples are enriched in the invasive tumor front. Shown here are *LAMA4*, *REST*, *BUB1*, and *MDM2* enriched in en bloc samples, and *CCL3* and *SEZ6* enriched in the Myriad samples. Gene names are color coded based on the pathways associated with (see also **Figure 6**).

Supplementary Figure 3 | Statistically enriched Gene Ontology terms associated with up or downregulated genes with enrichment Fisher Exact $p < 0.01$ (GO-Elite). Inferred interaction network of focal adhesion genes (direct interactions), Cytokine-cytokine receptor interactions (indirect interactions), and synaptic signaling genes (indirect interactions) were generated based on protein-protein interactions from pathway databases (WikiPathways, KEGG, BioGRID) using the software NetPerspective in AltAnalyze.

Supplementary Figure 4 | WikiPathway analyses in matched GBM 179 samples. Pathways implicated in GBM progression (e.g., PI3K-AKT, RTK/RAS, cell cycle progression, DNA repair) are shown for matched en bloc and Myriad samples from GBM179. Mutated genes are shown in red. Blue circles delineate non-overlapping genomic alterations identified in the two matched specimens for each patient.

Supplementary Figure 5 | WikiPathway analyses in matched GBM 199 samples. Pathways implicated in GBM progression (e.g., PI3K-AKT, RTK/RAS, cell cycle progression, DNA repair) are shown for matched en bloc and Myriad samples from GBM199. Mutated genes are shown in red. Blue circles delineate non-overlapping genomic alterations identified in the two matched specimens for each patient.

Supplementary Figure 6 | WikiPathway analyses in matched GBM 216 samples. Pathways implicated in GBM progression (e.g., PI3K-AKT, RTK/RAS, cell cycle progression, DNA repair) are shown for matched en bloc and Myriad samples from GBM216. Mutated genes are shown in red. Blue circles delineate non-overlapping genomic alterations identified in the two matched specimens for each patient.

Supplementary Table 1 | Identification of genomic "hot spots" in matched GBM samples. **(A,B)** Matched samples and corresponding PDX (when available) from each patients are shown in a different color in the chart (total of 13 patients). En bloc sample is designated–1 and Myriad samples is designated–2. GBM179-1X corresponds to the PDX generated from GBM179-1; GBM179-2X designates the PDX generated from GBM 179-2 tissue. Genomic DNA from matched samples was extracted from fresh frozen tissues and sequencing was performed using the MiSeq machine in conjunction with the Illumina tumor amplicon panel. The numbers shown in each cell represent allele frequencies (VAF). VAF between 0.1 and 1 are within the sequencer's detection limit. Concordance in VAF between matched specimens and with the corresponding PDX are also shown.

Supplementary Table 2 | Normalized gene expression values for 6 matched GBM patient samples (12 total) obtained by RNA Sequencing.

REFERENCES

1. Tamimi AF, Juweid M. Epidemiology and outcome of glioblastoma. In: De Vleeschouwer S, editor. *Glioblastoma*. Brisbane, AU: Codon Publications (2017). p. 143–53. doi: 10.15586/codon.glioblastoma.2017.ch8
2. Stupp R, Mason WP, van den Bent MJ, Weller M, Fisher B, Taphoorn MJB, et al. Radiotherapy plus concomitant and adjuvant temozolomide for glioblastoma. *N Engl J Med.* (2005) 352:987–96. doi: 10.1056/NEJMoa043330
3. Haj A, Doenitz C, Schebesch KM, Ehrensberger D, Hau P, Putnik K, et al. Extent of resection in newly diagnosed glioblastoma: impact of a specialized neuro-oncology care center. *Brain Sci.* (2018) 8:E5. doi: 10.3390/brainsci8010005
4. Lara-Velazquez M, Al-Kharboosh R, Jeanneret S, Vazquez-Ramos C, Mahato D, Tavanaiepour D, et al. Advances in brain tumor surgery for glioblastoma in adults. *Brain Sci.* (2017) 7:E166. doi: 10.3390/brainsci7120166
5. Shonka NA, Aizenberg MR. Extent of resection in glioblastoma. *Brain Sci.* (2017) 13:641–2. doi: 10.1200/JOP.2017.027599
6. William D, Mullins CS, Schneider B, Orthmann A, Lamp N, Krohn M, et al. Optimized creation of glioblastoma patient derived xenografts for use in preclinical studies. *J Transl Med.* (2017) 15:27. doi: 10.1186/s12967-017-1128-5
7. Patrizii M, Bartucci M, Pine SR, Sabaawy HE. Utility of glioblastoma patient-derived orthotopic xenografts in drug discovery and personalized therapy. *Front Oncol.* (2018) 8:23. doi: 10.3389/fonc.2018.00023
8. Zhou X, Zheng C, Shi Q, Li X, Shen Z, Yu R. Isolation, cultivation and identification of brain glioma stem cells by magnetic bead sorting. *Neural Regen Res.* (2012) 7:985–92. doi: 10.3969/j.issn.1673-5374.2012.13.004
9. McLaughlin N, Ditzel Filho LF, Prevedello DM, Kelly DF, Carrau RL, Kassam AB. Side-cutting aspiration device for endoscopic and microscopic tumor removal. *J Neurol Surg B Skull Base.* (2012) 73:11–20. doi: 10.1055/s-0032-1304834
10. Soroceanu L, Matlaf L, Khan S, Akhavan A, Singer E, Bezrookove V, et al. Cytomegalovirus immediate-early proteins promote stemness properties in glioblastoma. *Cancer Res.* (2015) 75:3065–76. doi: 10.1158/0008-5472.CAN-14-3307
11. Calapre L, Giardina T, Robinson C, Reid AL, Al-Ogaili Z, Pereira MR, et al. Locus-specific concordance of genomic alterations between tissue and plasma circulating tumor DNA in metastatic melanoma. *Mol Oncol.* (2019) 13:171–84. doi: 10.1002/1878-0261.12391
12. Soroceanu L, Murase R, Limbad C, Singer E, Allison J, Adrados I, et al. Id-1 is a key transcriptional regulator of glioblastoma aggressiveness and a novel therapeutic target. *Cancer Res.* (2013) 73:1559–69. doi: 10.1158/0008-5472.CAN-12-1943
13. Salomonis N, Schlieve CR, Pereira L, Wahlquist C, Colas A, Zambon AC, et al. Alternative splicing regulates mouse embryonic stem cell pluripotency and differentiation. *Proc Natl Acad Sci USA.* (2010) 107:10514–9. doi: 10.1073/pnas.0912260107
14. Olsson A, Venkatasubramanian M, Chaudhri VK, Aronow BJ, Salomonis N, Singh H, et al. Single-cell analysis of mixed-lineage states leading to a binary cell fate choice. *Nature.* (2016) 537:698. doi: 10.1038/nature19348
15. Singer E, Judkins J, Salomonis N, Matlaf L, Soteropoulos P, McAllister S, et al. Reactive oxygen species-mediated therapeutic response and resistance in glioblastoma. *Cell Death Dis.* (2015) 6:e1601. doi: 10.1038/cddis.2014.566
16. Nishikawa M, Inoue A, Ohnishi T, Kohno S, Ohue S, Matsumoto S, et al. Significance of glioma stem-like cells in the tumor periphery that express high levels of CD44 in tumor invasion, early progression, and poor prognosis in glioblastoma. *Stem Cells Int.* (2018) 2018:5387041. doi: 10.1155/2018/5387041
17. Cobbs C, Khan S, Matlaf L, McAllister S, Zider A, Yount G, et al. HCMV glycoprotein B is expressed in primary glioblastomas and enhances growth and invasiveness via PDGFR-alpha activation. *Oncotarget.* (2014) 5:1091–100. doi: 10.18632/oncotarget.1787
18. Rong Y, Brat DJ, Durden DL, Van Meir EG. 'Pseudopalisading' necrosis in glioblastoma: a familiar morphologic feature that links vascular pathology, hypoxia, and angiogenesis. *J Neuropathol Exp Neurol.* (2006) 65:529–39. doi: 10.1097/00005072-200606000-00001
19. Lu W, Chao T, Ruiqi C, Juan S, Zhihong LJ. Patient-derived xenograft models in musculoskeletal malignancies. *J Transl Med.* (2018) 16:107. doi: 10.1186/s12967-018-1487-6
20. Verhaak RGW, Hoadley KA, Purdom E, Wang V, Qi Y, Wilkerson MD, et al. Integrated genomic analysis identifies clinically relevant subtypes of glioblastoma characterized by abnormalities in PDGFRA, IDH1, EGFR, and NF1. *Cancer Cell.* (2010) 17:98–110. doi: 10.1016/j.ccr.2009.12.020.

21. Cancer Genome Atlas Research Network. Comprehensive genomic characterization defines human glioblastoma genes and core pathways. *Nature.* (2008) 455:1061–8. doi: 10.1038/nature07385
22. Wick W, Kessler T. New glioblastoma heterogeneity atlas — a shared resource. *Nat Rev Neurol.* (2018) 14:453–4. doi: 10.1038/s41582-018-0038-3
23. Darmanis S, Sloan SA, Croote D, Mignardi M, Chernikova S, Samghababi P, et al. Single-cell RNA-Seq analysis of infiltrating neoplastic cells at the migrating front of human glioblastoma. *Cell Rep.* (2017) 21:1399–410. doi: 10.1016/j.celrep.2017.10.030
24. Keskin DB, Anandappa AJ, Sun J, Tirosh I, Mathewson ND, Li S, et al. Neoantigen vaccine generates intratumoral T cell responses in phase Ib glioblastoma trial. *Nature.* (2019) 565:234–9. doi: 10.1038/s41586-018-0792-9
25. Sottoriva A, Spiteri I, Piccirillo SGM, Touloumis A, Collins VP, Marioni JC, et al. Intratumor heterogeneity in human glioblastoma reflects cancer evolutionary dynamics. *Proc Natl Acad Sci USA.* (2013) 110:4009–14. doi: 10.1073/pnas.1219747110
26. Patel AP, Tirosh I, Trombetta JJ, Shalek AK, Gillespie SM, Wakimoto H, et al. Single-cell RNA-seq highlights intratumoral heterogeneity in primary glioblastoma. *Science.* (2014) 344:1396–401. doi: 10.1126/science.1254257
27. Mecca C, Giambanco I, Donato R, Arcuri C. Targeting mTOR in glioblastoma: rationale and preclinical/clinical evidence. *Dis Mark.* (2018) 2018:9230479. doi: 10.1155/2018/9230479
28. Zhao HF, Wang J, Shao W, Wu CP, Chen ZP, To ST, et al. Recent advances in the use of PI3K inhibitors for glioblastoma multiforme: current preclinical and clinical development. *Mol Cancer.* (2017) 16:100. doi: 10.1186/s12943-017-0670-3
29. Akhavan D, Cloughesy TF, Mischel PS. mTOR signaling in glioblastoma: lessons learned from bench to bedside. *Neuro Oncol.* (2010) 12:882–9. doi: 10.1093/neuonc/noq052
30. Wahl M, Chang SM, Phillips JJ, Molinaro AM, Costello JF, Mazor T, et al. Probing the phosphatidylinositol 3-kinase/mammalian target of rapamycin pathway in gliomas: a phase 2 study of everolimus for recurrent adult low-grade gliomas. *Cancer.* (2017) 123:4631–9. doi: 10.1002/cncr.30909
31. Chen S, Le T, Harley BAC, Imoukhuede PI. Characterizing glioblastoma heterogeneity via single-cell receptor quantification. *Front Bioeng Biotechnol.* (2018) 6:92. doi: 10.3389/fbioe.2018.00092

9

Development and Validation of an IDH1-Associated Immune Prognostic Signature for Diffuse Lower-Grade Glioma

Xiangyang Deng [1], Dongdong Lin [1], Bo Chen [2], Xiaojia Zhang [1], Xingxing Xu [3], Zelin Yang [1], Xuchao Shen [1], Liang Yang [1], Xiangqi Lu [1], Hansong Sheng [1], Bo Yin [1], Nu Zhang [1] and Jian Lin [1*]*

[1] Department of Neurosurgery, The Second Affiliated Hospital and Yuying Children's Hospital of Wenzhou Medical University, Wenzhou, China, [2] The Second Clinical Medical College, Wenzhou Medical University, Wenzhou, China, [3] School of Basic Medical Sciences, Wenzhou Medical University, Wenzhou, China

***Correspondence:**
Nu Zhang
zhangnu65@163.com
Jian Lin
linjian32222@163.com

A mutation in the isocitrate dehydrogenase 1 (IDH1) gene is the most common mutation in diffuse lower-grade gliomas (LGGs), and it is significantly related to the prognosis of LGGs. We aimed to explore the influence of the IDH1 mutation on the immune microenvironment and develop an IDH1-associated immune prognostic signature (IPS) for predicting prognosis in LGGs. IDH1 mutation status and RNA expression were investigated in two different public cohorts. To develop an IPS, LASSO Cox analysis was conducted for immune-related genes that were differentially expressed between $IDH1^{wt}$ and $IDH1^{mut}$ LGG patients. Then, we systematically analyzed the influence of the IPS on the immune microenvironment. A total of 41 immune prognostic genes were identified based on the IDH1 mutation status. A four-gene IPS was established and LGG patients were effectively stratified into low- and high-risk groups in both the training and validation sets. Stratification analysis and multivariate Cox analysis revealed that the IPS was an independent prognostic factor. We also found that high-risk LGG patients had higher levels of infiltrating B cells, CD4+ T cells, CD8+ T cells, neutrophils, macrophages and dendritic cells, and expressed higher levels of CTLA-4, PD-1 and TIM-3. Moreover, a novel nomogram model was established to estimate the overall survival in LGG patients. The current study provides novel insights into the LGG immune microenvironment and potential immunotherapies. The proposed IPS is a clinically promising biomarker that can be used to classify LGG patients into subgroups with distinct outcomes and immunophenotypes, with the potential to facilitate individualized management and improve prognosis.

Keywords: lower-grade glioma, IDH1, mutation, immune prognostic signature, nomogram

INTRODUCTION

Gliomas are the most commonly occurring type of malignant primary tumor of the central nervous system, which arise from astrocytic, oligodendroglial, mixed oligoastrocytic, or neuronal-glial cells, and result in significant morbidity and mortality (1, 2). According to the WHO classification system based on the histological type, diffuse lower-grade gliomas (LGGs) have a grade of II or III (3).

Despite diverse natural course of this heterogeneous group, most LGGs will gradually evolve into higher-grade gliomas and eventually lead to death (4).

Some studies have indicated that key components of the immune response were significantly altered in gliomas, and subsequently led to immune evasion of tumors (5, 6). In addition to conventional treatment methods including surgery, radiotherapy and chemotherapy, immunotherapy is rapidly emerging as a promising treatment modality and works by evoking an anti-tumor immune response that inhibits immune evasion by the tumor. A number of immune-related parameters have been discovered to predict the outcomes of LGG patients (7, 8). However, there is still a lack of reliable biomarkers that can identify subsets of patients with potential sensitivity to immunotherapy. Moreover, few studies have systematically explored the immune microenvironment of LGG.

Based on the molecular profiles of gliomas, the mutation in the isocitrate dehydrogenase 1 (IDH1) gene has been identified to facilitate patient stratification and predict prognosis, along with other molecular markers including the 1p/19q co-deletion, methylguanine methyltransferase (MGMT) promoter methylation, tumor protein (TP) 53, and telomerase reverse transcriptase (TERT) promoters (9, 10). IDH1 encodes the cytosolic isocitrate dehydrogenase 1, an enzyme that catalyzes the oxidative decarboxylation of isocitrate to α-ketoglutarate and plays a critical role in cellular protection from oxidative stress (11, 12). Further studies have found this mutation to be present in up to 80% of LGG patients and was virtually absent in primary glioblastomas (13). More notably, research increasingly suggests that the IDH1 mutation conferred an immunologically quiescent phenotype (14–17). Berghoff et al. reported that the immunological tumor microenvironment was associated with IDH mutation status in gliomas. They found that IDH-mutant gliomas exhibit fewer tumor infiltrating lymphocytes (TILs) and show reduced expression of programmed death ligand 1 (PD-L1) protein compared to that in the wild-type counterparts, which may be at least in part due to differential PD-L1 gene promoter methylation levels (15). Bunse et al. also demonstrated that IDH-mutant gliomas display reduced T cell abundance and altered calcium signaling (17). Hence, we performed a comprehensive analysis to further explore the relationship between IDH1 mutation status and the immune response based on RNA sequencing (RNA-seq) data.

In the present study, we downloaded RNA-seq data from The Cancer Genome Atlas (TCGA) as a training set and from the Chinese Glioma Genome Atlas (CGGA) as a validation set. We systematically analyzed the influence of the IDH1 mutation on the immune microenvironment, and developed an immune prognostic signature (IPS) based on four IDH1-associated immune genes to classify patients into subgroups with distinct prognosis and immunophenotypes. We ascertained an independent role of this four-gene IPS and highlighted the potential value of the included genes to serve as therapeutic biomarkers. Furthermore, a reliable predictive nomogram model was designed to estimate overall survival (OS) for LGG patients.

MATERIALS AND METHODS

Gene Expression Datasets and Immune-Related Genes

The RNA-seq data of 511 LGG samples were obtained from the TCGA database as a training set. Information regarding the somatic mutation status and clinical dataset of the corresponding LGG patients were also downloaded from the TCGA website (https://portal.gdc.cancer.gov/repository). From the CGGA dataset (http://www.cgga.org.cn/), we downloaded RNA-seq data of 172 LGG samples as a validation set. In addition, a comprehensive immune-related gene set, identified to actively participate in the process of immune activity, was extracted from the Immunology Database and Analysis Portal (ImmPort) database (https://immport.niaid.nih.gov) (18). This was used to identify immune genes that were differentially expressed between patients with ($IDH1^{mut}$) and without IDH1 mutation ($IDH1^{wt}$).

Differential Expression Analysis

Differential expression analysis was conducted using the "DESeq2" R package (19). The log2 |fold change| > 1.5 and adj. $P < 0.05$ were set as the cut-off values to screen for differentially expressed genes.

Functional Enrichment Analysis

Metascape (http://metascape.Org) was used to perform functional and pathway enrichment analyses to explore the potential molecular mechanisms of the selected genes (20). Functional enrichment was conducted for Gene Ontology (GO) terms including the cellular component, biological process, and molecular function categories. The Kyoto Encyclopedia of Genes and Genomes (KEGG) pathways were also enriched. Only terms with a $P < 0.01$ and the number of enriched genes ≥3 were considered as significant and grouped into clusters based on their membership similarities. The most enriched term within a cluster was selected as the one to represent the cluster.

Construction of the Immune Prognostic Signature

Following quality filtering to exclude patients with missing survival information or a survival time of 0 days, there were 506 samples subjected to subsequent analysis. For further analysis, the transcriptome profiling of RNA measured by FPKM values was performed using the log2-based transformation. On the basis of the differentially expressed immune genes (DEIGs), Kaplan-Meier analysis was first performed to screen for prognostic genes in the TCGA set. These genes which were validated in CGGA were put into the Cox regression model with least absolute shrinkage and selection operator (LASSO) penalty for analysis using the "glmnet" R package (21–23). Finally, an IPS was constructed by weighting the Cox regression coefficients to calculate a risk score for each patient. Based on the optimal cut-off values obtained by the "survminer" R package, LGG patients were classified as low- and high-risk according to their risk score. To appraise the prognostic performance of the IPS, Kaplan-Meier analysis and the log-rank test were employed. Time-dependent receiver operating characteristic (ROC) curves were depicted to evaluate the sensitivity and specificity using the "timeROC" R package (24). Area under the curve (AUC) values were calculated from the ROC curves.

Principal Components Analysis (PCA) and Gene Set Enrichment Analysis (GSEA)

PCA was carried out using the "pca3d" R package to investigate gene expression patterns of grouped patients. GSEA (http://www.broadinstitute.org/gsea/index.jsp) was conducted between high- and low-risk phenotypes (25). A nominal $P < 0.05$ and a false discovery rate (FDR) < 0.25 were considered statistically significant.

TIMER Database Analysis

The TIMER database (https://cistrome.shinyapps.io/timer) is a comprehensive resource to analyze and visualize immune infiltrates among different cancer types (26). TIMER reanalyzes gene expression profiles, which includes 10,897 samples across 32 cancer types from TCGA to estimate six immune cell types in the tumor microenvironment, including B cells, CD4+ T cells, CD8+ T cells, macrophages, neutrophils, and dendritic cells (26). The data of immune infiltrate levels of LGG patients was extracted from the TIMER database to investigate the association with the IPS.

Development and Validation of the Nomogram

Univariate and multivariate Cox analyses were performed to assess the independent prognostic ability of the IPS. Then, a novel nomogram was generated based on the results of the multivariate Cox analysis using the "rms" R package and externally validated in the CGGA cohort. We conducted 1-, 3-, 5-year OS calibrations

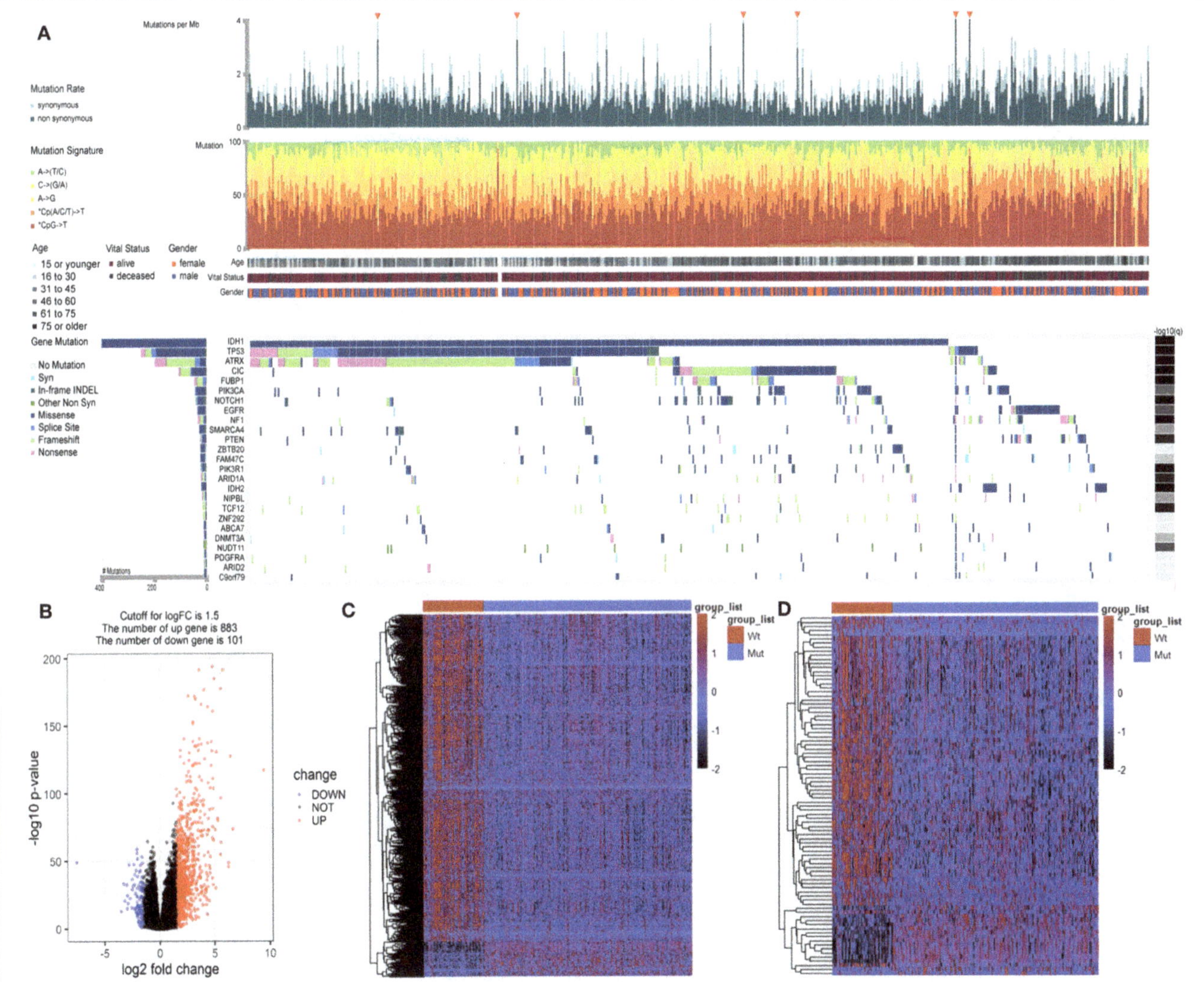

FIGURE 1 | Identified IDH1-associated immune genes. **(A)** Genomic landscape of LGG and the mutational signatures in the TCGA dataset, which were assayed on the FireBrowse platform. **(B)** Volcano plot of 984 genes differentially expressed between IDH1^{wt} and IDH1^{mut} patients. **(C)** Heatmap of genes differentially expressed between IDH1^{wt} and IDH1^{mut} patients. **(D)** Heatmap of immune genes differentially expressed between IDH1^{wt} and IDH1^{mut} patients.

to determine the predictive accuracy of the nomogram model. The concordance index (C-index) was used to evaluate the discrimination of the model. Bootstraps with 1,000 resamples were calculated to correct the C-index (27). In addition, the time-dependent ROC curves were plotted to illustrate the predictive performance. To assess the clinical utility of the nomogram, decision curve analysis (DCA) was employed to compare the benefits of different models.

Statistical Analysis

Heatmaps were generated using the "pheatmap" R package. A volcano plot and violin plots were generated using the "ggplot2" R package. OS was defined as the primary outcome. Statistical analyses of this study were conducted using the R software (version 3.5.2), GraphPad Prism (version 7.0.0), and SPSS software (version 24.0). A two-sided $P < 0.05$ was regarded as significant.

RESULTS

Identification of Differentially Expressed Immune Genes

In LGGs, the IDH1 mutation is the most common type of mutation (**Figure 1A**). Based on the DESeq2 algorithm, there were 984 genes identified that were differentially expressed between $IDH1^{wt}$ and $IDH1^{mut}$ patients, including 883 up-regulated and 101 down-regulated genes (**Figures 1B,C**). From this set of genes, 88 DEIGs were selected by the ImmPort database for further analysis (**Figure 1D**). As shown in **Figures 2A–C**, the DEIGs were mainly enriched in regulation of signaling receptor

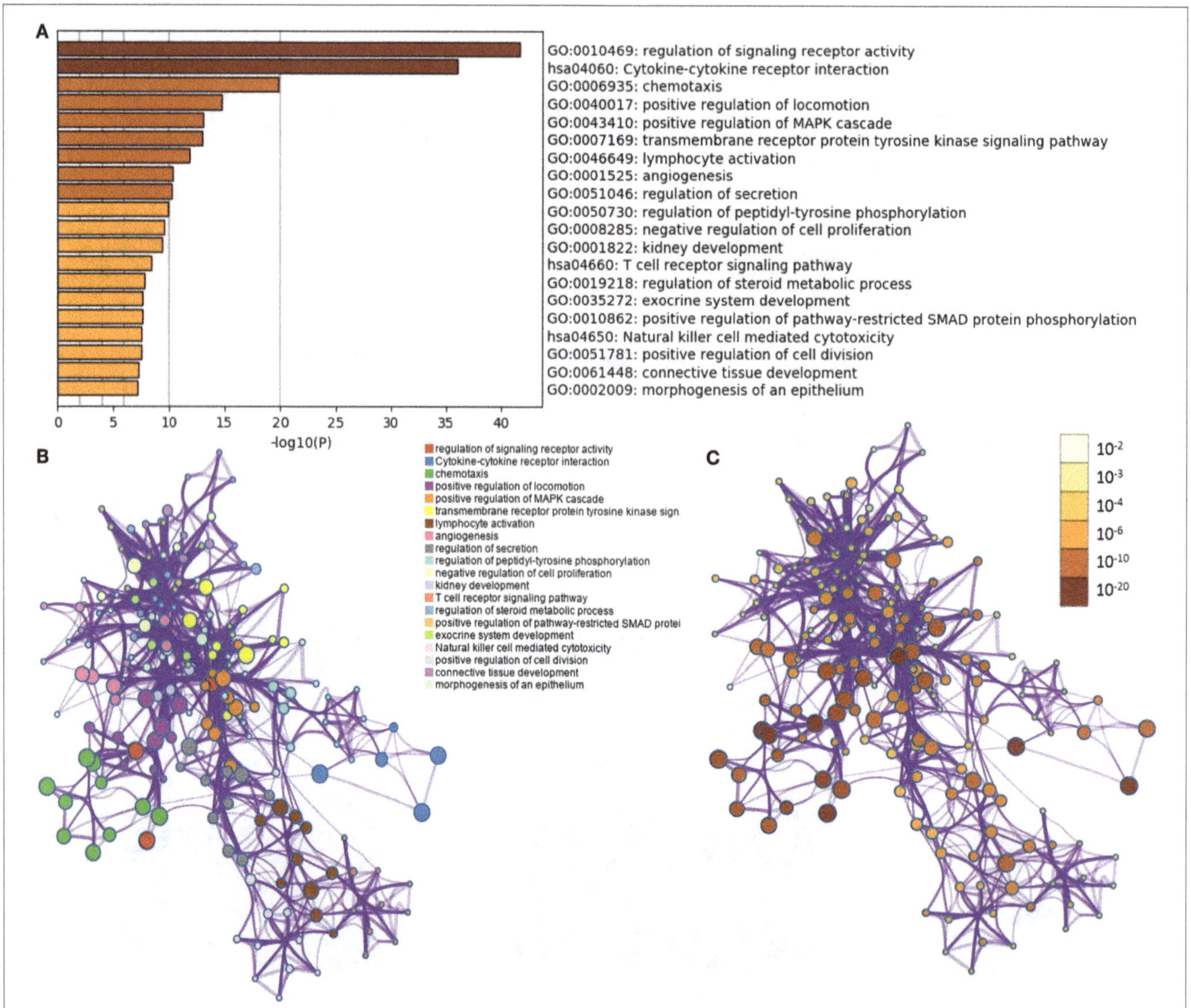

FIGURE 2 | Functional analysis of 88 IDH1-associated immune genes. **(A)** Heatmap of enriched terms across input gene lists, colored by *P*-values. Network of enriched terms: **(B)** colored by cluster ID, where nodes that share the same cluster ID are typically close to each other; **(C)** colored by *p*-value, where terms containing more genes tend to have a more significant *P*-value.

activity, chemotaxis, positive regulation of MAPK cascade, transmembrane receptor protein tyrosine kinase signaling pathway, lymphocyte activation (GO), and cytokine-cytokine receptor interaction (KEGG).

Construction of the Immune Prognostic Signature

Considering the differences in immune gene expression between $IDH1^{wt}$ and $IDH1^{mut}$ patients, we evaluated the prognostic value of DEIGs by Kaplan-Meier analysis. Log-rank tests were performed and revealed that 68 DEIGs were associated with prognosis. Using a cross validation with the CGGA set, 41 DEIGs were identified as showing significant correlation between gene expression and OS (**Supplementary Table 1**). Then, LASSO Cox analysis was performed to select genes with the best prognostic value and to build an IPS in the TCGA cohort (**Figures 3A,B**). Risk scores were calculated for each sample (risk score = 0.036*TNFRSF12A + 0.259*VAV3 + 0.104*TNFRSF11B

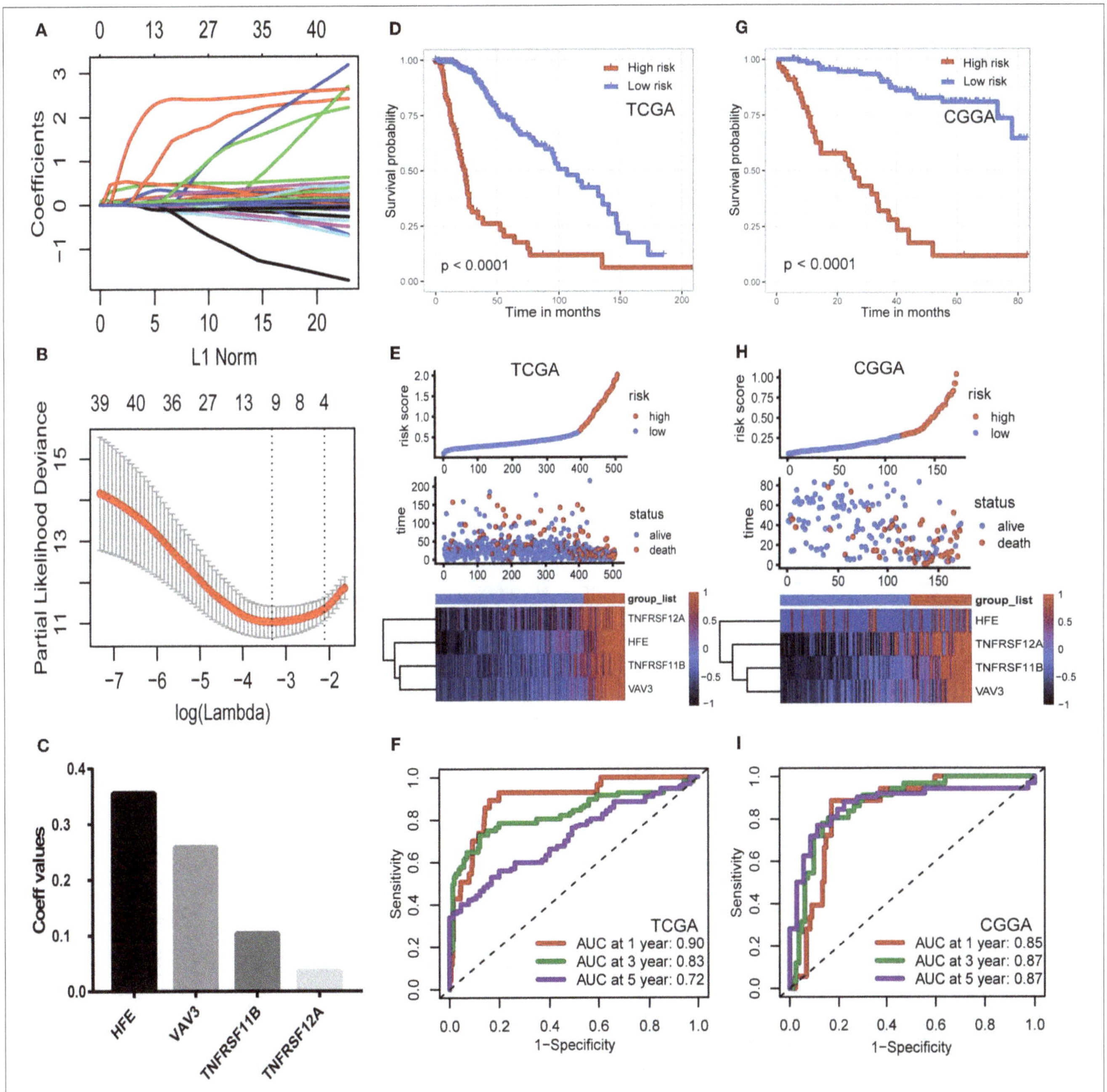

FIGURE 3 | Construction and validation of the immune prognostic signature. **(A,B)** LASSO Cox analysis identified four genes most correlated to overall survival in TCGA set. **(C)** Coefficient values for each of the four selected genes. **(D,G)** Kaplan-Meier curves of overall survival for LGG patients based on the IPS in TCGA cohort and CGGA cohort. **(E,H)** Risk scores distribution, survival status of each patient, and heatmaps of prognostic four-gene signature in TCGA and CGGA cohorts. **(F,I)** Time-dependent ROC curve analysis of the IPS.

+ 0.356*HFE, **Figure 3C**). Patients in the TCGA cohort then were assigned to a high- or low-risk group using the optimal cut-off value obtained with the "survminer" R package. The Kaplan-Meier analysis demonstrated that patients with a high-risk score were correlated with worse outcomes (**Figure 3D**). Risk score distribution and gene expression patterns are shown in **Figure 3E**. The time-dependent ROC curve analysis of the IPS in the TCGA cohort indicated a promising prognostic ability for OS (1-year AUC = 0.90, 3-year AUC = 0.83, 5-year AUC = 0.72, **Figure 3F**).

Validation of the Immune Prognostic Signature

To confirm that the IPS had a robust prognostic value, the same formula was applied to the CGGA set, which consisted of 172 LGG patients. Using the cut-off value obtained from the corresponding cohort, patients were divided into high- and low-risk groups. Consistent with the findings in the TCGA database, patients with high-risk scores had significantly worse OS than those with low-risk scores (**Figure 3G**). Risk score distribution and gene expression patterns are shown in **Figure 3H**. The time-dependent ROC analysis also showed that the IPS had high sensitivity and specificity (**Figure 3I**). AUC values were 0.85, 0.87, and 0.87 for 1-, 3-, and 5-year OS, revealing the high predictive value of the IPS for LGG patients.

Stratification Analyses

The IDH1 mutation is a stable marker for better prognosis in LGG. Stratification analyses were carried out to determine whether the predictive ability of the IPS would remain stable in distinct subgroups. As shown in **Figures 4A,B**, patients in the high-risk group showed worse survival compared to those in the low-risk group in both IDH1^{wt} and IDH1^{mut} subgroups. We also demonstrated that the IPS was still a powerful marker for predicting OS in patients with grade II or grade III tumors, younger or older, and male or female patients (**Figures 4C–H**).

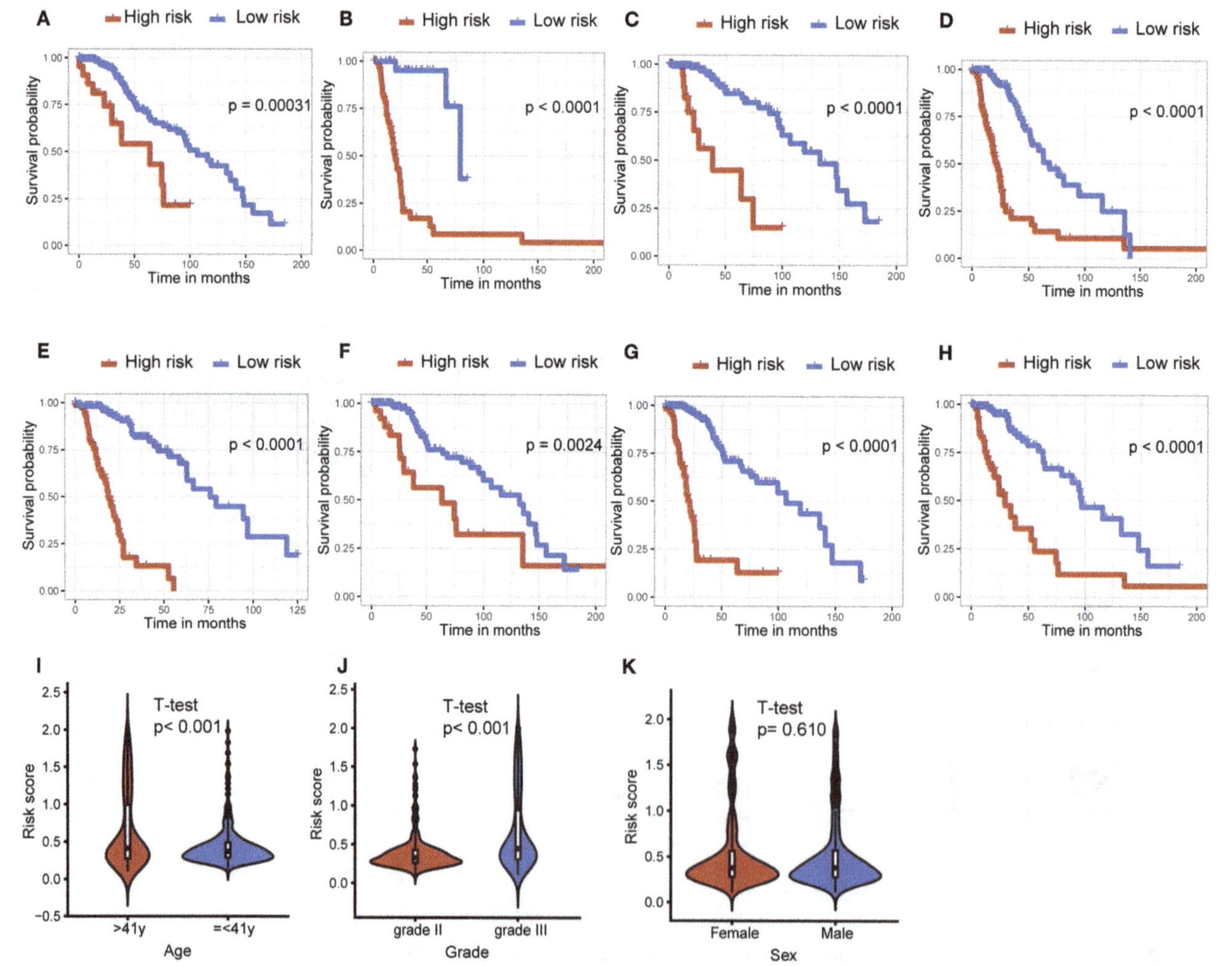

FIGURE 4 | Stratification analysis. The Kaplan–Meier analysis of the IPS grouping according to patients with **(A)** IDH1 mutant, **(B)** IDH1 wildtype, **(C)** grade II, **(D)** grade III, **(E)** > 41 years, **(F)** ≤ 41 years, **(G)** male, and **(H)** female. The risk score was group by **(I)** age, tumor grade **(J)**, and **(K)** sex.

Afterwards, we attempted to determine the statistical difference in the distribution of clinicopathological features between low- and high-risk groups. The risk scores distributed differently in stratified patients validating their association with the IPS. Patients with grade III tumor or at older ages exhibited a higher-risk level (**Figures 4I,J**). Whereas, there was no association between risk score and sex (**Figure 4K**).

High Risk Indicated an Enhanced Local Immune Phenotype

Considering different prognosis, we investigated differences between risk groups using RNA-seq data. Based on the genes comprising the IPS, PCA was performed and revealed that patients in high- or low-risk groups were distributed in discrete directions indicating differences in the immune phenotype (**Figure 5A**). GSEA was then conducted between the high- and low-risk groups, and more immune-related biological processes were found significantly enriched in the high-risk group, indicating that the high-risk score conferred an enhanced immune phenotype (**Figures 5B,C, Supplementary Table 2**).

Timer Database Analysis and Immune Checkpoints Analysis

Characterization of the immune infiltration landscape is important to explore the status of the immune microenvironment and investigate the tumor-immune interaction. We applied the TIMER tool to identify potential relationships between the IPS and infiltrating immune cells including B cells, CD4+ T cells, CD8+ T cells, neutrophils, macrophages and dendritic cells. As shown in **Figure 6A**, tumor-infiltrating immune cells were strongly interrelated and exhibited positive correlation with our IPS. Patients in the high-risk group had significantly higher proportions of infiltrating B cells, CD4+ T cells, CD8+ T cells, neutrophils, macrophages and dendritic cells than those in low-risk group (all $P < 0.05$, **Figure 6B**).

Immune checkpoints have been the subject of a wave of new studies for their important roles in immune regulation, and immune checkpoint blockade therapies are promising strategies in the treatment of cancer (28). Therefore, we investigated the relationship between the IPS and expression of critical immune checkpoints including PD-1, CTLA-4, LAG-3, TIM-3, and TIGIT. We found that the risk score showed a positive correlation with the expression of PD-1, CTLA-4, TIM-3, and TIGIT (**Figure 6C**). Among the risk groups, high-risk patients

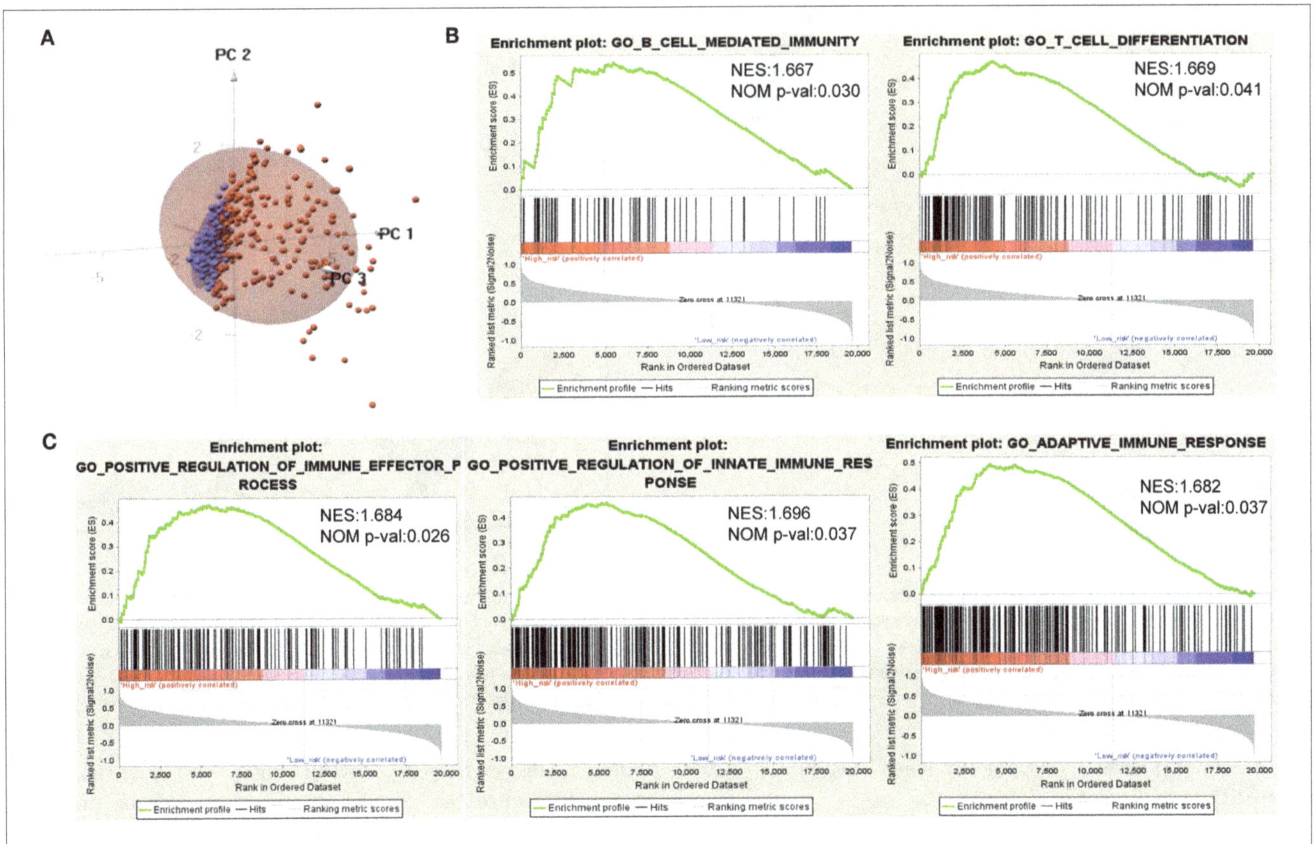

FIGURE 5 | Different immune phenotypes between high- and low-risk groups in TCGA cohort. **(A)** Principal components analysis of IDH1-associated immune genes between high- and low-risk groups. Blue color indicates low-risk patients, and red color represents high-risk patients. **(B,C)** Gene set enrichment analysis for comparing immune phenotype between high- and low-risk groups. Significant enrichment of five immune-related GO terms in high-risk group. FDR, false discovery rate; NES, normalized enrichment score.

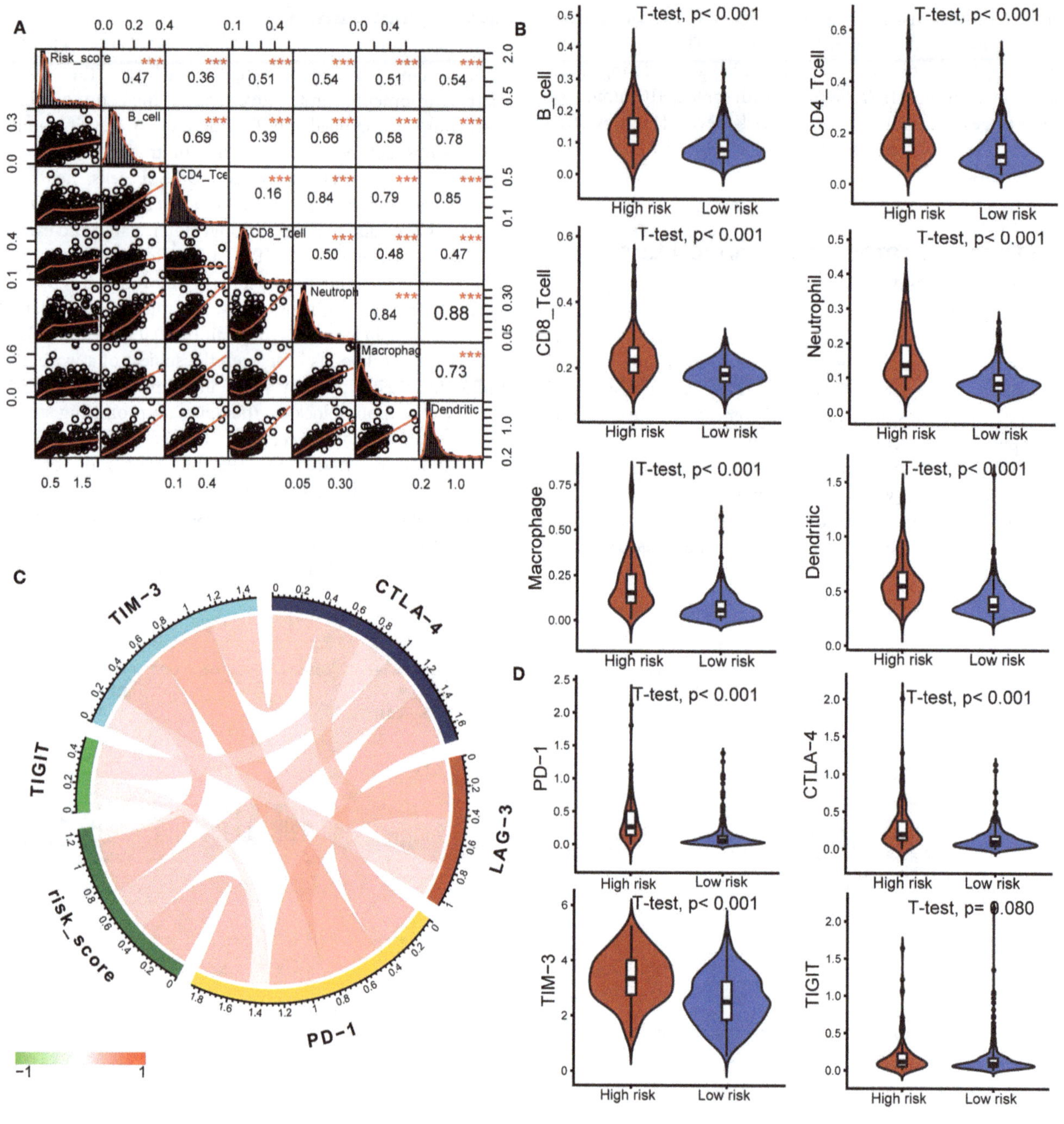

FIGURE 6 | Correlations of the IPS with infiltrating immune cell proportions and immune checkpoints. **(A)** Correlation of the risk score with infiltrating immune cell proportions. Pearson's correlation coefficient values with the level of significance were shown on the top of the diagonal. ***$P < 0.001$. **(B)** Violin plots visualizing significantly different immune cell proportions between high- and low-risk patients. **(C)** Correlation of the risk score with the expression of several crucial immune checkpoints **(D)** Violin plots visualizing significantly different immune checkpoints between high- and low-risk patients.

expressed higher levels of CTLA-4, PD-1, and TIM-3 (all $P < 0.05$, **Figure 6D, Supplementary Table 3**).

Functional Annotation of Prognostic DEIGs Between High- and Low-Risk Group

We identified 41 DEIGs validated in the CGGA database that were risk score-associated genes. These genes were differentially expressed between high- and low-risk LGG patients (**Figure 7A**). Similar to the results from the gene enrichment analysis of 88 DEIGs, these prognostic risk score-associated genes were mainly enriched in regulation of signaling receptor activity, cell chemotaxis, positive regulation of pathway-restricted SMAD protein phosphorylation, lymphocyte activation, positive regulation of MAPK cascade (GO), and

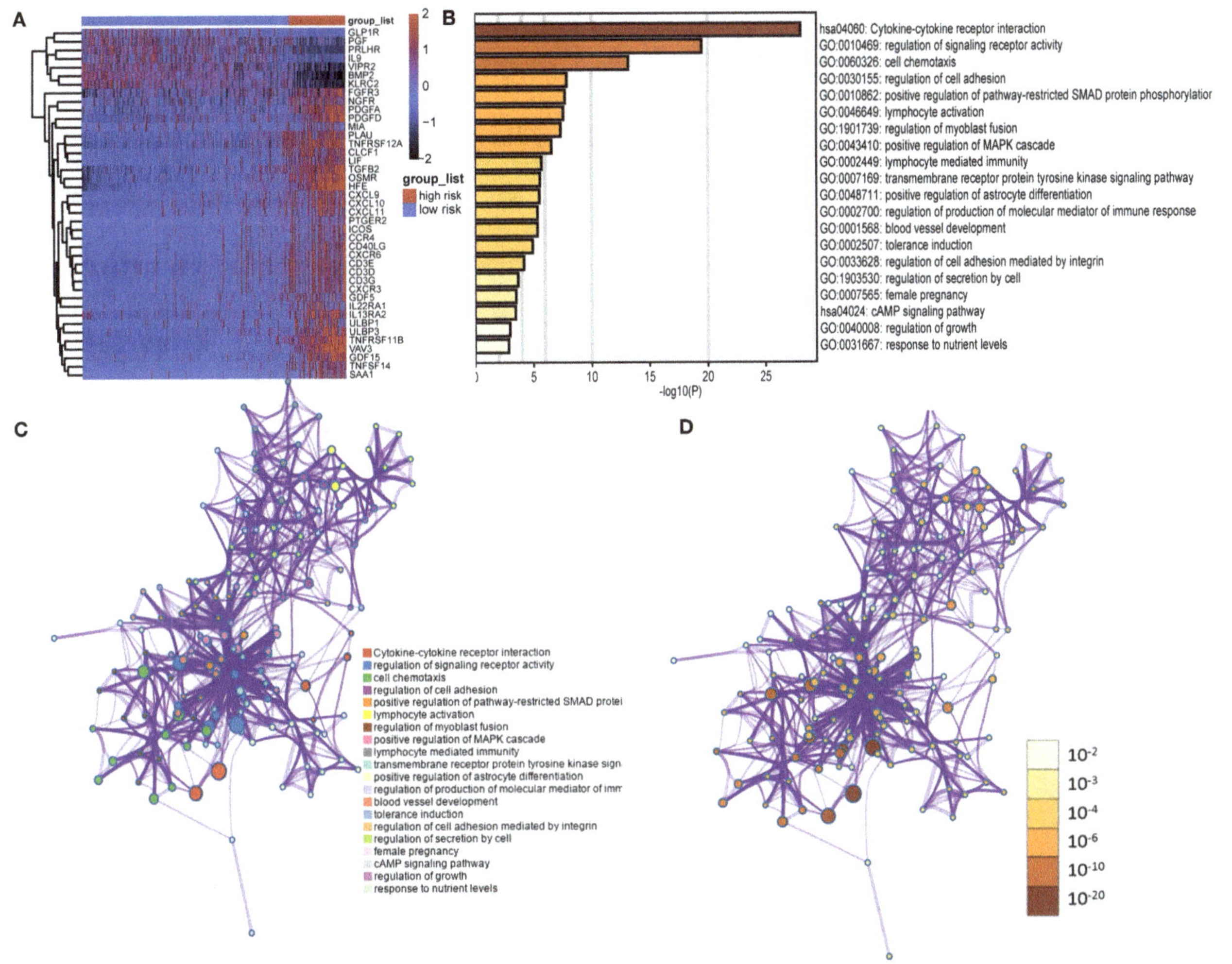

FIGURE 7 | Functional analysis of 41 risk score-associated genes. **(A)** Heatmap of IDH1-associated immune genes that were differentially expressed between patients with high- and low-risk scores. **(B)** Heatmap of enriched terms across input gene lists, colored by *P*-values. Network of enriched terms: **(C)** colored by cluster ID, where nodes that share the same cluster ID are typically close to each other; **(D)** colored by *P*-value, where terms containing more genes tend to have a more significant *P*-value.

cytokine-cytokine receptor interaction (KEGG, **Figures 7B–D**). This data thus provided a deeper understanding of the biological effects of the IPS.

IPS Was an Independent Predictive Marker of OS for LGG Patients

To examine whether the IPS was an independent prognostic factor for LGG patients, we first applied univariate Cox analysis and found that the IPS was significantly associated with OS [Hazard ratio (HR): 6.346, 95% confidence interval (CI): 5.436–9.078, $P < 0.001$; **Figure 8A**]. By adjusting for the available clinicopathological variables, multivariate Cox analysis revealed that the IPS was able to serve as an independent prognostic factor with a HR of 5.321 in the TCGA cohort (95% CI: 2.979–9.503, $P < 0.001$; **Figure 8A**). In addition, the same results were found in the CGGA cohort and indicated that the IPS had an independent role in predicting LGG survival (univariate: HR: 9.651, 95% CI: 5.266–17.685, $P < 0.001$; multivariate: HR:6.258, 95% CI: 2.825–13.864, $P < 0.001$; **Figure 8A**).

Establishment and Validation of an IPS-Based Nomogram Model

To provide a clinically associated quantitative method that could be employed to estimate OS for LGG patients, we developed a nomogram model in which the IPS integrated the two independent prognostic factors (age and grade; **Figure 8B**). The C-index values indicated favorable discrimination ability of the nomogram model (TCGA: C-index 0.839; CGGA: C-index 0.811). Calibration plots of observed vs. predicted probabilities of 1-, 3-, and 5-year OS demonstrated excellent concordance in both the TCGA (**Figure 8C**) and CGGA cohorts (**Figure 8D**). We then used time-dependent ROC curve analysis to compare the predictive accuracy between the nomogram model and individual predictors, including IPS, age, and

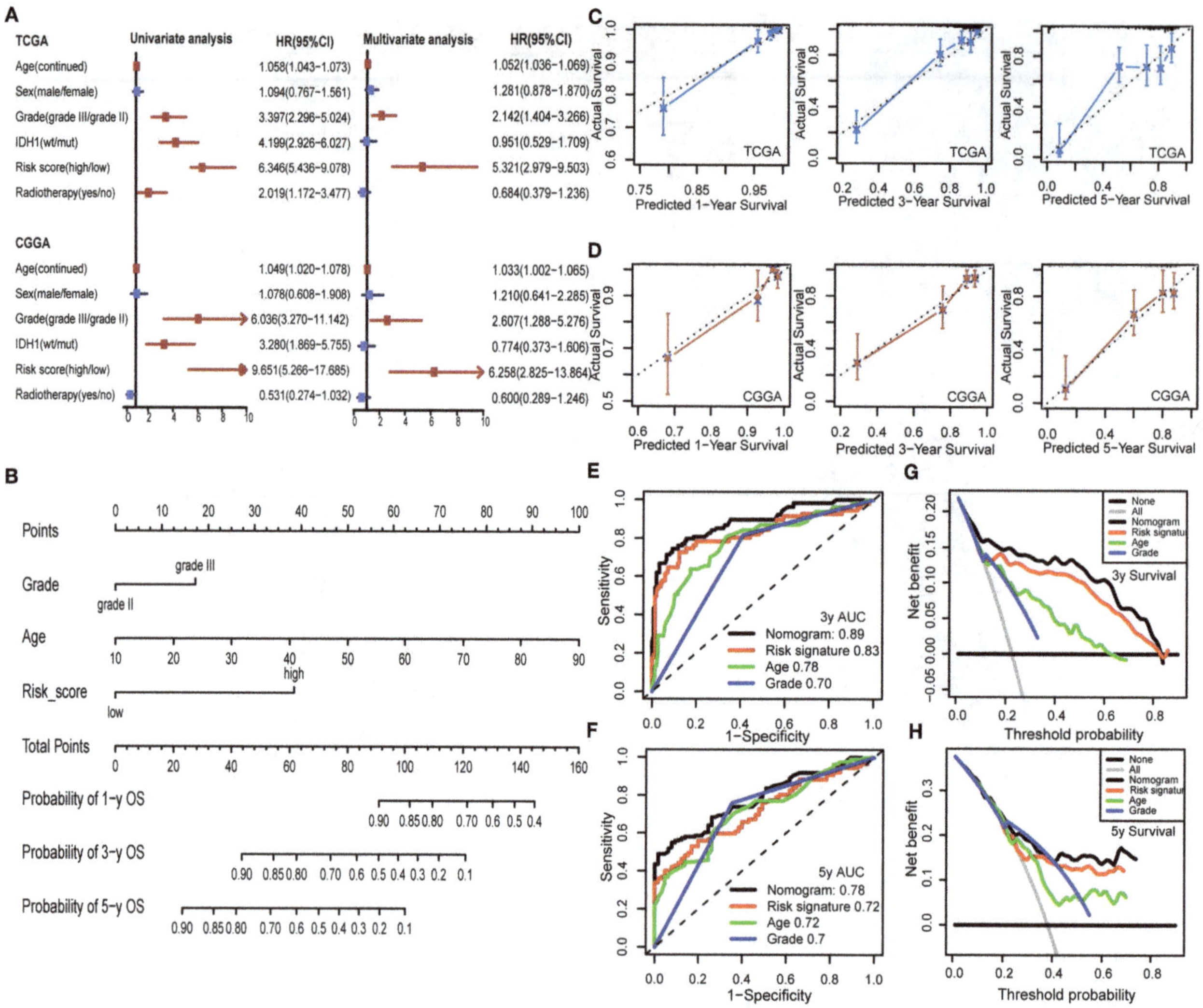

FIGURE 8 | Construction and validation of the nomogram model. **(A)** Univariate and multivariate Cox analyses indicated that IPS was significantly associated with OS in both TCGA and CGGA sets. Red indicates statistical significance, and blue indicates no statistical significance. **(B)** Nomogram model for predicting the probability of 1-, 3-, and 5-year OS in LGGs. **(C,D)** Calibration plots of the nomogram for predicting the probability of OS at 1, 3, and 5 years in TCGA and CGGA cohorts. **(E,F)** Time-dependent ROC curve analyses of the nomogram model, risk signature, age and tumor grade in TCGA cohort. **(G,H)** Decision curves of the nomogram predicting 3- and 5-year OS in TCGA cohort.

grade (**Figures 8E,F**). The nomogram model suggested higher prognostic accuracy at 3-and 5-year OS with a larger AUC. Ultimately, we attempted to determine the clinical benefit of the nomogram model and the corresponding scope of application via DCA. Compared with IPS, age and tumor grade, the nomogram mode revealed an enhanced net benefit with wider threshold probabilities and offered the best clinical utility (3-year OS: **Figure 8G**; 5-year OS: **Figure 8H**).

DISCUSSION

Although many new molecular markers have been identified, the IDH1 mutation remains the most stable, and is widely used in glioma studies (29). The discovery of IDH mutations in gliomas as compared to their IDH wildtype counterparts, plays a crucial part in the understanding of glioma biology. Mounting evidence reveals that the immunological tumor microenvironment of the gliomas differs based on their IDH1 mutation (15). However, the mechanism governing the association of IDH1 mutation with the immune microenvironment is yet to be studied.

In the current study, the role of IDH1 mutations in the regulation of immune phenotype in LGGs was comprehensively studied. An IDH1-associated IPS, which was significantly related to prognosis, was constructed based on a TCGA set, and validated in a CGGA set. The prognostic value of this four-gene IPS was also independent of the known strong prognostic factors, like IDH1 mutation, age, and tumor grade. In addition, the IPS enabled us to classify patients into subgroups with distinct outcomes and immunophenotypes, implying that it may be used to refine the current prognostic model and facilitate further stratification of patients. Therefore, we leveraged the complementary value of molecular and clinical characteristics, and integrated them to develop a novel nomogram model to provide superior survival prediction. Further bioinformatics analysis was conducted to better understand the biological function of these IDH1-associated immune prognostic genes.

The four genes included in our signature were HFE, VAV3, TNFRSF12A, and TNFRSF11B. Notably, there is no overlap between the IDH1-associated immune genes identified in the aforementioned studies. Moreover, these selected genes hold great promise to serve as novel molecular targets and improve patient management in the era of immunotherapy. The HFE gene encodes the HFE protein, an MHC I-like molecule that acts as an iron sensor in the body and is involved in iron metabolism (30). There is increasing evidence suggesting a role for HFE in antigen presentation with interactions between HFE and the antigen presentation pathway shown to impair antigen processing and T cell activation (31, 32). Previous studies have also demonstrated a relationship between HFE genotype and increased frequency of cancer. In patients with diffuse gliomas, HFE expression was associated with decreased survival (33). VAV3, a Rho-GTPase guanine nucleotide exchange factor, is widely expressed in multiple tissues and plays important roles in the formation of the cytoskeleton, cell differentiation, regulation of T and B cell signaling pathways, and oncogenesis (34, 35). Liu et al. demonstrated that high expression of VAV3 was related to poor survival in glioblastomas (36), whereas its effect on LGG prognosis was not identified previously. Furthermore, TNFRSF12A and TNFRSF11B are cytokine receptors belonging to the tumor necrosis factor receptor superfamily. Weller et al. explored the association between TNFRSF11B and Apo2L/TRAIL-based therapy in gliomas (37), but the underlying mechanisms of its involvement in tumor biology remains to be investigated. In our study, elevated expression of VAV3 and TNFRSF11B were found to be related to worse survival in LGGs for the first time.

Characterization of the immune infiltration landscape is of great significance in investigation of the cross-talk between tumors and immunity. Thus, we explored the correlation between the IPS and immune cell infiltration to reflect the status of the immune microenvironment in LGGs. On basis of the TIMER database, we found that the high-risk patients had higher infiltrating levels of B cells, CD4+ T cells, CD8+ T cells, neutrophils, macrophages, and dendritic cells. These results confirmed and expanded the finding that the heterogeneity of immune infiltration was crucial for LGG progression. The IPS could be used as a predictor for increased immune cell infiltration and may have significant clinical implications.

Currently, there are an unprecedented number of clinical trials evaluating the effects of immune checkpoint inhibitors in gliomas (38). Further analysis was conducted to explore the association between IPS and the expression of critical immune checkpoints. We found that high-risk patients had higher PD-1, CTLA-4, and TIM-3 expression in the tumor microenvironment suggesting that the immunosuppressive microenvironment partly led to worse survival of these patients. Thus, these patients might be more likely to benefit from immune checkpoint blockade therapies.

The current study provided novel insights into the LGG immune microenvironment and immunotherapies. The selected genes should be prioritized for functional and mechanistic studies to confirm the value of their clinical application. Moreover, a limitation of this study is its retrospective nature. Thus, further prospective studies are needed.

In summary, the IPS is a clinically promising biomarker that can be used to classify LGG patients into subgroups with distinct outcomes and immunophenotypes, with the potential to facilitate individualized management and improve prognosis. It also provides a novel way to elucidate the mechanism of the IDH1 mutation on prognosis from an immunological perspective.

AUTHOR CONTRIBUTIONS

XD and DL designed the study and wrote the initial draft of the manuscript. XD, BC, XZ, and XX contributed to data analysis. ZY, XS, LY, XL, HS, BY, NZ, and JL reviewed and edited the manuscript. All authors read and approved the manuscript.

FUNDING

This study was funded by the Public Welfare Projects of Science and Technology Department of Zhejiang Province (grant number 2015C33144).

ACKNOWLEDGMENTS

The authors would like to thank the ImmPort, TIMER, TCGA, and CGGA databases for the availability of the data.

REFERENCES

1. Ius T, Ciani Y, Ruaro ME, Isola M, Sorrentino M, Bulfoni M, et al. An NF-kappaB signature predicts low-grade glioma prognosis: a precision medicine approach based on patient-derived stem cells. *Neuro Oncol.* (2018) 20:776–87. doi: 10.1093/neuonc/nox234
2. Jang BS, Kim IA. A radiosensitivity gene signature and PD-L1 predict the clinical outcomes of patients with lower grade glioma in TCGA. *Radiother Oncol.* (2018) 128:245–53. doi: 10.1016/j.radonc.2018.05.003
3. Wesseling P, Capper D. WHO 2016 classification of gliomas. *Neuropathol Appl Neurobiol.* (2018) 44:139–50. doi: 10.1111/nan.12432
4. Liu X, Li Y, Li S, Fan X, Sun Z, Yang Z, et al. IDH mutation-specific radiomic signature in lower-grade gliomas. *Aging.* (2019) 11:673–96. doi: 10.18632/aging.101769
5. Gomez GG, Kruse CA. Mechanisms of malignant glioma immune resistance and sources of immunosuppression. *Gene Ther Mol Biol.* (2006) 10:133–46.
6. Wang Z, Wang Z, Zhang C, Liu X, Li G, Liu S, et al. Genetic and clinical characterization of B7-H3 (CD276) expression and epigenetic regulation in diffuse brain glioma. *Cancer Sci.* (2018) 109:2697–705. doi: 10.1111/cas.13744
7. Berghoff AS, Kiesel B, Widhalm G, Rajky O, Ricken G, Wohrer A, et al. Programmed death ligand 1 expression and tumor-infiltrating lymphocytes in glioblastoma. *Neuro Oncol.* (2015) 17:1064–75. doi: 10.1093/neuonc/nou307

8. Li G, Wang Z, Zhang C, Liu X, Cai J, Wang Z, et al. Molecular and clinical characterization of TIM-3 in glioma through 1,024 samples. *Oncoimmunology.* (2017) 6:e1328339. doi: 10.1080/2162402X.2017.1328339
9. Eckel-Passow JE, Lachance DH, Molinaro AM, Walsh KM, Decker PA, Sicotte H, et al. Glioma groups based on 1p/19q, IDH, and TERT promoter mutations in tumors. *N Engl J Med.* (2015) 372:2499–508. doi: 10.1056/NEJMoa1407279
10. Suzuki H, Aoki K, Chiba K, Sato Y, Shiozawa Y, Shiraishi Y, et al. Mutational landscape and clonal architecture in grade II and III gliomas. *Nat Genet.* (2015) 47:458–68. doi: 10.1038/ng.3273
11. Kloosterhof NK, Bralten LB, Dubbink HJ, French PJ, van den Bent MJ. Isocitrate dehydrogenase-1 mutations: a fundamentally new understanding of diffuse glioma? *Lancet Oncol.* (2011) 12:83–91. doi: 10.1016/S1470-2045(10)70053-X
12. Wefel JS, Noll KR, Rao G, Cahill DP. Neurocognitive function varies by IDH1 genetic mutation status in patients with malignant glioma prior to surgical resection. *Neuro Oncol.* (2016) 18:1656–63. doi: 10.1093/neuonc/now165
13. Philip B, Yu DX, Silvis MR, Shin CH, Robinson JP, Robinson GL, et al. Mutant IDH1 promotes glioma formation *in vivo*. *Cell Rep.* (2018) 23:1553–64. doi: 10.1016/j.celrep.2018.03.133
14. Zhang X, Rao A, Sette P, Deibert C, Pomerantz A, Kim WJ, et al. IDH mutant gliomas escape natural killer cell immune surveillance by downregulation of NKG2D ligand expression. *Neuro Oncol.* (2016) 18:1402–12. doi: 10.1093/neuonc/now061
15. Berghoff AS, Kiesel B, Widhalm G, Wilhelm D, Rajky O, Kurscheid S, et al. Correlation of immune phenotype with IDH mutation in diffuse glioma. *Neuro Oncol.* (2017) 19:1460–8. doi: 10.1093/neuonc/nox054
16. Kohanbash G, Carrera DA, Shrivastav S, Ahn BJ, Jahan N, Mazor T, et al. Isocitrate dehydrogenase mutations suppress STAT1 and CD8+ T cell accumulation in gliomas. *J Clin Invest.* (2017) 127:1425–37. doi: 10.1172/JCI90644
17. Bunse L, Pusch S, Bunse T, Sahm F, Sanghvi K, Friedrich M, et al. Suppression of antitumor T cell immunity by the oncometabolite (R)-2-hydroxyglutarate. *Nat Med.* (2018) 24:1192–203. doi: 10.1038/s41591-018-0095-6
18. Bhattacharya S, Andorf S, Gomes L, Dunn P, Schaefer H, Pontius J, et al. ImmPort: disseminating data to the public for the future of immunology. *Immunol Res.* (2014) 58:234–9. doi: 10.1007/s12026-014-8516-1
19. Love MI, Huber W, Anders S. Moderated estimation of fold change and dispersion for RNA-seq data with DESeq2. *Genome Biol.* (2014) 15:550. doi: 10.1186/s13059-014-0550-8
20. Zhou Y, Zhou B, Pache L, Chang M, Khodabakhshi AH, Tanaseichuk O, et al. Metascape provides a biologist-oriented resource for the analysis of systems-level datasets. *Nat Commun.* (2019) 10:1523. doi: 10.1038/s41467-019-09234-6
21. Tibshirani R. The lasso method for variable selection in the Cox model. *Stat Med.* (1997) 16:385–95. doi: 10.1002/(SICI)1097-0258(19970228)16:4<385::AID-SIM380>3.0.CO;2-3
22. Friedman J, Hastie T, Tibshirani R. Regularization paths for generalized linear models via coordinate descent. *J Stat Softw.* (2010) 33:1–22. doi: 10.18637/jss.v033.i01
23. Goeman JJ. L1 penalized estimation in the Cox proportional hazards model. *Biom J.* (2010) 52:70–84. doi: 10.1002/bimj.200900028
24. Heagerty PJ, Lumley T, Pepe MS. Time-dependent ROC curves for censored survival data and a diagnostic marker. *Biometrics.* (2000) 56:337–44. doi: 10.1111/j.0006-341X.2000.00337.x
25. Subramanian A, Tamayo P, Mootha VK, Mukherjee S, Ebert BL, Gillette MA, et al. Gene set enrichment analysis: a knowledge-based approach for interpreting genome-wide expression profiles. *Proc Natl Acad Sci USA.* (2005) 102:15545–50. doi: 10.1073/pnas.0506580102
26. Li T, Fan J, Wang B, Traugh N, Chen Q, Liu JS, et al. TIMER: a web server for comprehensive analysis of tumor-infiltrating immune cells. *Cancer Res.* (2017) 77:e108–10. doi: 10.1158/0008-5472.CAN-17-0307
27. Kiran M, Chatrath A, Tang X, Keenan DM, Dutta A. A prognostic signature for lower grade gliomas based on expression of long non-coding RNAs. *Mol Neurobiol.* (2018) 56:4786–98. doi: 10.1007/s12035-018-1416-y
28. Gu D, Ao X, Yang Y, Chen Z, Xu X. Soluble immune checkpoints in cancer: production, function and biological significance. *J Immunother Cancer.* (2018) 6:132. doi: 10.1186/s40425-018-0449-0
29. Cheng W, Ren X, Zhang C, Cai J, Han S, Wu A. Gene expression profiling stratifies IDH1-mutant glioma with distinct prognoses. *Mol Neurobiol.* (2017) 54:5996–6005. doi: 10.1007/s12035-016-0150-6
30. Hentze MW, Muckenthaler MU, Galy B, Camaschella C. Two to tango: regulation of Mammalian iron metabolism. *Cell.* (2010) 142:24–38. doi: 10.1016/j.cell.2010.06.028
31. de Almeida SF, Carvalho IF, Cardoso CS, Cordeiro JV, Azevedo JE, Neefjes J, et al. HFE cross-talks with the MHC class I antigen presentation pathway. *Blood.* (2005) 106:971–7. doi: 10.1182/blood-2004-12-4640
32. Reuben A, Phenix M, Santos MM, Lapointe R. The WT hemochromatosis protein HFE inhibits CD8(+) T-lymphocyte activation. *Eur J Immunol.* (2014) 44:1604–14. doi: 10.1002/eji.201343955
33. Weston C, Klobusicky J, Weston J, Connor J, Toms SA, Marko NF. Aberrations in the Iron regulatory gene signature are associated with decreased survival in diffuse infiltrating gliomas. *PLoS ONE.* (2016) 11:e0166593. doi: 10.1371/journal.pone.0166593
34. Chen X, Chen SI, Liu XA, Zhou WB, Ma RR, Chen L. Vav3 oncogene is upregulated and a poor prognostic factor in breast cancer patients. *Oncol Lett.* (2015) 9:2143–8. doi: 10.3892/ol.2015.3004
35. Shen Y, Zhang Y, Han Y, Su P, Gou M, Pang Y, et al. A novel Vav3 homolog identified in lamprey, lampetra japonica, with roles in lipopolysaccharide-mediated immune response. *Int J Mol Sci.* (2017) 18:2035. doi: 10.3390/ijms18102035
36. Liu JK, Lubelski D, Schonberg DL, Wu Q, Hale JS, Flavahan WA, et al. Phage display discovery of novel molecular targets in glioblastoma-initiating cells. *Cell Death Differ.* (2014) 21:1325–39. doi: 10.1038/cdd.2014.65
37. Naumann U, Wick W, Beschorner R, Meyermann R, Weller M. Expression and functional activity of osteoprotegerin in human malignant gliomas. *Acta Neuropathol.* (2004) 107:17–22. doi: 10.1007/s00401-003-0772-4
38. Hodges TR, Ott M, Xiu J, Gatalica Z, Swensen J, Zhou S, et al. Mutational burden, immune checkpoint expression, and mismatch repair in glioma: implications for immune checkpoint immunotherapy. *Neuro Oncol.* (2017) 19:1047–57. doi: 10.1093/neuonc/nox026

10

Inhibition of Sonic Hedgehog Signaling Suppresses Glioma Stem-Like Cells Likely Through Inducing Autophagic Cell Death

Hui-Chi Hung[1]*, Chan-Chuan Liu*[2]*, Jian-Ying Chuang*[3]*, Chun-Lin Su*[4*] *and Po-Wu Gean*[1,2,5*]

[1] Department of Pharmacology, College of Medicine, National Cheng-Kung University, Tainan, Taiwan, [2] Institute of Basic Medical Sciences, College of Medicine, National Cheng-Kung University, Tainan, Taiwan, [3] Graduate Institute of Neural Regenerative Medicine, College of Medical Science and Technology, Taipei Medical University, Taipei, Taiwan, [4] Division of Natural Sciences, Center for General Education, Southern Taiwan University of Science and Technology, Tainan, Taiwan, [5] Department of Biotechnology and Bioindustry Sciences, National Cheng-Kung University, Tainan, Taiwan

***Correspondence:**
Chun-Lin Su
tainandoctor@hotmail.com
Po-Wu Gean
powu@mail.ncku.edu.tw

Glioblastoma (GBM) often recurs after radio- and chemotherapies leading to poor prognosis. Glioma stem-like cells (GSCs) contribute to drug resistance and recurrence. Thus, understanding cellular mechanism underlying the growth of GSCs is critical for the treatment of GBM. Here GSCs were isolated from human U87 GBM cells with magnetic-activated cell sorting (MACS) using CD133 as a marker. The $CD133^+$ cells highly expressed sonic hedgehog (Shh) and were capable of forming tumor spheroids *in vitro* and tumor *in vivo*. Athymic mice received intracranial injection of luciferase transduced parental and $CD133^+$ GBM cells was utilized as orthotopic GBM model. Inhibited Shh by LDE225 delayed GBM growth *in vivo*, and downregulated Ptch1 and Gli1. $CD133^+$ cell proliferation was more sensitive to inhibition by LDE225 than that of $CD133^-$ cells. Treatment with LDE225 significantly reduced $CD133^+$-derived tumor spheroid formation. Large membranous vacuoles appeared in the LDE225-treated cells concomitant with the conversion of LC3-I to LC3-II. In addition, LDE225-induced cell death was mitigated in the presence of autophagy inhibitor 3-methyladenine (3-MA). Tumor growth was much slower in *Shh* shRNA-knockdown mice than in control RNA-transfected mice. Conversely, tumor growth was faster in Shh overexpressed mice. Furthermore, combination of LDE225 and rapamycin treatment resulted in additive effect on LC3-I to LC3-II conversion and reduction in cell viability. However, LDE225 did not affect the phosphorylated level of mTOR. Similarly, amiodarone, an mTOR-independent autophagy enhancer, reduced $CD133^+$ cell viability and tumor spheroid formation *in vitro* and exhibited anti-tumor activity *in vivo*. These results suggest that Shh inhibitor induces autophagy of $CD133^+$ cells likely through mTOR independent pathway. Targeting Shh signal pathway may overcome chemoresistance and provide a therapeutic strategy for patients with malignant gliomas.

Keywords: sonic hedgehog, glioblastoma, stem-like cells, autophagy, amiodarone

INTRODUCTION

Glioblastoma (GBM) is one of the most common and malignant subtype of brain tumors in adults (1). Although the incident rate is relatively low, GBM is very invasive that leads to rapid neurological destruction and a disproportionately high mortality. Despite the improvement of new surgical and radiation techniques, the median survival rate of patients with GBM is rather low (2, 3). A blood-brain-barrier permeable DNA alkylating agent temozolomide (4) is currently the first line chemotherapy for treating GBM. In clinics, combination of radiotherapy with temozolomide significantly prolongs the survival rate for GBM patients (5, 6). Unfortunately, tumor often regrows after radio- and chemotherapies (7, 8) resulting in poor prognosis (9, 10). The recurrence is caused at least in part, by the resistance of GBM to conventional chemo- and radio-therapies (11–14), highlighting an urgent necessity of designing new strategies for the treatment of GBM.

Sonic hedgehog (Shh) is a member of the hedgehog (Hh) family which functions as a chemical signal in transmitting information to the embryonic cells required for normal development. Shh plays a critical role in the regulation of vertebrate organogenesis and the development of brain and spinal cord including midbrain and ventral forebrain neuronal differentiation and proliferation, and many other parts of the body (15–18). Because of its role in embryonic development, aberrant or dysregulation of Shh signaling has been implicated in the initiation and/or maintenance of different types of tumor (19–21) including GBM (22). Consistent with these reports, Shh antagonists have been shown to possess anti-tumor activity in patients with basal cell carcinoma and medulloblastoma (21, 23, 24).

Cancer stem cells (CSCs) are cancer cells that possess the ability to replenish tumors through the self-renewal and differentiation into multiple cell types (25, 26). CSCs have been identified in the breast, colon, brain and other areas and can differentiate into all the cell phenotypes of the parental tumor (27, 28). CSCs are hypothesized to be associated with chemo- and radio-resistance that lead to recurrence of tumor formation. In this theory, conventional radio- and chemotherapies kill differentiated or differentiating cells which form the bulk of the tumor, while sparing CSCs. Therefore, targeting CSCs offers a promising approach to improve cancer treatment or even cure cancer (29). In the present study, we isolated glioma stem-like cells (GSCs) from human GBM cell line U87MG (U87) using CD133 as a marker. We found that Shh expression is higher in the $CD133^+$ cells than in the $CD133^-$ cells. LDE225, a smoothened antagonist (30, 31), delayed GBM growth *in vivo* and significantly reduced the number of tumor spheroids derived from $CD133^+$ cells. Furthermore, tumor growth was much slower in *Shh* knockdown mice suggesting that glioma growth may be dependent on a small population of $CD133^+$ cells that are regulated by the Shh pathway.

MATERIALS AND METHODS

Animals

The BALB/cAnN.Cg-Fox*n1*^{nu}/CrlNarl mice were purchased from the National Laboratory Animal Center (NLAC). Five mice were housed in a cage with controlled temperature (22 ±2°C) and humidity (55 ± 5%), kept on a 12 h light/dark cycle, and were given free access to water and food. Care and use of laboratory animals were in accordance with National Institutes of Health (NIH) guidelines. All the procedures were approved by the Institutional Animal Care and Use Committee of the College of Medicine, NCKU, with project approval number (#104064 and #107106).

Cell Culture

The human glioblastoma (GBM) cell lines U87MG (U87) was provided by Dr. Michael Hsiao (Genomics Research Center, Academia Sinica, Taiwan). GBM patient-derived cell line P#5 was developed by Dr. Jian Ying Chuang. Both cells were cultured in Dulbecco's Modified Eagle medium-high glucose (DMEM-high glucose, Caisson) supplemented with 10% fetal bovine serum (FBS, Sigma-Aldrich), 100 U/ml penicillin, and 0.1 mg/ml streptomycin (Caisson). All cells were maintained in a humidified incubator with 5% CO_2 at 37°C.

Isolation and Characterization of Cancer Stem Cells From Glioblastoma Cell Line

For magnetic-activated cell sorting (MACS) purification, fresh GBM and spheroids were dissociated, washed, and incubated either with PE conjugated CD133/2 or IgG2b (Miltenyi Biotech, 1:11) at a concentration of 10^8 nucleated cells per ml at room temperature for 15 min. EasySep? PE selection cocktail at 100 μl/ml cells was added and mixed down for more than 5 min. Magnetic cell separation was performed using manual FalconTM polystyrene round-bottom tubes and an EasySep? Magnet machine. Tube was removed from magnet and cells resuspended in an appropriate amount of desired medium. The $CD133^+$ cells were incubated in neural stem cells selection medium (NeuroCult^{TM} NS-A Basal Medium, NeuroCult^{TM} NS-A Proliferaction Supplement, bFGF 10 ng/mL, EGF 10 ng/mL, 20 μg/mL Heparin; STEMCELL, Canada) and gave rise to non-adherent spheres on Ultra Low Attachment Multiple Well Plates (CORNING). $CD133^+$ cells were initially allowed to form tumor spheroids in suspension culture, dissociated using Accutase (BD Biosciences) at 37°C for 30 min, and then split 1:3 to 1:5. The number of tumor spheroids formed by $CD133^+$ cells treated with or without LDE225 (25 μM) for 7 days in culture were determined with an Olympus DP72 image analysis system and Inverted fluorescence microscope Olympus IX71.

Cell Proliferation Assay

Cell proliferation was measured using WST1 [2-(4-iodophenyl)-3-(4-nitrophenyl)-5-(2,4-disulfophenyl)-2H-tetrazolium] assay (Clontech Laboratories, California, USA). The $CD133^+$ cells were seeded at a concentration of 8,000 cells/well in 200 μl culture medium containing various concentrations of LDE225 or cyclopamine (e.g., final concentration of 1–100 μM) into 96-well plates. The cells were incubated for 48 h at 37°C and 5% CO_2. WST-1 reagent (10 μl/well) was added, and cells were incubated for 1 h at 37°C and 5% CO_2. The absorbance of the product was measured at 440 nm with a microplate (ELISA) reader. The cell counts were determined by the percentage of the absorption relative to the vehicle-treated control culture.

Western Blotting Assay

Cell pellets were collected, centrifuged at 4,000 rpm and stored at −80°C. Drugs- or vehicle-treated cell pellets were lysed in a RIPA lysis buffer containing 50 mM Tris–HCl, pH 7.4, 150 mM NaCl, 1% Nonidet P-40, 0.25% sodium deoxycholate, 0.1% sodium dodecyl sulfate (SDS), protease inhibitor (Roche) and phosphatase inhibitor (Roche). Lysates were shaken at 40 rpm on ice for 1 h and then centrifuged at 12,000 rpm for 30 min at 4°C. The mouse brain tissues were homogenized in a lysis buffer (50 mM Tris-HCl, pH 7.5, 0.3 M sucrose, 5 mM EDTA and protease/phosphatase inhibitor cocktail (Roche, Nutley, USA). Supernatants were collected and then protein concentration was measured by Bradford assay. The protein was resuspended in 5X sample buffer (12.5 mM Tris, 25% glycerol, 4% SDS, 1.54% DTT, and 0.02% Bromophenol blue). The total protein was denatured at 95°C for 5 min. Protein electrophoresis on 15 or 8% SDS-polyacrylamide gel under 120 volt, and the separated protein was transferred to a PVDF membrane (Immunobilon transfer membranes, Millipore) by semi-dry transfer system (BIO-RAD) under 350 mA, 20 volt for 1.5 h. Membranes were incubated with blocking buffer (3% bovine serum albumin in PBS) for 1 h. Membranes were incubated with the following primary antibodies: rabbit anti-Shh (1:3,000, Millipore, Darmstadt, Germany), rabbit anti-P62 (1:2,000, Cell Signaling Technology, Danvers, USA), mouse anti-LC3 (1:2,000, MBL, Japan), mouse anti-CD133 (1:5,000, Millipore, Darmstadt, Germany), rabbit anti-Ptch1 (Protintech, Illinois, USA), rat anti-Gli1 (Sigma, Darmstadt, Germany) antibody overnight at 4°C, followed by treatment with HRP-conjugated secondary antibodies (Jackson ImmunoResearch Lab., West Grove, USA) for 1 h at room temperature. After three rinses with 0.3% Triton X-100 in PBS for 10 min each, the ECL-plus chemical reagents (PerkinElmer) were added to the membrane. Films (Fuji, Japan) were exposed at different time points to ensure the optimum density. The band intensities were analyzed for densitometry by using Windows Image-J version 1.29. The protein levels in all groups were expressed as a percentage of those in controls.

Immunofluorescent Staining

For immunostaining of tumor spheroids, $CD133^+$ cells were initially allowed to form spheroids in suspension culture for 7 days. The cells were then fixed with 4% paraformaldehyde in PBS pH 7.4 for 15 min at room temperature. The cells were then incubated for 1 h in blocking solution (1% bovine serum albumin), and then incubated in primary antibodies at 4°C overnight. The following primary antibodies were used: mouse anti-CD133 (1:100, Millipore, Darmstadt, Germany), rabbit anti-SOX-2 (1:1,000, Abcam, Cambridge, UK) and rabbit anti-Shh (1:200, Millipore, Darmstadt, Germany), rabbit anti-ALDH1A1 (Protintech, Illinois, USA), rat anti-ABCG2 (Santa Cruz, Texas, US), rabbit anti-LC3 (Novus, Colorado, US). After three rinses with PBS containing 0.1% Triton X-100 for 10 min each, the cells were incubated in secondary antibodies at room temperature for 1 h. The following secondary antibodies were used: Alexa Fluor®594-conjugated Goat-anti-rabbit IgG (Jackson ImmunoResearch Lab., West Grove, USA) and Alexa Fluor®488-conjugated Sheep-anti-mouse IgG and Alexa Fluor®488-conjugated Goat-anti-rat IgG (Jackson ImmunoResearch Lab., West Grove, USA). DAPI (4',6-diamidino-2-phenylindole) (1:1,000, Sigma-Aldrich, St. Louis, USA) dye was used as nuclear counterstain. The cells are washed in PBS containing 0.1% Triton X-100 three times for 10 min. The sections were cover-slipped with Prolong? gold anti-fade reagent (Life Technologies, Carlsbad, USA). Fluorescence signals were detected with a Leica DM 2500 microscope and MetaMorph image software used for counting the cells number.

JC-1 Mitochondrial Membrane Potential Assay

Early apoptosis was measured by using JC-1 Mitochondrial Membrane Potential assay (Cayman Chemical, Michigan, USA). The $CD133^+$ cells were seeded at a concentration of 5,000 cells/well in 100 μl culture medium containing 25 μM LDE225 or 0.1% DMSO as vehicle control into black 96-well plates. The cells were incubated for 48 h at 37°C and 5 % CO_2. JC-1 Staining solution (10 μl/well) was added, and cells were incubated for 30 min at 37°C and 5% CO_2. Plates were centrifuged at 300 × g at room temperature. The supernatant was removed, and JC-1 buffer was used to suspend JC-1 stained cells. The fluorescence intensity of J-aggregate and JC-1 monomer was measured with excitation and emission at 535/595 nm and 485/535 nm with a microplate (ELISA) reader. The ratio of J-aggregate and JC-1 was determined as early apoptosis.

Caspase-Glo® 3/7 Assay

The activity of caspase 3 and 7 was measured by using Caspase-Glo® 3/7 Assay (Promega, Wisconsin, US). The $CD133^+$ cells were seeded at a concentration of 1,000 cells/well in 100 μl culture medium containing 25 μM LDE225 or 0.1% DMSO as vehicle control into white 96-well plates. The cells were incubated for 48 h at 37°C and 5% CO_2. Caspase-Glo®3/7 Reagent (10 μl/well) was added, and cells were incubated for 1 h at 37°C and 5% CO_2. The luminescence was recorded with a microplate (ELISA) reader. The activity of caspase 3 and 7 was determined by the percentage of the luminescence signal relative to the control culture.

In vivo Intracranial Xenograft Animal Model and Bioluminescence Imaging

U87 GBM cells were transduced with lentiviral vector expressing GFP and firefly luciferase. GFP/Luc expressing cells were sorted out for further passages (FACS-Aria, BD Biosciences). For tumorigenesis, luciferase-expressing GBM cells were inoculated intracranially into the 8- to 10-week-old male nude mice

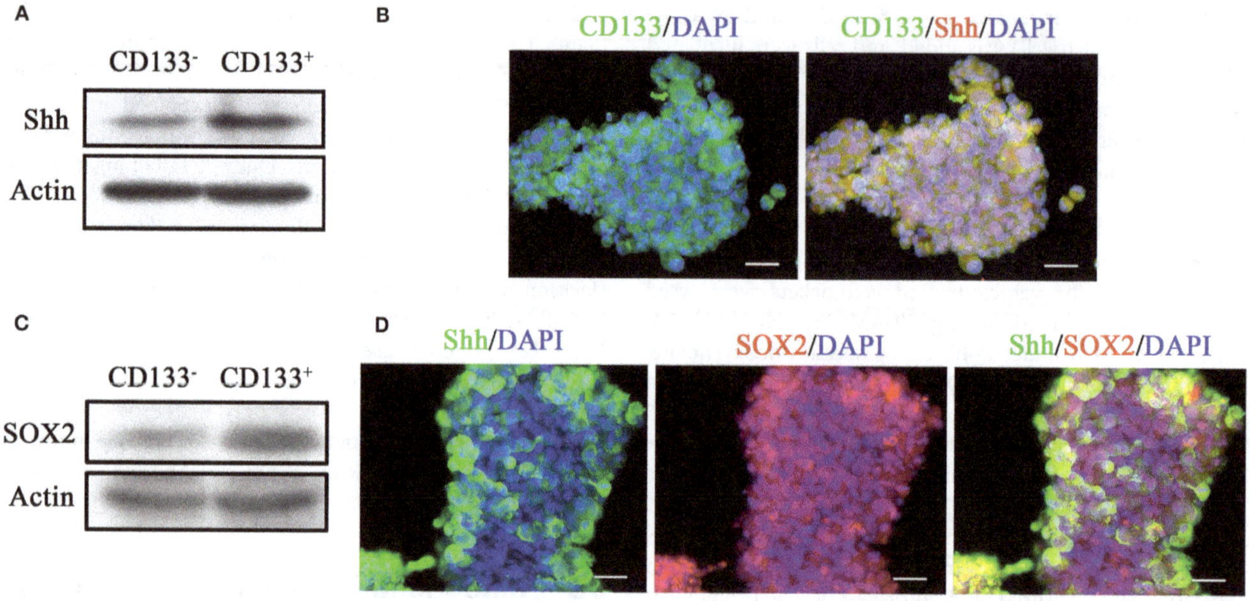

FIGURE 1 | Tumor spheroids derived from CD133+ cells exhibit higher level of Shh expression. **(A)** Expression of Shh in CD133+ and CD133− cells determined by Western blotting analysis. The CD133+ cells exhibited higher level of Shh expression. **(B)** Immunofluorescence staining of CD133 and Shh in tumor spheroids derived from CD133+ cells. CD133 and Shh were co-localized at tumor spheroids. **(C)** Expression of SOX2 in CD133+ and CD133− cells determined by Western blotting analysis. The CD133+ cells exhibited higher level of SOX2 expression. **(D)** Immunofluorescence staining of CD133, Shh, and SOX2 in tumor spheroids derived from CD133+ cells. CD133 and SOX2, Shh, and SOX2 were co-localized at tumor spheroids.

(BALB/cAnN-Foxnlnu/CrlNarl mice, National Laboratory Animal Center). Nude mice were anesthetized with chloral hydrate and placed on a stereotaxic device. Subsequently, a hamilton syringe with 30-gauge needle was mounted on a stereotaxic device, and luciferase-expressing GBM cells were injected into the left side of the brains, 1.5 mm caudal and lateral to the bregma, and at a depth of 3.5 to 4 mm. LDE225 (Cayman) was injected intraperitoneally injected at a dose of 20 mg/kg twice weekly. Tumor growth was monitored by IVIS spectrum Live Imaging System (IVIS-200, Xenogen) twice weekly. Before monitoring, mice were injected with 150 mg/kg D-luciferin (PerkinElmer), and simultaneously anesthetized with isoflurane. The results of luciferase radiance were quantitated by Live Imaging Software (Xenogen) and the results were analyzed by using GraphPad Prism software.

Shh shRNA Lentivirus Production

Production of lentivirus was initiated by triple transfection of HEK293T cells by a Lipofectamine® LTX Reagent (Life Technologies, Carlsbad, USA) method using small hairpin interfering RNA (shRNA) together with pCMV-dR8.91 and pMD2.G. The *Shh*-shRNA or scrambled shRNA conjugated on the vector of pLKO.1 with puromycin-resistant region was provided by National RNAi Core Facility (Institute of Molecular Biology, Academia Sinica, Taiwan). Cells were harvested 48 h later, medium containing lentiviruses filtered with 0.45 μm filters and viral particles were concentrated from the supernatant by Lenti-X™ Concentrator (Clontech Laboratories, Mountain View, USA) and purified to yield 1×10^8 transducing units/ml storing at −80°C until use. The target sequence of *Shh*-shRNA is described as follows: *Shh*-shRNA: 5′-GCGGAAGGTATGAAGG GAAGA-3′.

Shh-Over-Expression

To create lentiviruses over-expressing *Shh*, full-length *Shh* open reading frames (ORFs) (NM_000193; GenScript, New Jersey, USA) was amplified by PCR and was inserted into pLVX-IRES-ZsGreen1 expression vector (Clontech Laboratories, California, USA). The pLVX-NES1-IRES-ZsGreens1 vector encoding *Shh* (or empty vector) and the two packaging plasmids (pCMV-dR8.91 and pMD2.G) were co-transfected into HEK293T cells by lipofectamine® LTX Reagent (Life Technologies, Carlsbad, USA). Lentiviruses were harvested at 48 h after transfection, filter lentivirus supernatant through a 0.45 μm PVDF membrane filters, concentrated by Lenti-X™ Concentrator (Clontech Laboratories, Mountain View, USA), purified to yield 1×10^8 transducing units/ml and stored at −80°Cuntil use.

Statistical Analysis

Experiments were performed at least in triplicate. All results were presented as mean ± standard error of the mean (SEM). Independent experiments were analyzed by unpaired *t*-test. Two-way ANOVA was used to analyze the differences in tumor spheroids numbers *in vitro* and intracranial tumor growth *in vivo* at different times of treatment. Levels of $p < 0.05$ were considered to be of statistical significance.

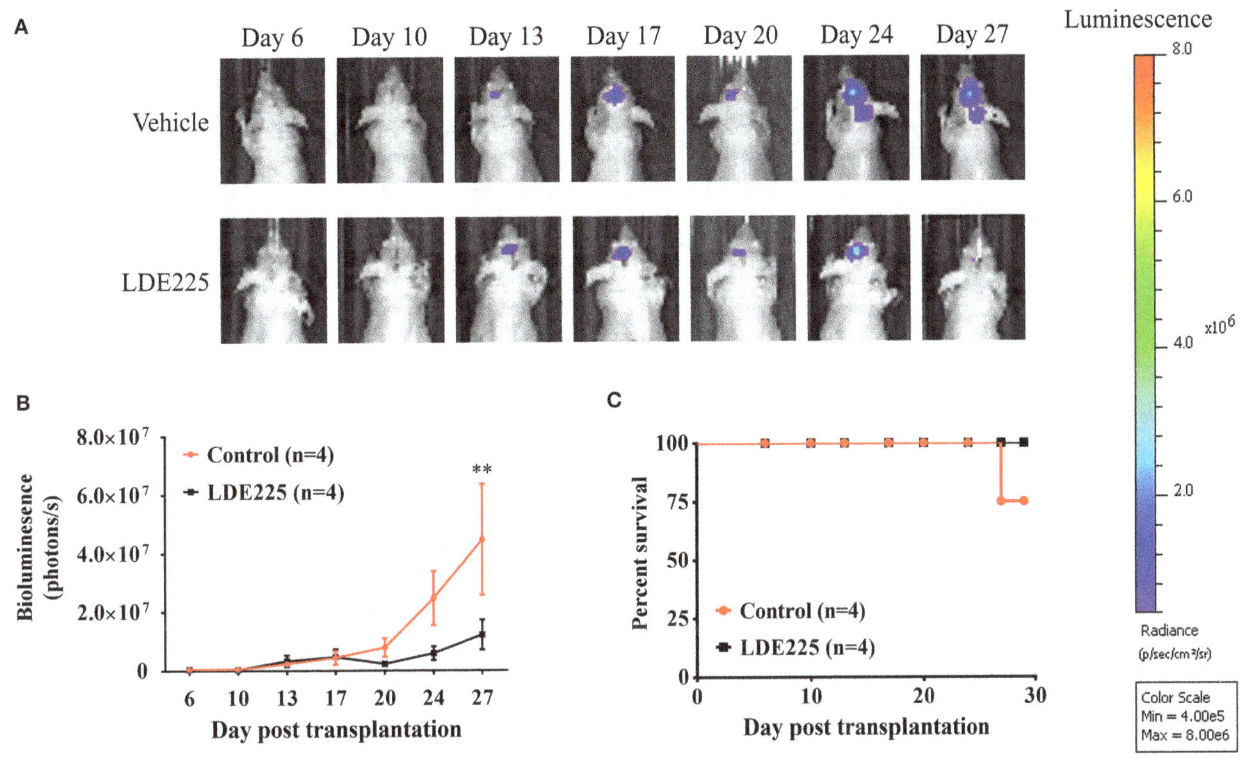

FIGURE 2 | LDE225 delays tumor growth in an intracranial tumor model. **(A)** Luc-expressing parental U87 cells (3 × 10^5 cells) were injected intracranially into athymic mice and tumor growth was monitored using the IVIS-200 imaging system. **(B)** Tumor growth was slower in LDE225 treated mice than in vehicle control mice. **p < 0.001 vs. vehicle control. **(C)** Kaplan–Meier analysis of LDE225 treatment on survival.

RESULTS

CD133 has been reported as a marker of human neural and brain tumor stem cells (32, 33). We previously have isolated cancer stem-like cells with CD133 from glioblastoma (GBM) cell lines using magnetic bead cell sorting (34). Then $CD133^+$ and $CD133^-$ cell populations were collected and cultured separately.

Shh Expression Is Higher in $CD133^+$ Cells

We examined Shh expression in $CD133^+$ and $CD133^-$ cells. Western blotting analysis showed that Shh expression was higher in the $CD133^+$ cells than in the $CD133^-$ cells (**Figure 1A**). Immunofluorescence staining revealed that most of $CD133^+$ cells were positive and co-localized with Shh (**Figure 1B**). SRY (sex determining region Y)-box 2 (SOX2) is a transcription factor that plays an important role in maintaining embryonic and neural stem cells (35, 36). **Figure 1C** showed that SOX2 expression was higher in the $CD133^+$ cells than in the $CD133^-$ cells.These Shh-positive cells were also co-immunolabeled with SOX2 (**Figure 1D**). ABCG2 is a member of the ATP-binding cassette (ABC) transporter superfamily. The expression level of ABCG2 has been implicated in multidrug resistance (MDR) in cancer chemotherapy and the ability of self-renewal which correlates with CD133 (37, 38). AlDH1A1 is a member of the highly conserved ALDH family that is observed in several cancer stem cells, and is often used to isolate and functionally characterize cancer stem cells (39). We also examined the expression of ABCG2 and AlDH1A1 by immunofluorescence in parental and $CD133^+$ cells. The expression of ABCG2 and ALDH1A1 is higher in $CD133^+$ cells than in parental cells (**Supplemental Figure 1**).

We used a potent and selective smoothened antagonist LDE225 (30) to determine the requirement of Shh signaling in the proliferation and tumor growth of GBM cell lines. We first confirmed the effect of LDE225 on tumor growth by using intracranial injection model. Luc-expressing parental U87 cells were injected intracranially into athymic mice and tumor growth was monitored using IVIS-200 imaging system. At day 7, LDE225 or DMSO as vehicle was injected intraperitoneally twice per week (20 mg/kg) into the mice and tumor growth was observed for 22 more days. Comparing with vehicle control, **Figure 2A** showed that LDE225 was able to delay tumor growth. A two-way ANOVA revealed a main effect of group (LDE225 vs. control) [$F_{(1,42)}$ =6.126, $p < 0.05$], interaction [$F_{(6,42)} =$ 2.297, $p = 0.0524$] and days after application [$F_{(6,42)} = 5.849$, $p < 0.001$] (**Figure 2B**). Kaplan–Meier analysis of the survival data of vehicle control and LDE225-treated mice displayed in **Figure 2C**. We also confirmed whether LDE225 inhibits Shh signal pathway. $CD133^+$ cells were treated with LDE225 (25 μM)

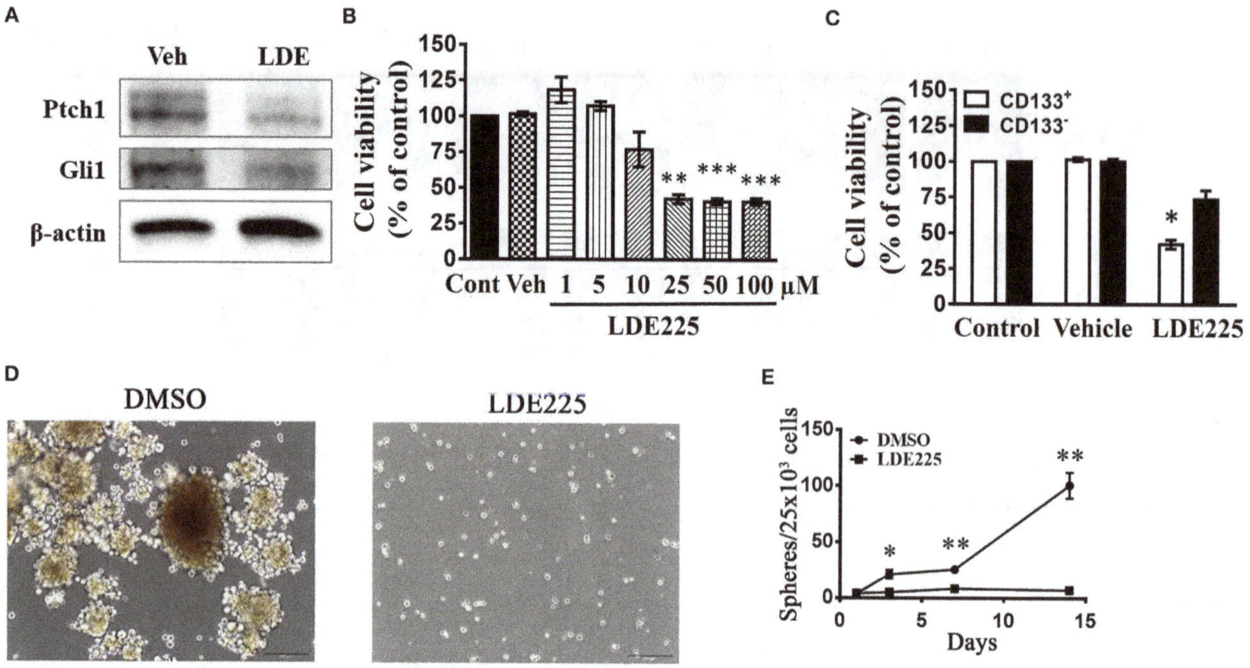

FIGURE 3 | Effects of Shh inhibitors LDE225 on the cell viability of CD133$^+$ and CD133$^-$ cells. **(A)** CD133$^+$ cells were treated with LDE-225 (25 μM) for 48 h and the expression of Patched1 and Gli1 was determined by the Western blotting analysis. LDE225 downregulated Patched1 and Gli1 in CD133$^+$ cells. **(B)** Concentration-dependent effect of LDE225 on the cell viability of CD133$^+$ cells. $^{**}p < 0.01$, $^{***}p < 0.001$ vs. vehicle. **(C)** CD133$^+$ and CD133$^-$ cells were treated with LDE225 (25 μM) for 48 h and cell viability was assessed using WST-1 assay. CD133$^+$ cells were more sensitive to LDE225 inhibition than that of CD133$^-$ cells. $^*p < 0.05$ vs. CD133$^-$ cells. **(D,E)** Effects of LDE225 (25 μM) on the number of tumor spheroids derived from CD133$^+$ cells. Primary tumor spheroids derived from CD133$^+$ were dissociated and cultured. They were then treated with LDE225 (25 μM) for the times as indicated in **(E)**. The medium was replaced every 2 days in the presence of LDE225. $^*p < 0.05$, $^{**}p < 0.01$ vs. Vehicle.

or vehicle for 48 h and the expression of Patch1 and Gli1 were determined by Western blotting analysis. As shown in **Figure 3A**, LDE225 downregulated the expression of PATCH1 and GLI1. Next, CD133$^+$ and CD133$^-$ cells were treated with LDE225 (25 μM) for 48 h and cell viability was assessed using WST-1 assay. Concentration dependent relationship estimated the IC_{50} of about 20 μM for LDE225 to reduce CD133$^+$ cell viability (**Figure 3B**), while IC_{50} of LDE225 was about 50 μM for parental cells (**Supplemental Figure 2A**). As shown in **Figure 3C**, CD133$^+$ cells were more sensitive to LDE225 inhibition than that of CD133$^-$ cells. At the concentration of 25 μM, LDE225 inhibited the proliferation of CD133$^+$ and CD133$^-$ cells by 57.57 ± 3.17% ($n = 3$) and 26.18 ± 6.22% ($n = 4$), respectively [$t_{(5)} = 4.013$, $p < 0.05$]. We also determined the effect of LDE225 on patient-derived cell line P#5 which displays various characteristics of GBM (40, 41). As illustrated in **Supplemental Figure 2B**, LDE225 inhibited cell viability with IC_{50} ~423 μM. Similar inhibition of CD133$^+$ was observed by another Shh inhibitor cyclopamine, which binds to and inactivates smoothened protein (42) ($IC_{50} \approx$ 100 μM, **Supplemental Figure 2C**). We determined the effect of Shh inhibition on self-renew capacity of CD133$^+$ cells (**Figure 3D**). CD133$^+$ cells were treated with LDE225 (25 μM) or vehicle and CD133$^+$-derived tumor spheroids were counted at 1, 3, 7, and 14 days. Treatment with LDE225 significantly reduced the number of tumor spheroids. A two-way ANOVA revealed a main effect of drug (LDE225 vs. vehicle) [$F_{(1,16)} = 100.9$, $p < 0.001$], interaction [$F_{(3,16)} = 44.27$, $p < 0.001$] and days after application [$F_{(3,16)} = 44.25$, $p < 0.001$] (**Figure 3E**).

Inhibition of Shh Induces Autophagy in CD133$^+$ Cells

In LDE225-treated cells, the observation by transmission electronic microscope showed the appearance of large membranous vacuoles in the cytoplasm which is a characteristic feature of cells undergoing autophagy (**Figure 4A**). In addition, LC3 is distributed in the autophagosome membrane (43). The conversion of LC3-I to LC3-II is a common biomarker for autophagy activation (44, 45). We determined the conversion of LC3-I to LC3-II with anti-LC3 antibody. Immunoblotting using lysates from LDE225 (25 μM)-treated CD133$^+$ cells revealed a significant increase in processed LC3-II [$t_{(5)} = 3.39$, $p < 0.05$] (**Figure 4B**). This was accompanied by the reduced expression of Mushashi-1, a RNA-binding protein selectively expressed in neural progenitor cells (46). The intensity of LC3 fluorescence punctate also increased after LDE225 treatment (**Figure 4C**). Furthermore, LDE225-induced cell death was rescued by autophagy inhibitor 3-methyladenine (3-MA) (47) (**Figure 4D**) suggesting that

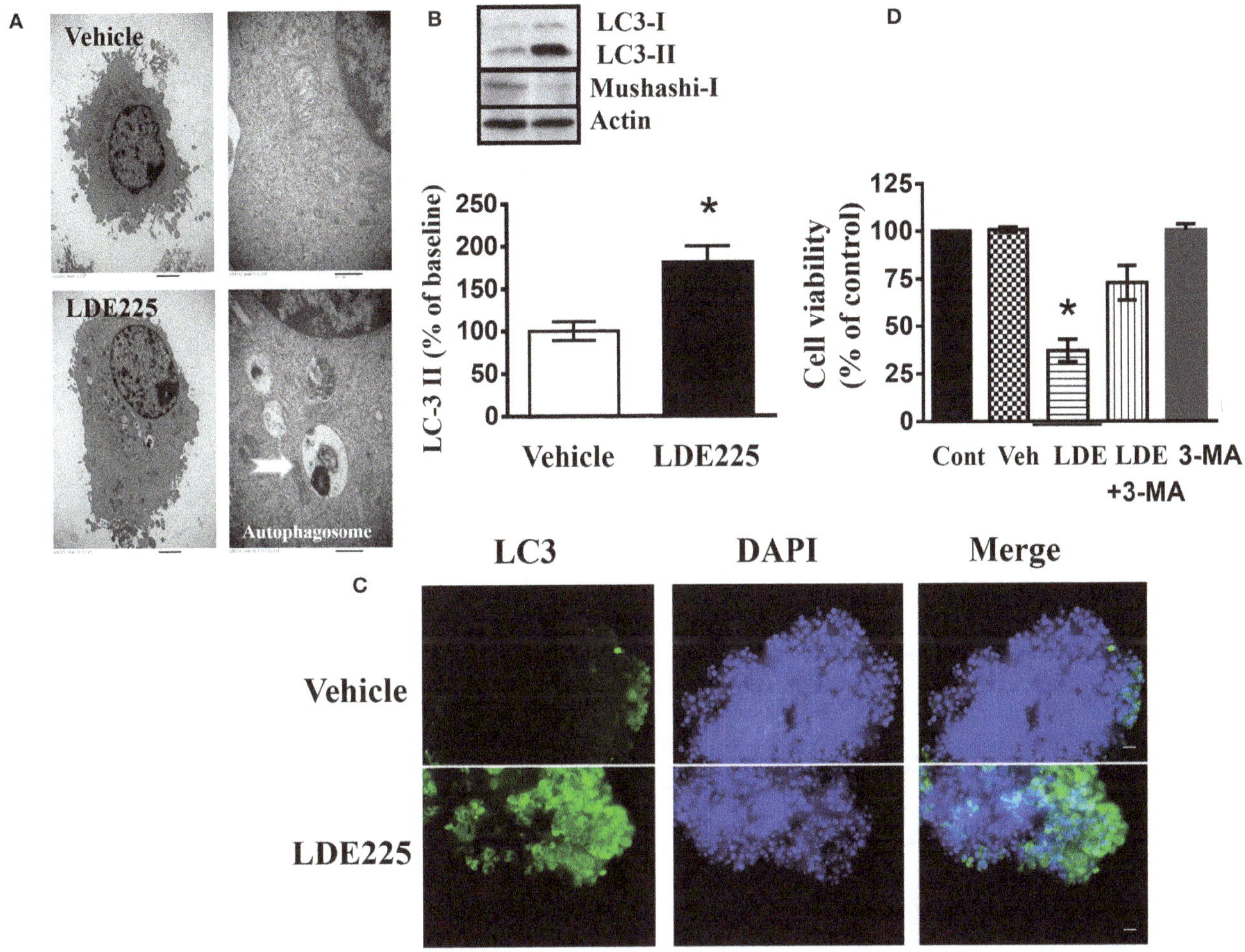

FIGURE 4 | LDE225 induces autophagy in the CD133$^+$ cells. **(A)** The graphs of transmission electron microscopy represented CD133$^+$ cells treated with LDE225 (25 µM) or vehicle for 48 h. Arrows indicate autophagosomes. **(B)** Western blot analysis of LC3-I/LC3-II and Mushashi-1 expression in the CD133$^+$ cells treated with LDE225 (25 µM) for 48 h. LDE225 induced conversion of LC3-I to LC3-II which was accompanied by the downregulation of Mushashi-1. **(C)** LC3 expression in CD133$^+$ cells treated with LDE225 (25 µM) or vehicle for 48 h. The fluorescence intensity of LC3 punctate increased after LDE225 treatment. **(D)** Block of LDE225-induced cell death by autophagy inhibitor 3-MA. CD133$^+$ cells were pretreated with 3-MA (3 µM) 1 h before the exposure to LDE225 (25 µM). Pretreatment with 3-MA attenuated LDE225-induced cell death. *$p < 0.05$.

autophagy plays a critical role in LDE225-induced cytotoxicity in CD133$^+$ cells.

We performed different apoptosis assays to evaluate whether LDE-induced cell death involves apoptosis. We used JC-1 mitochondrial membrane potential assay which measures the mitochondrial membrane potential as the indicator of cell health. Change in fluorescent property of JC-1 dye can be utilized to evaluate early apoptosis. CD133$^+$ cells were treated with LDE225 (25 µM) or 0.1% DMSO as vehicle control for 48 h. **Supplemental Figure 3A** shows that vehicle led to mitochondrial depolarization and decreased the ratio of J-aggregate/JC-1 monomer while that was not different between vehicle and LDE225 (25 µM) treatment. Caspase-Glo assay also revealed that Caspase 3/7 activity was not different between LDE225 and vehicle (**Supplemental Figure 3B**). These results suggest that LDE225-induced cell death likely was not mediated primarily through apoptosis.

Knockdown of Shh Slows Tumor Growth in an Intracranial Tumor Model

We clarified whether Shh plays a role in tumor growth under *in vivo* conditions using an orthotopic GBM model. To monitor intracranial tumor growth, we infected Luc-expressing CD133$^+$ cells with lentiviruses carrying the expression vector containing *Shh* shRNA. Transduced CD133$^+$ cells (8×10^4 cells) were injected intracranially into athymic mice and tumor growth was monitored using IVIS-200 imaging system. **Figure 5A** shows that tumor growth was much slower in *Shh* shRNA-knockdown mice than in control RNA-transfected mice. A two-way ANOVA revealed a main effect of group (*Shh* shRNA vs.

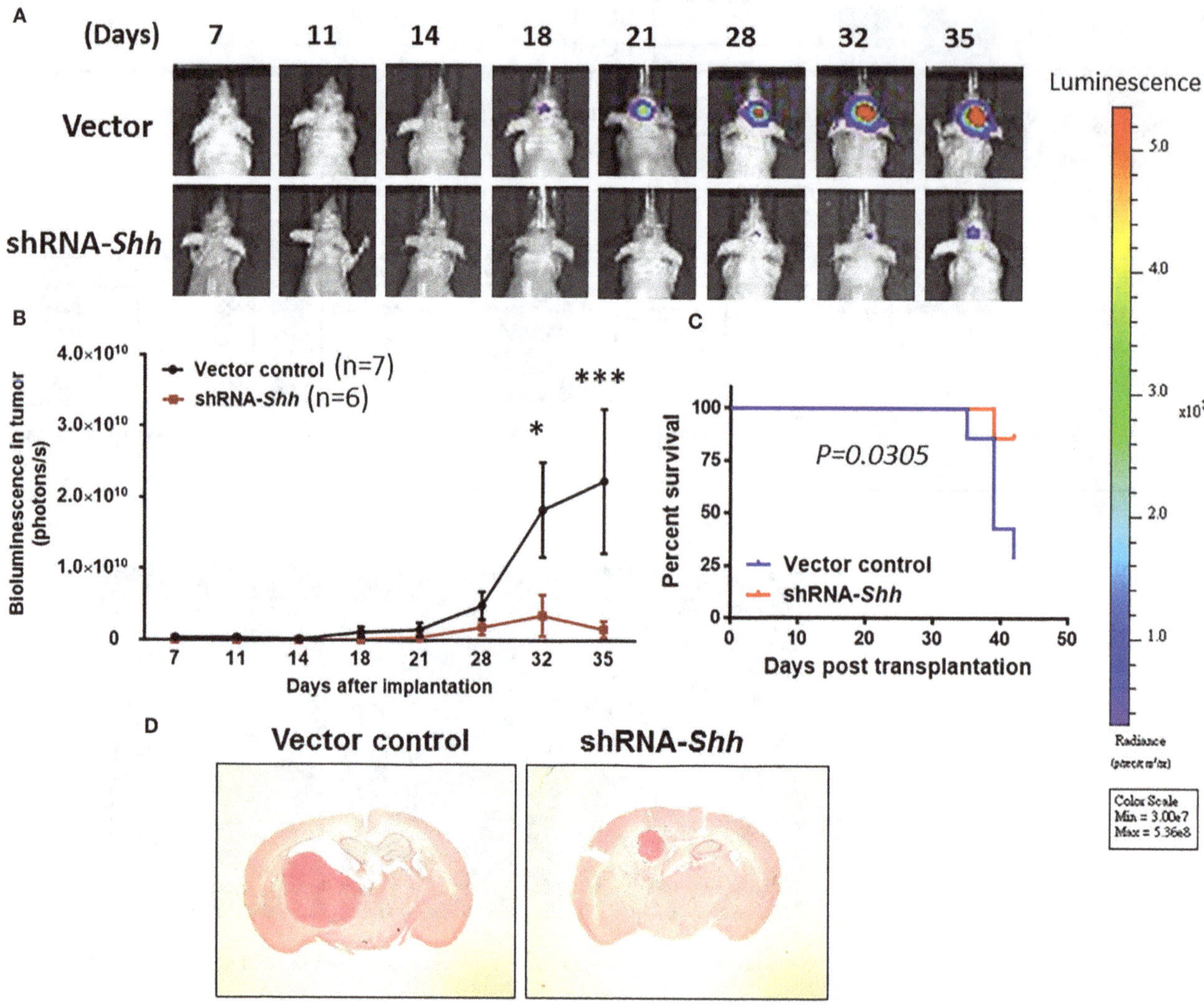

FIGURE 5 | Knockdown of Shh attenuates tumor growth in an intracranial tumor model. **(A)** Luc-expressing CD133$^+$ cells were infected with lentiviruses carrying the expression vector containing *Shh* shRNA. Transduced CD133$^+$ cells (8×10^4 cells) were injected intracranially into athymic mice and tumor growth was monitored using the IVIS-200 imaging system. **(B)** Tumor growth was much slower in *Shh* shRNA- transfected mice than in control RNA-transfected mice. $^*p < 0.05$, $^{***}p < 0.001$ vs. control RNA-transfected. **(C)** Kaplan–Meier analysis of *Shh* shRNA transfection on survival. **(D)** Brains of mice harboring tumors generated from control RNA-transfected mice and *Shh* shRNA-transfected mice and stained by H&E. Note that tumor in *Shh* shRNA-transfected mice was significantly larger than control RNA-transfected tumor.

control) [$F_{(1,11)} = 4.980, p < 0.05$], interaction [$F_{(7,77)} = 3.110, p < 0.01$] and days after application [$F_{(7,77)} = 4.853, p < 0.001$] (**Figure 5B**). Kaplan–Meier analysis of the survival data demonstrated a statistically significant difference ($p < 0.05$) in the median survival between vector control and *Shh* shRNA-treated mice (**Figure 5C**). Brain tumor growth was analyzed in coronal brain slices by H&E staining. As shown in **Figure 5D**, in comparison with vector control, shRNA-*Shh*-transfection generated significantly smaller intracranial tumor.

To examine whether knockdown of Shh affected autophagy and stemness *in vivo*, we examined the expression of LC3-II in *Shh* shRNA-treated mice. **Supplemental Figure 4** shows that the levels of Shh, CD133, mushashi-1 and SOX2 were lower whereas the conversion of LC3-I to LC3-II was higher in mice of Shh knockdown CD133$^+$ cells compared to CD133$^+$ cells of control mice. These results suggest that knockdown of *Shh* reduces stemness and GBM tumor growth.

Over-Expression of Shh Promotes Tumor Growth

To over-express Shh, we cloned the mouse *Shh* gene into parental U87 cells with lentiviruses carrying the expression vector containing *Shh* gene. The empty vector (LV-Vehicle) served as control. The LV-Shh or LV-vehicle transfected parental U87 GBM cells (8×10^4 cells) was injected intracranially into athymic mice. As shown in **Figures 6A,B**, tumor growth was much faster in LV-*Shh*-transfected mice than in LV-vehicle-transfected mice. A two-way ANOVA revealed a main effect

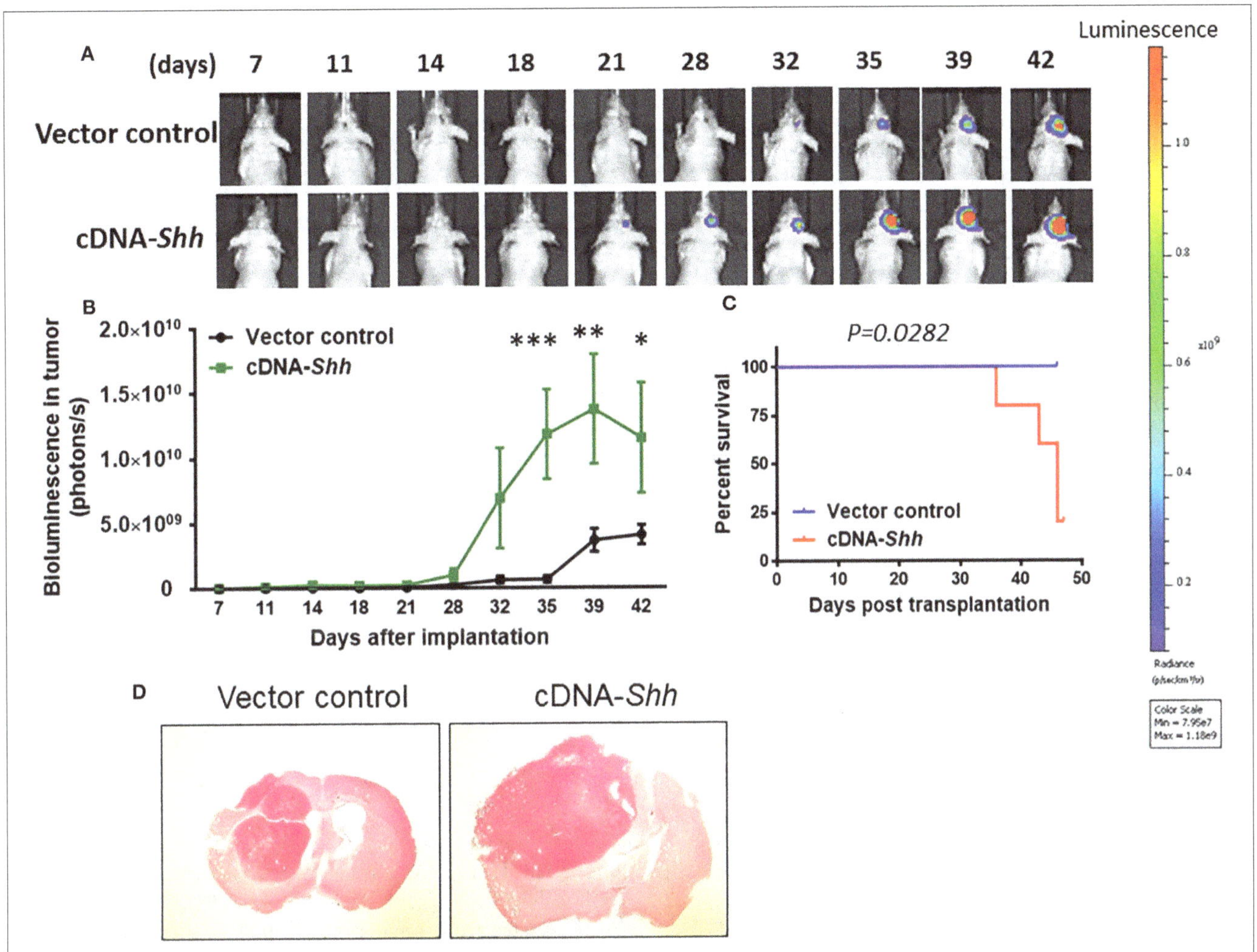

FIGURE 6 | Over-expression of Shh promotes tumor growth. **(A)** Shh overexpression in parental U87 cells was transduced by lentiviruses carrying the expression vector containing mouse *Shh* gene (LV-Shh). The empty vector (LV-Vehicle) served as control. The LV-Shh or LV-Vehicle infected U87 (8×10^4 cells) was injected intracranially into athymic mice. Tumor growth was monitored by IVIS-200 imaging system. **(B)** Tumor growth was much faster in LV-*Shh*-transfected mice than in LV-vehicle-transfected mice. $^*p < 0.05$, $^{**}p < 0.01$, $^{***}p < 0.001$ vs. vector control. **(C)** Kaplan–Meier analysis of over-expression of Shh transfection on survival. **(D)** Brains of mice harboring tumors generated from LV- Vehicle and LV-*Shh*-transfection and stained by H&E. Note that LV-*Shh*-transfection tumor was significantly larger than vector control tumor.

of group (LV-*Shh* vs. control) [$F_{(1,6)} = 7.665$, $p < 0.05$], interaction [$F_{(9,54)} = 4.022$, $p < 0.001$] and days after application [$F_{(9,54)} = 9.691$, $p < 0.001$]. Kaplan-Meier analysis of the survival data demonstrated a statistically significant difference ($p < 0.05$) in median survival between control and LV-*Shh*-treated mice (**Figure 6C**). Brain tumor size was analyzed in coronal brain slices. As shown in **Figure 6D**, in comparison with vector control, LV-*Shh*-transfection generated significantly larger intracranial tumor.

To examine whether over-expression of Shh affected autophagy and stemness *in vivo*, we examined the expression of LC3-II in LV-*Shh*-treated mice. **Supplemental Figure 5** shows that the levels of Shh, CD133, mushashi-1 and SOX2 were higher whereas the conversion of LC3-I to LC3-II was lower in Shh over-expression GBM compared to that of control. These results suggest that over-expression of *Shh* promotes cancer stemness and GBM tumor growth.

Additive Effect of Rapamycin and LDE225 on The Viability of $CD133^+$ Cells

Autophagy is negatively regulated by the mammalian target of rapamycin (mTOR) and can be induced by the mTOR inhibitor rapamycin (48–50). To confirm our hypothesis, we tested the effect of rapamycin on $CD133^+$ cells. Single treatment of $CD133^+$ cells with LDE225 (25 μM) or rapamycin (100 nM) inhibited the cell viability by 32.0 ± 7.9% ($n = 6$) and 24.6 ± 9.9% ($n = 6$), respectively. As shown in **Figure 7A**, combination of LDE225 and rapamycin resulted in 54.6 ± 3.3% ($n =$

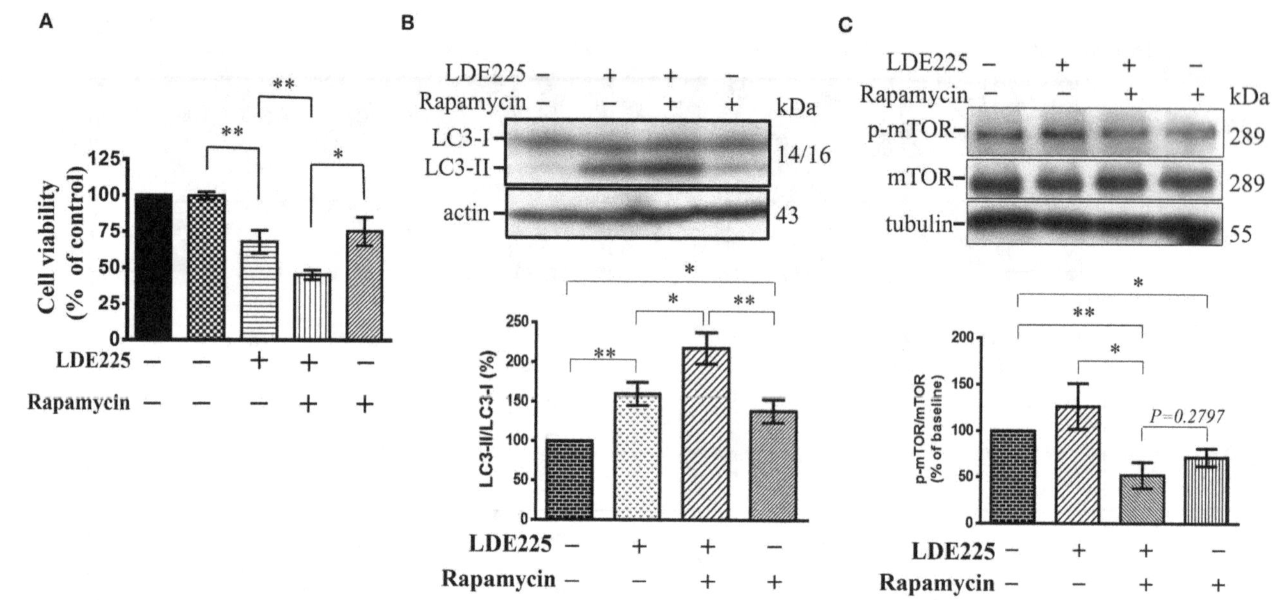

FIGURE 7 | LDE225 and rapamycin in combination additively reduces cell viability and induces conversion of LC3-I to LC3-II in $CD133^+$ cells. **(A)** $CD133^+$ cells were treated with LDE225 (25 μM) and rapamycin (100 nM) alone or in combination for 48 h and cell viability was assessed using WST-1 assay. **(B)** $CD133^+$ cells were treated with LDE225 (25 μM) and rapamycin (100 nM) alone or in combination for 48 h and the levels of LC3-I and LC3-II were measured by Western blotting analysis. **(C)** $CD133^+$ cells were treated with LDE225 (25 μM) and rapamycin (100 nM) alone or in combination for 48 h and the levels of p-mTOR and mTOR were measured by Western blotting analysis. Combined treatment with LDE225 and rapamycin reduced p-mTOR to the level not different from that treated with rapamycin alone (p = 0.2797). $^*p < 0.05$, $^{**}p < 0.01$.

6) inhibition ($p < 0.05$ vs. single treatment). Interestingly, combined treatment resulted in additive conversion of LC3-I to LC3-II. The conversion of LC3-I to LC3-II after LDE225 or rapamycin treatment was 159.8 ± 14.7% (n = 7) and 138.8 ± 14.5% (n = 7) of control, respectively. Combined treatment resulted in 217.7 ± 19.7% (n = 7) of control ($p < 0.05$ vs. LDE225, $p < 0.01$ vs. rapamycin) (**Figure 7B**).

Autophagy can also be induced through mTOR-independent pathway (50). We determined the effect of LDE225 (25 μM) on mTOR phosphorylation. LDE225 (25 μM) did not significantly influence the phosphorylated level of mTOR (p-mTOR) whereas rapamycin (100 nM) reduced it. Combined treatment with LDE225 and rapamycin reduced p-mTOR to the level not significantly different from treatment with rapamycin alone (p = 0.2797) (**Figure 7C**). Thus, it is likely that LDE225 induced autophagy through mTOR-independent pathway.

Amiodarone Reduces Stem-Like Cell Viability and Inhibits Tumor Formation

Amiodarone, a clinically used anti-arrhythmic drug, could induce autophagy via mTOR-independent signaling (51). We determined whether amiodarone reduced cancer stem-like cell viability *in vitro* and exhibited anti-tumor activity *in vivo*. $CD133^+$ cells were treated with amiodarone for 48 h and cell viability was assessed using WST-1 assay. As shown in **Figure 8A**, amiodarone dose-dependently reduced cell viability [$F_{(7,24)} = 16.71$, $p < 0.001$]. Immunoblotting using lysates from amiodarone (5 μM)-treated $CD133^+$ cells revealed a significant increase in processed LC3-II [$t_{(4)} = 4.3976$, $p < 0.05$] (**Figure 8B**). Furthermore, amiodarone-induced cell death was reversed by autophagy inhibitor 3-methyladenine (3-MA) (**Figure 8C**) suggesting that autophagy plays a critical role in amiodarone-induced cell death of $CD133^+$ cells. $CD133^+$ cells were treated with amiodarone (5 μM) or vehicle and $CD133^+$-derived tumor spheroids were counted at 1, 3, 7, and 14 days. Treatment with amiodarone significantly reduced the number of tumor spheroids [$t_{(4)} = 10.09$, $p < 0.001$, at 14 days culture] (**Figure 8D**).

We determined whether amiodarone inhibited tumor formation. Transduced $CD133^+$ cells (6×10^4 cells) were injected intracranially into athymic mice and tumor growth was monitored using IVIS-200 imaging system. At day 11, amiodarone was injected intraperitoneally once per day for 8 days (80 mg/kg) into the mice and tumor growth was observed for 17 more days. **Figure 9A** shows that tumor growth at day 35 was much slower in amiodarone-treated mice than in control vehicle-treated mice [$t_{(8)} = 2.758$, $p < 0.05$]. Brain tumor size was analyzed in coronal brain slices. As shown in **Figure 9B**, in comparison with vehicle control, amiodarone-treated mice generated significantly smaller intracranial tumor.

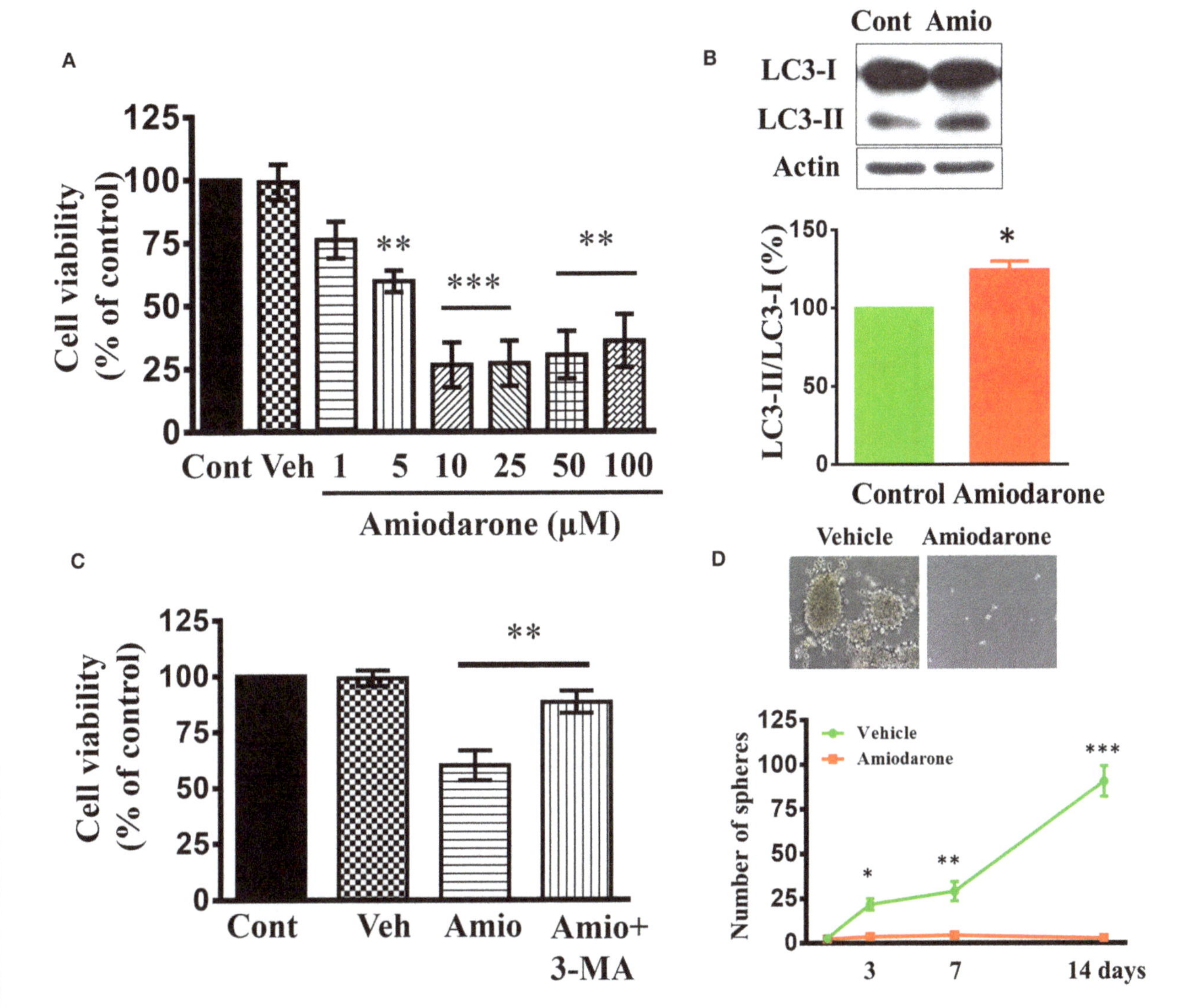

FIGURE 8 | Effects of amiodarone on the cell viability and tumor spheroid formation of $CD133^+$ cells. **(A)** Concentration-dependent effect of amiodarone on the cell viability of $CD133^+$ cells. $^{**}p < 0.01$, $^{***}p < 0.001$ vs. vehicle. **(B)** Western blot analysis of LC3-I and LC3-II expression in the $CD133^+$ cells treated with amiodarone (5 μM) for 48 h. **(C)** Block of amiodarone-induced cell death by autophagy inhibitor 3-MA. $CD133^+$ cells were pretreated with 3-MA (3 μM) 1 h before the exposure to amiodarone (5 μM). Pretreatment with 3-MA attenuated amiodarone-induced cell death. $^{**}p < 0.01$. **(D)** Effects of amiodarone (5 μM) on the number of tumor spheroids derived from $CD133^+$ cells. Primary tumor spheroids derived from $CD133^+$ were dissociated and cultured. They were then treated with amiodarone (5 μM) for the times as indicated. The medium was replaced every 2 days in the presence of amiodarone. $^{*}p < 0.05$, $^{**}p < 0.01$, $^{***}p < 0.001$ vs. Vehicle.

DISCUSSION

Roles of Shh Pathway in $CD133^+$ Cells-Derived Tumor Spheroid Formation and Tumorigenesis

We have isolated CD133-positive cells from human U87MG (U87) GBM cells using magnetic bead cell sorting (34). $CD133^+$-derived cell clones were able to grow *in vitro* in tumor spheroids and generate a tumor *in vivo* by intracranial cell injection in immunocompromised mice. The developmental signal transduction pathway mediated by Shh plays an important role during embryogenesis by regulating body patterning, cell proliferation and differentiation (52, 53). Activation of Shh has been causatively correlated with initiation and/or maintenance of cancer (54). In the present study, using Western blotting analysis and immunofluorescent staining, we showed that $CD133^+$ cells exhibited higher Shh expression compared to $CD133^-$ cells. Treatment with smoothened antagonist LDE225 significantly reduced the number of $CD133^+$ cells-derived tumor spheroids suggesting Shh signaling likely contributes to tumor spheroids formation *in vitro*. Silencing *Shh* gene with small hairpin interfering RNA inhibited tumor growth in an intracranial mouse model. Conversely, over-expression of *Shh* gene facilitated tumor

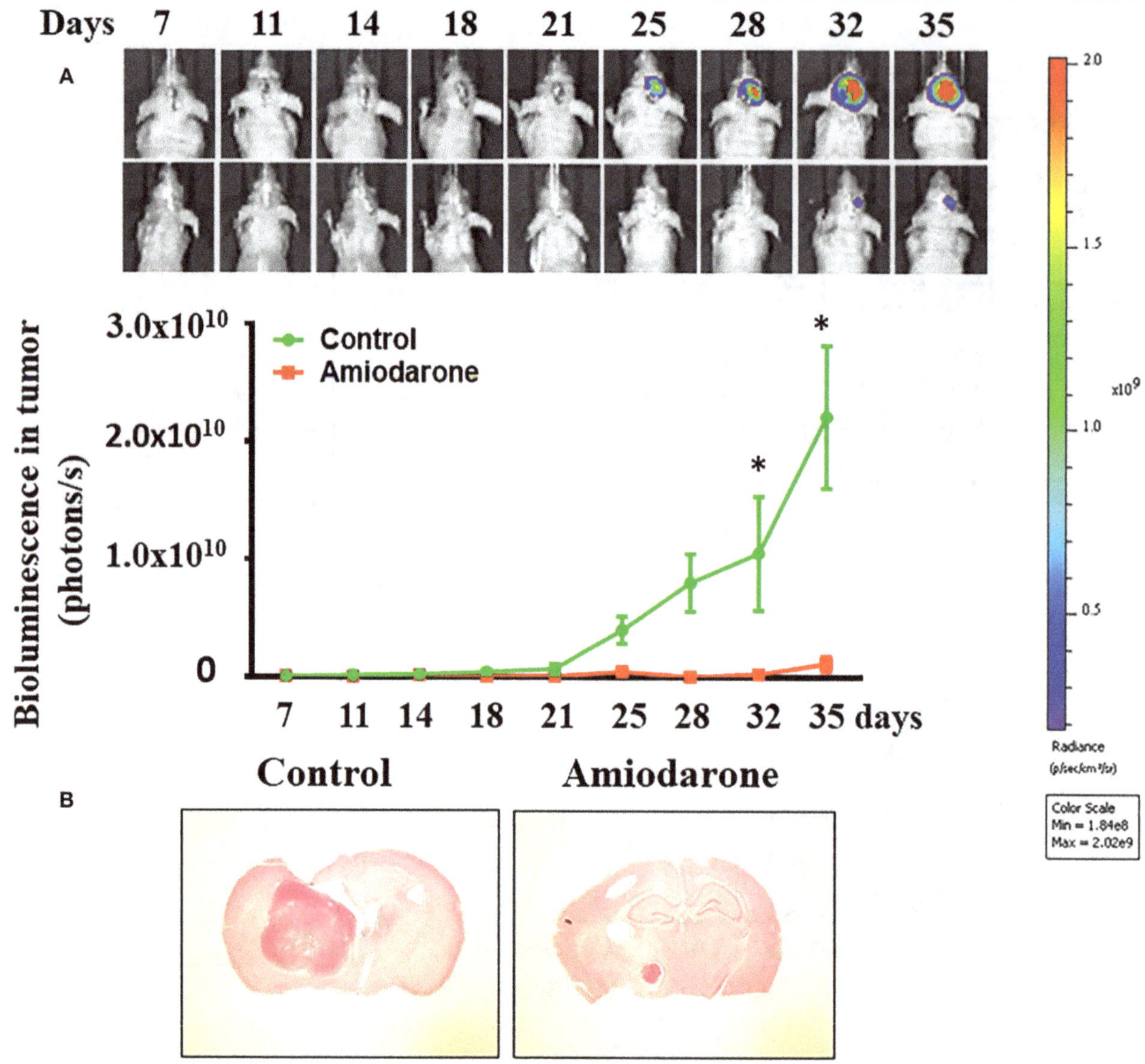

FIGURE 9 | Amiodarone slows tumor growth in an intracranial tumor model. **(A)** Transduced CD133$^+$ cells (6 × 10^4 cells) were injected intracranially into athymic mice and tumor growth was monitored using the IVIS-200 imaging system. At day 11, amiodarone was injected intraperitoneally once per day for 8 days (80 mg/kg) into the mice and tumor growth was observed for 17 more days. $^*p < 0.05$ vs. vehicle. **(B)** Amiodarone-treated mice generated significantly smaller intracranial tumor by H&E staining.

growth. Taken together, these results suggest that Shh signaling is involved in *in vitro* tumor spheroid formation and *in vivo* tumor growth.

Shh Inhibitor Reduces the Number of CD133$^+$-Derived Tumor Spheroids by Inducing Autophagy

The reports about the relationship between Shh and autophagy pathway in GBM are limited. One study in SHSY5Y cells showed that cyclopamine reduced serum starvation-induced LC3 positive cells but increased the levels of cleaved caspase 3 (54). They suggested that Shh inhibitor induced cell death by reducing autophagic processes concomitant with facilitating apoptotic cell death. In the present study, we demonstrated that LDE225 induced cell death in CD133$^+$ cells in a concentration-dependent manner with IC_{50} of ~20 µM. Similar inhibition of cell survival was observed after application of another Shh inhibitor cyclopamine. Electron microscopy examination revealed that, after exposure to LDE225, CD133$^+$ cells exhibited large membranous vacuoles in the cytoplasm that is a characteristic feature of cells undergoing autophagy. Further experiments of the conversion of LC3-I to LC3-II and attenuation of cell death by autophagy inhibitor 3-MA confirmed that

LDE225-induced autophagy in the CD133$^+$ cells. This study, in contrast to previous results, suggests that Shh inhibitor produces cytotoxicity in CD133$^+$ cells by inducing autophagic cell death.

To further test this hypothesis, we used rapamycin which is a mTOR inhibitor and is capable of inducing autophagy (49, 51). We found that rapamycin reduced CD133$^+$ cell viability. Interestingly, the effects of LDE225 and rapamycin were additive. Furthermore, LDE225 at the concentration that induced autophagy and reduced cell viability of CD133$^+$ cells did not affect the phosphorylated level of mTOR. Combined LDE225 and rapamycin failed to show further reduction of p-mTOR compared with rapamycin alone. These results suggest that LDE225 induces autophagy through mTOR-independent pathway. These findings also provide additional support that Shh regulation of autophagy plays an important role in the survival of GSCs. Thus, Shh pathway inhibitor could act as a sensitizer to increase efficiency of conventional chemotherapeutic agents in GBM by inducing cancer stem cell autophagic death.

Anti-tumorigenesis of Amiodarone

Amiodarone, a frequently prescribed anti-arrhythmic drugs in clinics, has been identified as a mTOR-independent autophagy enhancer (55, 56). If LDE225-induced cell death was mediated by the mTOR-independent autophagy, then amiodarone should produce similar effects as LDE225. Indeed, this was the case. Amiodarone reduced CD133$^+$ cell viability and tumor spheroid formation *in vitro* and exhibited anti-tumor efficacy *in vivo*.

In summary, there was a small percentage of human U87 GBM cells which were CD133-positive, exhibited cancer stem cell markers and were capable of forming tumor spheroids *in vitro* and tumor *in vivo*. These CD133$^+$ cells showed higher Shh expression and inhibition of Shh pathway with LDE225 reduced their survival and self-renew property. In LDE225-treated CD133$^+$ cells, there appeared large membranous vacuoles in the cytoplasm and the conversion of LC3-I to LC3-II. LDE225-induced cell death was reversed by autophagy inhibitor 3-MA, suggesting that LDE225-induced autophagic cell death in CD133$^+$ cells. Further, LDE225 did not affect the level of p-mTOR and combined LDE225 and rapamycin failed to show further reduction of p-mTOR when compared with rapamycin alone. Taken together, these results suggest that targeting Shh signal pathway may overcome chemoresistance and provide a therapeutic strategy for the treatment of malignant gliomas.

AUTHOR CONTRIBUTIONS

J-YC, C-LS, and P-WG contributed to the conception and design of the experiments. H-CH and C-CL performed the experiments and statistical analysis. C-LS and P-WG wrote the paper. All authors contributed to the article and approved the submitted version.

FUNDING

This study was supported by grants MOST 104-2320-B-006-007-MY3 and MOST-108-2320-B-006-008 from the Ministry of Sciences and Technology of Taiwan.

ACKNOWLEDGMENTS

We thank Dr. Yang-Kao Wang for providing lentiviral package plasmids, Dr. Shih-Chieh Lin for providing GFP/Luciferase plasmid, Dr. Min-Der Lai for correcting the grammar and scientific editing of the manuscript, and the Laboratory Animal Center, College ofMedicine, National Cheng Kung University and Taiwan Animal Consortium for the technical support in IVIS.

SUPPLEMENTARY MATERIAL

Supplemental Figure 1 | The differential expression of CD133 and cancer stem cell markers in parental GBM cells and tumor spheroids derived from CD133$^+$ cells. **(A)** Immunofluorescence staining of CD133, SOX2, ABCG2, and AIDH1A1 in parental U87 cells. **(B)** Immunofluorescence staining of ABCG2 and AIDH1A1 in tumor spheroids derived from CD133$^+$ cells.

Supplemental Figure 2 | The inhibitory effects of shh inhibition on cell proliferation. **(A)** Concentration-dependent effect of LDE225 on the cell viability of parental U87 cells. $^*p < 0.05$, $^{***}p < 0.001$ vs. vehicle. **(B)** Concentration-dependent effect of LDE225 on the cell viability of patient-derived P#5 cell line. $^*p < 0.05$, $^{***}p < 0.001$ vs. vehicle. **(C)** Concentration-dependent effect of cyclopamine on the cell viability of CD133$^+$ cells. $^*p < 0.05$, $^{***}p < 0.001$ vs. vehicle.

Supplemental Figure 3 | LDE225-induced cell death is not mediated primarily through apoptosis. CD133$^+$ cells were treated with LDE225 (25 μM) or vehicle for 48 h. **(A)** JC-1 assay detect the changes of mitochondria potential which is able to measure early apoptosis. Vehicle (0.1% DMSO) led to mitochondrial depolarization with the decreased ratio of J-aggregate/JC-1 monomer. There was not different from LDE225 (25 μM) treatment. **(B)** Caspase/Glo assay revealed the activity of Caspase 3/7. There was not different between LDE225 and vehicle treatment.

Supplemental Figure 4 | The conversion of LC3-I to LC3-II was enhanced in *Shh* shRNA transfection CD133$^+$-bearing mice. Tumor tissues were collected from *Shh* shRNA or vector-control transfection CD133$^+$-bearing mice. **(A)** The efficiency of *Shh* shRNA-mediated knockdown of Shh was confirmed by western blot analysis. **(B–D)** The levels of CD133 **(B)**, mushashi-1 **(C)**, and SOX2 **(D)** were lower in *Shh* shRNA transfection CD133$^+$-bearing mice. **(E)** The conversion of LC3-I to LC3-II was enhanced by *Shh* shRNA transfection. $^*p < 0.05$ vs. control.

Supplemental Figure 5 | The conversion of LC3-I to LC3-II was lower in Shh over-expression GBM-bearing mice. Tumor tissues were collected from LV-*Shh* or vector-control transfection GBM -bearing mice. **(A)** The efficiency of LV-*Shh*-mediated over-expression of Shh was confirmed by western blot analysis. **(B–D)** The levels of CD133 **(B)**, mushashi-1 **(C)**, and SOX2 **(D)** were higher in LV-*Shh* transfection GBM-bearing mice. **(E)** The conversion of LC3-I to LC3-II was reduced by LV-*Shh* transfection. $^*p < 0.05$, $^{**}p < 0.01$ vs. control.

REFERENCES

1. Jansen M, Yip S, Louis DN. Molecular pathology in adult gliomas: diagnostic, prognostic, and predictive markers. *Lancet Neurol.* (2010) 9:717–26. doi: 10.1016/S1474-4422(10)70105-8
2. Soderberg-Naucler C, Rahbar A, Stragliotto G. Survival in patients with glioblastoma receiving valganciclovir. *N Engl J Med.* (2013) 369:985–6. doi: 10.1056/NEJMc1302145
3. Wen PY, Kesari S. Malignant gliomas in adults. *N Engl J Med.* (2008) 359:492–507. doi: 10.1056/NEJMra0708126
4. Stevens MF, Hickman JA, Langdon SP, Chubb D, Vickers L, Stone R, et al.

Antitumor activity and pharmacokinetics in mice of 8-carbamoyl-3-methyl-imidazo[5,1-d]-1,2,3,5-tetrazin-4(3H)-one (CCRG 81045; M & B 39831), a novel drug with potential as an alternative to dacarbazine. *Cancer Res.* (1987) 47:5846–52.

5. Stupp R, Mason WP, van den Bent MJ, Weller M, Fisher B, Taphoorn MJ, et al. Radiotherapy plus concomitant and adjuvant temozolomide for glioblastoma. *N Engl J Med.* (2005) 352:987–96. doi: 10.1056/NEJMoa043330
6. Stupp R, Hegi ME, Mason WP, van den Bent MJ, Taphoorn MJ, Janzer RC, et al. Effects of radiotherapy with concomitant and adjuvant temozolomide versus radiotherapy alone on survival in glioblastoma in a randomised phase III study: 5-year analysis of the EORTC-NCIC trial. *Lancet Oncol.* (2009) 10:459–66. doi: 10.1016/S1470-2045(09)70025-7
7. Hou LC, Veeravagu A, Hsu AR, Tse VC. Recurrent glioblastoma multiforme: a review of natural history and management options. *Neurosurg Focus.* (2006) 20:E5. doi: 10.3171/foc.2006.20.4.2
8. Kioi M, Vogel H, Schultz G, Hoffman RM, Harsh GR, Brown JM. Inhibition of vasculogenesis, but not angiogenesis, prevents the recurrence of glioblastoma after irradiation in mice. *J Clin Invest.* (2010) 120:694–705. doi: 10.1172/JCI40283
9. Wong ET, Hess KR, Gleason MJ, Jaeckle KA, Kyritsis AP, Prados MD, et al. Outcomes and prognostic factors in recurrent glioma patients enrolled onto phase II clinical trials. *J Clin Oncol.* (1999) 17:2572–8. doi: 10.1200/JCO.1999.17.8.2572
10. Yung WK, Albright RE, Olson J, Fredericks R, Fink K, Prados MD, et al. A phase II study of temozolomide vs. procarbazine in patients with glioblastoma multiforme at first relapse. *Br J Cancer.* (2000) 83:588–93. doi: 10.1054/bjoc.2000.1316
11. Bao S, Wu Q, McLendon RE, Hao Y, Shi Q, Hjelmeland AB, et al. Glioma stem cells promote radioresistance by preferential activation of the DNA damage response. *Nature.* (2006) 444:756–60. doi: 10.1038/nature05236
12. Brada M, Hoang-Xuan K, Rampling R, Dietrich PY, Dirix LY, Macdonald D, et al. Multicenter phase II trial of temozolomide in patients with glioblastoma multiforme at first relapse. *Annals Oncol.* (2001) 12:259–66. doi: 10.1023/A:1008382516636
13. Frosina G. DNA repair and resistance of gliomas to chemotherapy and radiotherapy. *Mol Cancer Res.* (2009) 7:989–99. doi: 10.1158/1541-7786.MCR-09-0030
14. Schonberg DL, Lubelski D, Miller TE, Rich JN. Brain tumor stem cells: molecular characteristics and their impact on therapy. *Mol Aspects Med.* (2014) 39:82–101. doi: 10.1016/j.mam.2013.06.004
15. Ericson J, Morton S, Kawakami A, Roelink H, Jessell TM. Two critical periods of sonic hedgehog signaling required for the specification of motor neuron identity. *Cell.* (1996) 87:661–73. doi: 10.1016/S0092-8674008 1386-0
16. Chiang C, Litingtung Y, Lee E, Young KE, Corden JL, Westphal H, et al. Cyclopia and defective axial patterning in mice lacking sonic hedgehog gene function. *Nature.* (1996) 383:407–13. doi: 10.1038/383407a0
17. Wechsler-Reya RJ, Scott MP. Control of neuronal precursor proliferation in the cerebellum by sonic hedgehog. *Neuron.* (1999) 22:103–14. doi: 10.1016/S0896-6273(00)80682-0
18. Ruiz i Altaba A. Gli proteins and hedgehog signaling: development and cancer. *Trends Genet.* (1999) 15:418–25. doi: 10.1016/S0168-9525(99)01840-5
19. Kubo M, Nakamura M, Tasaki A, Yamanaka N, Nakashima H, Nomura M, et al. Hedgehog signaling pathway is a new therapeutic target for patients with breast cancer. *Cancer Res.* (2004) 64:6071–4. doi: 10.1158/0008-5472.CAN-04-0416
20. Katoh Y, Katoh M. Hedgehog target genes: mechanisms of carcinogenesis induced by aberrant hedgehog signaling activation. *Curr Mol Med.* (2009) 9:873–86. doi: 10.2174/156652409789105570
21. Gupta S, Takebe N, LoRusso P. Targeting the hedgehog pathway in cancer. *Ther Adv Med Oncol.* (2010) 2:237–50. doi: 10.1177/1758834010366430
22. Bar EE, Chaudhry A, Lin A, Fan X, Schreck K, Matsui W, et al. Cyclopamine-mediated hedgehog pathway inhibition depletes stem-like cancer cells in glioblastoma. *Stem Cells.* (2007) 25:2524–33. doi: 10.1634/stemcells.2007-0166
23. Rudin CM, Hann CL, Laterra J, Yauch RL, Callahan CA, Fu L, et al. Treatment of medulloblastoma with Hedgehog pathway inhibitor GDC-0449. *N Engl J Med.* (2009) 361:1202–5. doi: 10.1056/NEJMoa0902903
24. Von Hoff DD, Lorusso PM, Rudin CM, Reddy JC, Yauch RL, Tibes R, et al. Inhibition of the hedgehog pathway in advanced basal-cell carcinoma. *N Engl J Med.* (2009) 361:1164–72. doi: 10.1056/NEJMoa0905360
25. Chen J, Li Y, Yu TS, McKay RM, Burns DK, Kernie SG, et al. A restricted cell population propagates glioblastoma growth after chemotherapy. *Nature.* (2012) 488:522–6. doi: 10.1038/nature11287
26. Reya T, Morrison SJ, Clarke, MF, Weissman IL. Stem cells, cancer, and cancer stem cells. *Nature.* (2001) 414:105–11. doi: 10.1038/35102167
27. O'brien CA, Pollett A, Gallinger S, Dick JE. A human colon cancer cell capable of initiating tumour growth in immunodeficient mice. *Nature.* (2007) 445:106–10. doi: 10.1038/nature05372
28. Hemmati HD, Nakano I, Lazareff JA, Masterman-Smith M, Geschwind DH, Bronner-Fraser M, et al. Cancerous stem cells can arise from pediatric brain tumors. *Proc Natl Acad Sci USA.* (2003) 100:15178–83. doi: 10.1073/pnas.2036535100
29. Korkaya H, Wicha MS. Selective targeting of cancer stem cells: a new concept in cancer therapeutics. *BioDrugs.* (2007) 21:299–310. doi: 10.2165/00063030-200721050-00002
30. Jalili A, Mertz KD, Romanov J, Wagner C, Kalthoff F, Stuetz A, et al. NVP-LDE225, a potent and selective SMOOTHENED antagonist reduces melanoma growth *in vitro* and *in vivo*. *PLoS ONE.* (2013) 30:e69064. doi: 10.1371/journal.pone.0069064
31. Miller-Moslin K, Peukert S, Jain RK, McEwan MA, Karki R, lamas LL, et al. 1-amino-4-benzylphthalazines as orally bioavailable smoothened antagonists with antitumor activity. *J Med Chem.* (2009) 52:3954–68. doi: 10.1021/jm900309j
32. Singh SK, Clarke ID, Terasaki M, Bonn VE, Hawkins C, Squire J, et al. Identification of a cancer stem cell in human brain tumors. *Cancer Res.* (2003) 63:5821–8.
33. Pallini R, Ricci-Vitiani L, Montano N, Mollinari C, Biffoni M, Cenci T, et al. Expression of the stem cell marker CD133 in recurrent glioblastoma and its value for prognosis. *Cancer.* (2011) 117:162–74. doi: 10.1002/cncr.25581
34. Chang CH, Liu WT, Hung HC, Gean CY, Tsai HM, Su CL, et al. Synergistic inhibition of tumor growth by combination treatment with drugs against different subpopulations of glioblastoma cells. *BMC Cancer.* (2017) 17:905. doi: 10.1186/s12885-017-3924-y
35. Graham V, Khudyakov J, Ellis P, Pevny L. SOX2 functions to maintain neural progenitor identity. *Neuron.* (2003) 39:749–65. doi: 10.1016/S0896-6273(03)00497-5
36. Suh H, Consiglio A, Ray J, Sawai T, D'Amour KA, Gage FH. *In vivo* fate analysis reveals the multipotent and self-renewal capacities of Sox2+ neural stem cells in the adult hippocampus. *Cell Stem Cell.* (2007) 1:515–28. doi: 10.1016/j.stem.2007.09.002
37. Xu J, Peng H, Zhang JT. Human multidrug transporter ABCG2, a target for sensitizing drug resistance in cancer chemotherapy. *Curr Med Chem.* (2007) 14:689–701. doi: 10.2174/092986707780059580
38. Ma SA, Liu T, Jin Y, Wei J, Yang Y, Zhang H. ABCG2 is required for self-renewal and chemoresistance of CD133-positive human colorectal cancer cells. *Tumor Biol.* (2016) 37:12889–96. doi: 10.1007/s13277-016-5209-5
39. Silva IA, Bai S, McLean K, Yang K, Griffith K, Thomas D, et al. Aldehyde dehydrogenase in combination with CD133 defines angiogenic ovarian cancer stem cells that portend poor patient survival. *Cancer Res.* (2011) 71:3991–4001. doi: 10.1158/0008-5472.CAN-10-3175
40. Chang KY, Hsu TI, Hsu CC, Tsai SY, Liu JJ, Chou SW, et al. Specificity protein 1-modulated superoxide dismutase 2 enhances temozolomide resistance in glioblastoma, which is independent of O(6)-methylguanine-DNA methyltransferase. *Redox Biol.* (2017) 13:655–64. doi: 10.1016/j.redox.2017.08.005
41. Chang KY, Huang CT, Hsu TI, Hsu CC, Liu JJ, Chuang CK, et al. Stress stimuli induce cancer-stemness gene expression via Sp1 activation leading to therapeutic resistance in glioblastoma. *Biochem Biophys Res Commun.* (2017) 493:14–9. doi: 10.1016/j.bbrc.2017.09.095
42. Chen JK, Taipale J, Cooper MK, Beachy PA. Inhibition of hedgehog signaling by direct binding of cyclopamine to smoothened. *Genes Dev.* (2002) 6:2743–8. doi: 10.1101/gad.1025302
43. Kabeya Y, Mizushima N, Ueno T, Yamamoto A, Kirisako T, Noda T, et al. LC3, a mammalian homologue of yeast Apg8p, is localized in

autophagosome membranes after processing. *EMBO J.* (2000) 19:5720–8. doi: 10.1093/emboj/19.21.5720
44. Klionsky DJ, Cuervo AM, Seglen PO. Methods for monitoring autophagy from yeast to human. *Autophagy.* (2007) 3:181–206. doi: 10.4161/auto.3678
45. Li P, Du Q, Cao Z, Guo Z, Evankovich J, Yan W, et al. Interferon-γ induces autophagy with growth inhibition and cell death in human hepatocellular carcinoma (HCC) cells through interferon-regulatory factor-1 (IRF-1). *Cancer Lett.* (2012) 314:213–22. doi: 10.1016/j.canlet.2011.09.031
46. Kaneko Y, Sakakibara S, Imai T, Suzuki A, Nakamura Y, Sawamoto K, et al. Musashi 1: an evolutionarily conserved marker for CNS progenitor cells including neural stem cells. *Dev Neurosci.* (2000) 22:139–53. doi: 10.1159/000017435
47. Klionsky DJ, Abeliovich H, Agostinis P, Agrawal DK, Aliev G, Askew DS, et al. Guidelines for the use and interpretation of assays for monitoring autophagy in higher eukaryotes. *Autophagy.* (2008) 4:151–75. doi: 10.4161/auto.5338
48. Fleming A, Noda T, Yoshimori T, Rubinsztein DC. Chemical modulators of autophagy as biological probes and potential therapeutics. *Nat Chem Biol.* (2011) 7:9–17. doi: 10.1038/nchembio.500
49. Kim YC, Guan KL. mTOR: a pharmacologic target for autophagy regulation. *J Clin Invest.* (2015) 125:25–32. doi: 10.1172/JCI73939
50. Sarkar S, Ravikumar B, Floto RA, Rubinsztein DC. Rapamycin and mTOR-independent autophagy inducers ameliorate toxicity of polyglutamine-expanded huntingtin and related proteinopathies. *Cell Death Differ.* (2009) 16:46–56. doi: 10.1038/cdd.2008.110
51. Renna M, Jimenez-Sanchez J, Sarkar S, Rubinsztein DC. Chemical inducers of autophagy that enhance the clearance of mutant proteins in neurodegenerative diseases. *J Biol Chem.* (2010) 285:11061–7. doi: 10.1074/jbc.R109.072181
52. Ingham PW, Nakano Y, Seger C. Mechanisms and functions of Hedgehog signalling across the metazoa. *Nat Rev Genet.* (2011) 12:393–406. doi: 10.1038/nrg2984
53. Robbins DJ, Fei DL, Riobo NA. The hedgehog signal transduction network. *Sci Signal.* (2012) 5:re6. doi: 10.1126/scisignal.2002906
54. Milla LA, Gonzalez-Ramirez CN, Palma V. Sonic hedgehog in cancer stem cells: a novel link with autophagy. *Biol Res.* (2012) 45:223–30. doi: 10.4067/S0716-97602012000300004
55. Zhang L, Yu J, Pan H,Hu P, Hao Y, Cai W, et al. Small molecule regulators of autophagy identified by an image-based high-throughput screen. *Proc Natl Acad Sci USA.* (2007) 104:19023–8. doi: 10.1073/pnas.0709695104
56. Williams A, Sarkar S, Cuddon P, Ttofi EK, Saiki S, Siddiqi FH, et al. Novel targets for Huntington's disease in an mTOR-independent autophagy pathway. *Nat Chem Biol.* (2008) 4:295–305. doi: 10.1038/nchembio.79

11

Integrated Transcriptome Analyses and Experimental Verifications of Mesenchymal-Associated TNFRSF1A as a Diagnostic and Prognostic Biomarker in Gliomas

Biao Yang[1†], Yuan-Bo Pan[2†], Yan-Bin Ma[1] and Sheng-Hua Chu[1*]

[1] *Department of Neurosurgery, Shanghai Ninth People's Hospital Affiliated to Shanghai Jiao Tong University School of Medicine, Shanghai, China,* [2] *Department of Neurosurgery, Second Affiliated Hospital, School of Medicine, Zhejiang University, Hangzhou, China*

***Correspondence:**
Sheng-Hua Chu
shenghuachu@126.com

†*These authors have contributed equally to this work*

Gliomas are the most prevalent malignant primary brain tumors with poor outcome, and four different molecular subtypes (Mesenchymal, Proneural, Neural, and Classical) are popularly applied in scientific researches and clinics of gliomas. Public databases contain an abundant genome-wide resource to explore the potential biomarker and molecular mechanisms using the informatics analysis. The aim of this study was to discover the potential biomarker and investigate its effect in gliomas. Weighted gene co-expression network analysis (WGCNA) was used to construct the co-expression modules and explore the biomarker among the dataset CGGA mRNAseq_693 carrying 693 glioma samples. Functional annotations, ROC, correlation, survival, univariate, and multivariate Cox regression analyses were implemented to investigate the functional effect in gliomas, and molecular experiments *in vitro* were performed to study the biological effect on glioma pathogenesis. The brown module was found to be strongly related to WHO grade of gliomas, and KEGG pathway analysis demonstrated that TNFRSF1A was enriched in MAPK signaling pathway and TNF signaling pathway. Overexpressed TNFRSF1A was strongly related to clinical features such as WHO grade, and functioned as an independent poor prognostic predictor of glioma patients. Notably, TNFRSF1A was preferentially upregulated in the Mesenchymal subtype gliomas (Mesenchymal-associated). Knockdown of TNFRSF1A inhibited proliferation and migration of glioma cell lines *in vitro*. Our findings provide a further understanding of the progression of gliomas, and Mesenchymal-associated TNFRSF1A might be a promising target of diagnosis, therapy, and prognosis of gliomas.

Keywords: TNFRSF1A, subtype, prognosis, mesenchymal, proliferation, glioma

INTRODUCTION

Gliomas are the most prevalent malignant primary brain tumors (1). The origination of gliomas remains unclear, which are generally named according to the similar features to the normal glial cells (2). World Health Organization (WHO) gliomas are divided into low-grade gliomas (LGGs, grade I/II) and high-grade gliomas (HGGs, grade III/IV), respectively (3). Gliomas contain different

Central Nervous System (CNS) cancers that generated from the glial cells such as astrocytomas, anaplastic astrocytomas, and glioblastoma multiformes (GBMs). Among these different gliomas, GBMs (grade IV) account for 70% gliomas and represent the malignant tumor of gliomas with a poor overall survival (OS) time of 12–18 months (4). In 2016, molecular characteristics, including isocitrate dehydrogenase (IDH) mutation and 1p/19q codeletion, are included into the revised the classification of the CNS Tumors (5). With the rapid advances in the sequencing technology, personalized molecular subtypes were constructed and more molecular markers are identified. Based on a study of The Cancer Genome Atlas (TCGA), glioblastoma multiforme (GBM) were divided into four molecular subtypes: Proneural, Neural, Classical and Mesenchymal by using by abnormalities in PDGFRA, IDH1, EGFR, and NF1 (6). Additionally, a study found that low vimentin was a favorable prognostic biomarker with a better response to temozolomide therapy, and vimentin expression was also related to grade of glioma patients (7). These molecular subtypes and biomarkers promote the diagnostic accuracy as well as diagnostic effect and prognosis assessment in glioma patients. Moreover, the researches on the molecular subtypes and markers remain a hot topic area of gliomas.

Weighted gene co-expression network analysis (WGCNA) is a systems bioinformatics method used to construct co-expression modules by the different correlation patterns among genes and select the hub genes related to the certain clinical feature by the intra-modular connectivity (IC) (8). WGCNA has already been successfully utilized in many studies (9, 10). Using the genome-transcriptiomic data of gastric cancer (GC) cell lines from Cancer Cell Line Encyclopedia (CCLE), Xiang et al. found that upregulated COL12A1 and LOXL2 were associated with IDO1 expression, and further biological experiments verified that IDO1 and COL12A1 could synergistically improve GC metastasis (11). Zhang et al. adopted WGCNA and protein-protein interaction (PPI) analysis to reveal that Tgfβ2, Wnt9a, and Fgfr4 were the hub genes regulating the differentiation of aging satellite cells (12). Thus, WGCNA is good at identifying the potential biomarker and its mechanisms of diseases.

Tumor necrosis factor α (TNF-α) is a highly active cytokine participating in the signaling pathway of necrosis or apoptosis (13). TNF receptor (TNFR1) regulates cell survival, apoptosis and inflammation via activating TNF-induced NF-κB signaling pathway (14). TNF receptor superfamily member 1A (TNFRSF1A) is a member of the TNF receptor superfamily of proteins (15). TNFRSF1A polymorphism rs4149584 was found to alleviate the severity of multiple sclerosis patients by decreasing age at disease onset and retarding disease progression (16). TNFRSF1A also functions as a target gene of miR-29a promoting the apoptosis of AR42J cells in acute pancreatitis (14). A recent study found that a four-gene panel of CD44, ABCC3, TNFRSF1A, and MGMT could act as the prediction of GBM patients' therapy response (17). However, the role of TNFRSF1A in the development of gliomas still remains unclear.

In this study, TNFRSF1A was identified as a biomarker of molecular subtypes and an independent prognostic factor of gliomas based on the integrated bioinformatics analyses. TNFRSF1A is highly expressed in glioma tissues compared with normal brain tissues, and is related to poor prognosis of glioma patients. Knockdown of TNFRSF1A inhibited glioma cell proliferation and migration. These findings show that TNFRSF1A might be a significantly independent prognostic factor and a potential therapeutic target of gliomas.

MATERIALS AND METHODS

Downloading and Preprocessing of mRNA Data and Clinical Information

The glioma expression profiles with clinical information were downloaded from the Gene Expression Omnibus (GEO; http://www.ncbi.nlm.nih.gov/geo/) database, including GSE4271, GSE4290, GSE4412, GSE13041, and GSE68848. The GSE4271 and GSE4412 datasets were originated from GPL96, and the dataset GSE13041 with 267 samples included three platforms GPL96, GPL570, and GPL8300. And the dataset GSE4271 was used for correlation analyses between TNFRSF1A expression and microvascular proliferation or necrosis. And the two datasets GSE4290 and GSE68848 were generated from same microarray platform GPL570. In addition, RNA-seq data of LGGs and GBM were downloaded from The Cancer Genome Atlas (TCGA; http://cancergenome.nih.gov/). Moreover, three datasets with mRNA data and clinical information (containing molecular subtypes, WHO grade, IDH mutation, 1p/19q codeletion, and chemotherapy and radiotherapy status), including mRNA-array_301 with 301 glioma samples, mRNAseq_325 with 325 gliomas and mRNAseq_693 with 693 gliomas, were acquired from the Chinese Glioma Genome Altas (CGGA; http://www.cgga.org.cn/) database. Data preprocessing in different datasets were implemented. And all of these datasets were used to conduct correlation analyses between TNFRSF1A expression and clinical features (age, molecular subtypes, WHO grade and so on). Moreover, the datasets (mRNA-array_301, mRNAseq_325 and mRNAseq_693 of CGGA, GSE4271, GSE4412, GSE68848, TCGA_glioma, and TCGA_LGG) were used to perform survival and Cox regression analyses.

As we have previously described Molnar et al. (13), differentially expressed genes (DEGs) were identified between 504 HGG samples and 188 LGG samples in the dataset CGGA mRNAseq_693 using package Limma in R 3.5.0. And the expression profile of DEGs in CGGA mRNAseq_693 was used for WGCNA.

Additionally, Oncomine (https://www.oncomine.org) is an online database containing numerous available microarray data of the different tumors. Comparison statistical analysis of TNFRSF1A expression between brain/ CNS cancers and corresponding normal samples with the threshold of $P < 0.05$ and fold-change (FC)>0 was implemented using this tool (14). Gene Expression Profiling Interactive Analysis 2 (GEPIA2; http://gepia.cancer-pku.cn/index.html), based on the both TCGA and GTEx databases, is used to perform the correlation and survival analyses in this study (15). The Human Protein Atlas (HPA; https://www.proteinatlas.org), an immunohistochemistry-based expression data of the all proteins in normal and tumor samples, was used to determine the expression level of the protein TNFRSF1A in this study (16).

Construction of WGCNA

On the basis of the profile CGGA mRNAseq_693 carrying gene, weighted gene co-expression network was constructed using the WGCNA package in R (17). After cutting off the outliers, a proper soft-thresholding power (β) was determined to satisfy the scale-free topology, and then the adjacencies were turned into topological overlap matrix (TOM). The correlations between co-expression modules and clinical data (including age, subtypes, WHO grades and so on) were calculated by Pearson's correlation coefficient to explore the potentially biological value of the modules. Top 10 mRNAs with the highest IC in the interested module were selected as hub genes for the next analyses.

Functional Annotation for the Brown Module

For all mRNAs in the interested brown module, the Database for Annotation, Visualization and Integrated Discovery (DAVID, https://david.ncifcrf.gov/) v6.8 was used for functional enrichment analyses along with Gene Ontology (GO) and Kyoto Encyclopedia of Genes and Genomes (KEGG) pathway analyses (18, 19). The functional analysis results were displayed using the GOplot package in R (20). $P < 0.01$ was set as the cutoff criteria.

Cell Culture and RNA Interference

The human GBM cell lines (U87 and U251) were provided by Department of Neurosurgery, Shanghai Ninth People's Hospital Affiliated to Shanghai Jiao Tong University School of Medicine, and were cultured in Dulbecco's modified Eagle's medium (DMEM) supplemented with 10% fetal bovine serum (FBS) at 37°C in a 5% CO_2 atmosphere. And small interfering RNAs siRNAs specifically targeting TNFRSF1A (siRNA1, siRNA2, siRNA3), siRNA scrambled control (si-NC) were obtained from RiboBio (Guangzhou, China). qRT-PCR and western blotting was used to evaluate the specificity and efficacy of siRNAs and scrambled control.

RNA Extraction and Quantitative Real-Time Polymerase Chain Reaction (qRT-PCR)

In brief, total RNA was collected from cell lines using TRIzol reagent (Invitrogen, Carlsbad, CA, USA) for the reverse transcription reaction. GAPDH was used as an internal control. The primer sequences used were listed as below: TNFRSF1A, forward: 5′-TGCCATGCAGGTTTCTTTCT-3′, reverse: 5′-CACAACTTCGTGCACTCCAG-3′; GAPDH, forward: 5′-AGGTCGGAGTCAACGGATTT-3′, reverse: 5′-ATCTCGCTCCTGGAAGATGG-3′. The gene expression level was normalized to the internal control GAPDH. The relative expression level of TNFRSF1A was determined using the 2–ΔΔCt.

Western Blotting

As we have previously described Chen et al. (21), total protein samples were then separated by 15% SDS-PAGE and transferred onto PVDF membranes. Membranes were incubated overnight at 4°C after blocking with primary antibody anti-TNFRSF1A. Following washing and incubation, membranes were incubated with secondary antibody in TBST. Brands were detected using an enhanced chemiluminescence system.

Cell Counting Kit-8 (CCK-8) Assay

To explore cell proliferation ability, cells were cultured in 96-well plates with a density of 5 × 103 cells/well. CCK8 was performed according to the manufacture's instruction. After 4 h of incubation at 37°C in the presence of 5% CO_2, the absorbance of each well was measured at 450 nm by using a spectrophotometer at day 1, 2, 3, 4, 5, and 6 after initial plating.

Colony Formation Assay

According to the manufacture's instruction cells were inoculated and cultivated onto the 6-well plates (1 × 103 cells/well). The cells were then fixed with 4% paraformaldehyde for 30 min and stained with crystal violet for 30 min at room temperature. Final results were shown as an average of three independent assays.

Transwell Assay

Cell migration ability was conducted using Transwell assay. A total of 105 cells in FBS-free DMEM were added to the top chamber, while DMEM containing 10% FBS was added to the bottom chamber. After 24 h of incubation, the migrated cells were fixed with 100% methanol and stained with 0.5% crystal violet at room temperature. Images captured with a digital camera. The values for migration and invasion were obtained by counting three randomly selected fields.

Statistical Analyses

Statistical analyses were calculated by using SPSS 21.0 (San Diego, CA, USA), GraphPad Prism 7.0 (San Diego, CA, USA) or software R 3.5.0. The Pearson's correlation coefficient analysis was used to analyze the correlations. Comparisons of two groups were performed by unpaired student's t-test. Receiver operating characteristic (ROC) curves, and Cox regression analyses were implemented using R 3.5.0. Kaplane-Meier survival analysis was performed by GEPIA2 or R 3.5.0. Experimental data are displayed as the mean ± the standard deviation (SD), and $P < 0.05$ was considered to be statistically significant.

RESULTS

Construction of WGCNA

After difference analysis, a total of 1456 DEGs were identified between HGGs and LGGs with the cut-off criteria of $P < 0.05$ and $|\log2FC|>0.5$ using R language. Next, the expression profile of these DEGs was used to build the co-expression expression network using the WGCNA package in R. No outlier was identified (**Supplementary Figure 1**). The network topology was shown when different soft-thresholding powers (β) were set, and when the power was 5, the topology was roughly calculated being more than 0.85 (**Figures 1A,B**). Connectivity distribution and the scale-free topology were further analyzed. In fact, the scale-free topology (R^2) was 0.84 when $\beta = 5$ (**Figure 1C**), and on the other hand $R^2 = 0.9$ when $\beta = 6$ (**Figure 1D**). Clustering

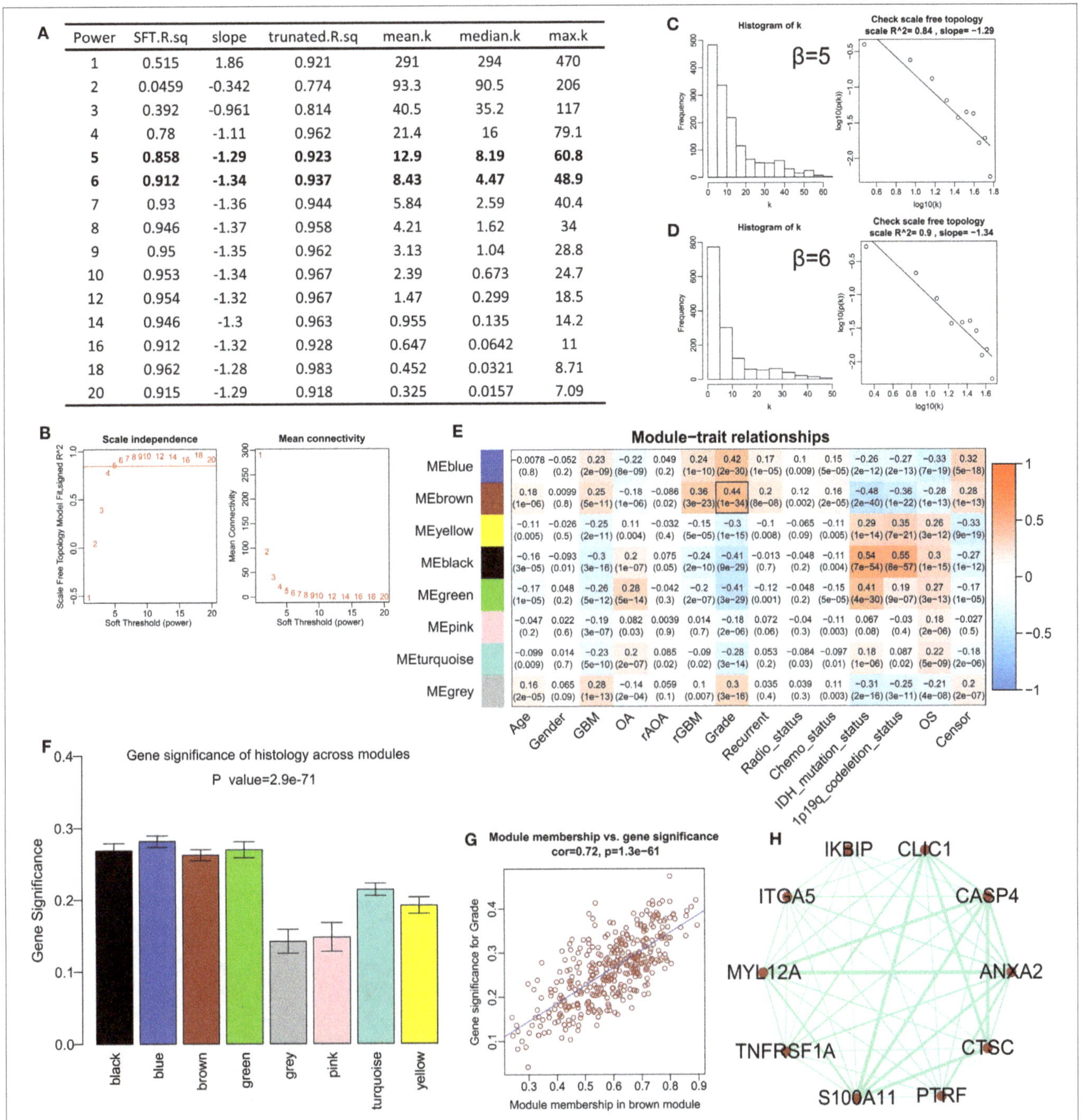

FIGURE 1 | Construction of the weighted gene co-expression network analysis in CGGA mRNAseq_693. **(A)** Table of network topology for various soft-thresholding powers (β). **(B)** Analyses of network topology for various soft-thresholding powers, and the scale-free topology were set as 0.85 roughly. **(C)** Histogram of connectivity distribution and checking the scale free topology ($R^2 = 0.84$) when $\beta = 5$. **(D)** Histogram of connectivity distribution and checking the scale-free topology ($R^2 = 0.9$) when $\beta = 6$. **(E)** Module-trait relationships. The brown module was strongly associated with the WHO grade. **(F)** Distribution of average gene significance and errors in different modules. **(G)** Scatter plots for correlations between module membership and gene significance in brown module. **(H)** The network for top 10 hub genes in brown module.

dendrogram of genes was shown in **Supplementary Figure 2**, and atotal of seven modules and a gray module were screened (**Figure 1E**). From the module-trait relationships in **Figure 1E**, the brown module consisted of 378 genes was found to be the most significant module related to WHO grade ($r = 0.44$, $P =$ 1e−34). The gene significances of the modules were shown in **Figure 1F**, and the correlation (correlation = 0.72, $P =$ 1.3e−61) was analyzed between module membership and gene significance of the brown module (**Figure 1G**). Top 10 genes with highest intra-modular connectivity was extracted as hub genes in brown module, including CLIC1, ANXA2, CASP4, ITGA5, MYL12A, S100A11, TNFRSF1A, CTSC, PTRF and IKBIP (**Figure 1H**).

Functional Enrichment Annotations of the Brown Module

GO analyses contained biological process (BP), molecular function (MF) and cell component (CC), and top 10 significant terms in each category were chosen using the online database DAVID in this study. The GO analysis results showed that all genes of the brown modules were significantly associated with extracellular matrix organization and immune response in BP (**Figure 2A**); extracellular space and extracellular exosome in CC (**Figure 2B**); and heparin binding and integrin binding in MF (**Figure 2C**). For the KEGG analysis, the genes with at least two terms, and the term which includes at least five genes are shown in this plot. Ultimately, seven signaling pathway terms were extracted, and TNFRSF1A was enriched in MAPK signaling pathway (**Figure 2D**).

TNFRSF1A Was Overexpressed and Related to Clinical Features in Gliomas

KEGG result showed that MAPK signaling pathway, which played an important role in the development of gliomas, contained 13 genes of this study. Additionally, TNFRSF1A was identified by merging of top 10 hub genes in brown module and these 13 genes of MAPK signaling pathway (**Supplementary Figure 3**). From the bodymap from the online tool GEPIA2 in **Figure 3A**, change fold of the median expression of TNFRSF1A between the brain tumor (red) and the corresponding normal brain (green) samples was obvious, which suggested that TNFRSF1A expression might have a significant difference between brain tumors and normal brain tissues. Furthermore, the TNFRSF1A expression prolife of various tumors from the GEPIA2 illustrated that TNFRSF1A was significantly overexpressed in four kinds of tumors compared with the corresponding normal samples, including GBM, LAML (acute myeloid leukemia), LGG and PAAD (pancreatic adenocarcinoma) (**Figure 3B**). The boxplots precisely revealed that TNFRSF1A expression was

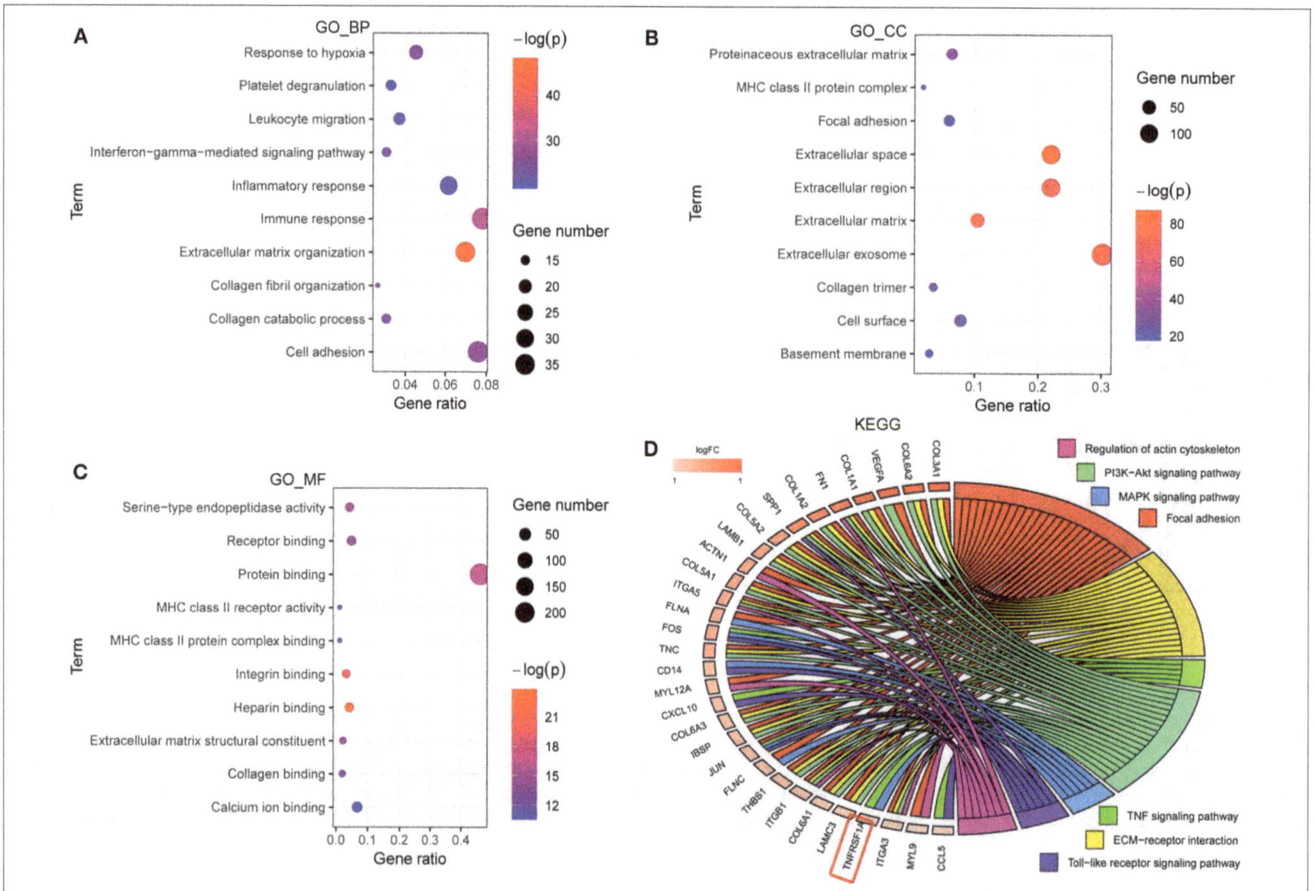

FIGURE 2 | The functional enrichment analyses of all genes in brown module. **(A–C)** The plots for the top 10 significant enrichment annotations of all genes in brown module for BP, CC and MF in GO, respectively. **(D)** KEGG analysis was visualized using the package GOplot in R. The plot included 7 KEGG pathway terms. The genes with at least two terms, and the term which includes at least five genes are shown in this plot. Log_2foldchange (logFC) represents the difference between high-grade gliomas and low-grade gliomas in the dataset CGGA mRNAseq_693. GO, Gene Ontology; BP, biological process; CC, cellular component; MF, molecular function; KEGG, Kyoto Encyclopedia of genes and genomes.

upregulated in gliomas (LGGs and GBMs) compared with the normal corresponding samples using the GEPIA2 (**Figure 3C**). Moreover, the comparison analyses across 6 datasets from the Oncomine database showed that TNFRSF1A in gliomas was significantly upregulated compared with normal samples with the cut-off of $P < 0.05$ and FC > 2 as well as gene rank = 10% (**Figure 3D**). On the other hand, TNFRSF1A expression increased in the order of control (normal brain) tissues, oligodendroglioma, astrocytoma, and GBM (**Figures 3E–G**). Interestingly, TNFRSF1A expression was upregulated in the order of control samples, LGGs and HGGs (**Figures 3H–J**). More importantly, the expression level of TNFRSF1A was positively associated with WHO grade in the eight datasets, including GSE4290, GSE68848, CGGA (mRNA-array_301, mRNAseq_325 and mRNAseq_693), TCGA_glioma, GSE4271 and GSE4412, respectively (**Figures 3I–P**). The clinical correlation analyses also showed that TNFRSF1A expression was significantly associated with histology (**Supplementary Tables 1–3, 5, 6**) and WHO grade (**Supplementary Tables 1–6**) of gliomas. Furthermore, ROC analysis found that TNFRSF1A was capable of predicting the pathological diagnosis of gliomas in GSE4290, GSE68848 and TCGA, respectively (AUC>0.7) (**Figures 4A–C**). Collectively, TNFRSF1A expression was upregulated in gliomas than normal samples, and related to glioma histology and WHO grade.

Besides, boxplots and clinical correlation analyses showed that TNFRSF1A expression was significantly associated with other clinical features, including age, microvascular proliferation, necrosis, chemotherapy and radiotherapy status, recurrence and KPS. Glioma samples with older age (≥60) or microvascular proliferation or necrosis or Chemo_status (chemotherapy status) or treatment and therapy status have higher TNFRSF1A expression compared with the corresponding samples (**Figures 4D–J**). As shown in **Figure 4K**, recurrent gliomas have higher expression level of TNFRSF1A than primary gliomas. The clinical correlation analyses of the six datasets showed that TNFRSF1A expression was significantly associated with age (**Supplementary Tables 1–3, 5, 6**), gender (**Supplementary Tables 4, 5**), microvascular proliferation (**Supplementary Table 4**), necrosis (**Supplementary Table 4**), chemo_status (**Supplementary Table 3**), Radio_status (radiotherapy status) (**Supplementary Table 1**), treatment and therapy status (**Supplementary Tables 5, 6**) and PRS_type (primary/ recurrent/ secondary) (**Supplementary Table 3**) of human patients with gliomas, and its expression had no significance with some clinical features such as gender (**Supplementary Tables 1–3, 6**), race (**Supplementary Tables 5, 6**), chemo_status (**Supplementary Tables 1, 2**), Radio_status (**Supplementary Tables 2, 3**), KPS (Karnofsky performance score) (**Supplementary Tables 5, 6**). Taken together, TNFRSF1A expression was upregulated in gliomas, increased as the advances of WHO grade, and was related to various clinical features (including age, microvascular proliferation, necrosis, chemotherapy and radiotherapy status, recurrence and KPS) in gliomas, suggesting that TNFRSF1A might be a potential target gene related to diagnosis, treatment and prognosis of gliomas.

TNFRSF1A Was a Novel Mesenchymal-Associated Biomarker in Molecular Classification of Gliomas

TCGA group classified HGGs into four subtypes: Classical, Mesenchymal, Neural and Proneural based on the molecular biomarkers such as 1p/19q codeletion and IDH mutation. Based on the datasets from GEO, TCGA and CGGA, TNFRSF1A could differentiate the various subtypes of gliomas, and more importantly, its expression level in Mesenchymal subtype gliomas was higher than other subtypes (**Figures 4L–P; Supplementary Tables 1, 4, 6**). Likewise, TNFRSF1A expression of gliomas carrying 1p/19q codeletion or IDH mutation was lower than the corresponding glioma samples (**Figures 4Q–V; Supplementary Tables 1–3**). Therefore, TNFRSF1A was a novel Mesenchymal-associated biomarker in molecular classification of gliomas.

TNFRSF1A Was an Independent Prognostic Indicator of OS in Gliomas

The Kaplan-Meier plots were performed to examine the relationship between the TNFRSF1A expression and OS of glioma patients. Prior to the analysis, glioma samples without survival information were cut off and obtained samples were classified into two groups: low expression group and high expression group, according to the median of TNFRSF1A expression. For the dataset CGGA mRNA-array_301, the low TNFRSF1A expression group (n = 149) had a favor prognosis of OS than the high expression (n = 149) (**Figure 5A**). Likewise, the high TNFRSF1A expression group (n = 156, 310, 39, 43, 142, 347, and 263 respectively) had a poor prognosis compared with the corresponding low group (n = 155, 309, 38, 42, 142, 346, and 263 respectively) in the other seven datasets, including CGGA (mRNAseq_325 and mRNAseq_693), GSE4271, GSE4412, GSE68848, TCGA_glioma, and TCGA_LGG, respectively (**Figures 5B–H**). Furthermore, glioma or LGG patients with high TNFRSF1A expression had a shorter disease-free survival (DFS) than the low expression group using GEPIA2 (**Figures 5I,J**). Thus, TNFRSF1A expression was associated with poor prognosis in gliomas.

Besides, whether TNFRSF1A expression was an independent prognostic indicator of OS was determined using the univariate and multivariate Cox regression analyses. In the dataset CGGA mRNA-array_301, univariate Cox regression analysis result revealed that a total of 10 factors were associated with OS of gliomas, including TNFRSF1A expression, age, WHO grade, PRS_type, histology, TCGA_subtypes, Radio_status, Chemo_status, IDH_mutation_status and 1p19q_codeletion_status (**Table 1**). However, multivariate analysis result illustrated that five factors were identified as independent prognostic indicators, including TNFRSF1A expression (P = 0.007, HR = 1.90, 95% CI = 1.19–3.01), WHO grade (P = 0.048, HR = 1.50, 95% CI = 1.00–2.25), TCGA_subtypes (P = 0.048, HR = 1.56, 95% CI = 1.00–2.42), Radio_status (P = 0.011, HR = 0.36, 95% CI = 0.16–0.79) and 1p19q_codeletion_status (P = 0.029, HR = 0.24, 95% CI = 0.07–0.87) (**Table 1**). Similarly in the another

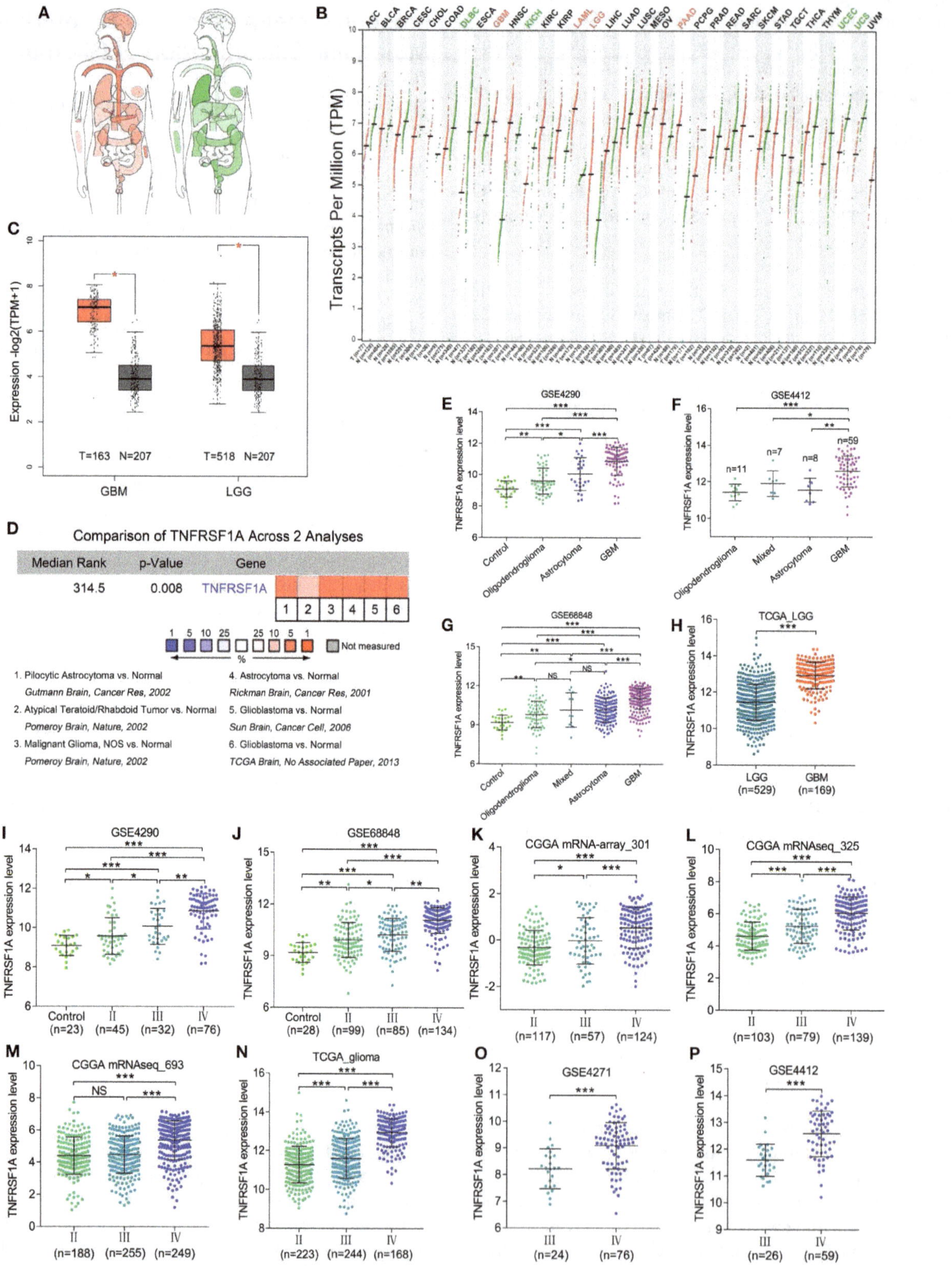

FIGURE 3 | The expression levels of TNFRSF1A in gliomas. **(A)** Bodymap for the median expression of TNFRSF1A in tumor (red) and normal (green) samples using GEPIA 2. **(B)** The TNFRSF1A expression profile across all tumor samples and paired normal tissues using GEPIA2. The red plot represents the tumor sample and the green one indicates the normal sample. The TNFRSF1A expression in tumor samples is significantly upregulated compared the corresponding normal tissues when

(Continued)

FIGURE 3 | the name of the tumor is red ($P < 0.05$); on the contrary, the green indicates that TNFRSF1A expression in the tumor samples is downregulated ($P < 0.05$). **(C)** TNFRSF1A expression in GBM and LGG samples was upregulated compared with the normal brain samples based on the TCGA normal and GTEx data from the online tool GEPIA2 ($P < 0.05$). **(D)** The comparison analyses across 6 datasets from the Oncomine database showed that TNFRSF1A in gliomas was significantly upregulated compared to normal samples with the cut-off of $P < 0.05$ and foldchange>2 as well as gene rank = 10%. **(E–H)** TNFRSF1A expression was analyzed in various histologies of gliomas. **(I–P)** The expression of TNFRSF1A is positively associated with WHO grades in the eight datasets, including GSE4290, GSE68848, CGGA (mRNA-array_301, mRNAseq_325 and mRNAseq_693), TCGA_glioma, GSE4271 and GSE4412, respectively. *$P < 0.05$; **$P < 0.01$; ***$P < 0.001$.

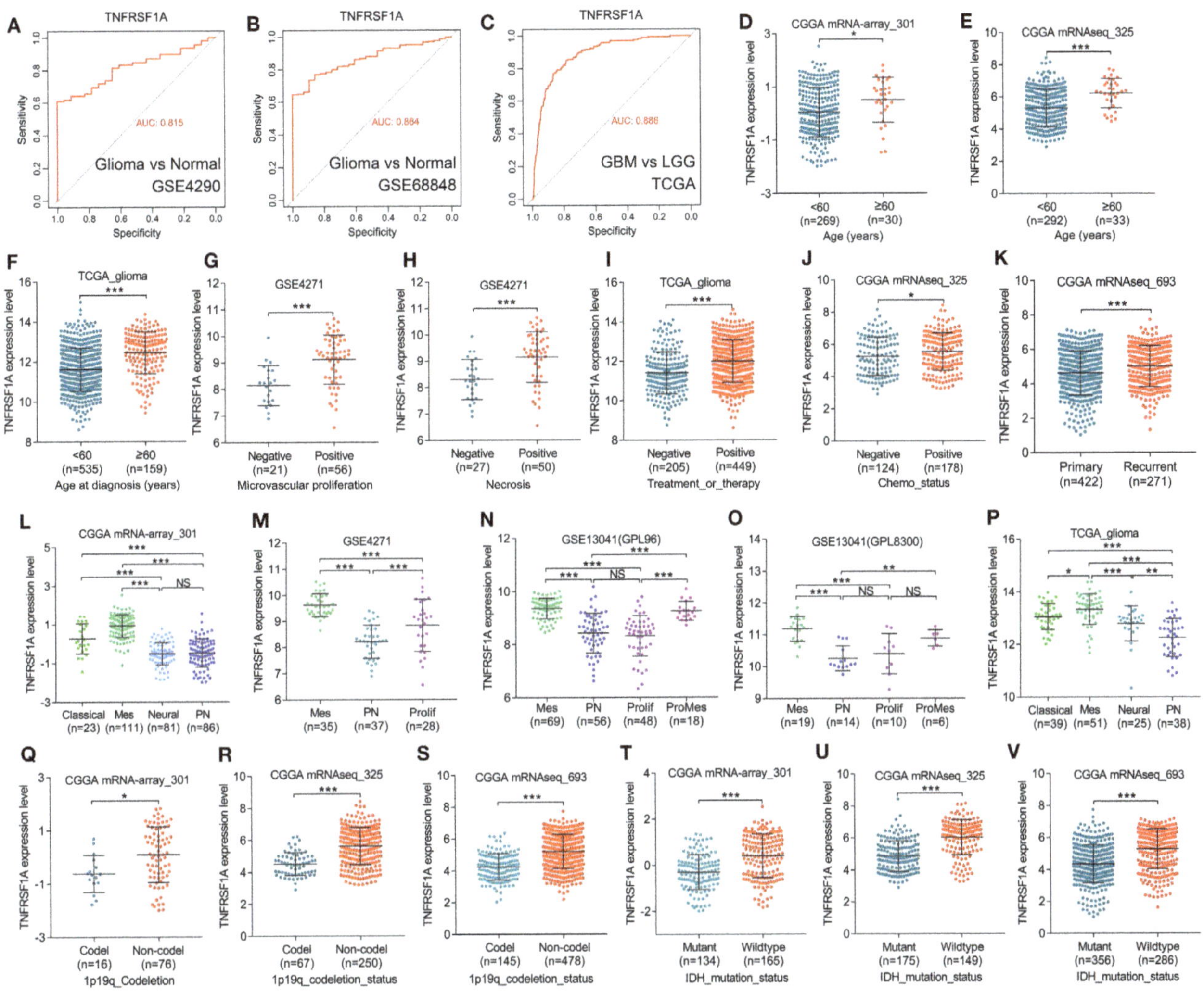

FIGURE 4 | TNFRSF1A expression was associated with clinical features and was a subtype-associated molecular biomarker in glioma patients. **(A–C)** ROC analysis found that TNFRSF1A was able to predict the pathological diagnosis of gliomas in GSE4290, GSE68848 and TCGA, respectively (AUC>0.7). **(D–J)** The relationships between TNFRSF1A expression and clinical features (including ages, microvascular proliferation, necrosis, chemotherapy, and therapy) were analyzed. **(K)** The expression of TNFRSF1A in recurrent gliomas was upregulated compared with primary samples in CGGA mRNAseq_693. **(L–P)** TNFRSF1A expression in different subtypes of gliomas was analyzed in the five datasets, including CGGA mRNA-array_301, GSE4271, GSE13041 (GPL96), GSE13041 (GPL8300), and TCGA_glioma, respectively. **(Q–V)** The associations between TNFRSF1A expression and molecular characteristics (1p/19q codeletion and IDH mutation) were determined in the datasets CGGA mRNA-array_301, mRNAseq_325 and mRNAseq_693, respectively. Mes, mesenchymal; Prolif, proliferative; PN, proneural; ProMes, proliferative and mesenchymal; Codel, 1p/19q codeletion; ROC, receiver operating characteristic; AUC, area under the curve. *$P < 0.05$; **$P < 0.01$; ***$P < 0.001$.

dataset CGGA mRNAseq_325, univariate analysis revealed that a total of 9 factors were associated with OS of gliomas, including TNFRSF1A expression, age, WHO grade, PRS_type, histology, Radio_status, Chemo_status, IDH_mutation_status and 1p19q_codeletion_status (**Table 2**). Multivariate result illustrated that six factors were identified as independent prognostic indicators, including TNFRSF1A expression (P = 0.049, HR = 1.16, 95% CI = 1.00–1.34), age (P = 0.013, HR = 1.02, 95% CI = 1.00–1.03), WHO grade ($P < 0.001$, HR = 2.04, 95% CI = 1.59–2.63), PRS_type (P =0.013, HR = 1.99,

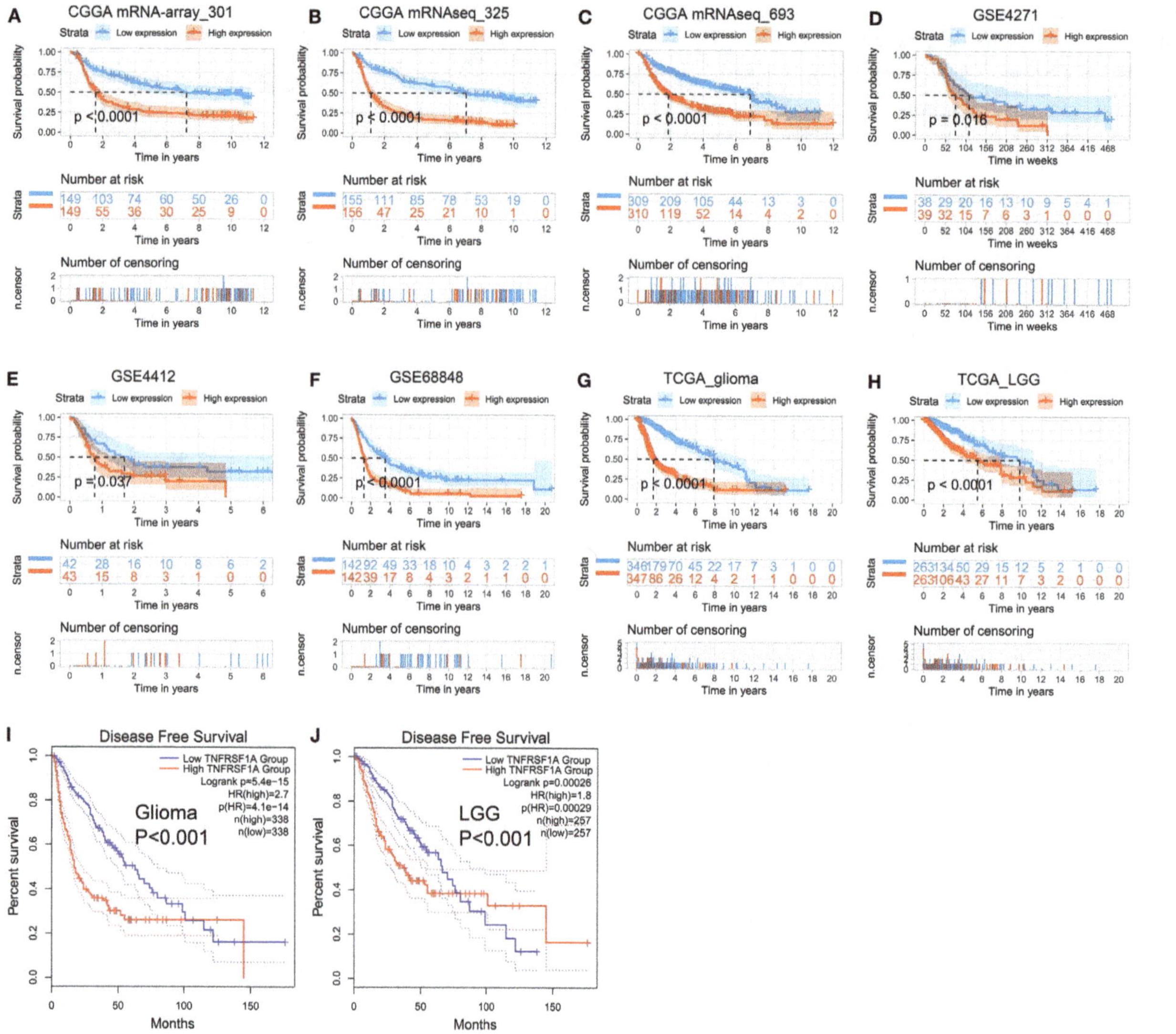

FIGURE 5 | TNFRSF1A expression is associated with poor prognosis of glioma patients. **(A–H)** The Kaplan-Meier plots of TNFRSF1A in the eight datasets, including CGGA (mRNA-array_301, mRNAseq_325, and mRNAseq_693), GSE4271, GSE4412, GSE68848, TCGA_glioma, and TCGA_LGG, respectively. **(I,J)** The glioma patients with high TNFRSF1A expression have shorter overall survival (OS) and disease-free survival (DFS) compared the low TNFRSF1A group using the GEPIA2. Red line indicates the high TNFRSF1A expression group and blue line represents the low TNFRSF1A expression group.

95% CI = 1.16–3.42), Chemo_status ($P = 0.036$, HR = 0.69, 95% CI = 0.49–0.98), and 1p19q_codeletion_status ($P < 0.001$, HR = 0.31, 95% CI = 0.18–0.55) (**Table 2**). Taken together, these results from the two datasets revealed that TNFRSF1A expression and WHO grade as well as 1p19q_codeletion_status were independent prognostic indicators of OS in gliomas.

Protein Expression of TNFRSF1A in Glioma Tissues Was Upregulated Compared to Normal Brain Tissues by IHC Staining From the HPA

Using the same antibody HPA004102 from the IHC-based HPA database, protein expression level of GNG5 protein increased in the order of normal brain tissue, LGG and HGG among different patients (**Figure 6**), which further confirmed the important role of TNFRSF1A in gliomas at the protein level.

Downregulation of TNFRSF1A Inhibited Glioma Cell Proliferation and Migration *in vitro*

To investigate the role of TNFRSF1A in glioma, TNFRSF1A was knocked down in U251 and U87. After transfection of glioma cells with si-NC or TNFRSF1A siRNAs, knockdown efficiency of TNFRSF1A siRNA2 was most obvious in both U251 and U87 (**Figure 7A**). Furthermore, TNFRSF1A expression was dramatically reduced at the protein level while TNFRSF1A

TABLE 1 | Cox regression analysis of TNFRSF1A expression as a survival indicator of gliomas in CGGA mRNA-array_301.

Parameter	Univariate analysis			Multivariate analysis		
	P	HR	95%CI	*P*	HR	95%CI
Age (≥60 vs. <60 years)	***P* < 0.001**	1.04	1.03–1.05	0.475	1.01	0.98–1.05
Gender (Male vs. Female)	0.164	1.24	0.92–1.67	NA	NA	NA
WHO grade (II vs. III vs. IV)	***P* < 0.001**	2.70	2.23–3.26	**0.048**	1.50	1.00–2.25
PRS_type (Primary vs. Recurrent vs. Secondary)	***P* < 0.001**	2.22	1.67–2.94	0.313	1.63	0.63–4.23
Histology (A vs. AA vs. AO vs. AOA vs. GBM vs. O vs. OA vs. rA vs. rAA vs. rAO vs. rAOA vs. rGBM vs. sGBM)	***P* < 0.001**	1.14	1.08–1.19	0.627	1.05	0.87–1.27
TCGA_subtypes (Classical vs. Mesenchymal vs. Neural vs. Proneural)	***P* < 0.001**	0.62	0.53–0.72	**0.048**	1.56	1.00–2.42
Radio_status (Positive vs. Negative)	**0.012**	0.58	0.37–0.89	**0.011**	0.36	0.16–0.79
Chemo_status (Positive vs. Negative)	**0.021**	1.43	1.05–1.94	0.425	0.76	0.39–1.49
IDH_mutation_status (Mutant vs. Wildtype)	***P* < 0.001**	0.38	0.28–0.52	0.639	0.82	0.35–1.90
1p19q_codeletion_status (Codel vs. Non-codel)	***P* < 0.001**	0.12	0.04–0.40	**0.029**	0.24	0.07–0.87
TNFRSF1A expression (High vs. low)	***P* < 0.001**	1.64	1.39–1.94	**0.007**	1.90	1.19–3.01

CGGA, the Chinese Glioma Genome Altas; WHO, World Health Organization; A, astrocytomas; AA, anaplastic astrocytomas; AO, anaplastic oligodendrogliomas; AOA, anaplastic oligoastrocytomas; GBM, glioblastoma multiforme; O, oligodendrogliomas; OA, oligoastrocytomas; rA, recurrent astrocytomas; rAA, recurrent anaplastic astrocytomas; rAO, recurrent anaplastic oligodendrogliomas; rAOA, recurrent anaplastic oligoastrocytomas; rGBM, recurrent glioblastoma multiforme; sGBM, secondary glioblastoma multiforme; TCGA, The Cancer Genome Atlas; NA, not analyze. The bold values is aimed to emphasize the parameter with P < 0.05.

TABLE 2 | Cox regression analysis of TNFRSF1A expression as a survival indicator of gliomas in CGGA mRNAseq_325.

Parameter	Univariate analysis			Multivariate analysis		
	P	HR	95%CI	*P*	HR	95%CI
Age (≥60 vs. <60 years)	***P* < 0.001**	1.03	1.02–1.04	**0.013**	1.02	1.00–1.03
Gender (Male vs. Female)	0.613	0.93	0.71–1.23	NA	NA	NA
WHO grade (II vs. III vs. IV)	***P* < 0.001**	2.74	2.28–3.30	***P* < 0.001**	2.04	1.59–2.63
PRS_type (Primary vs. Recurrent vs. Secondary)	***P* < 0.001**	2.12	1.75–2.57	**0.013**	1.99	1.16–3.42
Histology (A vs. AA vs. AO vs. AOA vs. GBM vs. O vs. OA vs. rA vs. rAA vs. rAO vs. rAOA vs. rGBM vs. rOA vs. sGBM)	***P* < 0.001**	1.12	1.08–1.16	0.559	0.97	0.88–1.07
Radio_status (Positive vs. Negative)	***P* < 0.001**	0.52	0.36–0.74	0.167	0.75	0.50–1.13
Chemo_status (Positive vs. Negative)	**0.004**	1.55	1.15–2.08	**0.036**	0.69	0.49–0.98
IDH_mutation_status (Mutant vs. Wildtype)	***P* < 0.001**	0.38	0.29–0.51	0.989	0.10	0.67–1.49
1p19q_codeletion_status (Codel vs. Non-codel)	***P* < 0.001**	0.17	0.10–0.28	***P* < 0.001**	0.31	0.18–0.55
TNFRSF1A expression (High vs. low)	***P* < 0.001**	1.60	1.43–1.79	**0.049**	1.16	1.00–1.34

CGGA, the Chinese Glioma Genome Altas; WHO, World Health Organization; A, astrocytomas; AA, anaplastic astrocytomas; AO, anaplastic oligodendrogliomas; AOA, anaplastic oligoastrocytomas; GBM, glioblastoma multiforme; O, oligodendrogliomas; OA, oligoastrocytomas; rA, recurrent astrocytomas; rAA, recurrent anaplastic astrocytomas; rAO, recurrent anaplastic oligodendrogliomas; rAOA, recurrent anaplastic oligoastrocytomas; rGBM, recurrent glioblastoma multiforme; rOA, recurrent oligoastrocytomas; sGBM, secondary glioblastoma multiforme; NA, not analyze. The bold values is aimed to emphasize the parameter with P < 0.05.

was knocked down using western blotting analysis (**Figure 7B**). Based on the CCK-8 assay, proliferative capacity of glioma cells transfected with TNFRSF1A siRNA2was significantly compared to those treated with si-NC (**Figures 7C,D**). The results of colony formation assay further demonstrated that colony numbers of glioma cells were significantly inhibited while TNFRSF1A was silencing (**Figure 7E**). As shown in **Figure 7F**, transwell assay showed that TNFRSF1A knockdown significantly reduced the migration of glioma cells. Taken together, downregulation of TNFRSF1A inhibited glioma cell proliferation and migration *in vitro*.

DISCUSSION

Gliomas are the most prevalent malignant primary brain tumors with poor survival prognosis (1), and according to abnormalities of several biomarkers GBMs are subgrouped into four molecular subtypes: Classical, Mesenchymal, Neural and Proneural, by the TCGA team (6). Owing to therapeutic resistance and high recurrent rate of gliomas, individual treatment based on the molecular biomarkers has gained more attentions (18). Recently, more transcriptome databases, such as TCGA, GEO and CGGA, have been constructed to be free to the public and provide

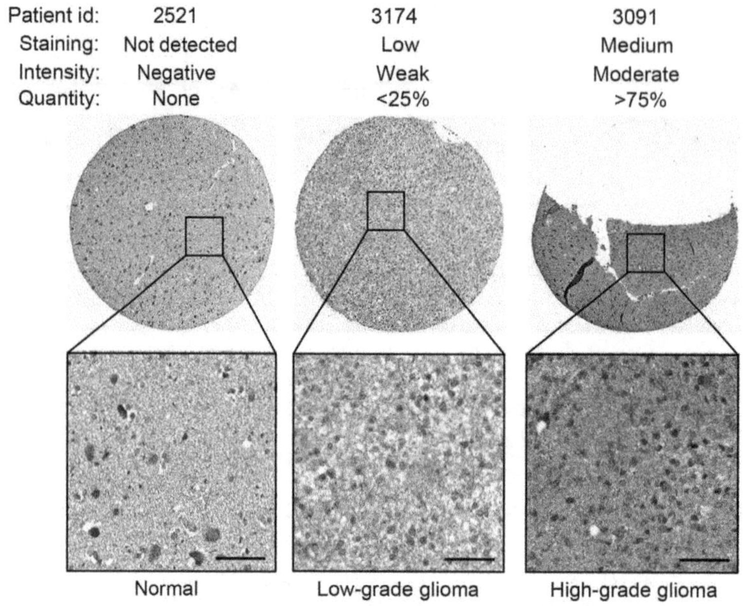

FIGURE 6 | IHC staining showed that TNFRSF1A expression increased in the order of normal brain tissue, low-grade glioma and high-grade glioma. Antibody TNFRSF1A was HPA004102, and representative TNFRSF1A staining images were shown. Scale bar, 50 μm.

abundant gene expression profiles and clinical information. In this study, an integrated bioinformatics analysis of the public databases found that the brown co-expression module and the biomarker TNFRSF1A was identified to be strongly related to WHO grade of gliomas. Further informatics analyses revealed that upregulated TNFRSF1A was significantly associated with clinical features, and functioned as an independent prognostic indicator of OS. Its effect and molecular mechanisms in glioma cell lines were verified using the biological experiments *in vitro*.

WGCNA, a system informatics method, is used to construct the network with scale-free distribution and is good at identifying the potential biomarker and its mechanisms of diseases. To date, there are also some similar researches on gliomas. For example, Xu et al. used WGCNA to screen four genes (OSMR, SOX21, MED10, and PTPRN) in the yellow module related to survival time and applied the Cox proportional hazards (PH) regression model to assess their prognostic significance (19). Likewise, Liang et al. identified a GBM-related module and adopted the Cox PH regression model to extract six prognostic lncRNAs like LINC00641 and LBX2-AS1 (20). A recent study have reported that an OS-associated module was identified and a lncRNA was screened by survival analyses based on the CGGA with 88 samples carrying compete clinical information (21). The three studies above adopted WGCNA to a co-expression module which related to survival time (or overall survival) or GBM, but there some limitations. One problem is that single survival time without status (including dead or alive) could not represent the exact survival time of tumor patients, and the ages at the diagnosis is the another factor related to the real survival time. Secondly, although GBM (glioma WHO IV) is the most serious pathology type of gliomas histologically, GBMs were classified into four subtypes (Classical, Mesenchymal, Neural and Proneural) (6) and different subtypes have different biological behaviors such as survival time from weeks to years (22). Also, when the module was selected based on the GBM diagnosis, there are only two events (Positive or Negative), which could not take full advantage of WGCNA because construction of co-expression modules depends on the patterns of the parameter changes. And in this study, we adopted WHO grade (I, II, III, and IV) of gliomas to investigate the co-expression modules. To a certain extent, this strategy could improve the risk stratification of different glioma patients according to the severity of gliomas and make best of WGCNA. Notably, the result of this study showed that the brown module was strongly related to WHO grade ($r = 0.44$, $P = 1e\text{-}34$), and no module was found to be associated with OS or GBM.

Moreover, glioma samples with some features (including older ages, high WHO grades, microvascular proliferation and necrosis) had a higher expression level of TNFRSF1A than the corresponding samples, suggesting that TNFRSF1A might be associated with poor prognosis. Furthermore, consistent with the above results, survival analyses and Cox regression analyses demonstrated that human patients with gliomas carrying high TNFRSF1A expression had a shorter OS or DFS than the low expression patients, and TNFRSF1A functioned as an independent prognostic indicator of OS. Thus, TNFRSF1A might be a novel biomarker of diagnosis, therapy, and prognosis related to progression of gliomas.

Besides, TNFRSF1A was verified to be associated to the molecular classification of gliomas, and it was highly upregulated in Mes subtype and downregualted in PN subtype of gliomas in this study. Compared with the translational histological

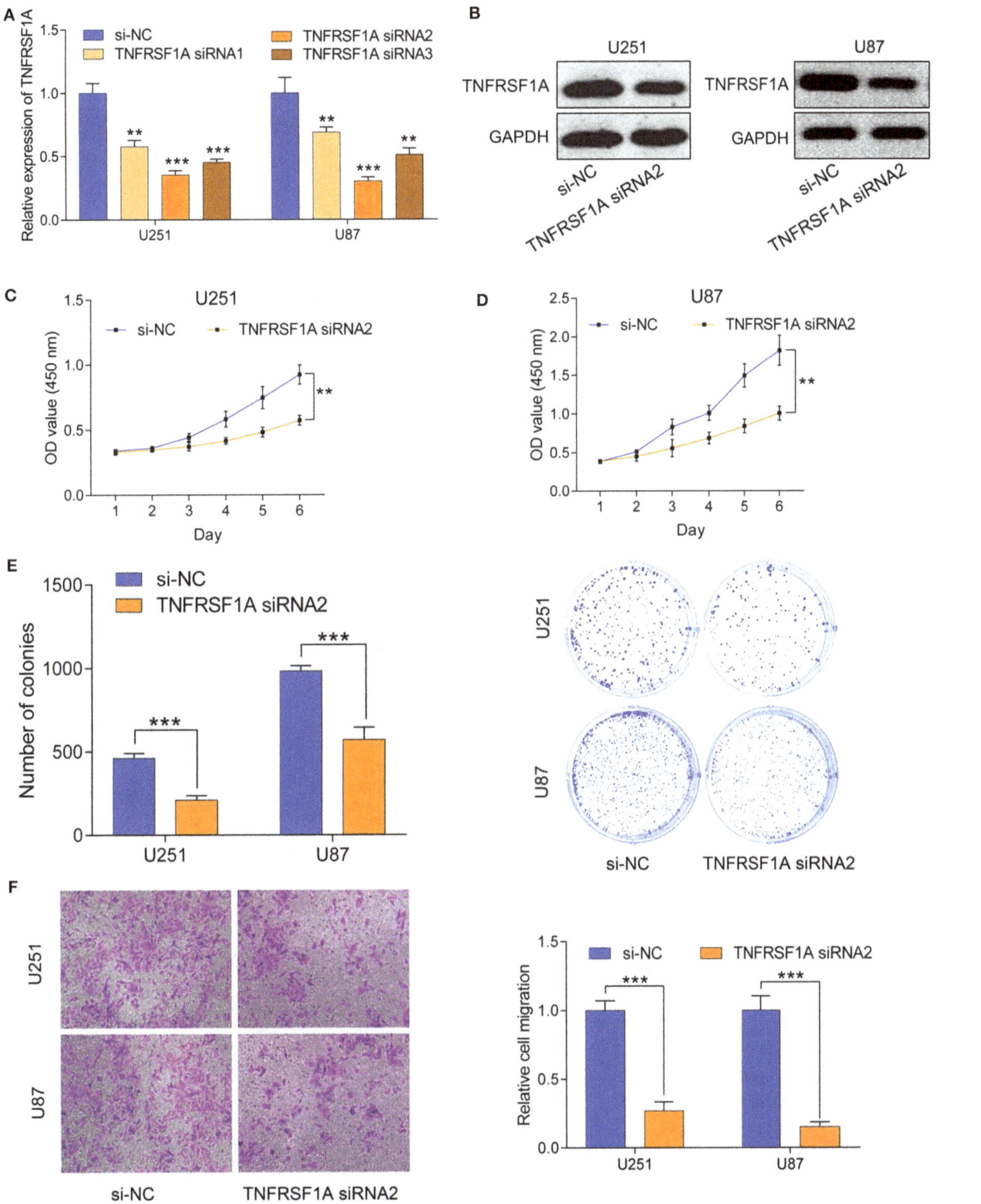

FIGURE 7 | Downregulation of TNFRSF1A inhibited glioma cell proliferation and migration *in vitro*. **(A)** Efficiency of siRNAs at the mRNA level was validated in U251 and U87 cells by qRT-PCR. And siRNA2 has highest efficiency and si-NC was used as control. **(B)** Expression levels of the protein TNFRSF1A in glioma cells transfected with siRNA2 or si-NC were examined by western blotting. **(C,D)** Effects of TNFRSF1A knockdown on glioma development were determined by Cell Counting Kit-8 assay in U251 and U87, respectively. **(E)** Proliferative capacity of TNFRSF1A knockdown in in U251 and U87 cells transfected with siRNA2 or si-NC by using colony formation assay. **(F)** Transwell migration assay was performed in U87 and U251 transfected with si-NC or TNFRSF1A siRNA2. Representative images of migration cells are displayed. The number of migration cells was counted and was inversely related to the expression levels of TNFRSF1A. **P < 0.01; ***P < 0.001.

classification, molecular classification highly took individual difference into account and added molecular characteristics to this classification. And glioma patients with molecular characteristics such as IDH mutation or 1p/19q codeletion had a lower expression level of TNFRSF1A than the glioma samples without these characteristics. From the above results that TNFRSF1A expression was an independent prognostic indicator related to poor prognosis in gliomas, therefore, gliomas with IDH mutation or 1p/19q codeletion had a longer survival time, which was consistent with the conclusions of the previous studies. A study with 941 malignant glioma samples found that the PN and Neural, and Classical and Mes subtypes frequently occurred in LGGs and HGGs, respectively (23). On the other hand, survival analyses demonstrated that the Mes subtype gliomas behaved a poor survival outcome and conversely the PN subtype gliomas displayed a better prognosis (23). Some previous studies found that IDH mutation was associated with 1p/19q codeletion (24), and glioma patients with IDH mutation had a longer median overall survival time than samples with IDH wildtype (25). Collectively, TNFRSF1A expression was significantly associated with the molecular characteristics and subtypes, and its overexpression was related to a poor prognosis, indicating that TNFRSF1A was a novel and promising Mesenchymal-associated biomarker in molecular subtypes of gliomas and might play critical roles in target therapy in the future.

KEGG enrichment analysis showed that TNFRSF1A could regulate the tumorignenesis of gliomas via activating the MAPK signaling pathway. Knockdown of TNFRSF1A suppressed glioma cells proliferation, migration and invasion *in vitro*, which further confirmed the important values of TNFRSF1A on glioma progression.

Overall, TNFRSF1A was identified by an integrated informatics analyses such as WGCNA, and transcriptome analyses further revealed that TNFRSF1A expression was upregulated in glioma samples compared with the normal brain samples. Moreover, the expression level of TNFRSF1A was associated with WHO grade and other clinical features such as molecular subtypes, and was found to serve as an independent prognostic indicator of OS in gliomas. Knockdown of TNFRSF1A suppressed the progression of glioma cell lines *in vitro*. These finding suggested that TNFRSF1A might be a promising biomarker of diagnosis, therapy and prognosis in Mesenchymal subtype gliomas.

AUTHOR CONTRIBUTIONS

S-HC and BY conceived and designed the study. BY performed the analysis procedures. Y-BP and Y-BM analyzed the results and contributed analysis tools. BY and S-HC contributed to the writing of the manuscript. All authors reviewed the manuscript.

FUNDING

This research was funded by Natural Science Foundation of Shanghai (Grant No. 19ZR1429800), Shanghai Jiao Tong University Medicine-Engineering Cross Research Foundation (Grant No. YG2015MS25) and the Research Foundation of Shanghai No. 3 People's Hospital Affiliated to Shanghai Jiao Tong University School of Medicine (Grant No. syz2015-015).

ACKNOWLEDGMENTS

This is a short text to acknowledge the contributions of specific colleagues, institutions, or agencies that aided the efforts of the authors.

SUPPLEMENTARY MATERIAL

Supplementary Figure 1 | Clustering dendrogram of samples to detect outliers.

Supplementary Figure 2 | Clustering dendrogram of genes among CGGA mRNAseq_693. The colored row below the dendrogram indicates module membership identified by the dynamic tree cut method, and different colors represent different modules respectively.

Supplementary Figure 3 | Venn diagram of the top 10 hub genes in brown module and the 13 genes of the MAPK signaling pathway. TNFRSF1A was the only common gene among the two cohorts.

Supplementary Table 1 | Correlation of TNFRSF1A with clinicopathologic features of glioma patients in CGGA mRNA-array_301.

Supplementary Table 2 | Correlation of TNFRSF1A with clinicopathologic features of glioma patients in CGGA mRNAseq_325.

Supplementary Table 3 | Correlation of TNFRSF1A with clinicopathologic features of glioma patients in CGGA mRNAseq_693.

Supplementary Table 4 | Correlation of TNFRSF1A with clinicopathologic features of glioma patients in GSE4271.

Supplementary Table 5 | Correlation of TNFRSF1A with clinicopathologic features of LGG patients in TCGA.

Supplementary Table 6 | Correlation of TNFRSF1A with clinicopathologic features of glioma patients in TCGA.

REFERENCES

1. Chen R, Smith-Cohn M, Cohen AL, Colman H. Glioma subclassifications and their clinical significance. *Neurotherapeutics.* (2017) 14:284–97. doi: 10.1007/s13311-017-0519-x
2. Modrek AS, Bayin NS, Placantonakis DG. Brain stem cells as the cell of origin in glioma. *World J Stem Cells.* (2014) 6:43–52. doi: 10.4252/wjsc.v6.i1.43
3. Louis DN, Ohgaki H, Wiestler OD, Cavenee WK, Burger PC, Jouvet A, et al. The 2007 WHO classification of tumours of the central nervous system. *Acta Neuropathol.* (2007) 114:97–109. doi: 10.1007/s00401-007-0243-4
4. D'Alessio A, Proietti G, Sica G, Scicchitano BM. Pathological and molecular features of glioblastoma and its peritumoral tissue. *Cancers.* (2019) 11:E469. doi: 10.3390/cancers11040469
5. Louis DN, Perry A, Reifenberger G, von Deimling A, Figarella-Branger D, Cavenee WK, et al. The 2016 World Health Organization classification of tumors of the central nervous system: a summary. *Acta Neuropathol.* (2016) 131:803–20. doi: 10.1007/s00401-016-1545-1
6. Verhaak RG, Hoadley KA, Purdom E, Wang V, Qi Y, Wilkerson MD, et al. Integrated genomic analysis identifies clinically relevant subtypes of glioblastoma characterized by abnormalities in PDGFRA, IDH1, EGFR, and NF1. *Cancer Cell.* (2010) 17:98–110. doi: 10.1016/j.ccr.2009.12.020

7. Lin L, Wang G, Ming J, Meng X, Han B, Sun B, et al. Analysis of expression and prognostic significance of vimentin and the response to temozolomide in glioma patients. *Tumour Biol.* (2016) 37:15333–9. doi: 10.1007/s13277-016-5462-7
8. Langfelder P, Horvath S. WGCNA: an R package for weighted correlation network analysis. *BMC Bioinform.* (2008) 9:559. doi: 10.1186/1471-2105-9-559
9. Pan S, Zhan Y, Chen X, Wu B, Liu B. Identification of biomarkers for controlling cancer stem cell characteristics in bladder cancer by network analysis of transcriptome data stemness indices. *Front Oncol.* (2019) 9:613. doi: 10.3389/fonc.2019.00613
10. Chen L, Peng T, Luo Y, Zhou F, Wang G, Qian K, et al. ACAT1 and metabolism-related pathways are essential for the progression of clear cell renal cell carcinoma (ccrcc), as determined by co-expression network analysis. *Front Oncol.* (2019) 9:957. doi: 10.3389/fonc.2019.00957
11. Xiang Z, Li J, Song S, Wang J, Cai W, Hu W, et al. A positive feedback between IDO1 metabolite and COL12A1 via MAPK pathway to promote gastric cancer metastasis. *J Exp Clin Cancer Res.* (2019) 38:314. doi: 10.1186/s13046-019-1318-5
12. Zhang W, Xu Y, Zhang L, Wang S, Yin B, Zhao S, et al. Synergistic effects of TGFbeta2, WNT9a, and FGFR4 signals attenuate satellite cell differentiation during skeletal muscle development. *Aging Cell.* (2018) 17:e12788. doi: 10.1111/acel.12788
13. Molnar L, Berki T, Hussain A, Nemeth P, Losonczy H. Detection of TNFalpha expression in the bone marrow and determination of TNFalpha production of peripheral blood mononuclear cells in myelodysplastic syndrome. *Pathol Oncol Res.* (2000) 6:18–23. doi: 10.1007/BF03032653
14. Borghini S, Fiore M, Di Duca M, Caroli F, Finetti M, Santamaria G, et al. Candidate genes in patients with autoinflammatory syndrome resembling tumor necrosis factor receptor-associated periodic syndrome without mutations in the TNFRSF1A gene. *J Rheumatol.* (2011) 38:1378–84. doi: 10.3899/jrheum.101260
15. Greco E, Aita A, Galozzi P, Gava A, Sfriso P, Negm OH, et al. The novel S59P mutation in the TNFRSF1A gene identified in an adult onset TNF receptor associated periodic syndrome (TRAPS) constitutively activates NF-κB pathway. *Arthritis Res Ther.* (2015) 17:93. doi: 10.1186/s13075-015-0604-7
16. Comabella M, Caminero AB, Malhotra S, Agullo L, Fernandez O, Reverter F, et al. TNFRSF1A polymorphisms rs1800693 and rs4149584 in patients with multiple sclerosis. *Neurology.* (2013) 80:2010–6. doi: 10.1212/WNL.0b013e318294b2d6
17. Wang F, Zheng Z, Guan J, Qi D, Zhou S, Shen X, et al. Identification of a panel of genes as a prognostic biomarker for glioblastoma. *EBioMed.* (2018) 37:68–77. doi: 10.1016/j.ebiom.2018.10.024
18. Lin L, Cai J, Jiang C. Recent advances in targeted therapy for glioma. *Curr Med Chem.* (2017) 24:1365–81. doi: 10.2174/0929867323666161223150242
19. Xu P, Yang J, Liu J, Yang X, Liao J, Yuan F, et al. Identification of glioblastoma gene prognosis modules based on weighted gene co-expression network analysis. *BMC Med Genom.* (2018) 11:96. doi: 10.1186/s12920-018-0407-1
20. Liang R, Zhi Y, Zheng G, Zhang B, Zhu H, Wang M. Analysis of long non-coding RNAs in glioblastoma for prognosis prediction using weighted gene co-expression network analysis, Cox regression, and L1-LASSO penalization. *Onco Targets Ther.* (2019) 12:157–68. doi: 10.2147/OTT.S171957
21. Chen X, Pan C, Xu C, Sun Y, Geng Y, Kong L, et al. Identification of survivalassociated key genes and long noncoding RNAs in glioblastoma multiforme by weighted gene coexpression network analysis. *Int J Mol Med.* (2019) 43:1709–22. doi: 10.3892/ijmm.2019.4101
22. Yang Q, Wang R, Wei B, Peng C, Wang L, Hu G, et al. Candidate biomarkers and molecular mechanism investigation for glioblastoma multiforme utilizing WGCNA. *Biomed Res Int.* (2018) 2018:4246703. doi: 10.1155/2018/4246703
23. Lin N, Yan W, Gao K, Wang Y, Zhang J, You Y. Prevalence and clinicopathologic characteristics of the molecular subtypes in malignant glioma: a multi-institutional analysis of 941 cases. *PLoS ONE.* (2014) 9:e94871. doi: 10.1371/journal.pone.0094871
24. Yan H, Parsons DW, Jin G, McLendon R, Rasheed BA, Yuan W, et al. IDH1 and IDH2 mutations in gliomas. *Curr Neurol Neurosci Rep.* (2009) 360:765–73. doi: 10.1056/NEJMoa0808710

12

MiR-9-5p Inhibits Glioblastoma Cells Proliferation Through Directly Targeting FOXP2 (Forkhead Box P2)

Hongbo Zhang[1,2†], *Yuntao Li*[3,4†], *Yinqiu Tan*[3†], *Qi Liu*[5], *Shuting Jiang*[3], *Dongyuan Liu*[3], *Qianxue Chen*[3*] *and Shizhong Zhang*[1,2*]

[1] *Department of Neurosurgery, Zhujiang Hospital, Southern Medical University, Guangzhou, China,* [2] *Guangdong Provincial Key Laboratory on Brain Function Repair and Regeneration, The National Key Clinic Specialty, The Engineering Technology Research Center of Education Ministry of China, The Neurosurgery Institute of Guangdong Province, Southern Medical University, Guangzhou, China,* [3] *Department of Neurosurgery, Renmin Hospital of Wuhan University, Wuhan, China,* [4] *Department of Neurosurgery, Huzhou Central Hospital, Zhejiang University School of Medicine, Huzhou, China,* [5] *Department of Rheumatology, The Third Affiliated Hospital of Sun Yat-sen University, Guangzhou, China*

Correspondence:
Qianxue Chen
chenqx666@whu.edu.cn
Shizhong Zhang
zhangshizhong@smu.edu.cn

† *These authors have contributed equally to this work*

Glioblastoma (GBM) is the most malignant tumor in the central nervous system and the treatment is still unsatisfactory because the mechanism of the disease remains unclear. The abnormal expression of miRNAs and its target proteins play a crucial role in the development of glioblastoma. In this study, we demonstrated that high expression of miR-9-5p and low expression of forkhead box P2 (FOXP2) were related with better outcome in patients with GBM, and down regulated FOXP2 expression was able to inhibit glioma cells proliferation by cell cycle arrest. Furthermore, we found that FOXP2 was the target protein of miR-9-5p in luciferase assay. The results of this study suggest a novel regulatory mechanism that miR-9-5p can inhibit glioma cells proliferation by downregulating FOXP2.

Keywords: miR-9-5p, FOXP2, glioblastoma, proliferation, glioma

INTRODUCTION

Glioblastoma (GBM) is one of the most malignant tumors in adult central nervous system. With the development of modern medical technology, it is possible to remove the tumor through surgical resection followed by chemoradiation. However, it is still a challenge to completely cure due to the strong invasive and proliferative nature of GBM. In the past decade, the prognosis and treatment for GBM have not improved significantly, but there have been important gains in our understanding on genetic alterations associated with gliomagenesis, and the gene targeting therapy might be promising for glioblastoma (1, 2).

MicroRNAs (miRNA) are a class of small non-coding RNAs and usually regulate the expression of target functional proteins through the interaction with 3′ untranslated regions (3′-UTRs) of mRNA, thus regulating the physiological and pathological processes. In the past few decades, miRNAs have been widely studied as important molecules in tumor progression, among which, the abnormal expression of miR-9 can be found in many malignancies. Interests of miR-9 have been grown with the aim of using it as a diagnostic and prognostic marker for tumors (1–3).

MiR-9 as a tumor promoter promotes the metastasis and invasion of non-small cell lung cancer (NSCLC) cells by inhibiting the expression of E-cadherin (4, 5). On the other hand, miR-9 functions as a tumor inhibitor suppressing cell proliferation and invasive ability through the SDF-1/CXCR4 pathway in epithelial ovarian cancer (6). The miR-9 can also induce cell arrest and apoptosis of oral squamous cell carcinoma via CDK 4/6 pathway (7), or down-regulate TNFAIP8 to inhibit the gastric cancer cell proliferation (8). In glioma, miR-9 inhibits glioma cells growth through various signals and promote apoptosis (9, 10). In the EGFRvIII pathway, miR-9 plays a negative role on tumorigenic capacity (11). Low expression of miR-9-3p results in a high level of Herpud1, which may protect against apoptosis in glioma (12). Over expressed miR-9 in U87 and U251 cells increases apoptosis by structural maintenance of chromosomes 1A (SMC1A) (13). It is also reported that miR-9 can reduce cell migration and the invasion of Glioblastoma cell lines through MAPK14 pathway (14). However, other researches showed different results. For example, Wu et al. found increased expression of microRNA-9 predicts an unfavorable prognosis in human Glioma (15). However, its important to note that the researches made no distinguishing between miR-9, miR-9-3p, or miR-9-5p in various tumors reported functions of miR-9.

Forkhead box P2 (FOXP2) was first found as a transcription factor involved in speech and language acquisition (16). Recently, abnormal expression of FOXP2 was found in kinds of tumors. However, the results are still controversial. Studies showed downregulation of FOXP2 in breast cancer, hepatocellular carcinoma and gastric cancer biopsies (16–18), while overexpression of FPXP2 was found in multiple myelomas, MGUS (Monoclonal Gammopathy of Undetermined Significance), several subtypes of lymphomas, osteosarcoma, neuroblastomas, and ERG fusion-negative prostate cancers (19–21).

Our previous work demonstrated miR-9-5p was a positive marker for prognosis in GBM, while FOXP2 a negative marker. FOXP2 is predicted as a direct target of miR-9-5p. In this study, miR-9-5p inhibited cell proliferation in 3 GMB cell lines *in vitro*. Reverse test was used to prove FOXP2 as a key point in miR-9-5p inhibiting GBM cells proliferation. Finally, we identified miR-9-5p inhibit tumor growth in mouse model by reducing FOXP2 expressing.

Combining these results, we conclude that miR-9-5p, through directly downregulating FOXP2 and inhibiting proliferation, is a tumor suppressor in GBM.

MATERIALS AND METHODS

GBM Tissue Collection

All the 110 samples were collected from March 2015 to April 2017 in the Department of Neurosurgery of Renmin Hospital of Wuhan University (Wuhan, China) and Department of neurosurgery, Zhujiang Hospital of Southern Medical University (Guangzhou, China). All the tumor samples were pathologically diagnosed as glioblastoma. The study was approved by local Ethics Committee of Wuhan University and Zhujiang hospital of Southern Medical University.

Cells and Cell Culture

Three human glioblastoma-derived cancer cell lines, U251, A118MG, and U87MG, were used in the study. The cells were purchased from the Cell Bank Type Culture Collection of Chinese Academy of Sciences, and were cultured in DMEM (Gibco) containing 10% fetal bovine serum (Gibco) and 1% penicillin-streptomycin (Sigma-Aldrich) at a temperature of 37°C and a humidified atmosphere of 5% CO_2.

DNA and RNA Transfection

Human FOXP2 (GenBank ID: NM_148898) full length cDNA was subcloned into a pcDNA3.1 vector to generate expression construct. All cell lines in this study were transfected with plasmids by using Lipofectamine 3000 (Thermo Fisher, USA) according to the manufacturers' protocols. FOXP2 small interfering ribonucleic acid (siRNA) (5′GACAGGCAGTTAACACTTAAT3′) and a non-specific si-RNA (as a negative control) transfections were conducted in non-serum-containing conditions using Lipofectamine 3000. All si-RNAs were used at a final concentration of 20 nM. Has-miR-9-5p mimics (5′UCUUUGGUUAUCUAGCUGUAUGA3′), negative control miRNA mimics (miR-ctrl mimics), and inhibitor (5′AGAAACCAAUAGAUCGACAUACU′3) were constructed by RiboBio (Guangzhou, China). Transfections were conducted in non-serum-containing conditions using Lipofectamine 3000 according to the manufacturer's instructions.

Western Blot

Cell lysates were prepared by sonicating cells briefly in a modified RIPA buffer (0.1% SDS, 50 mM Tris-HCl, pH 7.5, 150 mM NaCl, 0.1% sodium deoxycholate, 1% Nonidet P-40) with proteinase and phosphatase inhibitors. BCA protein assay (TaKaRa) was used for protein quantifying. The antibody used were as follows: anti-FOXP2 (Abcam, ab16046, USA), anti-p21 (Abcam, ab109520, USA), Goat anti-Rabbit, and Goat anti-Mouse infrared dye secondary antibodies (800 CW), which were purchased from LI-COR Biosciences (Lincoln, NE, USA). Proteins were visualized with Odyssey Bioanalyzer (LI-COR).

Real Time PCR

Total RNAs of human tissues and cells were extracted using TRIzol reagent (Invitrogen). Quantitative real-time PCR technology was used to measure the miR-9-5p expression by using the All in-One miRNA qRT-PCR Detection Kit (GeneCopoeia, Rockville,MD, USA). hsa-miR-9-5p forward primer: 5′TGCGCTCTTTGGTTATCTAGCTG3′; reverse primer: 5′CCAGTGCAGGGTCCGAGGTATT3′; U6 forward primer: 5′CGCTTCGGCAGCACATATAC 3′; reverse primer: 5′AAATATGGAACGCTTCACGA3′. All qRT-PCR processes and analyses were carried out using Applied Biosystems 7500 Fast Real-Time PCR system (Life Technologies). Relative expression of miRNA and mRNA was calculated using the $2^{-\Delta\Delta CT}$ method.

Luciferase Reporter Assay

Candidate targets and its putative binding site of miR-9-5p were predicted by miRNA database (http://www.microrna.org/microrna/home.do). The 3′UTR of FOXP2, containing the wild-type or mutant miR-9-5p binding sequence, was cloned into the pMIRREPORT vector (Ambion, USA). U251 cells were cultured in 24-well plates and transfected with 0.1 μg of luciferase reporter vectors with miR-9-5p mimics or miR-ctrl mimics. The pRL-TK vector (Promega, USA) containing Renilla luciferase was also co-transfected for normalization in all experiments. Cells were harvested 48 h after transfection, and Firefly and Renilla luciferase activities were measured using the Dual-Luciferase Reporter Assay System (Promega) according to the manufacturer's protocol.

Cell Proliferation Assay

U251, A118MG, and U87MG cell growth was measured 24, 48, and 72 h after transfection with FTL si-RNA by using the Cell Counting Kit-8 (CCK-8; Dojindo Molecular Technologies, Inc., Rockville, MD, USA), according to the manufacturer's protocol. On average, six replicates for each time point were statistically analyzed. EdU assay was also used to measure the cell growth, Cell-Light EdU Apollo488 *in vitro* Flow Cytometry Kit (20T) (RiboBio, China) was used according to the manufacturer's instructions.

Flow Cytometry

Transfected glioma cells were trypsinized and fixed in 70% icecold ethanol at 20°C overnight. After centrifugation and wash with phosphate-buffered saline (PBS), the cells were suspended in propidium iodide (PI) working solution (50 mg/ml PI, 0.2 mg/ml RNase A, and 0.1% Triton X-100) for 30 min at 37°C. Twenty thousand cells were harvested and analyzed by FACS Calibur flow cytometry (BD Biosciences, USA).

Tumor Formation Assay in a Nude Mouse Model

U251 cells were collected at a concentration of 2×10^7 cells/mL and 0.1 ml was subcutaneously injected into either side of the armpit of male BALB/c nude mice (4–5 weeks old) the next day. Mice were purchased from Shanghai Experimental Animal Center of the Chinese Academy of Sciences (Shanghai, China). AgomiR-9-5p [micrON hsa-miR-9-5p agomiR was purchased from RiboBio (GuangZhou, China)] or agomiR control were injected into tumor at 1 nmol every 4 days for 4 times after transplanted. Tumor volumes and weights were measured every 4 days and tumor volumes were calculated using the following equation: $V = 0.5 \times D \times d2$ (V, volume; D, longest diameter; d, diameter perpendicular to the longest diameter). On the 20th day after injection, mice were killed, and the subcutaneous growth of each tumor was examined. Primary tumors were excised and tumor tissues were used to perform qPCR analysis of miR-9-5p levels. ***This study was carried out in strict accordance with the recommendations in the Guide for the Care and Use of Laboratory Animals of the National Institutes of Health. The protocol was approved by the Committee on the Ethics of Animal Experiments of the Southern Medical University.***

Statistical Analysis

Data were expressed as mean ± standard error. Statistical analysis was performed with SPSS 20.0 software. Differences between means were assessed by student's *t*-test for normal distribution

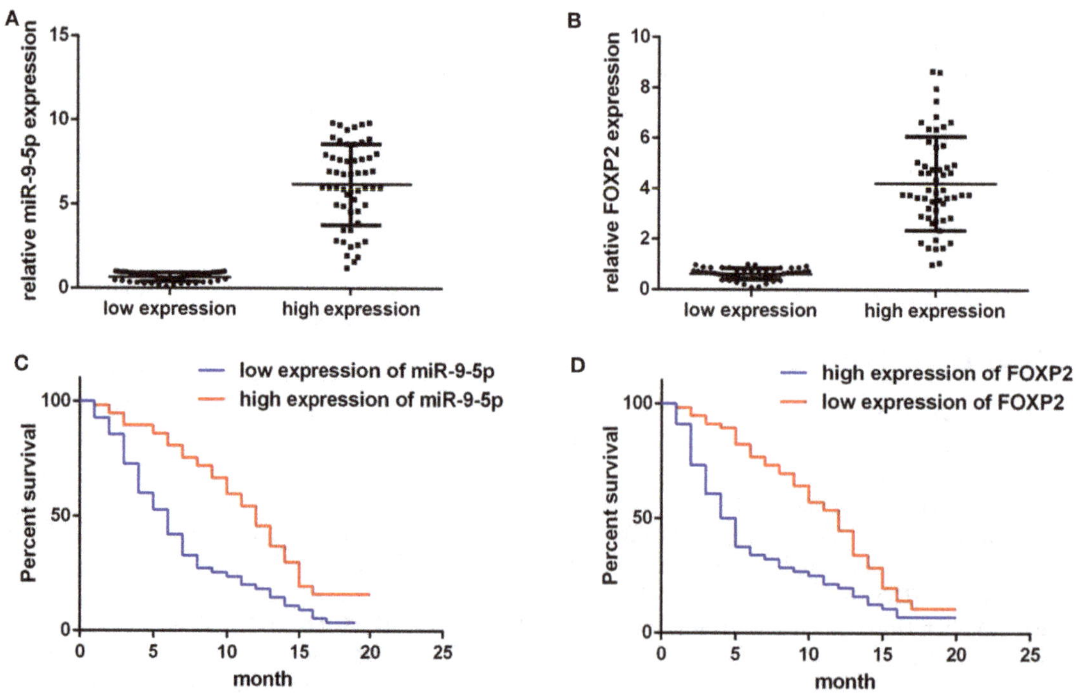

FIGURE 1 | The expression of miR-9-5p and FOXP2 in glioblastoma and patients' survival. **(A)** Cases are divided into two groups according to the expression of miR-9-5p in GBM. **(B)** Cases are divided into two groups according to the expression of FOXP2 in GBM. **(C)** Kaplan-Meir survival curve analysis reveals that lower miR-9-5p predicts poorer survival (110 GBM patients). **(D)** Kaplan-Meir survival curve analysis reveals that higher FOXP2 predicts poorer survival (110 GBM patients).

data, or Mann–Whitney U-test for non-normal distribution data. In multiple comparisons, one-way analysis of variance (ANOVA) was used. Pearson's test was used to detect the correction of two groups and compare quantitative values of expression. Survival curves were plotted by the Kaplan-Meier method and compared by log-rank test. A value of $P < 0.05$ was considered statistically significant.

RESULTS

Expression of miR-9-5p and FOXP2 in GBM and Clinical Features

To detect the expression of miR-9-5p and FOXP2 in GBM, 110 GBM samples with complete clinical and follow-up survey data were collected for this study. According to the expression level of miR-9-5p or FOXP2, cases were

TABLE 1 | Clinical features and relative expression of miR-9 in glioblastoma (110 cases).

Clinical variables	Num	miR-9 relative expression		X^2/H	P value
		High expression	Low expression		
Total	110	**55**	**55**		
Gender					
Male	51	27 (49.1)	24 (43.6)	0.329	0.566
Female	59	28 (50.9)	31 (56.9)		
Age (y)					
<50	48	22 (40.0)	26 (47.3)	0.591	0.442
>50	61	33 (60.0)	29 (52.7)		
Recurrences					
Yes	44	16 (29.1)	28 (50.9)	5.455	0.020
No	66	39 (70.9)	27 (49.1)		
Onset time (m)					
≤12	43	18 (32.7)	25 (45.5)	1.871	0.171
>12	67	37 (67.3)	30 (54.5)		
Num of lobes involved					
Single	64	40 (72.7)	24 (43.6)	9.565	0.002
Multiple	46	15 (27.3)	31 (56.4)		
Pre-op KPS score					
≥80	59	33 (60.0)	26 (47.3)	1.791	0.181
<80	51	22 (40.0)	29 (52.7)		
Post-op KPS score					
≥80	658	431 (53.4)	27 (46.6)	10.584	0.445
<80	452	124 (46.2)	328 (53.8)		
Tumor size					
<3 cm	35	17 (30.9)	18 (32.7)	3.251	0.197
3–5 cm	45	19 (34.5)	26 (47.3)		
>5 cm	30	19 (34.5)	11 (20.0)		
Adjuvant therapy					
Yes	52	23 (41.8)	29 (52.7)	1.313	0.252
No	58	32 (58.2)	26 (47.3)		
Degree of tumor resection					
Totally	30	12 (21.8)	18 (32.7)	0.157	0.692[a]
Most partially/partially	54	33 (60.0)	21 (38.1)		
Biopsy	26	10 (18.2)	16 (29.1)		
Survivals					
<6 m	37	10 (18.2)	27 (49.1)	15.209	<0.001
6–12 m	29	14 (25.5)	15 (27.3)		
>12 m	44	31 (56.4)	13 (23.6)		

Pre-op, pre-operative; Post-op, post-operative; Num, number.
[a]Degree of tumor resection is a hierarchical variable was used by the Kruskal Wallis H-test of non-parametric test.

TABLE 2 | Clinical features and relative expression of FOXP2 in glioblastoma (110 cases).

Clinical variables	Num	FOXP2 relative expression		X^2/H	P value
		High expression	Low expression		
Total	**110**	**55**	**55**		
Gender					
Male	52	27 (49.1)	25 (45.5)	0.146	0.702
Female	58	28 (50.1)	30 (54.5)		
Age (y)					
<50	52	28 (50.9)	24 (43.6)	0.584	0.445
>50	58	27 (49.1)	31 (56.4)		
Recurrences					
Yes	59	38 (69.1)	21 (38.2)	10.565	0.001
No	51	17 (30.9)	34 (61.8)		
Onset time (m)					
≤12	68	42 (76.4)	26 (47.3)	9.860	0.002
>12	42	13 (23.6)	29 (52.7)		
Num of lobes involved					
Single	56	32 (58.2)	24 (43.6)	2.328	0.127
Multiple	54	23 (41.8)	31 (56.4)		
Pre-op KPS score					
≥80	59	36 (65.5)	23 (41.8)	6.178	0.013
<80	51	19 (34.5)	32 (58.2)		
Post-op KPS score					
≥80	62	30 (54.5)	32 (58.2)	0.148	0.701
<80	48	25 (45.5)	23 (41.8)		
Tumor size					
<3 cm	34	11 (20.0)	23 (41.8)	6.972	0.031
3–5 cm	38	20 (36.4)	18 (32.7)		
>5 cm	38	24 (43.6)	14 (25.5)		
Adjuvant therapy					
Yes	98	50 (90.9)	48 (87.3)	0.374	0.541
No	12	5 (9.1)	7 (12.7)		
Degree of tumor resection[b]					
Totally	43	21 (38.2)	22 (40.0)	0.085	0.771[a]
Most partial/partial excision	43	24 (43.6)	19 (34.5)		
Biopsy	24	10 (18.2)	14 (25.5)		
Survivals					
<6 m	45	35 (63.6)	10 (18.2)	23.793	<0.001
6–12 m	29	10 (18.2)	19 (34.5)		
>12 m	36	10 (18.2)	26 (47.3)		

Pre-op, pre-operative; Post-op, post-operative; Num, number.
[a]Chi-square test with continuous correction was adopted and the minimum expected value was 4.1.
[b]Degree of tumor resection is a hierarchical variable was used by the Kruskal Wallis H-test of non-parametric test.

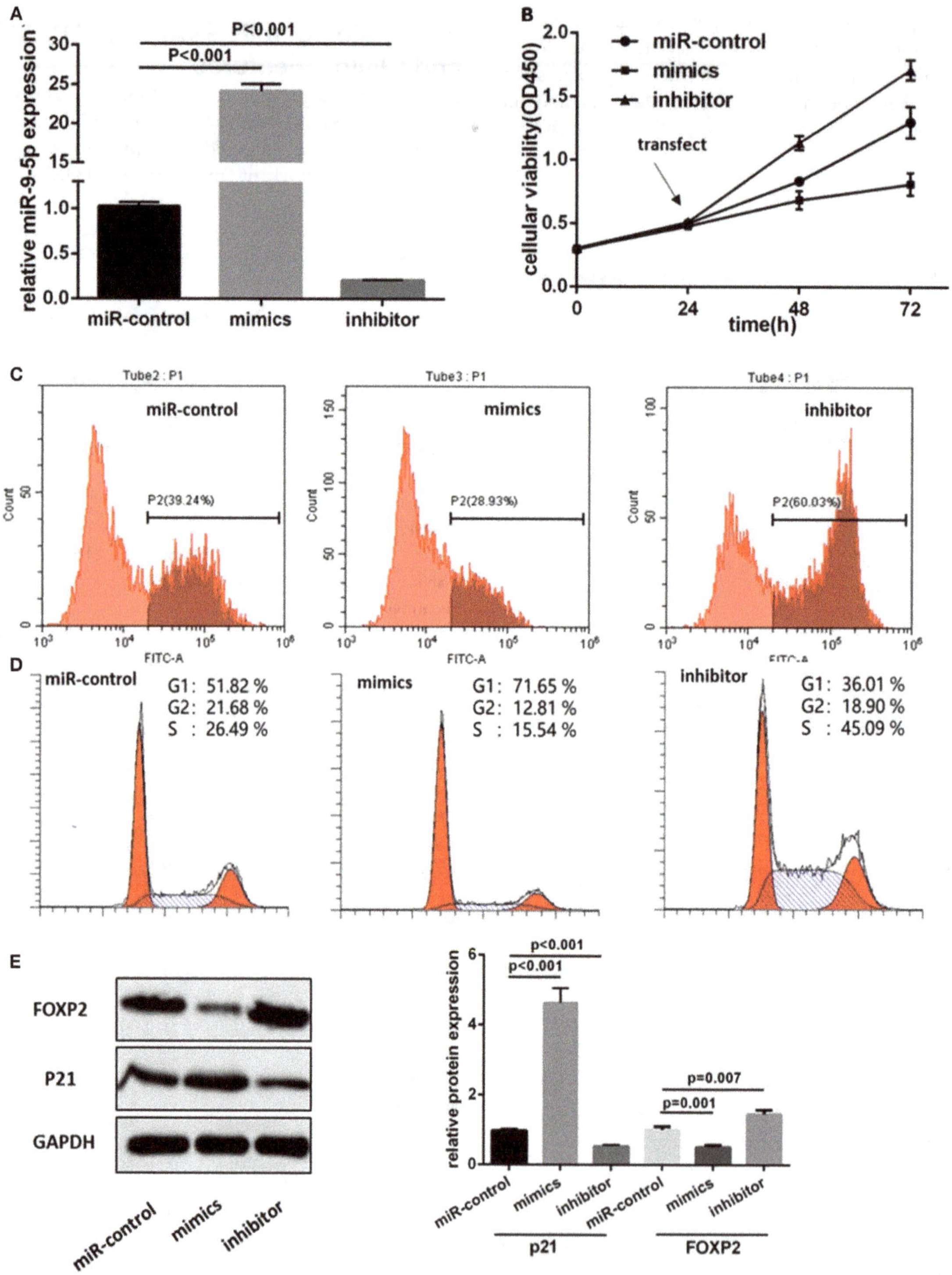

FIGURE 2 | MiR-9-5p inhibits GBM cell growth through cell cycle arrest *in vitro*. **(A)** Expression of miR-9-5p in U251 cell transfected with miRNA. **(B,C)** CCK-8 **(B)** and EdU **(C)** show that high expression of miR-9-5p inhibits cell growth while low expression leads to the opposite effect. **(D)** Cell cycle is arrested in cells with high expression of miR-9-5p analyzed by Flow cytometry. **(E)** Over expression of miR-9-5p leads to down regulation of FOXP2 ($p = 0.001$) and up regulation of p21 ($p = 0.001$); while the inhibited miR-9-5p leads to up regulation of FOXP2 ($p = 0.003$) and down regulation of p21 ($p < 0.001$).

divided into high expression group and low expression group (**Figures 1A,B**). The clinical features and relative expression of miR-9-5p and FOXP2 are presented in **Tables 1**, **2**. The cases with high expression of miR-9-5p and low expression of FOXP2 showed higher overall survival rate (**Figures 1C,D**).

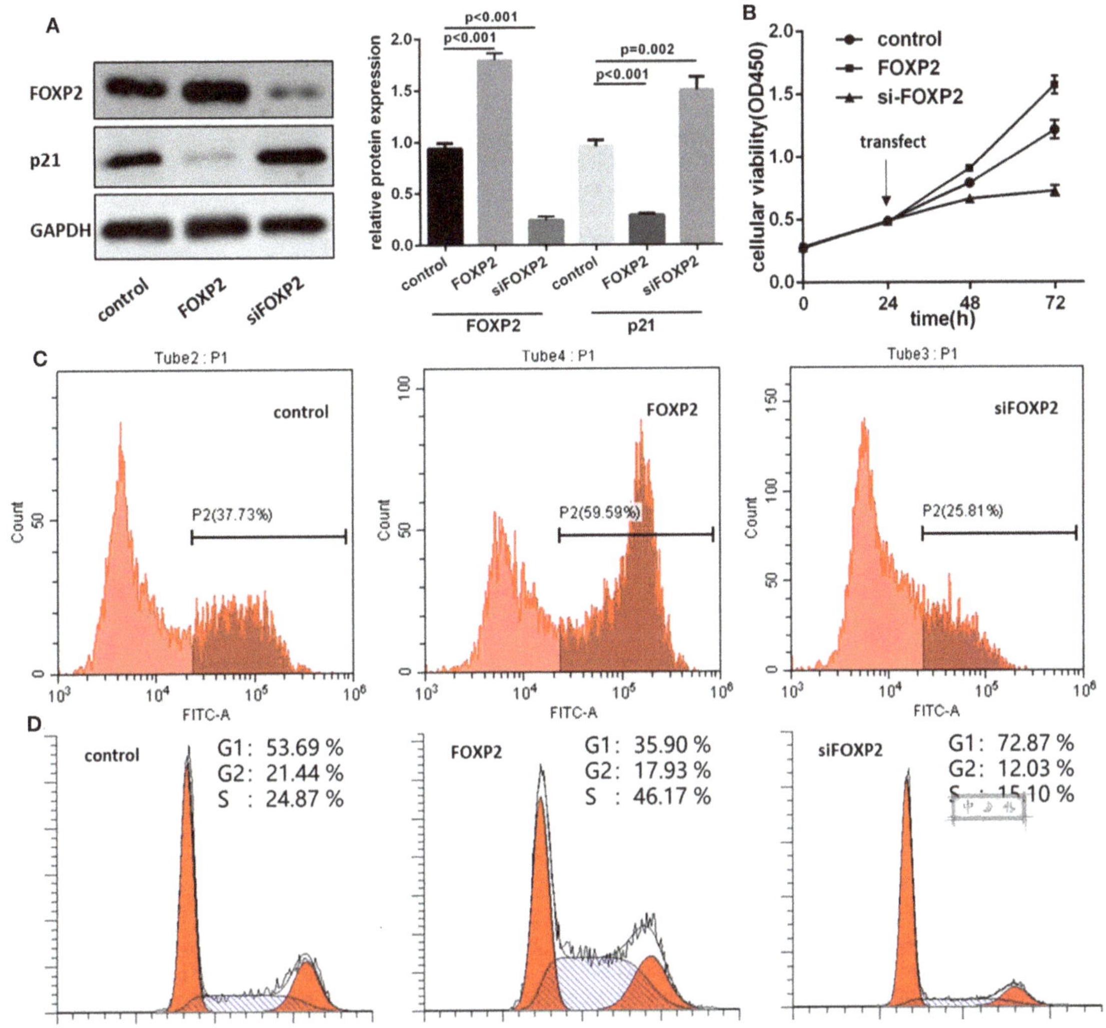

FIGURE 3 | FOXP2 is a positive regulator of U87MG cell proliferation. **(A)** pcDNA3.1-FOXP2 and siRNA transfection is used to regulate the FOXP2 expression in U251 cell. Western blot shows that FOXP2 expresses as expected ($p < 0.001$). Upregulated FOXP2 leads to low expression of p21 ($p < 0.001$) and down regulated FOXP2 leads to high expression of p21 ($p = 0.002$). **(B,C)** CCK-8 **(B)** and EdU **(C)** shows high expression of FOXP2 contributes to cell proliferation while low expression leads to the opposite effect. **(D)** Cell cycle is arrested in cells with low expression of miR-9-5p analyzed by Flow cytometry.

miR-9-5p Was a Negative Regulator of GBM Cell Proliferation

We transfected the miR-9-5p mimics, inhibitor and mi-control into the U251 and U118MG cell, and q-PCR assay showed miR-9-5p expression were significantly different (**Figure 2A**). CCK-8 assay was used to observe the proliferation change. Comparing with the cells transfected with mi-control, the cellular viability of the groups transfected with mimics and inhibitor was significantly decreased and increased, respectively (**Figure 2B**). Flow cytometry was used in EdU assay, and the results showed that less marked cells were detected in the group transfected with mimics, while more in the group with inhibitor (**Figure 2C**). The expression level of miR-9-5p had a significant influence on G1 phase (**Figure 2D**). Further, we detected proteins functioning in the cell cycle process though Western blot assay, and the expression of p21 was significantly higher in miR-9-5p (**Figure 2E**).

FOXP2 Was a Positive Regulator of GBM Cell Proliferation

To demonstrate that FOXP2 exerts positive effects on GBM cell proliferation, we intervened in the expression of FOXP2 (**Figure 3A**). Similar assays were used to analyze the cell proliferation, cell cycle and cell cycle associated proteins. Results showed that low expression of FOXP2 slowed down the cell proliferation (**Figures 3B,C**) and G1 arrested (**Figure 3D**) and inhibited p21 high expression (**Figure 3A**).

miR-9-5p Directly Regulated FOXP2 Expression

Figure 3A shows a significant, negative relationship between the expression of FOXP2 and miR-9-5p. In GBM cells, miR-9-5p mimics resulted in FOXP2 down regulation, while the inhibitor exert a opposite effect (**Figure 2E**). Luciferase reporter assay

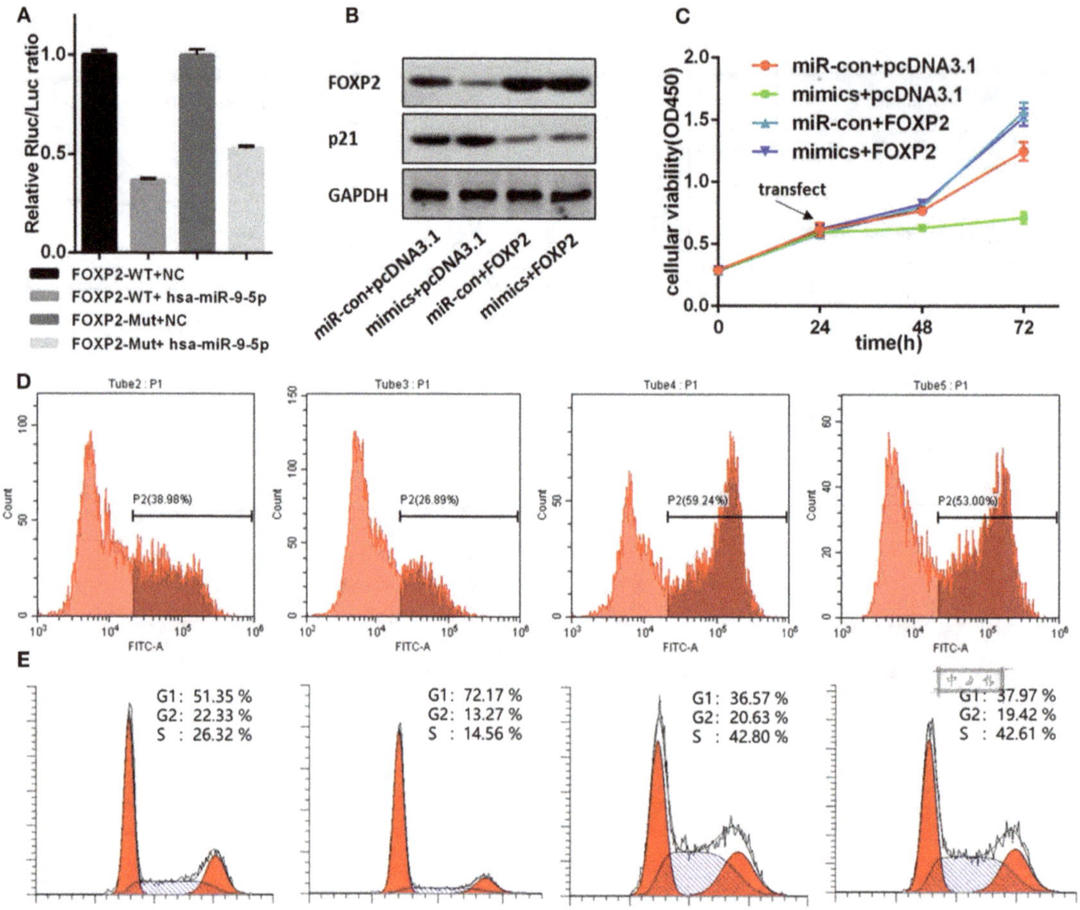

FIGURE 4 | FOXP2 is indispensable for miR-9-5p suppressing U87MG cell proliferation. **(A)** Luciferase reporter assay suggests FOXP2 is the direct target of miR-9-5p. **(B)** Western bolt shows that the DNA transfection hold back the down regulation of FOXP2. Further, the up regulation of p21 caused by miR-9-5p is also restrained. **(C,D)** CCK-8 **(C)** and EdU **(D)** show that cell proliferation inhibition caused by miR-9-5p is restrained by stable expression of FOXP2. **(E)** Cell cycle arrest is blocked by the stable FOXP2.

suggested that FOXP2 was the direct target of miR-9-5p (**Figure 4A**).

FOXP2 Was Indispensable for miR-9-5p Suppressing Tumor Growth

We re-expressed FOXP2 in the U251 cell with high level miR-9-5p by DNA transfection, and the result showed that the original cell proliferation inhibition and the cell cycle arrest caused by miR-9-5p were changed (**Figures 4C–E**). Further, western blot showed no difference in p21 between cells with high level miR-9-5p and the control group (**Figure 4B**).

miR-9-5p Up-Regulation Inhibited GBM Growth *in vivo*

To further investigate whether the level of miR-9-5p expression could inhibit GBM growth *in vivo*, we inoculated U251 cell into male nude mice, and injected miR-9-5p mimics or mi-control (as control) into their tail vein. Twenty-one days after injection, all mice developed xenograft tumors at the injection site and the tumor size of the mimics group was significantly smaller compared with that of the control group (**Figure 5A**). Moreover, the growth of tumors was significantly slower in the mimics group than that in the mi-control group (**Figure 5A**). The injected group showed a higher expression of miR-9-5p (**Figure 5B**), a lower expression of FOXP2 expression and higher p21 (**Figure 5C**).

DISCUSSION

A better understanding of key pathways driving glioma growth and development has the potential to improve the treatment of GBM. Previous studies have demonstrated that high expression of miR-9 led to lower survival rate in patients with high grade (WHO III IV) glioma (15). However, opposite results were presented in other studies. Participating in mutant EGFR signaling, the most common abnormal signaling in GBM, suppressed miR-9 expression increased GBM cells proliferation (11, 22). On the basis of the malignant behavior, Glioma

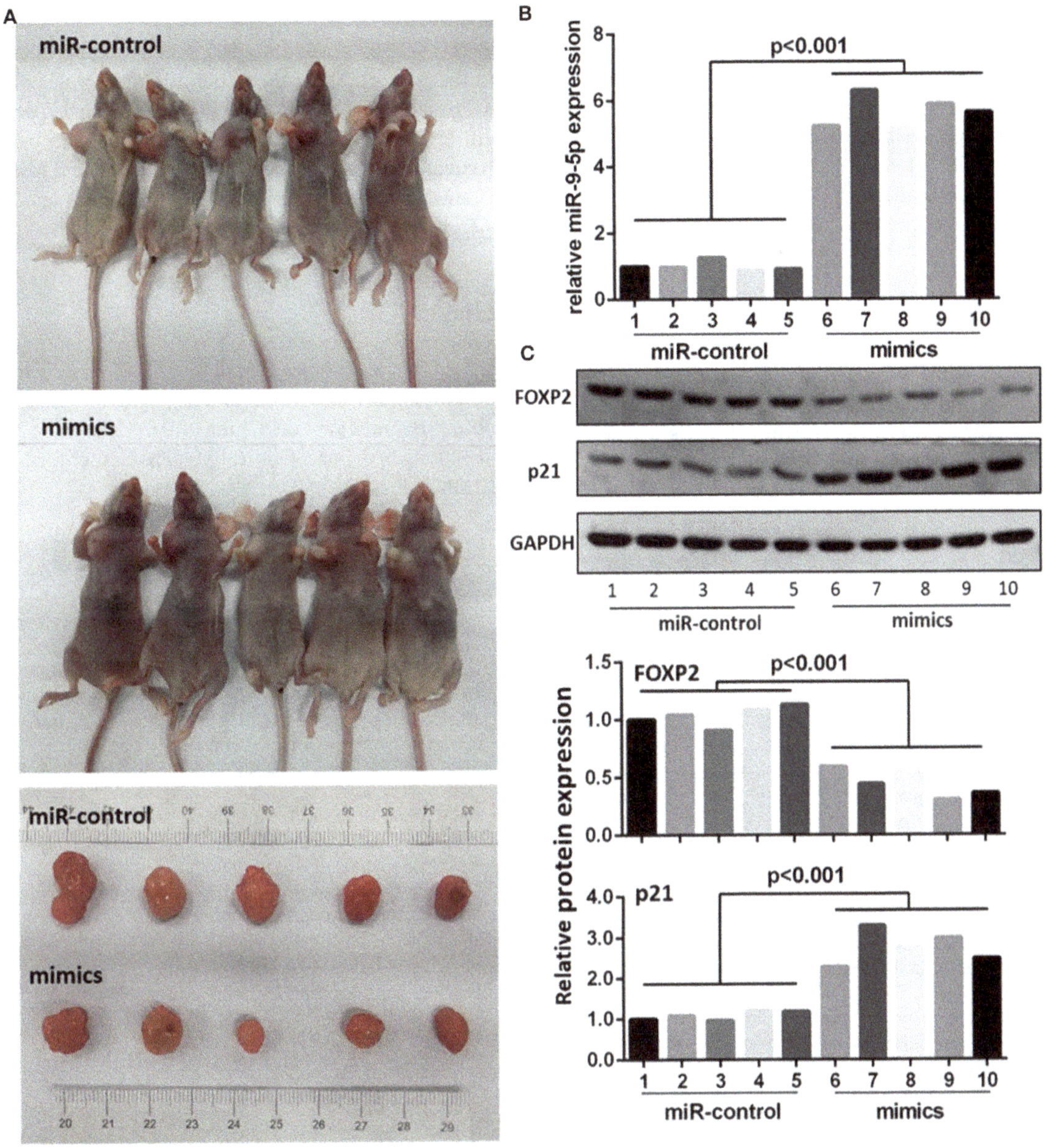

FIGURE 5 | MiR-9-5p inhibits tumor growth *in vivo*. **(A)** Mice injected with miR-9-5p mimics have smaller tumors compared with control group. **(B)** q-PCR shows that miR-9-5p expression of mimics group is extremely higher than that of control group ($p < 0.001$). **(C)** Western blot shows that in mimics group, FOXP2 expression is lower ($p < 0.001$) and p21 expression is higher ($p < 0.001$).

is mainly divided into two types according to WHO I–IV classification (23, 24). In this study, we found that low expression of miR-9-5p led to poor prognosis while high miR-9-5p expression inhibited tumor growth by cell cycle arrest. Similar results were found in neck cancer cells (25).

For the past few years, researches have demonstrated the involvement of FOXP2 in oncogenesis (26), but it exerts opposite function in different cancers. In neuroblastomas, multiple myelomas and several subtypes of lymphomas, FOXP2 is overexpressed (19, 20, 27). In the present study, we demonstrated that FOXP2 was a tumor promoter, and it was able to accelerate the cell cycle and increase the proliferation of GBM cells. It has been reported that FOXP2 functions in neurogenesis in embryonic development (28). FOXP2 null mutant mice developed cerebellar hypoplasia (29). Consider the important effects of FOXP2 on central nervous system, we presume that once unbalanced, it may lead to GBM oncogenesis. A previous study has found that the downregulation of FOXP2 in TP53 associated glioma cell apoptosis (30), which probably indicates that FOXP2 acts as a cancer-promoting gene in GBM.

In the clinical data, FOXP2 was relatively high expressed in recurrent GBM. It is widely considered that chemotherapy resistance is a vital factor leading to GBM recurrence. FOXP2 was reported to directly target the adenosine triphosphate (ATP)-binding cassette (ABC) family proteins such as ABCA6 and ABCG2, which were transporters expelling chemical compounds (31–33). This might be a mechanism in chemotherapy resistance of GBM and a reason for why relatively high expression of FOXP2 was found in recurrent GBM.

CONCLUSION

In this study, we confirmed that the high expression of miR-9-5p, which down regulated FOXP2, was able to suppress the proliferation of GBM via p21-dependent cell cycle arrest both *in vivo* and *in vitro*. It suggests a potential pathway of miR-9-5p-FOXP2 signal which may be applied to GBM therapy in the future.

AUTHOR CONTRIBUTIONS

HZ and YL planned and designed the experimental scheme and the initial draft of the paper, tumor sample collection, and performed experiment. YT, QL, SJ, and DL participated in the cell culture, microRNA extraction experiments, and participated in the collation of experimental data, statistics, and results analysis. QC and SZ were fully responsible for the implementation and supervision of the subject.

FUNDING

This study was supported by China postdoctoral science foundation (2018M640802 to HZ), and the National Natural Science Foundation of China (81671240 to SZ), and the Guangdong Provincial Clinical Medical Center for Neurosurgery (2013B020400005 to SZ).

REFERENCES

1. Tang J, Li Y, Liu K, Zhu Q, Yang WH, Xiong LK, et al. Exosomal miR-9-3p suppresses HBGF-5 expression and is a functional biomarker in hepatocellular carcinoma. *Minerva Med.* (2018) 109:15–23. doi: 10.23736/S0026-4806.17.05167-9
2. Moridikia A, Mirzaei H, Sahebkar A, Salimian J. MicroRNAs: potential candidates for diagnosis and treatment of colorectal cancer. *J Cell Physiol.* (2018) 233:901–13. doi: 10.1002/jcp.25801
3. Cui Y, Xue Y, Dong S, Zhang P. Plasma microRNA-9 as a diagnostic and prognostic biomarker in patients with esophageal squamous cell carcinoma. *J Int Med Res.* (2017) 45:1310–7. doi: 10.1177/03000605177 09370
4. Zhou B, Xu H, Xia M, Sun C, Li N, Guo E, et al. Overexpressed miR-9 promotes tumor metastasis via targeting E-cadherin in serous ovarian cancer. *Front Med.* (2017) 11:214–22. doi: 10.1007/s11684-017-0518-7
5. Wang H, Wu Q, Zhang Y, Zhang HN, Wang YB, Wang W. TGF-beta1-induced epithelial-mesenchymal transition in lung cancer cells involves upregulation of miR-9 and downregulation of its target, E-cadherin. *Cell Mol Biol Lett.* (2017) 22:22. doi: 10.1186/s11658-017-0053-1
6. He L, Zhang L, Wang M, Wang W. miR-9 functions as a tumor inhibitor of cell proliferation in epithelial ovarian cancer through targeting the SDF-1/CXCR4 pathway. *Exp Ther Med.* (2017) 13:1203–8. doi: 10.3892/etm.2017.4118
7. Shang A, Lu WY, Yang M, Zhou C, Zhang H, Cai ZX, et al. miR-9 induces cell arrest and apoptosis of oral squamous cell carcinoma via CDK 4/6 pathway. *Artif Cells Nanomed Biotechnol.* (2018) 46:1754–62. doi: 10.1080/21691401.2017.1391825
8. Gao HY, Huo FC, Wang HY, Pei DS. MicroRNA-9 inhibits the gastric cancer cell proliferation by targeting TNFAIP8. *Cell Prolif.* (2017) 50:e12331. doi: 10.1111/cpr.12331
9. Peng Z, Ying L. Effects of TNFalpha on cell viability, proliferation and apoptosis of glioma cells U251. *J Buon.* (2014) 19:733–41.
10. Song Y, Mu L, Han X, Li Q, Dong B, Li H, et al. MicroRNA-9 inhibits vasculogenic mimicry of glioma cell lines by suppressing Stathmin expression. *J Neurooncol.* (2013) 115:381–90. doi: 10.1007/s11060-013-1245-9
11. Gomez GG, Volinia S, Croce CM, Zanca C, Li M, Emnett R, et al. Suppression of microRNA-9 by mutant EGFR signaling upregulates FOXP1 to enhance glioblastoma tumorigenicity. *Cancer Res.* (2014) 74:1429–39. doi: 10.1158/0008-5472.CAN-13-2117
12. Yang L, Mu Y, Cui H, Liang Y, Su X. MiR-9-3p augments apoptosis induced by H2O2 through down regulation of Herpud1 in glioma. *PLoS ONE.* (2017) 12:e174839. doi: 10.1371/journal.pone.0174839
13. Zu Y, Zhu Z, Lin M, Xu D, Liang Y, Wang Y, et al. MiR-9 promotes apoptosis via suppressing SMC1A expression in GBM cell lines. *Curr Chem Genom Transl Med.* (2017) 11:31–40. doi: 10.2174/2213988501711010031
14. Ben-Hamo R, Zilberberg A, Cohen H, Efroni S. hsa-miR-9 controls the mobility behavior of glioblastoma cells via regulation of MAPK14 signaling elements. *Oncotarget.* (2016) 7:23170–81. doi: 10.18632/oncotarget.6687
15. Wu Z, Wang L, Li G, Liu H, Fan F, Li Z, et al. Increased expression of microRNA-9 predicts an unfavorable prognosis in human glioma. *Mol Cell Biochem.* (2013) 384:263–8. doi: 10.1007/s11010-013-1805-5
16. Yan X, Zhou H, Zhang T, Xu P, Zhang S, Huang W, et al. Downregulation of FOXP2 promoter human hepatocellular carcinoma cell invasion. *Tumour Biol.* (2015) 36:9611–9. doi: 10.1007/s13277-015-3701-y
17. Cuiffo BG, Campagne A, Bell GW, Lembo A, Orso F, Lien EC, et al. MSC-regulated microRNAs converge on the transcription factor FOXP2 and promote breast cancer metastasis. *Cell Stem Cell.* (2014) 15:762–74. doi: 10.1016/j.stem.2014.10.001
18. Jia WZ, Yu T, An Q, Yang H, Zhang Z, Liu X, et al. MicroRNA-190 regulates FOXP2 genes in human gastric cancer. *Onco Targets Ther.* (2016) 9:3643–51. doi: 10.2147/OTT.S103682
19. Wong KK, Gascoyne DM, Soilleux EJ, Lyne L, Spearman H, Roncador G, et al. FOXP2-positive diffuse large B-cell lymphomas exhibit a poor response to R-CHOP therapy and distinct biological signatures. *Oncotarget.* (2016) 7:52940–56. doi: 10.18632/oncotarget.9507
20. Khan FH, Pandian V, Ramraj S, Natarajan M, Aravindan S, Herman TS, et al. Acquired genetic alterations in tumor cells dictate the development of high-risk neuroblastoma and clinical outcomes. *BMC Cancer.* (2015) 15:514. doi: 10.1186/s12885-015-1463-y
21. Gascoyne DM, Spearman H, Lyne L, Puliyadi R, Perez-Alcantara M, Coulton L, et al. The Forkhead transcription factor FOXP2 is required for regulation of p21WAF1/CIP1 in 143B osteosarcoma cell growth arrest. *PLoS ONE.* (2015) 10:e128513. doi: 10.1371/journal.pone.0128513
22. Frederick L, Wang XY, Eley G, James CD. Diversity and frequency of epidermal growth factor receptor mutations in human glioblastomas. *Cancer Res.* (2000) 60:1383–7.
23. Morgan LL. The epidemiology of glioma in adults: a "state of the science" review. *Neuro Oncol.* (2015) 17:623–4. doi: 10.1093/neuonc/nou358
24. Olar A, Aldape KD. Using the molecular classification of glioblastoma to inform personalized treatment. *J Pathol.* (2014) 232:165–77. doi: 10.1002/path.4282
25. Hersi HM, Raulf N, Gaken J, Folarin N, Tavassoli M. MicroRNA-9 inhibits growth and invasion of head and neck cancer cells and is a predictive biomarker of response to plerixafor, an inhibitor of its target CXCR4. *Mol Oncol.* (2018) 12:2023–41. doi: 10.1002/1878-0261.12352

26. Herrero MJ, Gitton Y. The untold stories of the speech gene, the FOXP2 cancer gene. *Genes Cancer.* (2018) 9:11–38. doi: 10.18632/genesandcancer.169
27. Campbell AJ, Lyne L, Brown PJ, Launchbury RJ, Bignone P, Chi J, et al. Aberrant expression of the neuronal transcription factor FOXP2 in neoplastic plasma cells. *Br J Haematol.* (2010) 149:221–30. doi: 10.1111/j.1365-2141.2009.08070.x
28. Tsui D, Vessey JP, Tomita H, Kaplan DR, Miller FD. FoxP2 regulates neurogenesis during embryonic cortical development. *J Neurosci.* (2013) 33:244–58. doi: 10.1523/JNEUROSCI.1665-12.2013
29. Shu W, Cho JY, Jiang Y, Zhang M, Weisz D, Elder GA, et al. Altered ultrasonic vocalization in mice with a disruption in the Foxp2 gene. *Proc Natl Acad Sci USA.* (2005) 102:9643–8. doi: 10.1073/pnas.0503739102
30. Seznec J, Weit S, Naumann U. Gene expression profile in a glioma cell line resistant to cell death induced by the chimeric tumor suppressor-1 (CTS-1), a dominant-positive variant of p53–the role of NFkappaB. *Carcinogenesis.* (2010) 31:411–8. doi: 10.1093/carcin/bgp319
31. Hedditch EL, Gao B, Russell AJ, Lu Y, Emmanuel C, Beesley J, et al. ABCA transporter gene expression and poor outcome in epithelial ovarian cancer. *J Natl Cancer Inst.* (2014) 106:dju149. doi: 10.1093/jnci/dju149
32. Dlugosz A, Janecka A. ABC transporters in the development of multidrug resistance in cancer therapy. *Curr Pharm Des.* (2016) 22:4705–16. doi: 10.2174/1381612822666160302103646
33. Mao Q, Unadkat JD. Role of the breast cancer resistance protein (BCRP/ABCG2) in drug transport–an update. *AAPS J.* (2015) 17:65–82. doi: 10.1208/s12248-014-9668-6

13

LCTL is a Prognostic Biomarker and Correlates with Stromal and Immune Infiltration in Gliomas

*Jun Su[1], Qianquan Ma[2], Wenyong Long[1], Hailin Tang[3], Changwu Wu[1], Mei Luo[1], Xiangyu Wang[1], Kai Xiao[1], Yang Li[1], Qun Xiao[1], Chi Zhang[1], Haoyu Li[1] and Qing Liu[1,4]**

[1] Department of Neurosurgery, Xiangya Hospital, Central South University, Changsha, China, [2] Department of Neurosurgery, Peking University Third Hospital, Peking University, Beijing, China, [3] Sun Yat-sen University Cancer Center, State Key Laboratory of Oncology in South China, Collaborative Innovation Center for Cancer Medicine, Guangzhou, China, [4] Institute of Skull Base Surgery & Neuro-oncology at Hunan, Changsha, China

***Correspondence:**
Qing Liu
liuqingdr@csu.edu.cn

Immune evasion in glioma strongly correlates with clinical outcomes; however, the molecular mechanisms driving the maintenance of immunosuppression remain largely unknown. Recently studies demonstrate that Klothos are aberrantly expressed in several cancers and are potential therapeutic targets in cancers. However, their roles are still unclear in glioma. Here, we show that *LCTL* is highly expressed in gliomas and that its expression is regulated by DNA methylation status at the promoter. *LCTL* expression is also found to be significantly associated with high tumor aggressiveness and poor outcomes for glioma patients. Mechanistically, results suggested that *LCTL* might play an important immunosuppressive role by recruiting immunosuppressive cells and regulating tumor-associated macrophages polarization, T cell exhaustion, and epithelial–mesenchymal transition through FGF signaling in glioma. Our results establish *LCTL* as a key biomarker for prognosis that could be considered a potential epigenetic and immunotherapeutic target for treatment.

Keywords: *Klotho*, *LCTL*, immune infiltration, methylation, FGF signaling, glioma

INTRODUCTION

Gliomas are the most common primary tumors of the central nervous system and account for nearly 75% of malignant brain tumors in adults, of which glioblastoma multiform (GBM) is categorized as the most malignant subtype (1, 2). Despite current standard multimodal treatment, including maximal safe resection followed by combined radio-chemotherapy, the median survival time for patients with glioma is still <2 years (3, 4). Glioma resistant to advanced therapeutic strategies has been widely reported as a consequence of distinct metabolic mechanisms and the complicated immunosuppressive microenvironment that surrounds the tumor niche (5, 6). With advancements in molecular biology, a number of significant genetic alterations (IDH mutation, 1p/19q codeletion, H3ys27Met, and RELA-fusion) are now associated with heterogeneous tumor histology and are clinically significant based on the revised 2016 World Health Organization (WHO) classification (7). Strengthening the knowledge of such molecular alterations will ultimately contribute to a more comprehensive understanding of the diagnosis, classification, and treatment of gliomas. From this perspective, it is urgent to identify novel molecular targets and biomarkers to develop efficient therapeutic strategies.

Klotho was originally identified as an anti-aging gene in 1997 (8). The *Klotho* family comprises three classic members, namely *Klotho (KL)*, *βKlotho (KLB)*, and *γKlotho* (also referred as *LCTL*) (9). All of these three genes encode transmembrane proteins, belonging to glycosidase family 1 and sharing structural similarities to β-glycosidases. However, the critical residues required for enzymatic activity are not conserved in any of the Klotho proteins (10), which indicates that their biological function is independent of glycosidase activity. Klothos proteins are known as essential cofactors that participate in interactions between fibroblast growth factors (FGFs) and fibroblast growth factor receptors (FGFRs) (9, 11). FGF and FGFRs regulate a wide range of biological functions including cell fate, angiogenesis, immunity, and metabolism, and are aberrantly activated during carcinogenesis (12, 13). In addition, recent studies have demonstrated aberrant expression of *Klothos* in several cancers including breast cancer, lung cancer, and hepatocellular carcinoma (9, 14–17). Most studies indicate that *KL* functions as a tumor suppressor and modulates several signaling pathways such as insulin-like growth factor-1 (IGF-1), FGF, and Wnt/β-Catenin (18, 19). However, the role of *KLB* in cancer is controversial. Poh et al. (17) reported that it is up-regulated and associated with FGFR4 signaling in hepatocellular carcinoma. In contrast, Ye et al. (20) reported *KLB* is down-regulated in this disease and regulates Akt/GSK-3β/cyclin D1 signaling. Although mounting evidence suggests potential connections between the *klotho* family and tumor development, the role of *LCTL* in tumorigenesis is still uncertain. Recently, Trost et al. (9) reported that *LCTL* is a potential oncogene in triple negative breast cancer and that it is necessary for resistance to increased oxidative damage. *LCTL* was also reported to be associated with cell proliferation, apoptosis, and epithelial-mesenchymal transition (EMT) in urothelial carcinoma of the bladder (21). However, the role and clinical importance of Klothos is still unclear with respect to glioma.

In this study, we first performed differential gene expression analysis of Klothos comparing the TCGA databases for glioma and normal brain tissues via a bioinformatics approach. We found of *Klotho* genes, only *LCTL* met the preset thresholds of differential expression. Further analysis revealed that the expression of *LCTL* is significantly elevated in gliomas compared to that in normal brain tissues, and that it is strictly associated with pathologic and molecular characteristics of different mutants. Moreover, by analyzing certain prognostic outcomes, *LCTL* was found to be associated with overall survival time in patients with glioma. Similar to that with KL, DNA methylation of the *LCTL* promoter can silence its endogenous expression. After identifying that high *LCTL* expression might lead to glioma progression, we further investigated its potential biological role in glioma based on gene ontology (GO) analysis and observed that it is markedly involved in tumor-associated immune responses in this disease. Further analysis revealed that increased *LCTL* expression is particularly associated with various immunosuppressive behaviors such as the recruitment of suppressive immune cells, secretion of cytokines, and transformation to tumor-promoting phenotype via FGF signaling, which in turn impairs normal immunosurveillance and leads to disease progression.

MATERIALS AND METHODS

Data Sets and Human Tissue Samples

The Patient clinical annotation and gene expression data used in this study were obtained from publicly available databases. The TCGA lower grade glioma and glioblastoma (GBMLGG) dataset, which included genomic data and phenotypic data, was obtained from the University of California, Santa Cruz, Xena browser (https://xenabrowser.net/). The genomic data set contained DNA methylation and gene expression RNAseq (IlluminaHiSeq) data, whereas the phenotype dataset contained demographic, clinical, pathological, and IDH status. An additional data set was obtained from the Gene Expression Omnibus (GEO) GSE16011 (n = 284), which includes lower grade glioma and glioblastoma; and the data are also available on the R2: Genomics Analysis and Visualization Platform (http://r2.amc.nl).

In addition, we obtained glioma tissue samples from 45 patients (15 grade II, 15 grade III, and 15 grade IV glioma) and 15 normal brain tissue samples from the Department of Neurosurgery, Xiangya Hospital, Hunan, China. This study was approved by the Ethics Committee of Xiangya Hospital, Central South University and informed consent was obtained from all the patients. Tissues were frozen in RNAlater (Ambion) in liquid nitrogen and stored until total RNAs were extracted.

Differential Expression Analysis

Gene Differential gene expression analysis was performed using the online database Gene Expression Profiling Interactive Analysis (GEPIA). GEPIA (22) is an interactive web platform for gene expression analysis, which includes 9,736 tumors and 8,587 normal samples from TCGA and GTEx databases and its gene expression data have been re-computed from raw RNA-Seq data based on the UCSC Xena project and a uniform pipeline for solving the imbalance between tumor and normal data. The preset differential thresholds were p-value < 0.05 and $|\log_2 FC| > 1$. Based on differential analysis, the expression data are first log2(TPM + 1)-transformed and the log2FC is defined as median (tumor)—median (normal). Only genes that meet the preset thresholds are considered differentially expressed.

Gene Expression Analysis

Gene expression data from TCGA were generated using the Illumina HiSeq 2000 RNA Sequencing platform, and this dataset shows gene-level transcription estimates, as log2(x + 1)-transformed RSEM normalized counts. Gene expression data from GSE16011 was generated using an Affymetrix Gene Chip Human Genome U133 Plus 2.0 Array. In addition, *LCTL* expression in diverse cancers was analyzed via Tumor Immune Estimation Resource (TIMER, http://cistrome.org/TIMER/) (23).

Analysis of Genetic Alterations and DNA Methylation

The Genetic alterations analysis was performed using The cBioPortal for Cancer Genomics (http://cbioportal.org), which provides a web resource to explore, visualize, and analyze multidimensional cancer genomics data (24). DNA promoter methylation data (Methylation 450k), similar to gene expression data, were also downloaded from UCSC Xena browser. Pearson correlation analysis of gene expression and DNA methylation was performed and evaluated via R language.

Survival Analysis

Kaplan–Meier survival analysis and the Cox proportional hazard model were used to estimate the prognostic value of *LCTL* based on TCGA GBMLGG data using R language packages (survival and survminer). Kaplan–Meier survival analysis for the GSE16011 data set was generated by the R2: Genomics Analysis and Visualization Platform.

Gene Ontology (GO) Enrichment Analysis

Gene ontology enrichment analysis was performed by The Database for Annotation, Visualization and Integrated Discovery (DAVID, https://david.ncifcrf.gov/), an online software, to identify GO categories by their biological processes, molecular functions, and cellular components (25). Enriched ontological terms with $P < 0.05$ were regarded as statistical significance.

Analysis of Stromal and Immune Infiltration

ESTIMATE (Estimation of STromal and Immune cells in MAlignant Tumor tissues using Expression) algorithm was described by Yoshihara (26) to assess the presence of stromal cells and the infiltration of immune cells in tumor samples, and its predictive ability has been validated in large and independent data sets. The ESTIMATE algorithm generates three scores as follows: stromal score (positively correlating with the presence of stroma in tumor tissue), immune score (positively correlating with the level of immune cells infiltrations in tumor tissue), and estimate score (which infers and negatively correlates with tumor purity). xCell, reported by Aran (27) to estimate the enrichment of cell types, can estimate 64 cell types, spanning multiple adaptive and innate immune cells, hematopoietic progenitors, epithelial cells, and extracellular matrix cells derived from expression profiles. The scores, calculated by the ESTIMATE algorithm, were downloaded from https://bioinformatics.mdanderson.org/estimate/. The pre-calculated TCGA data based on xCell was downloaded from http://xcell.ucsf.edu/. Then the correlation between *LCTL* expression and ESTIMATE scores and 64 cell types from the TCGA glioma dataset were analyzed using R language.

Protein-Protein Interaction (PPI) Analysis

The Search Tool for the Retrieval of Interacting Genes (STRING), an online database, was used to identify proteins that can interact with *LCTL* and construct PPI networks for this protein, immunosuppressive cell recruitment factors, immunosuppressive factors, factors promoting M2 differentiation, and markers of T cell exhaustion and EMT.

Cell Lines and Culture

The human glioma cell lines (U87, U251, SF126, SF767, A172, and SHG-44) and the normal glial cell line HEB were obtained from Sun Yat-Sen University Cancer Center. All the cell lines were cultured in DMEM with 10% FBS and antibiotics (100 μg/ml penicillin and 100 μg/ml streptomycin), and maintained in standard culture condition.

RNA Extraction and Real-Time PCR

Total RNA was extracted from cell lines or human tissues by Trizol reagent (Invitrogen) according to the manufacturer's protocol. Then, total RNA was quantified and 1 μg of RNA was reverse-transcribed with the Reverse Transcription Kit (Thermo Fisher Scientific). Q-PCR was performed using SYBR Premix Ex Taq II (Takara Bio). β-Actin mRNA was used to normalize the expression of genes. Primers are described in **Supplementary Table S1**.

Statistical Analysis

Statistical computations and the creation of figures were performed with several packages (ggplot2, survival, survminer, corrplot) in the statistical software environment R, version 3.5.3 (http://www.r-project.org).

RESULTS

LCTL mRNA Expression Levels in Gliomas and Other Cancers

To assess the differential expression of *Klotho* genes in gliomas and normal brain tissues, the online database GEPIA was used. Results showed that there was no significant difference in the expression of *KL* between gliomas and normal brain tissues ($p > 0.05$, **Supplementary Figure S1A**). Even though the expression of *KLB* was significantly downregulated in glioma compared to levels in normal brain tissue ($p < 0.05$, **Supplementary Figure S1B**), it was still not a differentially expressed, as the $|\log_2 FC|$ value was <1. Interestingly, among *Klotho* genes, only *LCTL* met the preset criterion and was significantly upregulated in both brain lower grade glioma (LGG) and GBM, as compared to levels in normal tissue ($p < 0.05$, **Figure 1A**). We further analyzed the expression of this gene in different grades of glioma and found that its level significantly increases with WHO grades based on the TCGA dataset (**Figure 1B**, left). Further, this result was validated by the GSE16011 dataset (**Figure 1B**, right). In addition, *LCTL* expression was significantly upregulated in the mesenchymal subtype compared with other three respective molecular subtypes in the TCGA dataset (**Figure 1C**). To further validate these findings, Q-PCR was performed in cell lines and our 45 gliomas samples. The results showed that *LCTL* was upregulated in glioma cell lines compared with that in normal glial cell line (**Figure 1D**), its expression level was higher in glioma tissues than that in normal brain tissues (**Figure 1E**), and the expression level of *LCTL*

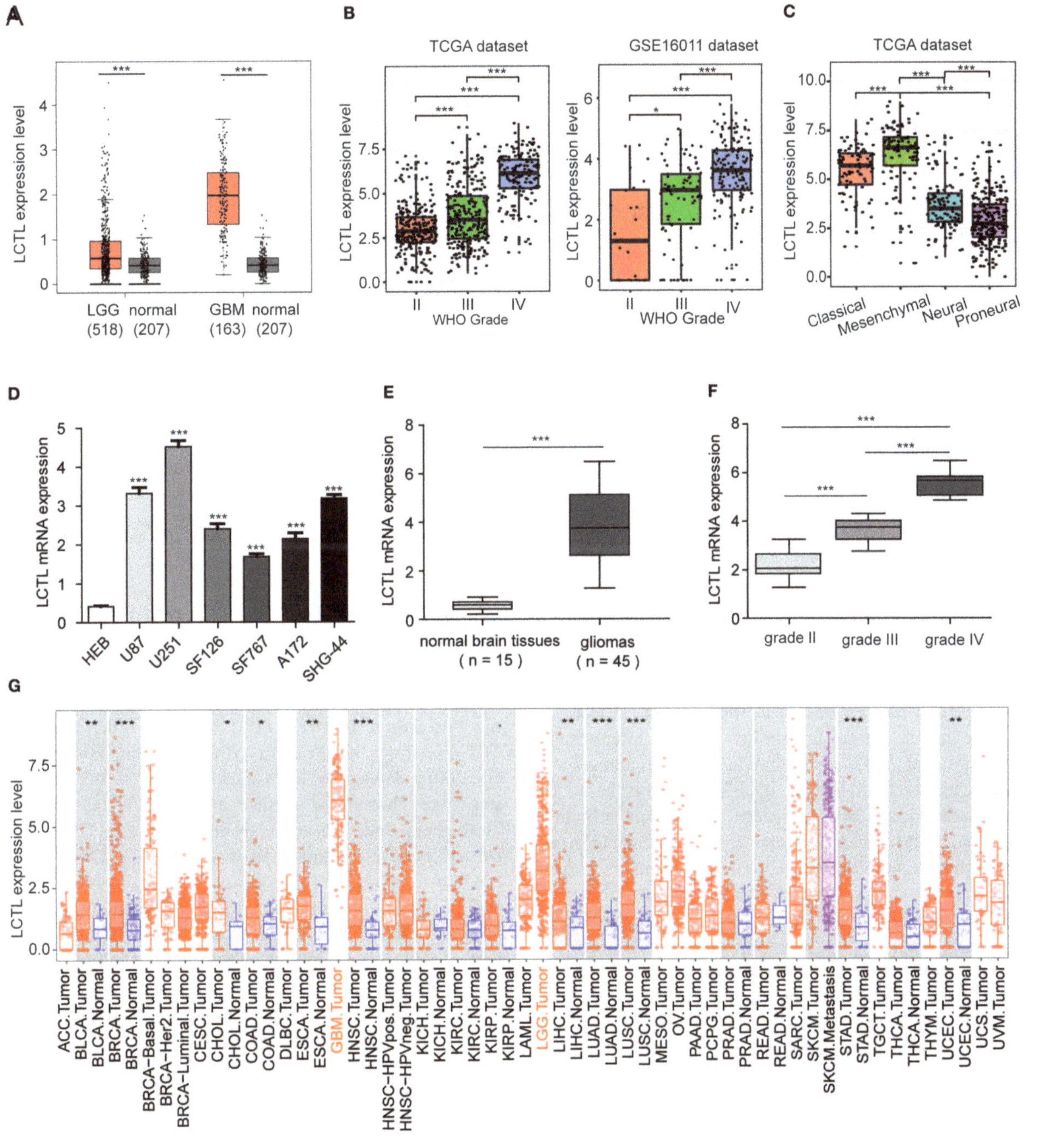

FIGURE 1 | *LCTL* is highly expressed in gliomas and significantly associated with tumor aggressiveness. **(A)** Differential expression of *LCTL* in brain lower grade glioma (LGG) and glioblastoma (GBM) compared to levels in normal brain tissues. **(B)** *LCTL* expression in glioma of WHO grade II–IV based on both TCGA and GSE16011 datasets. **(C)** *LCTL* expression pattern in different molecular subtypes of glioma (classical, mesenchymal, neural, proneural) in the TCGA dataset. **(D)** The mRNA expression level of *LCTL* in glioma cell lines and the normal glial cell line HEB by Q-PCR. **(E)** Validation of aberrant mRNA expression of *LCTL* in 45 gliomas compared to 15 normal brain tissues via Q-PCR. **(F)** *LCTL* expression in glioma of WHO grade II–IV based on our patient samples. **(G)** Expression of *LCTL* in multiple cancers as determined by TIMER analysis. ACC, Adrenocortical carcinoma; BLCA, Bladder Urothelial Carcinoma; BRCA, Breast invasive carcinoma; CESC, Cervical squamous cell carcinoma and endocervical adenocarcinoma; CHOL, Cholangiocarcinoma; COAD, Colon adenocarcinoma; DLBC, Lymphoid Neoplasm Diffuse Large B-cell Lymphoma; ESCA, Esophageal carcinoma; GBM, Glioblastoma multiforme; HNSC, Head and Neck squamous cell carcinoma; KICH, Kidney Chromophobe; KIRC, Kidney renal clear cell carcinoma; KIRP, Kidney renal papillary cell carcinoma; LAML, Acute Myeloid Leukemia; LGG, Brain Lower Grade Glioma; LIHC, Liver hepatocellular carcinoma; LUAD, Lung adenocarcinoma; LUSC, Lung squamous cell carcinoma; MESO, Mesothelioma; OV, Ovarian serous cystadenocarcinoma; PAAD, Pancreatic adenocarcinoma; PCPG, Pheochromocytoma and Paraganglioma; PRAD, Prostate adenocarcinoma; READ, Rectum adenocarcinoma; SARC, Sarcoma; SKCM, Skin Cutaneous Melanoma; STAD, Stomach adenocarcinoma; TGCT, Testicular Germ Cell Tumors; THCA, Thyroid carcinoma; THYM, Thymoma; UCEC, Uterine Corpus Endometrial Carcinoma; UCS, Uterine Carcinosarcoma; UVM, Uveal Melanoma. $^{**}P < 0.01$, $^{***}P < 0.001$.

positively correlated with WHO grade of gliomas (**Figure 1F**). Moreover, an analysis of *LCTL* expression in multiple human cancer types via TIMER showed that the expression levels were highest in GBM, following by skin cutaneous melanoma (SKCM) and LGG (**Figure 1G**). These results indicated that *LCTL* is significantly up regulated in glioma and several other cancers.

LCTL Expression Is Associated With Glioma Patient Outcomes

Since the expression of *LCTL* was found to be aberrantly expressed in gliomas and to correlate with histological grade and molecular subtype, we further studied its prognostic value. For this, Kaplan–Meier survival analysis was performed to evaluate the predictive effects of this gene using both TCGA and GSE16011 datasets. Results indicated that high *LCTL* expression is not only significantly associated with poor prognosis in glioma patients (**Figures 2A,B**), but also in patients with high grade glioma (**Figures 2C,D**). Recently, increasing evidence has suggested recurrent point mutations in isocitrate dehydrogenase genes (*IDH1* and *IDH2*) occur in specific types of glioma (28). Although tumors exhibit identical histologies, the outcome for IDH-mutant (IDH-Mut) diffuse gliomas is better than that with IDH-wildtype (IDH-Wt) disease (29). Further, in the latest version of the WHO Classification of Central Nervous System Tumors published in 2016, IDH mutations were adopted as a decisive marker for glioma classification (30). Currently, this is widely used clinically as a strong prognostic marker for glioma patients. Interestingly, we also found that *LCTL* expression in IDH-Wt gliomas was significantly higher than that in IDH-Mut tumors based on TCGA dataset (**Figure 2E**), consistent with results obtained from the GSE16011 dataset (**Figure 2F**). Simultaneously, we wondered whether *LCTL* could be an independent prognostic marker for glioma and performed univariate and multivariate Cox regression analysis based on the TCGA dataset. Univariate analysis revealed that *LCTL* expression, patient age at diagnosis, WHO grade, and IDH status, were significantly associated with overall survival. Based on multivariate analysis, the expression of *LCTL* was also a significant predictive factor after adjusting for the aforementioned clinical factors (**Table 1**). Taken together, *LCTL* is an independent prognostic factor, and high expression indicates poor clinical outcome for glioma patients.

Promoter DNA Methylation Regulates *LCTL* mRNA Expression

It is widely recognized that both genetic alterations (mutations, loss of heterozygosity, deletions, insertions, aneuploidy, etc.) and epigenetic alterations (DNA methylation, non-coding RNAs, transcription factors, etc.) equally contribute to carcinogenesis (31). Whereas, the former perturb normal patterns of gene expression, which is dependent on changes to normal DNA sequences, the latter result in the inappropriate silencing or activation of cancer-associated genes without changing DNA sequences (32). Interestingly, after the analysis of genetic alterations by cBioPortal, we found no genetic alterations including mutations and putative copy-number alterations in *LCTL* in TCGA Merged Cohort of LGG and GBM (**Supplementary Table S2**). Next, we investigated epigenetic alterations of *LCTL*, and especially promoter DNA methylation. After integrating TCGA glioma datasets, we identified 593 patients with both *LCTL* expression and DNA methylation data. The *LCTL* DNA methylation beta values at cg00686404 were significantly higher in the low *LCTL* expression group than in the high *LCTL* expression group (**Figure 3A**). Meanwhile, the beta values at cg00686404 were negatively correlated with *LCTL* mRNA expression (Pearson's $r = -0.682$, $p < 2.2e\text{-}16$; **Figure 3B**). Consistently, an analysis of DNA methylation at cg25923629 generated similar results (**Figures 3C,D**). To further validate our previous results, we next analyzed the predictive value of *LCTL* promoter DNA methylation for glioma patients and found that patients with high levels had significantly better prognosis than those with low levels (**Figures 3E,F**, $p < 0.0001$). In summary, these results indicate that the expression of *LCTL* is likely regulated by DNA methylation of its promoter, and that this epigenetic modification might also represent a potential prognostic marker for glioma patients.

LCTL Related GO Functional Enrichment in Glioma

To further clarify the biologic role of *LCTL* in glioma, GO enrichment analysis was performed. First, we analyzed the correlation between *LCTL* and all other genes in the TCGA dataset by Pearson correlation analysis and in the GSE16011 dataset by R2. Genes with $|R| > 0.5$ in both data sets were chosen for further analysis. Finally, we obtained 2091 genes and 161 genes from TCGA and GSE16011 gene lists, respectively (**Supplementary Table S3**). Then, we probed the bio-function of these genes by GO analysis in DAVID Bioinformatics Resources 6.8 (**Supplementary Tables S4, S5**) and found that genes that were tightly correlated with *LCTL* expression in TCGA and GSE16011 datasets were enriched in 66 biological processes terms (the top 15 terms are shown in **Figure 4A** left, *p*-value < 0.01) and nine terms (**Figure 4A** right, *p*-value < 0.01), respectively. When comparing the two lists of GO terms, we found that genes closely related with *LCTL* were involved in the immune response and inflammatory response for both TCGA and GSE16011 datasets. Regarding molecular function, these genes were mainly enriched in protein binding (**Supplementary Figures S1C,D**). Moreover, cell component analysis indicated enrichment predominantly occurred at the extracellular region (**Supplementary Figures S1E,F**), which indicated that these genes might play a vital role in the tumor microenvironment (TME) of glioma. Importantly, the majority of genes that were enriched in immune response and inflammatory response in the TCGA dataset were significantly positively correlated with *LCTL* expression (**Figure 4B** and **Supplementary Figure S2**). Collectively, these findings suggest that *LCTL* participates in regulating the tumor immune environment.

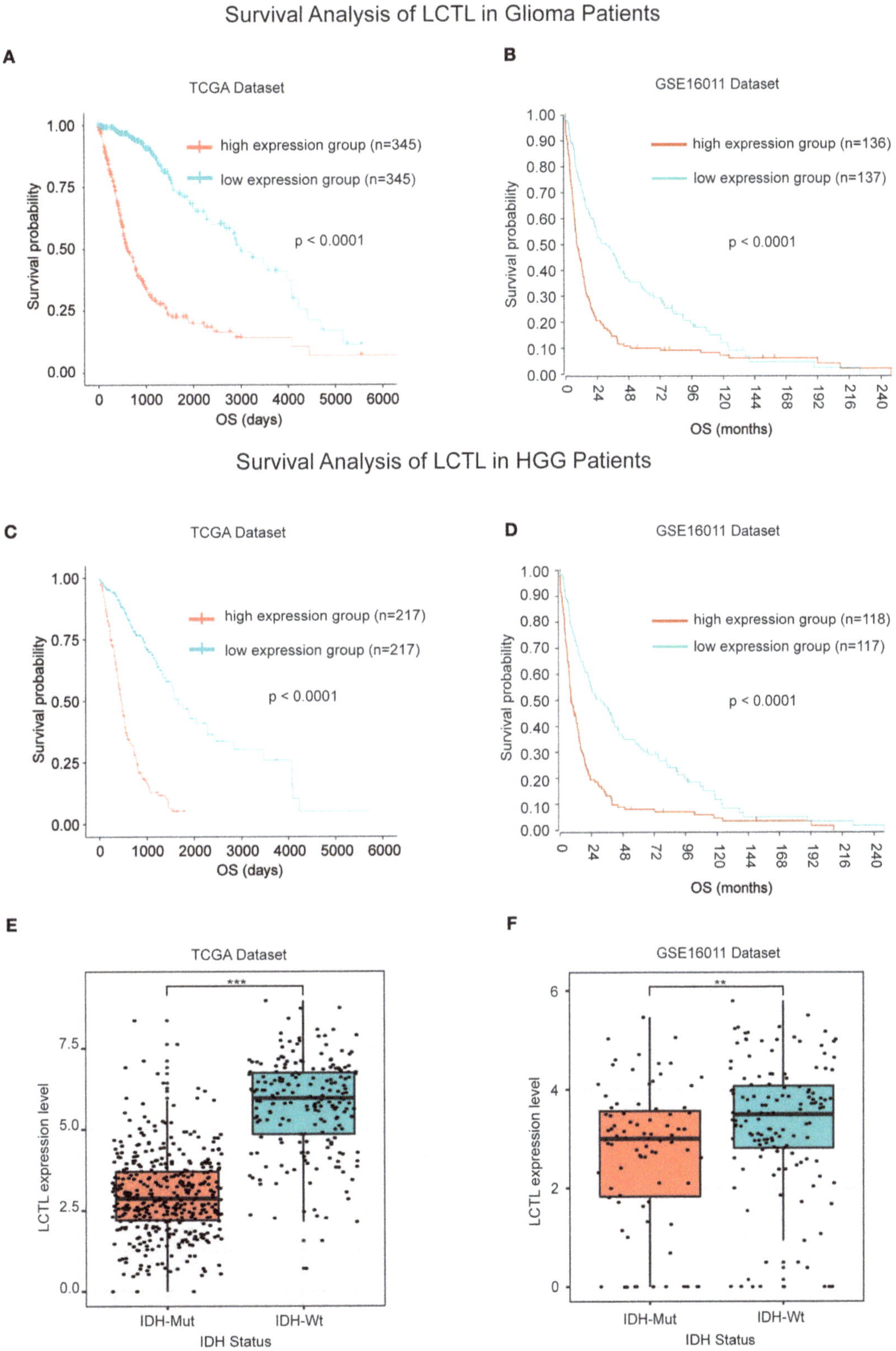

FIGURE 2 | *LCTL* is a prognostic factor for glioma patients. **(A,B)** Kaplan–Meier survival analysis showing that high *LCTL* expression predicts poor prognosis for glioma patients based on both the TCGA and GSE16011 datasets. **(C,D)** Kaplan–Meier survival analysis showing that high *LCTL* expression predicts poor prognosis for high grade glioma (HGG) patients in both the TCGA and GSE16011 datasets. **(E,F)** The expression of *LCTL* is significantly higher in IDH-Wt gliomas than that in IDH-Mut disease based on both the TCGA and GSE16011 datasets. $^{**}P < 0.01$, $^{***}P < 0.001$, t-test.

TABLE 1 | Univariate and multivariate analysis of clinical prognostic parameters based on the TCGA Dataset.

Variable	Univariate analysis			Multivariate analysis		
	HR	95% CI	*p*	HR	95% CI	*p*
LCTL	1.685	1.562–1.816	<0.001	1.167	1.051–1.296	<0.01
Age	1.072	1.061–1.083	<0.001	1.035	1.022–1.047	<0.001
WHO grade	10.670	7.815–14.56	<0.001	1.983	1.352–2.907	<0.001
IDH status	9.991	7.425–13.440	<0.001	3.577	2.317–5.523	<0.001
Gender	1.113	0.848–1.461	0.4	1.228	0.930–1.619	0.147

LCTL Expression Is Correlated With Stromal and Immune Cell Infiltration in Gliomas

Infiltrating stromal and immunes cells, which form the major normal cells component of tumors, play an important role in cancer biology and perturb tumor signaling based on molecular studies (26). Considering the results of GO analysis, we next explored whether *LCTL* expression is associated with immune infiltration in glioma. First, we examined the association between *LCTL* expression and ESTIMATE scores. Results revealed that *LCTL* expression was significantly positively correlated with stromal score, immune score, and ESTIMATE score in both LGG (**Figure 5A**) and GBM patients (**Figure 5B**), suggesting that it has a marked influence on stromal and immune cell infiltration. Since the immune and stromal scores were, respectively, generated based on their gene signatures (26), we therefor performed Q-PCR to investigate the association between mRNA expression of *LCTL* and typical genes of immune and stromal scores in our 45 glioma samples. The results demonstrated that mRNA expression of *LCTL* significantly correlated with that of selected typical genes (top genes correlated with immune and stromal scores in TCGA GBMLGG cohort, **Supplementary Figure S3**). To further determine which cell types play a predominant role in this process, we next analyzed the correlation between *LCTL* expression and 64 non-cancerous cell types, as estimated by xcells, based on TCGA glioma patients. The results showed that there were 39 cell types that significantly correlated with *LCTL* expression (**Figure 5C** and **Table 2**, Spearman's *r*, BH-adjust *p*-value < 0.05), among which, 25 types were positively correlated, whereas 14 types were negatively correlated. These cells types comprised seven lymphoid, 11 myeloid cells, eight stromal, five stem, and eight other cell types. Notably, the majority of myeloid cells, stromal cells, stem cells, and other cells were positively correlated with *LCTL* expression; however, most lymphoid cells were negatively correlated. These findings strongly indicate that *LCTL* plays a specific role in stromal and immune cell infiltration in gliomas.

LCTL Correlates With Immunosuppressive Properties

Since *LCTL* was found to be positively related to immunosuppressive cells, such as M2 macrophages and neutrophils, among others, but was negatively correlated with anti-tumor immune cells such as CD8+ T cells, we hypothesized that this gene could be involved in the immunosuppressive properties of glioma. To confirm this, we performed correlation analysis of *LCTL* expression and critical factors that recruit myeloid-derived suppressor cells, tumor-associated macrophages (TAMs), and tumor-associated neutrophils, as well as the immunosuppressive factors secreted by these cells (**Figures 6A,B**). *LCTL* was found to be significantly positively correlated with the majority of immunosuppressive cell recruitment factors [reviewed in (5)] and immunosuppressive factors [reviewed in (5, 33)]. TAMs can be divided into the "classically activated" M1 phenotype and the "alternatively activated" M2 phenotype (34). It is the M2 phenotype of TAMs that contributes to the immunosuppressive tumor environment (35). Indeed, key factors [CSF-1,CCL2, IL-4, IL-6, IL-10, TGFβ, reviewed in (5)] that drive M2 phenotype differentiation were found to be closely related to *LCTL* expression (**Figure 6C**). It is well-established that T cell exhaustion occurs in humans with cancer and that exhausted T cells in the TME lead to cancer immune evasion (36). Exhausted T cells express high levels of inhibitory receptors including PD-1, CTLA-4, TIM-3, LAG-3, BTLA, and TIGIT [reviewed in (36)]. To further substantiate these findings, we next analyzed the correlation between *LCTL* and inhibitory receptors of exhausted T cells (**Figure 6D**). Our GO enrichment analysis suggested that *LCTL* might be involved in TME, from which various pro-invasion signals can control EMT (37). Further, *LCTL* can promote EMT, as recently reported for bladder cancer (21). Consistently, we found significant correlations between *LCTL* and common EMT biomarkers, except CDH1 and KRT1 (**Figure 6E**). Specifically, *LCTL* expression was positively related to mesenchymal cell markers and negatively correlated with epithelial cell markers. Furthermore, we selected 14 genes, which showed the most correlation with *LCTL* in the TCGA dataset, from abovementioned immunosuppressive factors to validate the correlation between *LCTL* and immunosuppressive properties in our 45 glioma samples by Q-PCR. The results show that *LCTL* expression significantly correlated with the expression of these 14 genes at mRNA level (**Supplementary Figure S4**). Importantly, we found that *LCTL* can directly interact with several proteins, especially FGFRs and FGFs, via PPI analysis (**Supplementary Figure S5A**). Interestingly, via associations with FGFs and FGFRs, *LCTL* could indirectly interact with immunosuppressive factors, recruitment factors, M2 phenotype-driving factors, and markers of exhausted T cells and EMT (**Figure 6F** and **Supplementary Figure S5B**). Therefore, our

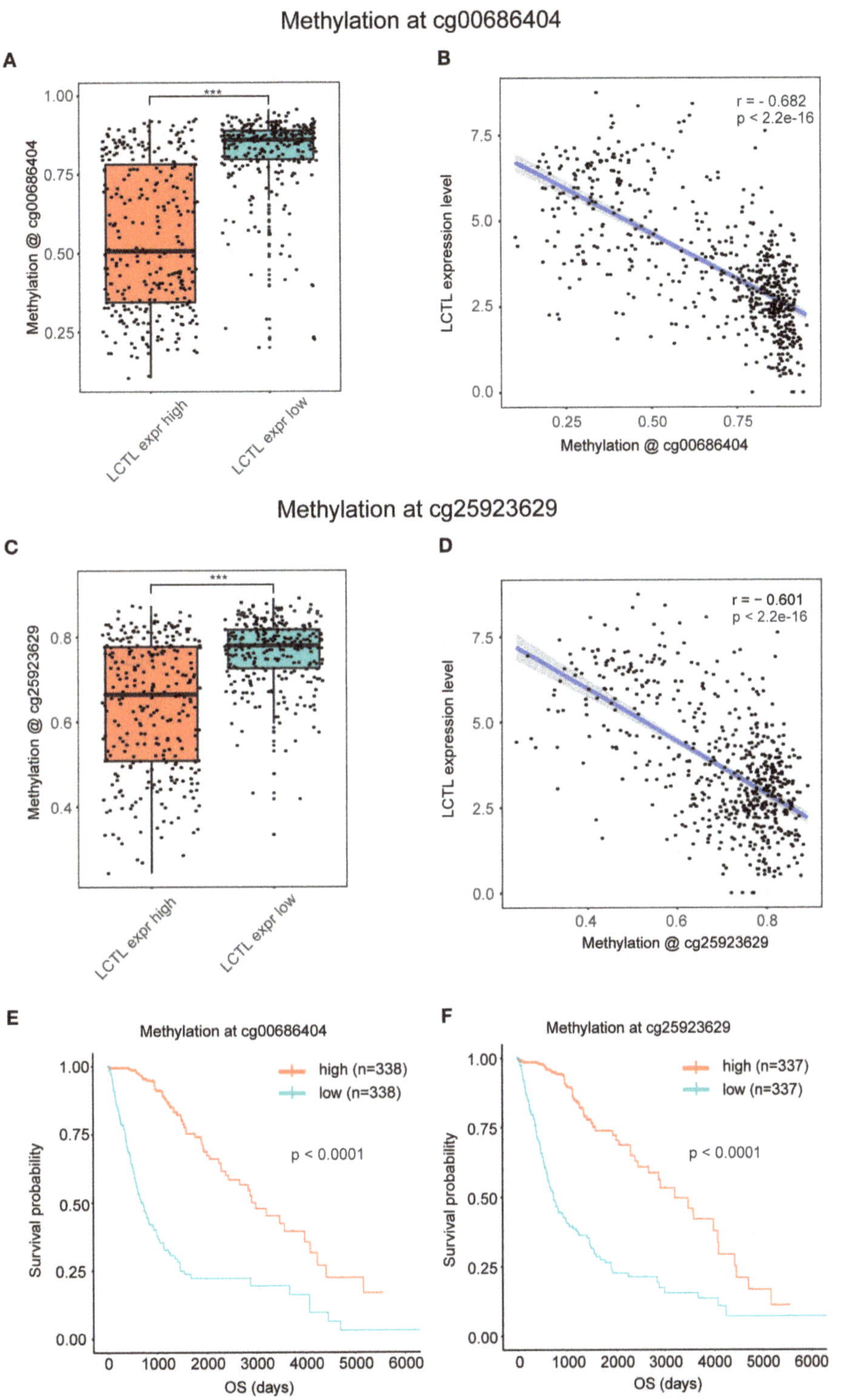

FIGURE 3 | Promoter DNA methylation regulates *LCTL* mRNA expression and correlates with glioma patient prognosis. **(A)** Comparison of DNA methylation beta values at cg0686404. **(B)** Correlation between *LCTL* mRNA expression and promoter DNA methylation at the probe cg00686404. **(C)** Comparison of DNA methylation beta values at cg25923629. **(D)** Correlation between *LCTL* mRNA expression and promoter DNA methylation at the probe cg25923629. **(E)** Association between the promoter DNA methylation value of *LCTL* at cg0686404 overall survival time for glioma patients. **(F)** Association between the promoter DNA methylation value of *LCTL* at cg25923629 and overall survival time for glioma patients. ****P* < 0.001, t-test.

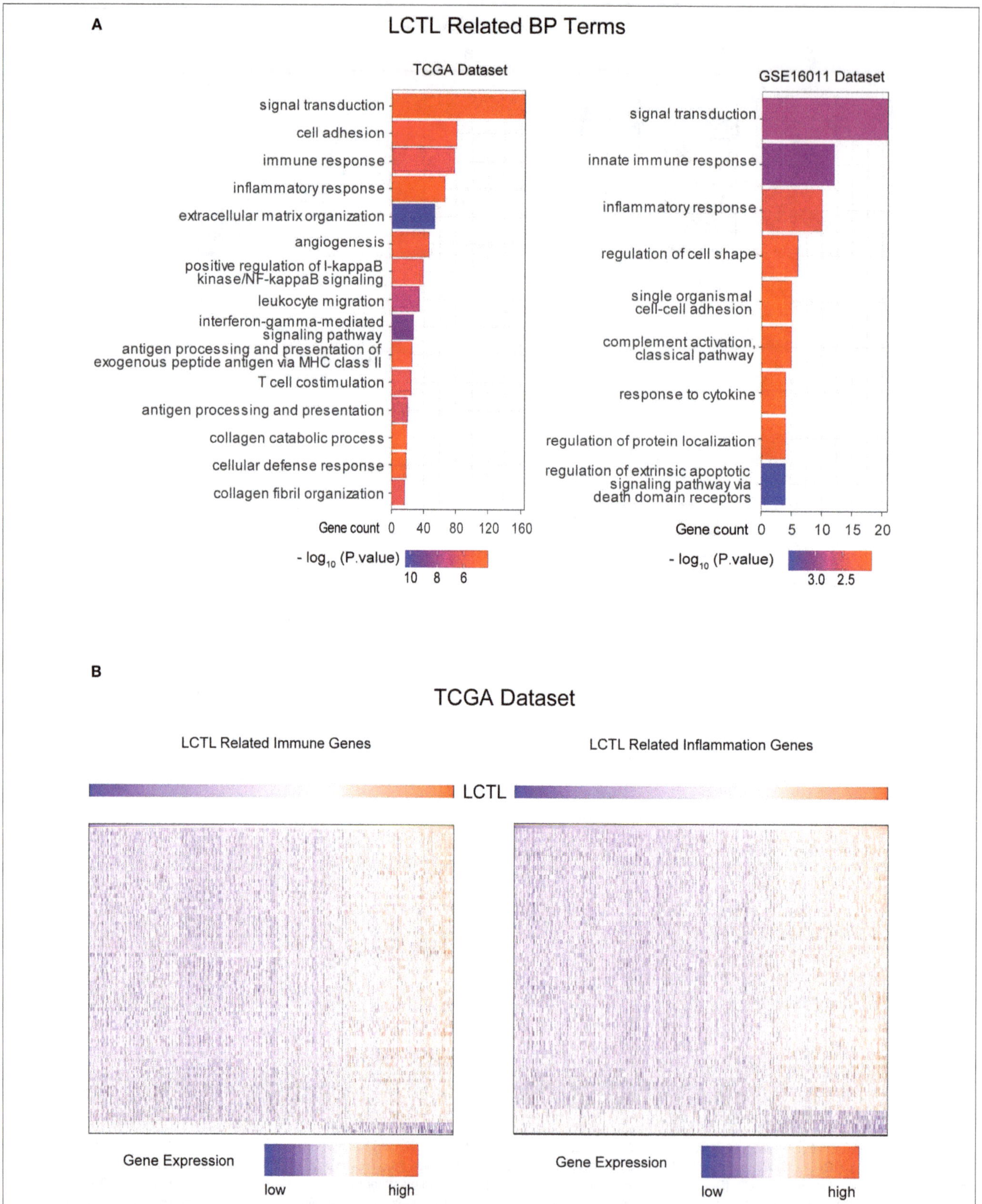

FIGURE 4 | *LCTL* is related to specific gene ontology (GO) terms in glioma. **(A)** Results of BF (biological function) terms analyzed by DAVID based on the TCGA and GSE16011datasets. **(B)** Most immune response and inflammatory response related genes were significantly positively correlated with *LCTL*.

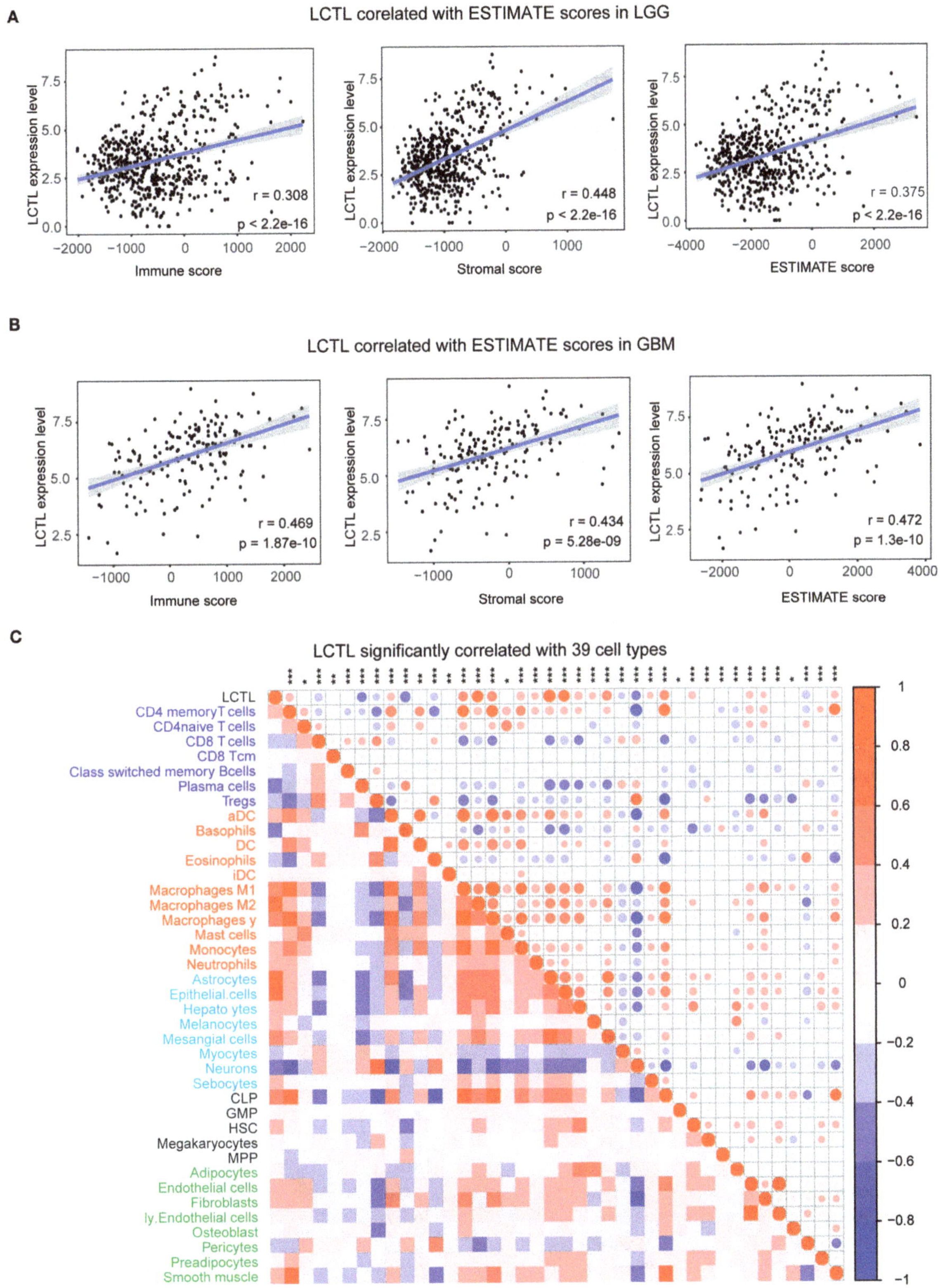

FIGURE 5 | Correlation between *LCTL* expression and ESTIMATE algorithm/xcells scores in glioma. **(A)** *LCTL* expression was positively correlated with immune score, stromal score and ESTIMATE score in lower grade glioma (LGG) patients. **(B)** *LCTL* expression was positively correlated with immune score, stromal score and ESTIMATE score in glioblastoma (GBM) patients. **(C)** *LCTL* expression was significantly correlated with 39 cell types, as calculated by xcells in glioma. *$P < 0.05$, **$P < 0.01$, ***$P < 0.001$.

TABLE 2 | Correlation ship between *LCTL* and 64 types of non-cancerous cells.

xCells	Category	*r* value (Spearman)	CI adjust	Ajust. *P*. val (BH)
Plasma cells	Lymphoids	−0.453	−0.573~−0.312	2.69E-33
CD8+T cells	Lymphoids	−0.346	−0.482~−0.193	5.81E-19
CD4+ memory T cells	Lymphoids	0.336	0.183~0.473	6.99E-18
Tregs	Lymphoids	−0.279	−0.423~−0.121	1.89E-12
Class switched memory B cells	Lymphoids	−0.18	−0.333~−0.017	1.28E-05
CD8+ Tcm	Lymphoids	−0.128	−0.285~0.036	2.90E-03
CD4+ naive T cells	Lymphoids	0.093	−0.252~0.072	3.91E-02
Th2 cells	Lymphoids	0.071	−0.093~0.232	1.30E-01
NK cells	Lymphoids	−0.059	−0.220~0.105	2.25E-01
CD4+ Tcm	Lymphoids	−0.059	−0.220~0.106	2.31E-01
CD8+ Tem	Lymphoids	0.056	−0.108~0.217	2.59E-01
CD8+ naive T cells	Lymphoids	0.041	−0.123~0.203	4.39E-01
B cells	Lymphoids	0.034	−0.130~0.196	5.36E-01
naive B cells	Lymphoids	−0.031	−0.193~0.133	5.73E-01
Th1 cells	Lymphoids	−0.031	−0.193~0.133	5.80E-01
Memory B cells	Lymphoids	0.016	−0.147~0.179	7.87E-01
CD4+ T cells	Lymphoids	−0.015	−0.178~0.148	8.01E-01
Tgd cells	Lymphoids	0.010	−0.154~0.173	8.84E-01
CD4+Tem	Lymphoids	−0.007	−0.170~0.156	9.15E-01
pro B cells	Lymphoids	−0.006	−0.169~0.157	9.29E-01
Natural killer T cells (NKT)	Lymphoids	0.000	−0.163~0.163	9.97E-01
Macrophages M2	Myeloids	0.618	0.506~0.710	5.99E-69
Basophils	Myeloids	−0.559	−0.662~−0.436	6.81E-54
Macrophages y	Myeloids	0.460	0.320~0.579	1.87E-34
Macrophages M1	Myeloids	0.436	0.294~0.559	1.04E-30
Monocytes	Myeloids	0.365	0.215~0.499	3.64E-21
Eosinophils	Myeloids	−0.321	−0.460~−0.167	2.17E-16
Activated dendritic cells (aDC)	Myeloids	0.312	0.157~0.452	1.81E-15
Neutrophils	Myeloids	0.256	0.096~0.402	1.51E-10
Immature DC (iDC)	Myeloids	0.126	−0.037~0.284	3.23E-03
Denritic cells (DC)	Myeloids	0.125	−0.039~0.282	3.67E-03
Mast cells	Myeloids	−0.092	−0.251~0.072	4.11E-02
Xonventional dendritic cells (cDC)	Myeloids	−0.035	−0.197~0.129	5.24E-01
Plasmacytoid dendritic cells (pDC)	Myeloids	−0.025	−0.188~0.138	6.59E-01
Astrocytes	Others	0.681	0.583~0.760	3.58E-89
Epithelial cells	Others	0.601	0.486~0.696	1.89E-64
Mesangial cells	Others	0.464	0.326~0.583	3.22E-35
Neurons	Others	−0.420	−0.546~−0.276	2.18E-28
Hepatocytes	Others	0.361	0.210~0.495	1.25E-20
Melanocytes	Others	0.257	0.098~0.404	1.09E-10
Myocytes	Others	−0.226	−0.375~−0.065	2.14E-08
Sebocytes	Others	0.222	0.061~0.372	3.91E-08
Keratinocytes	Others	0.031	−0.133~0.193	5.79E-01
Common lymphoid progenitors (CLP)	Stem cells	0.466	0.327~0.584	1.86E-35
Hematopoietic stem cells (HSC)	Stem cells	0.317	0.162~0.457	6.06E-16
Multipotent rogenitors (MPP)	Stem cells	−0.169	−0.323~−0.006	4.72E-05
Megakaryocytes	Stem cells	0.159	−0.005~0.314	1.42E-04
Granulocyte-macrophage progenitorGMP	Stem cells	0.100	−0.065~0.259	2.50E-02
Platelets	Stem cells	−0.030	−0.192~0.134	5.91E-01

(Continued)

TABLE 2 | Continued

xCells	Category	*r* value (Spearman)	CI adjust	Ajust. *P*. val (BH)
Common myeloid progenitors (CMP)	Stem cells	0.021	−0.142~0.184	7.15E-01
Megakaryocyte–erythroid progenitors (MEP)	Stem cells	0.009	−0.154~0.172	8.96E-01
Erythrocytes	Stem cells	−0.005	−0.168~0.159	9.48E-01
Pericytes	Stromal cells	−0.396	−0.525~−0.249	4.61E-25
Smooth muscle	Stromal cells	0.316	0.161~0.456	6.93E-16
Endothelial cells	Stromal cells	0.290	0.133~0.433	2.20E-13
Fibroblasts	Stromal cells	0.213	0.051~0.363	1.56E-07
Preadipocytes	Stromal cells	0.199	0.037~0.351	1.06E-06
ly Endothelial cells	Stromal cells	0.193	0.031~0.345	2.39E-06
Adipocytes	Stromal cells	0.142	−0.022~0.298	8.01E-04
Osteoblast	Stromal cells	−0.110	−0.269~0.054	1.18E-02
mv Endothelial cells	Stromal cells	0.080	−0.084~0.240	8.21E-02
Skeletal muscle	Stromal cells	−0.046	−0.208~0.118	3.66E-01
Mesenchymal stem cells (MSC)	Stromal cells	−0.044	−0.206~0.120	3.98E-01
Chondrocytes	Stromal cells	0.032	−0.132~0.194	5.67E-01

study identifies *LCTL* as a regular of the TME in glioma, which functions by recruiting and promoting immunosuppressive cells to secrete immunosuppressive factors, in addition to regulating M2 transformation, T cell exhaustion, and EMT via the FGF signaling pathway; this is thought to ultimately facilitate tumor immune evasion, resulting in poor outcomes for glioma patients.

DISCUSSION

Glioma patient prognosis remains poor, which is clinically frustrating (3, 4). Even with intensive therapies, most GBM patients relapse very soon due to the highly aggressive nature of this disease. Recently, immunotherapy has shown promise for the treatment of many cancers including glioma. However, the widespread application of immunotherapy is difficult, which is attributed to autoimmune-like side effects (38, 39). One potential therapeutic strategy is to develop immunotherapy against glioma by targeting overexpressed proteins that play an essential role in immunosuppression. Our present study first identified a novel function for *LCTL* in promoting aggressive behavior and leading to immune evasion.

Originally, *Klotho*, the first identified member of the *Klotho* family, was discovered as an anti-aging gene in 1997 (8). Recently, both *Klotho* and *βKlotho* have been reported to be aberrantly expressed in several cancers (40). Although some studies have demonstrated the abnormal expression of *LCTL* in different cancers, its function was previously unclear. In this study, we found that the expression of *LCTL* is not only abnormally upregulated, but also significantly associated with WHO grade, molecular subtype, and IDH status in glioma. Furthermore, our study showed that *LCTL* is an independent prognostic marker for glioma patients and that high levels of *LCTL* expression predict poor outcome. DNA methylation, the main epigenetic modification, is also involved in the pathogenesis of cancer (41, 42). Accordingly, the methylation of promoters of certain genes involved in key biological pathways in glioma has been widely reported (43). For example, promoter methylation of the O6-methylguanine-DNA methyltransferase (*MGMT*) gene occurs in ~40% of glioma patients and is clinically used as a biomarker of response to alkylating agents (44). Because DNA methylation is potentially reversible, it is a potential target for cancer treatment. Actually, the Food and Drug Administration (FDA) has approved DNA methylation inhibitors and histone deacetylase inhibitors for cancer monotherapy (45). Here, we found that the endogenous expression of *LCTL* is regulated by promoter DNA methylation rather than genetic alterations in glioma. Moreover, *LCTL* promoter methylation levels were found to have predictive value for glioma patients, which is similar to results found for mRNA levels. Taken together, *LCTL* is a good candidate prognostic and therapeutic target for glioma patient.

Immunotherapy is rapidly becoming the newest and the most promising pillar of malignancy treatment, with the potential to harness the potency of and active the host immune system. However, the TME including stromal cells, inflammatory cells, vasculature, and ECM, usually prevents effective lymphocyte initiation, reduces their infiltration, and suppresses infiltrating effector cells, which contributes to host failure in rejecting tumors (46). It is thus of great importance to explore novel molecular biomarkers and targets that play critical roles in the TME. Here, we conducted GO analysis with two different large datasets, and the results strongly suggested that *LCTL* is involved in the regimenting immunity and the TME in glioma. Furthermore, we found that *LCTL* expression significantly correlates with non-cancerous cells, mainly stromal and immune cells, in glioma via two methods, namely the ESTIMATE algorithm and xcell. Interestingly, these infiltratimg cells such as M2 macrophages and neutrophils, among others, are mainly considered immunosuppressive cells based on previous studies. Moreover, the correlation between *LCTL* expression and marker genes encoding immunoregulatory factors, as well as exhausted T cells, imply a role for *LCTL* in regulating tumor immunology in glioma. On the one hand, *LCTL* expression was significantly positively correlated with cytokines or chemokines that recruit immunosuppressive

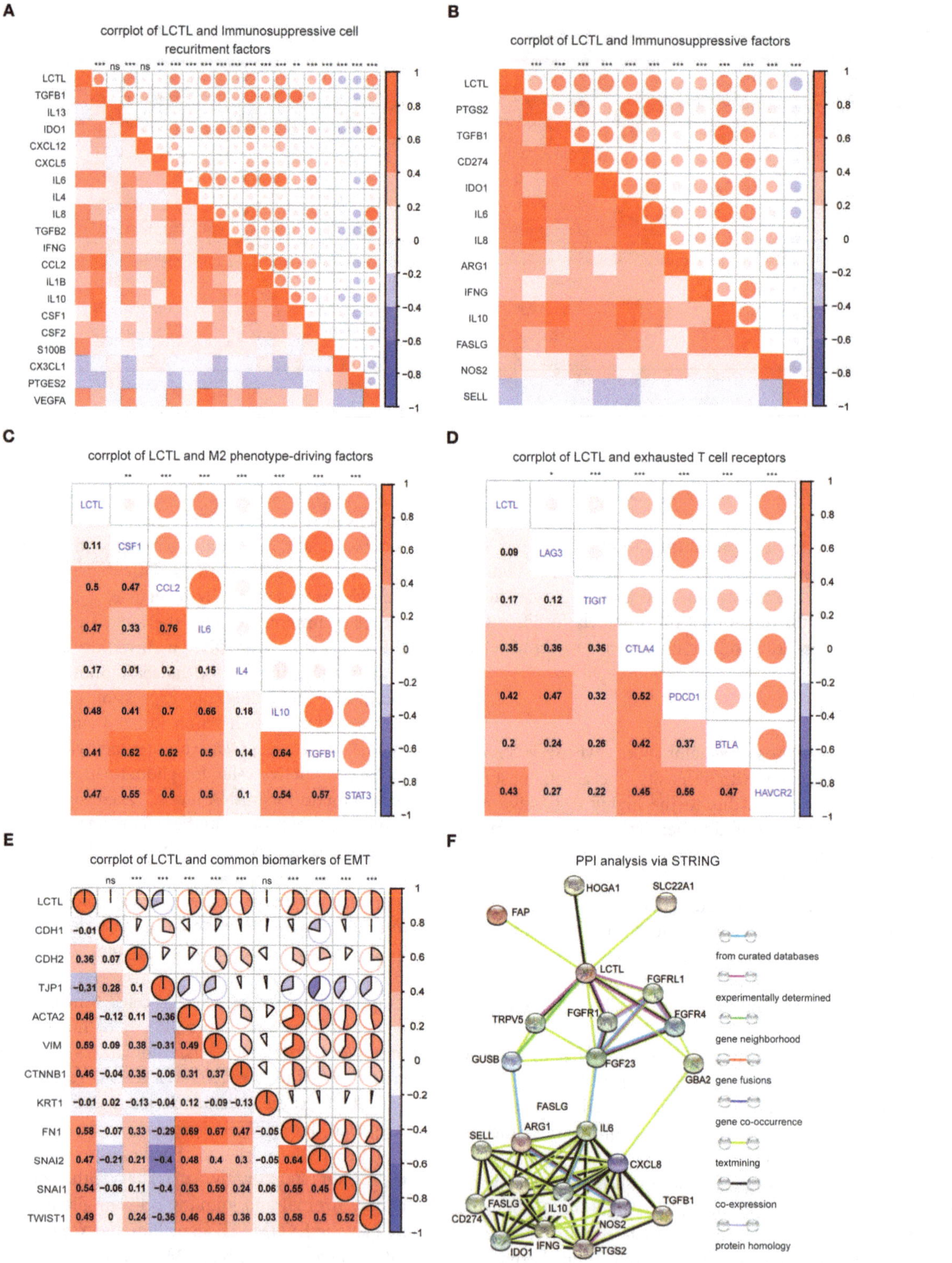

FIGURE 6 | *LCTL* correlates with immunosuppressive properties and promotes epithelial-mesenchymal transition (EMT). **(A)** Correlation between *LCTL* and immunosuppressive cell recruitment factors. **(B)** Correlation between *LCTL* and immunosuppressive factors secreted by myeloid-derived suppressor cells (MDSCs), tumor-associated macrophages (TAMs) and tumor-associated neutrophils (TANs). **(C)** Correlation between *LCTL* and M2 phenotype-driving factors. **(D)** Correlation between *LCTL* and exhausted T cell receptors. **(E)** Correlation between *LCTL* and common biomarkers of epichelial-mesenchymal transition (EMT). **(F)** Protein-protein interaction (PPI) analysis of the network linking *LCTL* and immunosuppressive factors. $^{*}P < 0.05$, $^{**}P < 0.01$, $^{***}P < 0.001$, $^{ns}P > 0.05$.

cells, such as myeloid-derived suppressor cells, TAMs, and tumor-associated neutrophils, as well as immunosuppressive factors secreted by these cells. On the other hand, *LCTL* was found to be positively associated with factors that drive M2 phenotype differentiation, which suggests a potential regulatory role for *LCTL* in TAMs polarization. In addition, our results indicate that *LCTL* can induce T cell exhaustion. Recently, accumulating evidence has demonstrated that cross-talk between EMT-associated factors and the TME might facilitate tumor immune escape (47). Accordingly, *LCTL* was found to promote bladder cancer EMT (21). In glioma, we also found that *LCTL* expression is positively related to mesenchymal cell markers and negatively correlated with epithelial cell markers. Thus, we propose that this gene might be involved in regulation of the immunosuppressive microenvironment by recruiting and promoting immunosuppressive cells to secrete immunosuppressive factors, regulating M2 polarization, promoting EMT, and inducing T cell exhaustion in glioma, finally facilitating tumor immune evasion.

Mechanistically, *LCTL* might regulate the immunity in glioma through FGF signaling pathway. FGFR dysfunction is widely found in cancers and FGF biology is involved in many effects in a myriad of cell types, and is a key component of the tumor environment (48). In addition, increasing evidence suggests that FGF signaling can influence the recruitment and activity of TAMs. For example, the activation of inducible FGFR1 in mammary cells causes their transformation and induces the secretion of factors to recruit TAMs (49, 50). Furthermore, FGF2 secreted from esophageal cancer cells promotes macrophage migration and survival through FGFR1 signaling (51). Moreover,

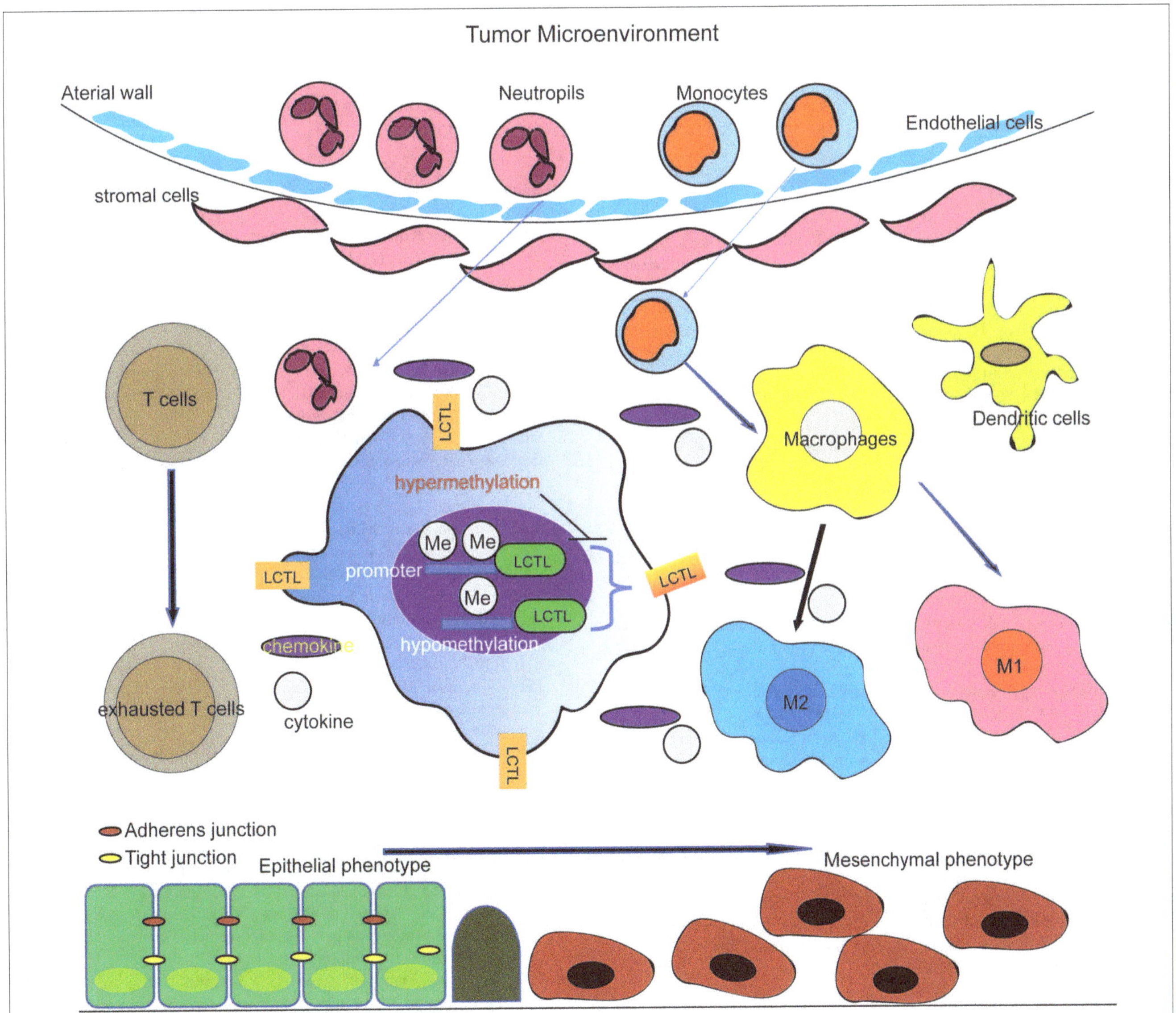

FIGURE 7 | Working model of the effect of *LCTL* in the glioma microenvironment. *LCTL* is highly expressed in glioma, regulated by DNA promotor methylation and acts an immunosuppressive role via interacting with some immunosuppressive factors in glioma TME.

by cooperating with proinflammatory cytokines, FGF2 can also promote the expression of adhesion molecules by endothelial cells, thus contributing to the recruitment of circulating immune cells to the tumor (52). Indeed, a recent study demonstrated that *Klotho* regulates immune invasion in the cenral nervous system and inhibits thioredoxin-interacting protein-dependent activation of the NLRP3 inflammasome in macrophages via FGF23 signaling (53). It has also been determined that *LCTL* can interact efficiently with FGFR1b, FGFR-1c, FGFR2c, and FGFR-4 (11). In our study, we found that *LCTL* can interact with FGFR1, FGFRL1, FGFR4, and FGF23 through PPI analysis. Interestingly, this analysis also revealed that *LCTL* plays an immunoregulatory role that is dependent on FGF signaling.

Based on our findings, we propose a working modal wherein *LCTL*, which is highly expressed in glioma and regulated by DNA methylation at its promoter, facilitates the recruitment of and immunosuppressive cells and promote the secretion of immunosuppressive factors by these cells. This further regulates M2 transformation, T cell exhaustion in glioma, and EMT, finally augmenting tumor immune evasion (**Figure 7**). Our findings provide opportunities to explore novel therapeutic approaches based on the epigenetic targeting of *LCTL*. Further, this gene might be an ideal target for immunotherapy against gliomas.

AUTHOR CONTRIBUTIONS

JS analyzed the data, performed computational coding, and wrote the manuscript. QM and WL involved in design of study, manuscript editing. HT performed the Q-PCR experiments and analyzed the results. CW, ML, XW, KX, YL, QX, CZ, and HL collected the data and samples. QL involved in design of study, manuscript review and editing, supervision of the entire work. All authors had approved the final manuscript.

FUNDING

This study was supported by grants from the National Natural Science Foundation of China (No. 81802974).

ACKNOWLEDGMENTS

We gratefully thank China Scholarship Council for supporting JS (201706370050).

REFERENCES

1. Ostrom QT, Gittleman H, Liao P, Vecchione-Koval T, Wolinsky Y, Kruchko C, et al. CBTRUS Statistical Report: Primary brain and other central nervous system tumors diagnosed in the United States in 2010-2014. *Neuro Oncol.* (2017) 19(suppl_5), v1–88. doi: 10.1093/neuonc/nox158
2. Yi X, Cao H, Tang H, Gong G, Hu Z, Liao W, et al. Gliosarcoma: a clinical and radiological analysis of 48 cases. *Eur Radiol.* (2019) 29:429–38. doi: 10.1007/s00330-018-5398-y
3. Wen PY, Kesari S. Malignant gliomas in adults. *N Engl J Med.* (2008) 359:492–507. doi: 10.1056/NEJMra0708126
4. Stupp R, Hegi ME, Mason WP, van den Bent MJ, Taphoorn MJ, Janzer RC, et al. Effects of radiotherapy with concomitant and adjuvant temozolomide versus radiotherapy alone on survival in glioblastoma in a randomised phase III study: 5-year analysis of the EORTC-NCIC trial. *Lancet Oncol.* (2009) 10:459–66. doi: 10.1016/S1470-2045(09)70025-7
5. Ma Q, Long W, Xing C, Chu J, Luo M, Wang HY, et al. Cancer stem cells and immunosuppressive microenvironment in glioma. *Front Immunol.* (2018) 9:2924. doi: 10.3389/fimmu.2018.02924
6. Huang J, Liu F, Liu Z, Tang H, Wu H, Gong Q, et al. Immune checkpoint in glioblastoma: promising and challenging. *Front Pharmacol.* (2017) 8:242. doi: 10.3389/fphar.2017.00242
7. Lapointe S, Perry A, Butowski NA. Primary brain tumours in adults. *Lancet.* (2018) 392:432–46. doi: 10.1016/S0140-6736(18)30990-5
8. Kuro-o M, Matsumura Y, Aizawa H, Kawaguchi H, Suga T, Utsugi T, et al. Mutation of the mouse klotho gene leads to a syndrome resembling ageing. *Nature.* (1997) 390:45–51. doi: 10.1038/36285
9. Trost N, Pena-Llopis S, Koirala S, Stojan J, Potts PR, Fon Tacer K, et al. gammaKlotho is a novel marker and cell survival factor in a subset of triple negative breast cancers. *Oncotarget.* (2016) 7:2611–28. doi: 10.18632/oncotarget.6006
10. Ito S, Fujimori T, Hayashizaki Y, Nabeshima Y. Identification of a novel mouse membrane-bound family 1 glycosidase-like protein, which carries an atypical active site structure. *Biochim Biophys Acta.* (2002) 1576:341–5. doi: 10.1016/S0167-4781(02)00281-6
11. Fon Tacer K, Bookout AL, Ding X, Kurosu H, John GB, Wang L, et al. Research resource: Comprehensive expression atlas of the fibroblast growth factor system in adult mouse. *Mol Endocrinol.* (2010) 24:2050–64. doi: 10.1210/me.2010-0142
12. Tanner Y, Grose RP. Dysregulated FGF signalling in neoplastic disorders. *Semin Cell Dev Biol.* (2016) 53:126–35. doi: 10.1016/j.semcdb.2015.10.012
13. Katoh M. Therapeutics targeting fgf signaling network in human diseases. *Trends Pharmacol Sci.* (2016) 37:1081–96. doi: 10.1016/j.tips.2016.10.003
14. Ligumsky H, Rubinek T, Merenbakh-Lamin K, Yeheskel A, Sertchook R, Shahmoon S, et al. Tumor suppressor activity of klotho in breast cancer is revealed by structure-function analysis. *Mol Cancer Res.* (2015) 13:1398–407. doi: 10.1158/1541-7786.MCR-15-0141
15. Chen B, Wang X, Zhao W, Wu J. Klotho inhibits growth and promotes apoptosis in human lung cancer cell line A549. *J Exp Clin Cancer Res.* (2010) 29:99. doi: 10.1186/1756-9966-29-99
16. Shu G, Xie B, Ren F, Liu DC, Zhou J, Li Q, et al. Restoration of klotho expression induces apoptosis and autophagy in hepatocellular carcinoma cells. *Cell Oncol.* (2013) 36:121–9. doi: 10.1007/s13402-012-0118-0
17. Poh W, Wong W, Ong H, Aung MO, Lim SG, Chua BT, et al. Klotho-beta overexpression as a novel target for suppressing proliferation and fibroblast growth factor receptor-4 signaling in hepatocellular carcinoma. *Mol Cancer.* (2012) 11:14. doi: 10.1186/1476-4598-11-14
18. Wolf I, Levanon-Cohen S, Bose S, Ligumsky H, Sredni B, Kanety H, et al. Klotho: a tumor suppressor and a modulator of the IGF-1 and FGF pathways in human breast cancer. *Oncogene.* (2008) 27:7094–105. doi: 10.1038/onc.2008.292
19. Liu H, Fergusson MM, Castilho RM, Liu J, Cao L, Chen J, et al. Augmented Wnt signaling in a mammalian model of accelerated aging. *Science.* (2007) 317:803–6. doi: 10.1126/science.1143578
20. Ye X, Guo Y, Zhang Q, Chen W, Hua X, Liu W, et al. betaKlotho suppresses tumor growth in hepatocellular carcinoma by regulating Akt/GSK-3beta/cyclin D1 signaling pathway. *PLoS ONE.* (2013) 8:e55615. doi: 10.1371/journal.pone.0055615
21. Hori S, Miyake M, Tatsumi Y, Morizawa Y, Nakai Y, Onishi S, et al. Gamma-Klotho exhibits multiple roles in tumor growth of human bladder cancer. *Oncotarget.* (2018) 9:19508–24. doi: 10.18632/oncotarget.24628
22. Tang Z, Li C, Kang B, Gao G, Li C, Zhang Z. GEPIA: a web server for cancer and normal gene expression profiling and interactive analyses. *Nucleic Acids Res.* (2017) 45:W98–102. doi: 10.1093/nar/gkx247
23. Li B, Severson E, Pignon JC, Zhao H, Li T, Novak J, et al. Comprehensive analyses of tumor immunity: implications for cancer immunotherapy. *Genome Biol.* (2016) 17:174. doi: 10.1186/s13059-016-1028-7
24. Gao J, Aksoy BA, Dogrusoz U, Dresdner G, Gross B, Sumer SO, et al. Integrative analysis of complex cancer genomics and clinical profiles using the cBioPortal. *Sci Signal.* (2013) 6:pl1. doi: 10.1126/scisignal.2004088

25. Jiao X, Sherman BT, Huang da W, Stephens R, Baseler MW, Lane HC, et al. DAVID-WS: a stateful web service to facilitate gene/protein list analysis. *Bioinformatics.* (2012) 28:1805–6. doi: 10.1093/bioinformatics/bts251
26. Yoshihara K, Shahmoradgoli M, Martinez E, Vegesna R, Kim H, Torres-Garcia W, et al. Inferring tumour purity and stromal and immune cell admixture from expression data. *Nat Commun.* (2013) 4:2612. doi: 10.1038/ncomms3612
27. Aran D, Hu Z, Butte AJ. xCell: digitally portraying the tissue cellular heterogeneity landscape. *Genome Biol.* (2017) 18:220. doi: 10.1186/s13059-017-1349-1
28. Yan H, Parsons DW, Jin G, McLendon R, Rasheed BA, Yuan W, et al. IDH1 and IDH2 mutations in gliomas. *N Engl J Med.* (2009) 360:765–73. doi: 10.1056/NEJMoa0808710
29. Hartmann C, Hentschel B, Tatagiba M, Schramm J, Schnell O, Seidel C, et al. Molecular markers in low-grade gliomas: predictive or prognostic? *Clin Cancer Res.* (2011) 17:4588–99. doi: 10.1158/1078-0432.CCR-10-3194
30. Komori T. The 2016 WHO classification of tumours of the central nervous system: the major points of revision. *Neurol Med Chir.* (2017) 57:301–11. doi: 10.2176/nmc.ra.2017-0010
31. Kagohara LT, Stein-O'Brien GL, Kelley D, Flam E, Wick HC, Danilova LV, et al. Epigenetic regulation of gene expression in cancer: techniques, resources and analysis. *Brief Funct Genomics.* (2018) 17:49–63. doi: 10.1093/bfgp/elx018
32. Herceg Z, Hainaut P. Genetic and epigenetic alterations as biomarkers for cancer detection, diagnosis and prognosis. *Mol Oncol.* (2007) 1:26–41. doi: 10.1016/j.molonc.2007.01.004
33. Motz GT, Coukos G. Deciphering and reversing tumor immune suppression. *Immunity.* (2013) 39:61–73. doi: 10.1016/j.immuni.2013.07.005
34. Mantovani A, Locati M. Tumor-associated macrophages as a paradigm of macrophage plasticity, diversity, and polarization: lessons and open questions. *Arterioscler Thromb Vasc Biol.* (2013) 33:1478–83. doi: 10.1161/ATVBAHA.113.300168
35. Hambardzumyan D, Gutmann DH, Kettenmann H. The role of microglia and macrophages in glioma maintenance and progression. *Nat Neurosci.* (2016) 19:20–7. doi: 10.1038/nn.4185
36. Jiang Y, Li Y, Zhu B. T-cell exhaustion in the tumor microenvironment. *Cell Death Dis.* (2015) 6:e1792. doi: 10.1038/cddis.2015.162
37. Jung HY, Fattet L, Yang J. Molecular pathways: linking tumor microenvironment to epithelial-mesenchymal transition in metastasis. *Clin Cancer Res.* (2015) 21:962–8. doi: 10.1158/1078-0432.CCR-13-3173
38. Han SJ, Zygourakis C, Lim M, Parsa AT, Immunotherapy for glioma: promises and challenges. *Neurosurg Clin N Am.* (2012) 23:357–70. doi: 10.1016/j.nec.2012.05.001
39. Anderson AC. Tim-3: an emerging target in the cancer immunotherapy landscape. *Cancer Immunol Res.* (2014) 2:393–8. doi: 10.1158/2326-6066.CIR-14-0039
40. Zhou X, Wang X. Klotho: a novel biomarker for cancer. *J Cancer Res Clin Oncol.* (2015) 141:961–9. doi: 10.1007/s00432-014-1788-y
41. Zeng WJ, Yang YL, Liu ZZ, Wen ZP, Chen YH, Hu XL, et al. Integrative analysis of DNA methylation and gene expression identify a three-gene signature for predicting prognosis in lower-grade gliomas. *Cell Physiol Biochem.* (2018) 47:428–39. doi: 10.1159/000489954
42. Baylin SB, Jones PA. A decade of exploring the cancer epigenome - biological and translational implications. *Nat Rev Cancer.* (2011) 11:726–34. doi: 10.1038/nrc3130
43. Feng J, Zhang Y, She X, Sun Y, Fan L, Ren X, et al. Hypermethylated gene ANKDD1A is a candidate tumor suppressor that interacts with FIH1 and decreases HIF1alpha stability to inhibit cell autophagy in the glioblastoma multiforme hypoxia microenvironment. *Oncogene.* (2019) 38:103–19. doi: 10.1038/s41388-018-0423-9
44. Esteller M, Garcia-Foncillas J, Andion E, Goodman SN, Hidalgo OF, Vanaclocha V, et al. Inactivation of the DNA-repair gene MGMT and the clinical response of gliomas to alkylating agents. *N Engl J Med.* (2000) 343:1350–4. doi: 10.1056/NEJM200011093431901
45. Raynal NJ, Da Costa EM, Lee JT, Gharibyan V, Ahmed S, Zhang H, et al. Repositioning FDA-approved drugs in combination with epigenetic drugs to reprogram colon cancer epigenome. *Mol Cancer Ther.* (2017) 16:397–407. doi: 10.1158/1535-7163.MCT-16-0588
46. Tang H, Qiao J, Fu YX. Immunotherapy and tumor microenvironment. *Cancer Lett.* (2016) 370:85–90. doi: 10.1016/j.canlet.2015.10.009
47. Terry S, Savagner P, Ortiz-Cuaran S, Mahjoubi L, Saintigny P, Thiery JP, et al. New insights into the role of EMT in tumor immune escape. *Mol Oncol.* (2017) 11:824–46. doi: 10.1002/1878-0261.12093
48. Clayton NS, Wilson AS, Laurent EP, Grose RP, Carter EP. Fibroblast growth factor-mediated crosstalk in cancer etiology and treatment. *Dev Dyn.* (2017) 246:493–501. doi: 10.1002/dvdy.24514
49. Schwertfeger KL, Xian W, Kaplan AM, Burnett SH, Cohen DA, Rosen JM. A critical role for the inflammatory response in a mouse model of preneoplastic progression. *Cancer Res.* (2006) 66:5676–85. doi: 10.1158/0008-5472.CAN-05-3781
50. Bohrer LR, Schwertfeger KL. Macrophages promote fibroblast growth factor receptor-driven tumor cell migration and invasion in a CXCR2-dependent manner. *Mol Cancer Res.* (2012) 10:1294–305. doi: 10.1158/1541-7786.MCR-12-0275
51. Takase N, Koma Y, Urakawa N, Nishio M, Arai N, Akiyama H, et al. NCAM- and FGF-2-mediated FGFR1 signaling in the tumor microenvironment of esophageal cancer regulates the survival and migration of tumor-associated macrophages and cancer cells. *Cancer Lett.* (2016) 380:47–58. doi: 10.1016/j.canlet.2016.06.009
52. Zittermann SI, Issekutz AC. Basic fibroblast growth factor (bFGF, FGF-2) potentiates leukocyte recruitment to inflammation by enhancing endothelial adhesion molecule expression. *Am J Pathol.* (2006) 168:835–46. doi: 10.2353/ajpath.2006.050479
53. Zhu L, Stein LR, Kim D, Ho K, Yu GQ, Zhan L, et al. Klotho controls the brain-immune system interface in the choroid plexus. *Proc Natl Acad Sci USA.* (2018) 115:E11388–96. doi: 10.1073/pnas.1808609115

14

LncRNAs Predicted to Interfere with the Gene Regulation Activity of *miR-637* and *miR-196a-5p* in GBM

Jingfang Zheng[1], *Zhiying Su*[2], *Yang Kong*[3,4], *Qingping Lin*[1], *Hongli Liu*[1], *Yanlong Wang*[1*] *and Jian Wang*[3,4*]

[1] *Department of Gynecology, Women and Children's Hospital, School of Medicine, Xiamen University, Xiamen, China,* [2] *Department of Reproductive Medicine, Women and Children's Hospital, School of Medicine, Xiamen University, Xiamen, China,* [3] *Department of Neurosurgery, Qilu Hospital of Shandong University and Institute of Brain and Brain-Inspired Science, Shandong University, Jinan, China,* [4] *Translational Cancer Research Group, Department of Biomedicine, University of Bergen, Bergen, Norway*

Correspondence:
Yanlong Wang
xmfy_wyl@126.com
Jian Wang
jian.wang@uib.no

Rigorous molecular characterization of biological systems has uncovered a variety of gene variations underlying normal and disease states and a remarkable complexity in the forms of RNA transcripts that exist. A recent concept, competitive endogenous RNA, suggests that some non-coding RNAs can bind to miRNAs to modulate their role in gene expression. Here, we used several platforms, integrating mRNA, non-coding RNAs and protein data to generate an RNA-protein network that may be dysregulated in human glioblastoma multiforme (GBM). Publicly available microarray data for mRNA and miRNA were used to identify differentially expressed miRNAs and mRNAs in GBM relative to non-neoplastic tissue samples. Target miRNAs were further selected based on their prognostic significance, and the intersection of their target gene set with the differentially expressed gene set in Venn diagrams. Two miRNAs, miR-637 and miR-196a-5p, were associated with poor and better prognosis, respectively, in GBM patients. Non-coding RNAs, ENSG00000203739/ENSG00000271646 and TPTEP1, were predicted to be miRNA target genes for miR-637 and miR-196a-5p and positively correlated with the selected mRNA, CYBRD1 and RUFY2. A local protein interaction network was constructed using these two mRNAs. Predictions based on the ENSG00000203739/ENSG00000271646-miR-637-CYBRD1 and TPTEP1-miR-196a-5p-RUFY2 regulation axes indicated that the two proteins may act as an oncogene and tumor suppressor, respectively, in the development of GBM. These results highlight competitive endogenous RNA networks as alternative molecular therapeutic targets in the treatment of the disease.

Keywords: lncRNA, mRNA, GBM, molecular datasets, network

INTRODUCTION

Glioblastoma multiforme (GBM) is the most aggressive central nervous system tumor in adults, and the prognosis is bleak. Conventional therapies, including surgery, radiotherapy, and chemotherapy with temozolomide have not resulted in significant improvement in the survival outcomes of patients with GBM. Median overall survival is 15–23 months, and 5-year survival is <6% (1). Causes of poor prognosis include invasive tumor growth in an essential organ that cannot be thoroughly removed, the presence of the blood-brain barrier (BBB), their intrinsic resistance to the induction of cell death, tumor heterogeneity and a complex pathogenesis. The basis for this behavior is the simultaneous corruption of many genes which results in the lack of a single, targetable oncogenic pathway, and thus, significant challenges in systemic therapy.

Answers for treatment are thought to be buried in the molecular datasets accumulating since 2006 when The Cancer Genome Atlas (TCGA) team, sponsored by the National Cancer Institute (NCI), published DNA copy number, gene expression, and DNA methylation analysis for 206 GBMs. Rigorous analysis of these data has led to some critical insights in the development of human gliomas. GBMs can now be classified as one of four molecular subtypes based on transcriptome expression data: classical, neural, mesenchymal, and proneural. Subsequent analysis of the methylation status of DNA promoter regions in 272 GBMs revealed two major glioma-CpG island methylation phenotypes (glioma-CpG island methylator phenotype, or G-CIMP and non-G-CIMP types). Finally, a total 1,122 gliomas samples were divided into *IDH* mutated and wild type tumors based on analysis of the multi-dimensional histological data.

Non-coding RNAs have also become part of the story. A collection of dysregulated lncRNAs, including hundreds of candidate onco- and tumor-suppressor lncRNAs, have been identified in the context of 14 different tumor types (2). Recurrent hypomethylation of 1,006 lncRNA genes in cancer, including *EPIC1* (epigenetically-induced lncRNA1) has also been described (3). *EPIC1* promotes cell-cycle progression by interacting with MYC, enhancing luminal B breast cancer cell growth *in vitro* and *in vivo*.

The expanding landscape for RNA transcript types has triggered additional theories about gene regulation. A recent concept, competitive endogenous RNA (ceRNA), represents a novel regulatory mechanism between non-coding and coding RNAs. The theory suggests that lncRNAs, cirRNAs, and pseudogenes can act as "molecular sponges" to compete for miRNAs and effectively modulate their functions. The competition for miRNAs is mediated by miRNA binding sites or miRNA response elements (4). This creative hypothesis is supported by an increasing number of experimental results.

With the development of high-throughput gene sequencing and chip technology, analyzing molecular data has become an extremely meaningful but challenging task. An increasing number of R language packages and bioinformatics analysis tools have become more user friendly for a broader range of investigators. Here, we used some of these tools to analyze miRNA and mRNA datasets to determine where they might converge in the development of human GBM. Our results led us to two miRNAs, *miR-196a-5p* and *miR-637*, their target mRNAs encoding a putative oncogene and tumor suppressor, and non-coding RNAs regulating the miRNA activity. We show how a fundamental biological question, which genes and miRNAs are differentially expressed in human GBM, can provide the basis for the construction of a molecular network including RNAs and proteins that might drive aspects of GBM development. Such "excavation" of molecular datasets is the key for the advancement of novel therapies in the treatment of the disease.

MATERIALS AND METHODS

Microarray Data

MicroRNA expression profiles in GSE25631 from the publicly available NCBI GEO database, which had been collected using the Illumina GPL8179 platform (Human v2 microRNA Expression Beadchip), were analyzed. The GSE25631 dataset includes 82 primary GBM surgical specimens and 5 non-neoplastic brain tissue samples from areas surrounding arteriovenous malformations as controls. mRNA expression profiles were obtained from the GSE4290 dataset (5), which is based on the Affymetrix GPL570 platform (HG U133 Plus 2.0 Array). The GSE4290 dataset includes 79 GBM samples and 23 non-neoplastic brain tissue samples from epilepsy patients as controls. To validate our results, GSE90604 and GSE65626, two microRNA expression datasets, were also analyzed.

Analysis to Identify Differentially Expressed microRNAs and Differentially Expressed Genes (DEGs)

Analysis using GEO2R, a webtool available from the NCBI, was performed to detect differentially expressed microRNAs and DEGs between GBM and non-neoplastic control samples. Details of the R script of GEO2R are provided in the **Supplementary Material.** Adjusted *P*-values were used to reduce the false positive rate using the Benjamini and Hochberg false discovery rate method by default (6, 7). $P < 0.05$ and $|\text{logFC}| \geq 2$ were set as the cutoff values.

Identification of Target Genes of Candidate microRNAs

Cytoscape, open-source software for the integration of molecular interaction network data, was used to visualize the relationship between microRNAs and differentially expressed genes (DEGs). CyTargetLinker (8), a plug-in for Cytoscape, was used to identify microRNA-target genes (MTGs), based on experimentally validated microRNA-target interaction (MTIs) files stored in miRTarBase (9), a database containing miRNA-target interactions. In general, the collected MTIs in miRTarBase have been validated experimentally using luciferase assays, western blots, microarrays and next-generation sequencing.

GO and KEGG Pathway Enrichment Analysis for MTGs of Candidate microRNAs and DEGs

Kyoto Encyclopedia of Genes and Genomes (10) (KEGG) pathway analysis was performed to identify potential functions of the MTGs of the candidate microRNAs and DEGs. Gene ontology analysis (GO), a common useful method for annotating genes and identifying characteristic biological attributes, including biological processes, molecular functions, and cellular components, for high-throughput genome or transcriptome data (11), was performed on DEGs. Metascape (http://metascape.org), a web-based online bioinformatics resource that aims to provide tools for the functional interpretation of large lists of genes or proteins (12), was also used to identify function of

MTGs and to conduct GO and KEGG pathway enrichment (13) on DEGs derived in our analysis. The enriched KEGG pathways of MTGs were visualized using ClueGO+Cluepedia, a plug-in that visualizes the non-redundant biological terms for large clusters of genes in a functionally grouped network (14). For DEGs, visualization of the biological processes, molecular functions, cellular components and pathways was performed using Excel and R ggplot2 packages.

Identification of Hub Genes Among DEGs

Protein names encoded by DEGs were imported into STRING (https://string-db.org/) to obtain a protein-protein interaction (PPI) network (15). CentiScaPe 2.2 was used to analyze nodes in the network (16). Genes with the highest degrees of connectivity were selected as hub genes. Analysis of the core genes can represent whether the chip results are consistent with GBM.

Identification of Candidate Genes Regulated by DEGs and MTGs

Venn diagrams (17) were used to identify the intersection between *miR-196a-5p* target and GBM down-regulated genes, as well as between *miR-637* target and GBM up-regulated genes. Gene Expression Profiling Interactive Analysis (GEPIA; http://gepia.cancer-pku.cn/index.html), a newly developed interactive web server, was used to analyze differences in expression between tumor and normal samples using RNA sequencing data (18). A boxplot was generated to visualize the relationship.

Identification of Target Non-coding RNAs of Candidate microRNAs

Analysis using LncBase v.2 was performed to predict the target non-coding RNAs of differentially expressed microRNAs in GBM (19). To acquire high confidence target non-coding RNAs, the threshold was set at > 0.9, and the tissue was confined to brain. Target non-coding RNAs of candidate genes, including lncRNAs, cirRNAs, and pseudogenes, were chosen based on a positive relationship with candidate genes in the data collected from TCGA GBMs on the Tanric website (20). The expression of target non-coding RNAs and candidate genes was set to a positive correlation above moderate levels (correlation coefficient > 0.4, *P*-value < 0.01). The intersection between candidate genes and predicted target non-coding RNAs was made.

PPI Network Extension and Establishment of the Competitive Endogenous RNA (ceRNA) Hypothesis

Protein names encoded by candidate genes were imported into STRING, a database of known and predicted protein-protein interactions (https://string-db.org/) (21). PPI networks were extended until the proteins from our analysis connected with each other. Candidate microRNA and non-coding RNAs were then mapped to the network.

RESULTS

Identification of Differentially Regulated Candidate miRNAs in GBM

Analysis of the GSE25631 dataset yielded a total of 67 differentially expressed miRNAs ($P < 0.05$ and $|\text{logFC}| \geq 2$) between GBM and non-neoplastic brain. Of these miRNAs, 27 were up-regulated and 40 were down-regulated in GBM relative to control samples (**Figure 1A**). We examined the prognostic value of 10 miRNAs with the most significant fold changes in expression (**Table 1**), using OncoLnc, a tool for interactively exploring survival correlations coupled to expression data for mRNAs, miRNAs, or lncRNAs. Two of these miRNAs, *miR-196a-5p* and *miR-637*, were associated with overall survival (OS; **Figures 1B,C**). High expression of *miR-196a-5p* in GBMs (HR = 0.196, $P = 0.000795$) was associated with worse OS in patients (**Figure 1D**), while high expression of *miR-637* (HR = −0.634, $P = 0.045$) was associated with better OS in patients (**Figure 1E**). Because the statistical difference in OS using *miR-637* was not significant, we selected multiple cutoff values for verification. The results are shown in **Supplementary Figure 1**. The expression of *miR-196-5p* and *miR-637* was also verified in the TCGA database. The expression of *miR-196-5p* was consistent with the results obtained with the GSE25631 dataset. However, compared with the control group, *miR-637* was not significantly reduced in GBM from the TCGA (**Supplementary Figures 2A,B**).

KEGG Enrichment Analysis Links *miR-196-5p* and *miR-637* to Pathways Involved in Cancer

To understand the possible function of *miR-196-5p* and *miR-637* in the development of GBM, KEGG pathway enrichment analysis of their target genes was performed. KEGG analysis was performed on the *miR-196-5p* and *miR-637* target genes ($n = 356$) identified using Cytoscape (**Figure 1F**). The results revealed these genes to be associated with several pathways involved in disease development, including small cell lung cancer, proteoglycans in cancer, Parkinson's disease, viral carcinogenesis, prostate cancer, chronic myeloid leukemia, the Hedgehog signaling pathway, glioma, microRNAs in cancer, and the cell cycle (**Figure 1G**). We further validated the results using the open-source pathway database REACTOME (https://reactome.org/) (**Supplementary Figures 3A,B**) (22).

Identification of Differentially Expressed Genes (DEGs) and Enrichment Analysis

To identify differentially expressed genes in GBM relative to non-neoplastic brain, we performed analysis on the GSE4290 dataset containing mRNA expression profiles (5). A total of 1,170 differentially expressed genes were detected; 397 were up-regulated and 773 were down-regulated in GBM samples relative to non-neoplastic brain tissue (**Figure 2A**). To associate function with the DEGs, we performed GO (**Figure 2B**) and KEGG pathway analysis (**Figure 2C**). DEGs were found to be enriched in biological processes (BP, **Figure 2B**) involving the regulation of neurogenesis, plasma membrane

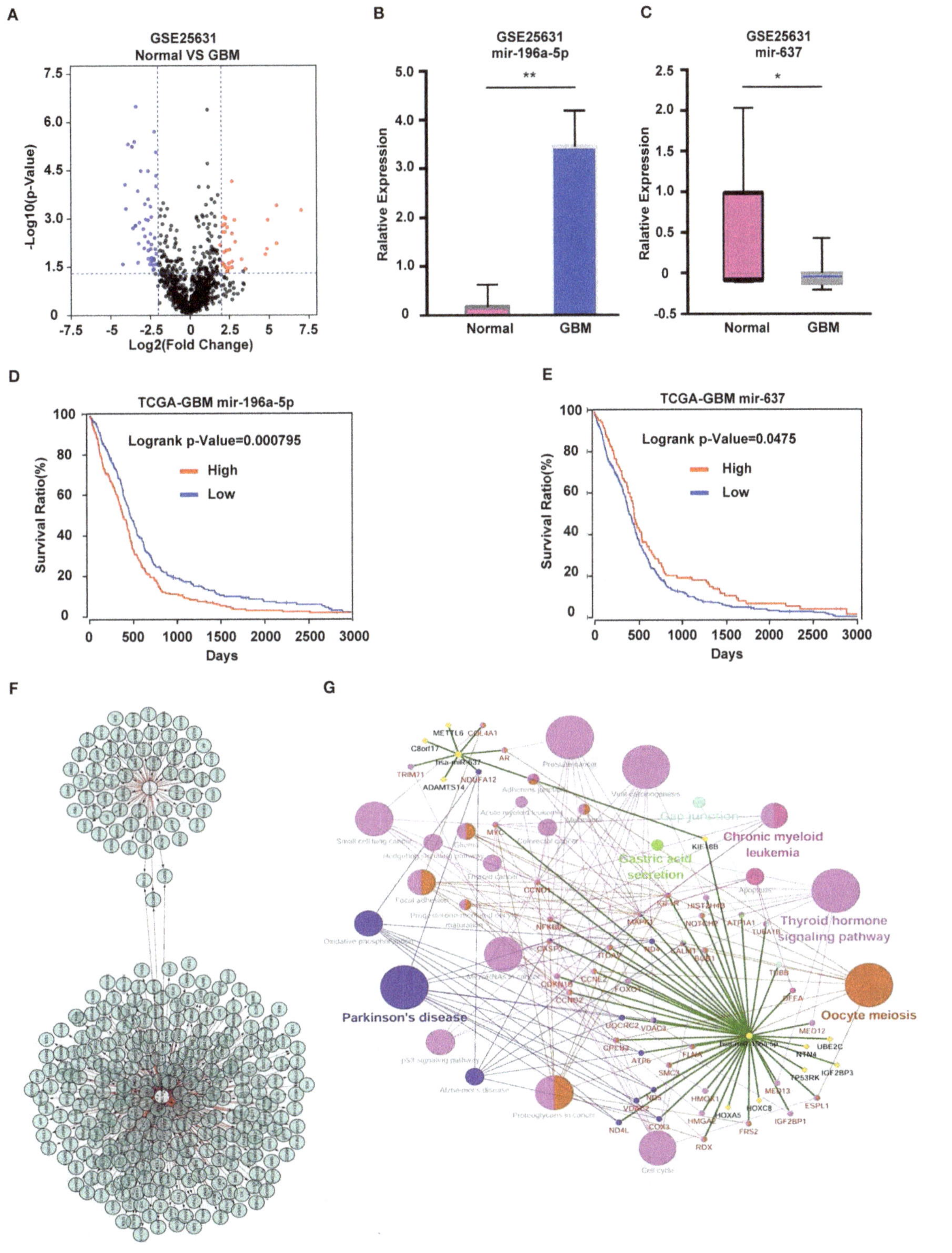

FIGURE 1 | Identification of candidate miRNAs and prediction of their target genes. **(A)** Volcano plot compiled using expression data obtained from the publicly available dataset GSE25631. Red and blue dots represent up-regulated and down-regulated differentially expressed microRNAs, respectively ($P < 0.05$, $|\log FC| \geq 2$). **(B)** The expression of *miR-196a-5p* and **(C)** *miR-637* in GBM relative to non-neoplastic brain tissue samples. **(D)** Prognostic value of *miR-196a-5p* **(E)** and *miR-637* in GBM based on the TCGA database. **(F)** Predicted target genes of *miR-196-5p* and *miR-637*. **(G)** KEGG pathway enrichment analysis of target genes of *miR-196-5p* and *miR-637*. Figures in **(F,G)** were designed using the open source software Cytoscape 3.6.1 and its plugin or app CyTargetLinker, ClueG+Cluepedia. Data are shown as the mean ± standard deviation. $^{*}P < 0.05$; $^{**}P < 0.01$ vs. control samples.

TABLE 1 | Top 10 differentially expressed miRNAs in GSE25631.

miRNA_ID	*P*-value	Log_2FC
hsa-miR-196a-5p	4.38E-04	5.599188
hsa-miR-558	6.37E-03	5.553814
hsa-miR-144	1.19E-03	5.045044
hsa-miR-106a	9.89E-03	4.979875
hsa-miR-637	2.93E-02	−4.14014
hsa-miR-876-3p	9.70E-05	−3.97221
hsa-miR-1224-5p	5.50E-06	−3.78824
hsa-miR-518e	4.09E-02	3.611791
hsa-miR-138-2-3p	6.31E-06	−3.54098
hsa-miR-203	2.13E-03	−3.45736

bounded cell projection morphogenesis, cell morphogenesis involved in neuron differentiation, neurotransmitter secretion, and regulation of neurogenesis. They were also enriched in molecular functions (MF, **Figure 2B**) involving ion channel activity, protein kinase activity, and cell adhesion molecule binding. Based on cellular components (CC, **Figure 2B**), DEGs were found to be located in the synapse, the vesicle membrane, the perinuclear region of the cytoplasm, and the extracellular matrix. KEGG pathway enrichment analysis linked DEGs to processes involving the synaptic vesicle cycle, pathways in cancer, PI3K-Akt signaling, proteoglycans in cancer, and Ras signaling. These results suggest that these DEGs may play a role in promoting tumor progression through their function.

Analysis of DEGs Interaction Network and Acquisition of Hub Genes

Using the STRING protein databases, we generated a PPI network for the top 20 hub genes with the highest degrees of connectivity (**Figure 2D**). The top 20 included genes known to promote the development of human cancer. *CDK1*, *CCNB2*, and *CDC20* (23) are involved in the regulation of the cell cycle. *EGFR* and *VEGFA* have been reported to promote GBM proliferation and invasion. *TOP2A*, *BUB1*, *NDC80*, and *TTK* participate in mitosis. *BIRC5* is a member of the inhibitor of apoptosis (IAP) gene family, which prevents apoptotic cell death. Finally, *HMMR* encodes a protein involved in cell motility.

Identification of Candidate Genes Regulated by *miR-196-5p/miR-637*

To identify DEGs that may be regulated by *miR-196-5p/miR-637*, we generated a venn diagram illustrating the intersection between the target genes of *miR-196-5p/miR-637* and the DEGs (**Figure 3A**). Among the genes appearing in the intersection of the two datasets were *CYBRD1* and *RUFY2* (**Table 2**). Expression levels were high and low for *CYBRD1* and *RUFY2*, respectively, in GBM, corresponding with activity as a putative oncogene or tumor suppressor gene. The expression of these two genes was also related to the OS of patients (**Figures 3B,C**). High expression of *CYBRD1* was related to poor survival whereas high expression of *RUFY2* was associated with better survival. The differential mRNA expression of *CYBRD1* and *RUFY2* was consistent with results obtained using the expression data from the TCGA GBMs (**Figures 3D,E**). We also analyzed the relationship between the expression of *CYBRD1/RUFY2* and *MGMT/IDH* status within TCGA GBM samples. Neither mRNA exhibited significant differences between methylated/unmethylated *MGMT* and wild-type/mutant *IDH* in tumors (**Supplementary Figure 4**). Finally, a heatmap based on mRNA expression data of intersection genes from GSE4290 illustrates the differential expression of the two genes between GBM and non-neoplastic samples (**Figure 3F**).

Identification of Non-coding RNAs Involved in the Regulation of *miR-196-5p/miR-637* and *CYBRD1/RUFY2*

To determine whether any non-coding RNAs might be involved in the regulation of *CYBRD1* and *RUFY2*, we generated a diagram to reveal the intersection between predicted target ncRNAs of *miR-196a-5p/miR-637* and non-coding RNAs which are positively related to these two genes (**Figure 3G**). Three ncRNAs, *ENSG00000203739*, *ENSG00000271646*, and *ENSG00000100181*, emerged from the analysis, and high expression of *ENSG00000203739* and *ENSG00000271646* was associated with poor prognosis in GBM using Log-Rank models (**Figures 3H,I**). The survival curve for the third ncRNA, *ENSG00000100181*, was only statistically significant in the Cox model for GBM and low grade glioma (**Figures 3J,K**).

The official symbol of *ENSG00000100181* is *TPTEP1*, which is also known as *psiTPTE22*. psiTPTE22-HERV has been reported to be epigenetically silenced by DNA methylation in cancers of the kidney, liver, lung, and stomach (24–26). We were therefore interested in the possibility that *TPTEP1* expression might differ on the basis of GBM molecular subtype. Using the TCGA database, we found expression of *TPTEP1* to be significantly higher in the G-CIMP subtype relative to the other molecular subtypes. As patients with G-CIMP subtype tumors in general have a better prognosis, low-expression of *TPTEP1* in non-G-CIMP subtypes may be consistent with a role as a tumor suppressor gene (**Figure 3L**). Therefore, we believe the role of *TPTEP1* in the pathogenesis of GBM warrants further investigation.

A Competitive Endogenous RNA (ceRNA) Regulation Network Involving *TPTEP1*, CYBRD1, and RUFY2 Built in GBM

Using the String database, we constructed a local protein network between the proteins CYBRD1 and RUFY2 (**Figure 4**). We then integrated the ncRNAs. In this network, high-expression of *ENSG00000203739/ENSG00000271646* was predicted to promote GBM proliferation and invasion by suppressing *miR-637* which leads to increased expression of CYBRD1, a putative oncogene. Loss of *TPTEP1* however leads to increased levels of *miR-196a-5p*/to adsorpt/bind to *miR-196a-5p*. When overexpressed, *miR-196a-5p* impedes translation of RUFY2, a putative tumor suppressor protein. Thus, dysregulation of these ncRNAs can lead to progression of GBM through gain and loss of the CYBRD1 and RUFY2, respectively.

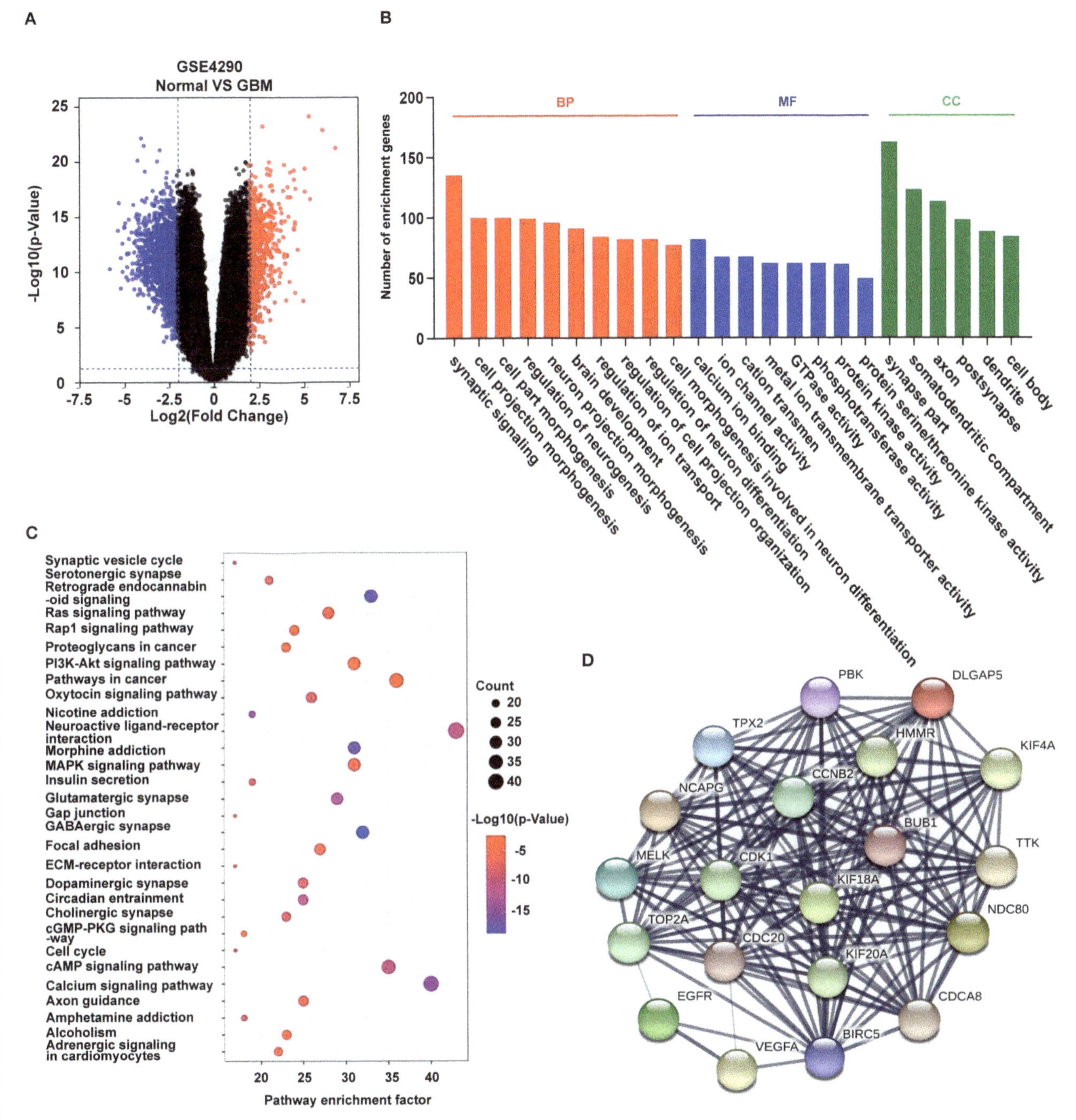

FIGURE 2 | GO function and KEGG pathway enrichment analysis of DEGs and hub genes in GSE4290. **(A)** Volcano plot derived using the data in GSE4290. Red and blue dots represent up-regulated and down-regulated DEGs, respectively ($P < 0.05$ plus $|\log FC| \geq 2$). **(B)** Statistically enriched biological processes, molecular functions, and cellular components identified using GO function analysis of the DEGs. **(C)** Top 30 enriched pathways identified using KEGG pathway analysis of DEGs in GSE4290. **(D)** Top 20 hub genes predicted from the DEGs. These hub genes were representative genes involved in occurrence and progression of GBM. The figure in **(D)** was designed using the open source software Cytoscape3.6.1 and its plugin or the app STRING.

The local PPI network also included the proteins EFNA5, EFNB2, ACTR2, EPHA3. Many of these proteins are implicated in GBM development. EFNA5, for example, is a member of the ephrin gene family, which participates in late stage nervous system development and differentiation. EFNB2 plays an important role in physiological and pathological angiogenesis, and its role in tumor vessel development has been extensively studied. EFNB2 has been shown to mediate perivascular invasion of glioblastoma stem-like cells (27). ACTR2 is known to be a major constituent of the ARP2/3 complex, which is located at the cell surface and is essential for cell shape and motility through lamellipodial actin assembly and protrusion. Overexpression of

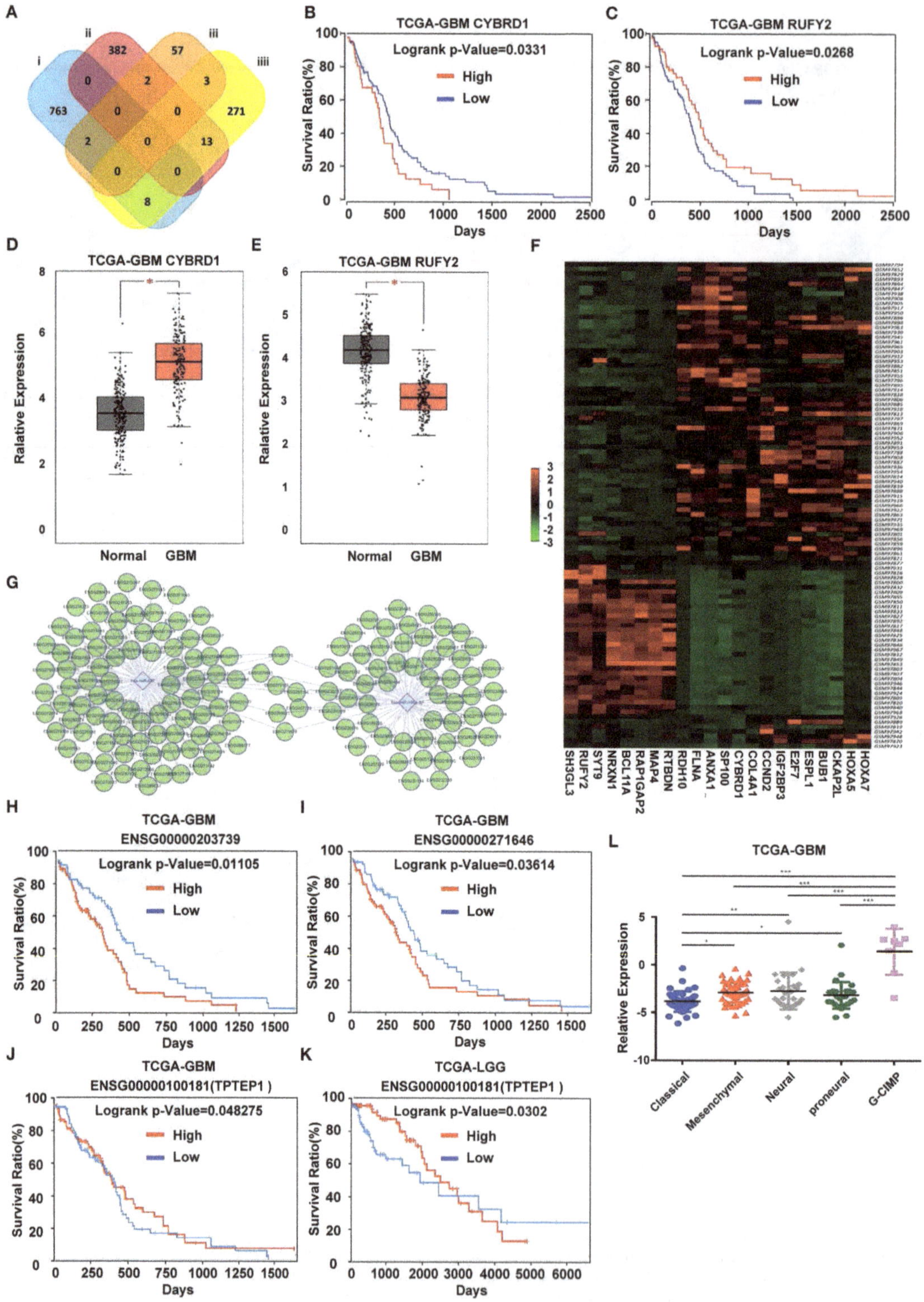

FIGURE 3 | Identification of candidate genes and construction of a ceRNA network. **(A)** Venn diagrams showing the intersection between predicted target genes of *miR-196-5p/miR-637* and DEGs. Kaplan-Meier plots showing the prognostic value of **(B)** *CYBRD1* and **(C)** *RUFY2* in GBM based on the TCGA database. The expression of **(D)** *CYBRD1* and **(E)**. *RUFY2* in GBM relative to non-neoplastic brain tissue samples in the TCGA database. **(F)** Heatmap displaying differential expression of intersecting genes between the GBM and control groups in GSE4290. **(G)** Target non-coding RNAs of *miR-196-5p* and *miR-637*. Kaplan-Meier plots showing the prognostic value of **(H)** *ENSG00000203739* and **(I)** *ENSG00000271646* in GBM, and *ENSG00000100181* (*TPTEP1*) in **(J)** GBM and **(K)** LGG based on the TCGA database. **(L)** Expression of *TPTEP1* in GBM molecular subtypes based on the TCGA database. The figure in **(A)** was designed using the open source software Cytoscape3.6.1. Data are shown as the mean ± standard deviation. $^{*}P < 0.05$; $^{**}P < 0.01$; $^{***}P < 0.001$ vs. control samples.

TABLE 2 | Intersection of non-coding RNAs involved in the regulation of miR-196-5p/miR-637 and CYBRD1/RUFY2.

MicroRNA	Prediction score	Non-coding RNA	Gene	Correlation coefficient	*P*-value
hsa-miR-637	1	ENSG00000203739	CYBRD1	0.401	3.17E-07
hsa-miR-637	0.999	ENSG00000246263	CYBRD1	0.425	5.35E-08
hsa-miR-637	0.999	ENSG00000254154	CYBRD1	0.417	9.96E-08
hsa-miR-637	0.999	ENSG00000271646	CYBRD1	0.445	1.09E-08
hsa-miR-637	0.998	ENSG00000272908	CYBRD1	0.403	2.89E-07
has-196a-5p	0.904	ENSG00000100181	RUFY2	0.421	2.78E-05

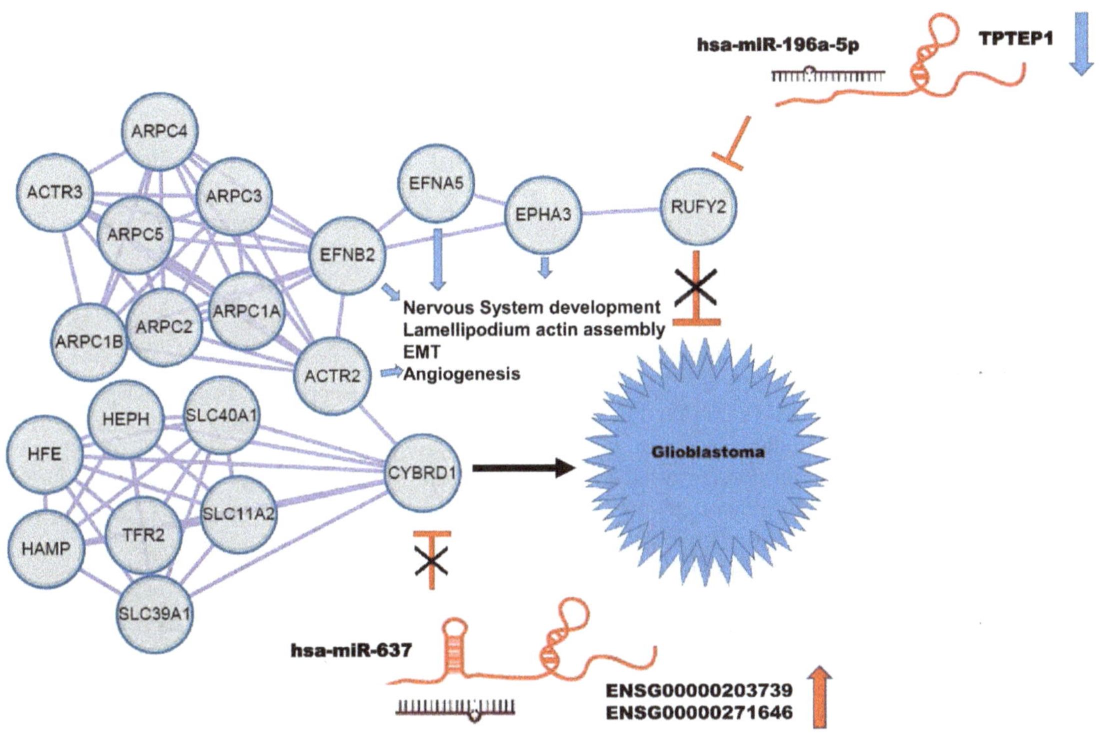

FIGURE 4 | Construction of a ceRNA regulation network in GBM based on differentially expressed miRNAs and DEGs. CeRNA network where gray circles represent predicted proteins. High-expression of *ENSG00000203739/ENSG00000271646* promotes GBM proliferation and invasion by suppressing *miR-637* and promoting expression of the putative oncogene *CYBRD1*. Down-regulation of *TPTEP1* fails to adsorb/bind to *miR-196a-5p*. The overexpression of *miR-196a-5p* impedes translation of the putative tumor suppressor RUFY2. Dysregulation at both points in the network potentially contributes to progression of GBM. EFNA5, FNB2, ACTR2, EPHA3 also act as putative oncogenes.

ARP2 has been shown to promote gastric cancer cell migration and invasion. In contrast, ARP2 knockdown suppressed cell motility (28). Finally, *EPHA3* is frequently overexpressed in GBM and in particular, in the mesenchymal molecular subtype, which also shows a more aggressive phenotype in patients (29). Importantly, *EPHA3* is highly expressed on the tumor-initiating cell population in glioma, which potentially maintains tumor cells in a less differentiated state by modulating mitogen-activated protein kinase signaling.

The results, therefore, could be consistent with a regulatory network composed of ceRNA plus the interactive proteins CYBRD1 and RUFY2 and involved in the proliferation and invasion of GBM.

DISCUSSION

The challenge today is in analyzing burgeoning molecular datasets in ways that will yield biologically and clinically meaningful insights into the development and treatment of human disease. In the current study, we explored the integration of RNA and protein datasets to identify pathways regulating the development of human GBM. We first analyzed standard array data to identify differentially expressed microRNAs and mRNAs in GBM relative to non-neoplastic brain tissue controls using the data contained in the StarBase, LncBase, Tanric, and TCGA databases. Based on the theory of ceRNA, we found potential ncRNA regulatory pathways involving an oncogene and a tumor suppressor, *ENSG00000203739/ENSG00000271646-miR-637*-CYBRD1 and *TPTEP1-miR-196a-5p*-RUFY2, and constructed a local PPI network which might contribute to proliferation and invasion of GBM.

Experimental results are consistent with some of our predictions. First, Boult et al. have reported that CYBRD1 was overexpressed in the progression of Barrett's metaplasia to adenocarcinoma and this change are associated with increased iron deposition (30). Brookes et al. also confirmed that the increased expression in iron import proteins, including CYBRD1, was associated with progression to colorectal cancer (31). However, other studies showed that high CYBRD1 expression has been associated with increased metastasis- and/or relapse-free survival in breast cancer (32). In functional experiments, CYBRD1 inhibited phosphorylation of FAK and the focal adhesion pathway which is involved in migration and invasion. The reasons for these discrepancies include differences in pathogenesis and the shift between proliferation and migration in tumors. Second, *miR-196a* has been reported to function as a putative oncogene in many cancers. *MiR-196a* is significantly upregulated in GBM, and high levels of *miR-196a* are positively related to the malignant progression of gliomas (33). Third, *miR-196a-5p* promotes proliferation and suppresses apoptosis in GBM cells both *in vitro* and *in vivo* by targeting IkBa (34). *MiR-196a-5p* also interacts directly with the 3'UTR of *ZMYND11* and promotes the growth of GBM cells (35). Finally, *miR-637* has been reported to be a tumor suppressor gene in diverse human cancers, such as gastric (36), ovarian (37) and colorectal cancers (38). Results in human glioma are consistent with a function as a tumor suppressor; expression levels of *miR-637* were significantly reduced in clinical glioma tissues compared with normal brain tissues (39). Moreover, these studies revealed that *miR-637* directly binds AKT1 and inhibits glioma cell growth, migration and invasion *in vitro* and *in vivo*. These data support the feasibility of our approach.

There are however deficiencies in our strategy. First, excluding function as a "molecular sponge," the mode of action of lncRNAs can be roughly divided into the following categories: signal, guide and scaffold. Second, due to the complexity of molecular mechanisms regulating disease development and the limitations of our analytical methods, many important molecules involved in GBM remain unidentified. Third, we input more processed TCGA data into our analysis, which may result in the loss of a more comprehensive perspective. Finally, because many algorithms are based on computer models, many prediction results cannot be achieved in real-life experiments.

Significant effort to analyze and integrate such large amounts of molecular data are taking place worldwide. Researchers funded by the National Institutes of Health (NIH), for example, have completed a comprehensive genomic analysis known as the PanCancer Atlas. This project published a total of 27 top bioinformatics papers. These articles are undoubtedly innovative and encouraging. But such efforts are merely the beginning. Here, we laid the groundwork for a new strategy to explore the complicated molecular mechanisms underlying the development of GBM or other diseases. The next important step is to verify our approach using functional experiments to confirm our model in **Figure 4**.

AUTHOR CONTRIBUTIONS

JZ, YK, and JW contributed to the conception of the study. JZ and YK contributed to experimental technology and experimental design. JZ, ZS, YK, QL, and HL performed the data analyses. JZ, YK, and JW wrote the manuscript. YW and JW supervised the study.

FUNDING

This work was supported by the Department of Science & Technology of Shandong Province (2017CXGC1502, GG201809170226, and ZR2017MH116), the Jinan Science and Technology Bureau of Shandong Province (2019GXRC006), Helse-Vest, the University of Bergen, the Norwegian Cancer Society, and the Norwegian Research Council.

SUPPLEMENTARY MATERIAL

Supplementary Figure 1 | Survival curves for the upper 20% of patients with high hsa-miR-637 expression in comparison with the lower 20%, 30%, 40%, 50%, 60%, 70%, and 80% of patients with low hsa-miR-637 expression **(A–G)**. Survival curve for the upper 30% of patients with high hsa-miR-637 expression in comparison with the lower 30% of patients with low hsa-miR-637 expression **(H)**

Supplementary Figure 2 | The expression of **(A)** *miR-196a-5p*, **(B)** *miR-637*, **(C)** *CYBRD1* and **(D)** *RUFY2* in GBMs and normal tissues in the TCGA database. $^{***}P < 0.001$ vs. control sample.

Supplementary Figure 3 | (A) PPI network generated using the REACTOME database. **(B)** The PPI network consists of top 300 DEGs in GSE4290.

Supplementary Figure 4 | Relationship between the expression of *CYBRD1/RUFY2* and *MGMT/IDH* status within TCGA GBM samples. The expression of *CYBRD1* in **(A)** methylated/unmethylated *MGMT* and **(B)** wild-type/mutant *IDH* tumors. The expression of *RUFY2* in **(C)** methylated/unmethylated MGMT and **(D)** wild-type/mutant *IDH* tumors.

REFERENCES

1. Ostrom QT, Gittleman H, Xu J, Kromer C, Wolinsky Y, Kruchko C, et al. CBTRUS statistical report: primary brain and other central nervous system tumors diagnosed in the United States in 2009-2013. *Neuro Oncol.* (2016) 18:v1–75. doi: 10.1093/neuonc/now207
2. Chiu HS, Somvanshi S, Patel E, Chen TW, Singh VP, Zorman B, et al. Pan-cancer analysis of lncRNA regulation supports their targeting of cancer genes in each tumor context. *Cell Rep.* (2018) 23:297–312.e12. doi: 10.1016/j.celrep.2018.03.064
3. Cui X, Morales RT, Qian W, Wang H, Gagner JP, Dolgalev I, et al. Hacking macrophage-associated immunosuppression for regulating glioblastoma angiogenesis. *Biomaterials.* (2018) 161:164–78. doi: 10.1016/j.biomaterials.2018.01.053
4. Salmena L, Poliseno L, Tay Y, Kats L, Pandolfi PP. A ceRNA hypothesis: the rosetta stone of a hidden RNA language? *Cell.* (2011) 146:353–8. doi: 10.1016/j.cell.2011.07.014
5. Sun L, Hui AM, Su Q, Vortmeyer A, Kotliarov Y, Pastorino S, et al. Neuronal and glioma-derived stem cell factor induces angiogenesis within the brain. *Cancer Cell.* (2006) 9:287–300. doi: 10.1016/j.ccr.2006.03.003

6. Feser WJ, Fingerlin TE, Strand MJ, Glueck DH. Calculating average power for the Benjamini-Hochberg procedure. *J Stat Theory Appl.* (2009) 8:325–52.
7. Madar V, Batista S. FastLSU: a more practical approach for the Benjamini-Hochberg FDR controlling procedure for huge-scale testing problems. *Bioinformatics.* (2016) 32:1716–23. doi: 10.1093/bioinformatics/btw029
8. Shannon P, Markiel A, Ozier O, Baliga NS, Wang JT, Ramage D, et al. Cytoscape: a software environment for integrated models of biomolecular interaction networks. *Genome Res.* (2003) 13:2498–504. doi: 10.1101/gr.1239303
9. Chou CH, Shrestha S, Yang CD, Chang NW, Lin YL, Liao KW, et al. Mirtarbase update 2018: a resource for experimentally validated microRNA-target interactions. *Nucleic Acids Res.* (2018) 46:D296–302. doi: 10.1093/nar/gkx1067
10. Du J, Yuan Z, Ma Z, Song J, Xie X, Chen Y. KEGG-PATH: Kyoto encyclopedia of genes and genomes-based pathway analysis using a path analysis model. *Mol Biosyst.* (2014) 10:2441–7. doi: 10.1039/C4MB00287C
11. Gene Ontology C. Gene Ontology Consortium: going forward. *Nucleic Acids Res.* (2015) 43:D1049–56. doi: 10.1093/nar/gku1179
12. Tripathi S, Pohl MO, Zhou Y, Rodriguez-Frandsen A, Wang G, Stein DA, et al. Meta- and orthogonal integration of influenza "OMICs" data defines a role for UBR4 in virus budding. *Cell Host Microbe.* (2015) 18:723–35. doi: 10.1016/j.chom.2015.11.002
13. Shirolkar A, Chakraborty S, Mandal T, Dabur R. Unbiased plasma metabolomics reveal the correlation of metabolic pathways and Prakritis of humans. *J Ayurveda Integr Med.* (2017) 9:113–22. doi: 10.1016/j.jaim.2017.05.002
14. Bindea G, Galon J, Mlecnik B. CluePedia Cytoscape plugin: pathway insights using integrated experimental and *in silico* data. *Bioinformatics.* (2013) 29:661–3. doi: 10.1093/bioinformatics/btt019
15. Szklarczyk D, Morris JH, Cook H, Kuhn M, Wyder S, Simonovic M, et al. The STRING database in 2017: quality-controlled protein-protein association networks, made broadly accessible. *Nucleic Acids Res.* (2017) 45:D362–8. doi: 10.1093/nar/gkw937
16. Scardoni G, Tosadori G, Faizan M, Spoto F, Fabbri F, Laudanna C. Biological network analysis with CentiScaPe: centralities and experimental dataset integration. *F1000Res.* (2014) 3:139. doi: 10.12688/f1000research.4477.1
17. Pathan M, Keerthikumar S, Ang CS, Gangoda L, Quek CY, Williamson NA, et al. FunRich: an open access standalone functional enrichment and interaction network analysis tool. *Proteomics.* (2015) 15:2597–601. doi: 10.1002/pmic.201400515
18. Tang Z, Li C, Kang B, Gao G, Li C, Zhang Z. GEPIA: a web server for cancer and normal gene expression profiling and interactive analyses. *Nucleic Acids Res.* (2017) 45:W98–102. doi: 10.1093/nar/gkx247
19. Paraskevopoulou MD, Vlachos IS, Karagkouni D, Georgakilas G, Kanellos I, Vergoulis T, et al. DIANA-LncBase v2: indexing microRNA targets on non-coding transcripts. *Nucleic Acids Res.* (2016) 44:D231–8. doi: 10.1093/nar/gkv1270
20. Li J, Han L, Roebuck P, Diao L, Liu L, Yuan Y, et al. TANRIC: an interactive open platform to explore the function of lncRNAs in cancer. *Cancer Res.* (2015) 75:3728–37. doi: 10.1158/0008-5472.CAN-15-0273
21. Szklarczyk D, Franceschini A, Wyder S, Forslund K, Heller D, Huerta-Cepas J, et al. STRING v10: protein-protein interaction networks, integrated over the tree of life. *Nucleic Acids Res.* (2015) 43:D447–52. doi: 10.1093/nar/gku1003
22. Haw R, Stein LD. Using the reactome database. *Curr Protoc Bioinformatics.* (2004) Chapter 8:Unit 8.7. doi: 10.1002/0471250953.bi0807s7
23. Belinky F, Nativ N, Stelzer G, Zimmerman S, Iny Stein T, Safran M, et al. PathCards: multi-source consolidation of human biological pathways. *Database.* (2015) 2015:bav006. doi: 10.1093/database/bav006
24. Esteller M, Herman JG. Cancer as an epigenetic disease: DNA methylation and chromatin alterations in human tumours. *J Pathol.* (2002) 196:1–7. doi: 10.1002/path.1024
25. Norwood MS, Lupo PJ, Chow EJ, Scheurer ME, Plon SE, Danysh HE, et al. Childhood cancer risk in those with chromosomal and non-chromosomal congenital anomalies in Washington state: 1984-2013. *PLoS ONE.* (2017) 12:e0179006. doi: 10.1371/journal.pone.0179006
26. Liang Q, Ding J, Xu R, Xu Z, Zheng S. The novel human endogenous retrovirus-related gene, psiTPTE22-HERV, is silenced by DNA methylation in cancers. *Int J Cancer.* (2010) 127:1833–43. doi: 10.1002/ijc.25213
27. Sun Y, Shang Y, Ren G, Zhou L, Feng B, Li K, et al. Coronin3 regulates gastric cancer invasion and metastasis by interacting with Arp2. *Cancer Biol Ther.* (2014) 15:1163–73. doi: 10.4161/cbt.29501
28. Krusche B, Ottone C, Clements MP, Johnstone ER, Goetsch K, Lieven H, et al. EphrinB2 drives perivascular invasion and proliferation of glioblastoma stem-like cells. *Elife.* (2016) 5:e14845. doi: 10.7554/eLife.14845
29. Day BW, Stringer BW, Al-Ejeh F, Ting MJ, Wilson J, Ensbey KS, et al. EphA3 maintains tumorigenicity and is a therapeutic target in glioblastoma multiforme. *Cancer Cell.* (2013) 23:238–48. doi: 10.1016/j.ccr.2013.01.007
30. Boult J, Roberts K, Brookes MJ, Hughes S, Bury JP, Cross SS, et al. Overexpression of cellular iron import proteins is associated with malignant progression of esophageal adenocarcinoma. *Clin Cancer Res.* (2008) 14:379–87. doi: 10.1158/1078-0432.CCR-07-1054
31. Brookes MJ, Hughes S, Turner FE, Reynolds G, Sharma N, Ismail T, et al. Modulation of iron transport proteins in human colorectal carcinogenesis. *Gut.* (2006) 55:1449–60. doi: 10.1136/gut.2006.094060
32. Lemler DJ, Lynch ML, Tesfay L, Deng Z, Paul BT, Wang X, et al. DCYTB is a predictor of outcome in breast cancer that functions via iron-independent mechanisms. *Breast Cancer Res.* (2017) 19:25. doi: 10.1186/s13058-017-0814-9
33. Huang F, Tang J, Zhuang X, Zhuang Y, Cheng W, Chen W, et al. MiR-196a promotes pancreatic cancer progression by targeting nuclear factor kappa-B-inhibitor alpha. *PLoS ONE.* (2014) 9:e87897. doi: 10.1371/journal.pone.0087897
34. Zhang J, Zheng F, Yu G, Yin Y, Lu Q. MiR-196a targets netrin 4 and regulates cell proliferation and migration of cervical cancer cells. *Biochem Biophys Res Commun.* (2013) 440:582–8. doi: 10.1016/j.bbrc.2013.09.142
35. Yang JP, Yang JK, Li C, Cui ZQ, Liu HJ, Sun XF, et al. Downregulation of ZMYND11 induced by miR-196a-5p promotes the progression growth of GBM. *Biochem Biophys Res Commun.* (2017) 494:674–80. doi: 10.1016/j.bbrc.2017.10.098
36. Guan EC, Xu XG, Xue FX. Circ-NOTCH1 acts as a sponge of miR-637 and affects the expression of its target gene Apelin to regulate gastric cancer cell growth. *Biochem Cell Biol.* (2019). doi: 10.1139/bcb-2019-0079. [Epub ahead of print].
37. Zhang M, Xia B, Xu Y, Zhang Y, Xu J, Lou G. Circular RNA (hsa_circ_0051240) promotes cell proliferation, migration and invasion in ovarian cancer through miR-637/KLK4 axis. *Artif Cells Nanomed Biotechnol.* (2019) 47:1224–33. doi: 10.1080/21691401.2019.1593999
38. Wang L, Jiang F, Xia X, Zhang B. LncRNA FAL1 promotes carcinogenesis by regulation of miR-637/NUPR1 pathway in colorectal cancer. *Int J Biochem Cell Biol.* (2019) 106:46–56. doi: 10.1016/j.biocel.2018.09.015
39. Que T, Song Y, Liu Z, Zheng S, Long H, Li Z, et al. Decreased miRNA-637 is an unfavorable prognosis marker and promotes glioma cell growth, migration and invasion via direct targeting Akt1. *Oncogene.* (2015) 34:4952–63. doi: 10.1038/onc.2014.419

15

Therapeutic Prospects of mRNA-Based Gene Therapy for Glioblastoma

Xiangjun Tang[1,2,3†], *Shenqi Zhang*[1†], *Rui Fu*[2], *Li Zhang*[2], *Kuanming Huang*[2], *Hao Peng*[2], *Longjun Dai*[2,4*] and *Qianxue Chen*[1*]

[1] *Department of Neurosurgery, Renmin Hospital of Wuhan University, Wuhan, China,* [2] *Department of Neurosurgery, Taihe Hospital, Hubei University of Medicine, Shiyan, China,* [3] *Department of Neurosurgery, Affiliated Hospital of Xi'an Jiaotong, University Health Science Center, Xi'an, China,* [4] *Department of Surgery, University of British Columbia, Vancouver, BC, Canada*

***Correspondence:**
Longjun Dai
ljdai@mail.ubc.ca
Qianxue Chen
chenqx666@whu.edu.cn

† These authors have contributed equally to this work

The treatment of glioblastoma has been a big challenge for decades in the oncological field mainly owing to its unique biological characteristics, such as high heterogeneity, diffusing invasiveness, and capacity to resist conventional therapies. The mRNA-based therapeutic modality holds many superior features, including easy manipulation, rapid and transient expression, and adaptive convertibility without mutagenesis, which are suitable for dealing with glioblastoma's complexity and variability. Synthetic anticancer mRNAs carried by various vehicles act as the ultimate attackers of the tumor across biological barriers. In this modality, specifically targeted glioblastoma treatment can be guaranteed by adding targeting molecules at certain levels. The choice of mRNA-bearing vehicle and administration method is a fully patient-tailored selection. This review covers the advantages and possible limitations of mRNA-based gene therapy, the *in vitro* synthesis of mRNA, the feasible methods for synthetic mRNA delivery and clinical therapeutic prospects of mRNA-based gene therapy for glioblastoma.

Keywords: mRNA, gene therapy, glioblastoma, patient-tailored, targeting molecules

BACKGROUND

Glioblastoma multiforme (GBM) is the most common and aggressive primary brain tumor with inferior prognosis. GBM is thought to arise from the neuroglial stem or progenitor cells and has been defined by WHO as a grade IV glioma (1, 2). It is recurrent in almost all patients (3). GBM affects 3–4 people out of every 100,000 per year, with a sustained and highly significant incidence rise across all ages (4, 5). The outcomes for treating GBM retain gloomy, though surgical techniques and adjuvant therapies have progressively developed for decades. GBM remains a virtually incurable disease, resulting in a death rate of greater than 95% within 5 years of diagnosis (6). The main reasons that GBM is challenging to treat relate both the restriction of surgical resection and the resistance to irradiation and chemotherapy (7). Not only the drugs were prevented to enter into gliomas' cells by blood-brain barrier (BBB) and brain-tumor barrier (BTB) in the brain, but also the complexity of tumor composition and diffusing invasiveness have hindered the better effective treatment for over three decades (8, 9). There is an urgent need for advancement in treatment strategies to improve outcomes for GBM patients. Since Wolff et al. pioneered the concept of nucleic acid based therapy, reporting functional protein expression in target organs after the direct injection of plasmid DNA or mRNA (10), gene therapy has held a great potential to provide a viable alternative to conventional treatments toward effectively overcoming cancer progression in GBM (11).

Till now, four main types of vectors have been widely used in gene-related therapy, including plasmids, viral vectors, cosmids, and artificial chromosomes. Viral vectors used for gene therapy are associated with severe safety issues (12, 13). Meanwhile, low transfection efficiency and the potential to induce mutations limited the development of non-viral DNA vectors (14). Recent research reported that novel stabilized mRNA constructs have become more attractive alternatives to the most commonly used DNA-based plasmid (pDNA) (15, 16), mainly due to their ease of manipulation and safety in clinical applications. This review discusses the advantages and possible limitations of mRNA-based gene therapy, the feasible methods for mRNA-based gene delivery and clinical therapeutic prospects of mRNA-based gene therapy for glioblastoma.

THE BENEFICIAL ASPECTS OF mRNA-BASED GENE TRANSFER

Synthetic mRNA has emerged as an efficient gene transfection tool, and a wide range of therapeutic applications have been developed (17). Prolonged intracellular persistence of mRNA is a basic prerequisite for synthetic mRNA to be effectively used in gene therapy. mRNA-based gene have significantly enhanced translational efficience of foreign mRNA in host cells, mainly owe to the discovery of 5′mRNA anti-reverse cap analogs (ARCA), the insertion of additional untranslated regions, and poly(A) tails (15, 18–20). To summarize, compared with pDNA delivery in gene therapy, mRNA-based gene treatment has more significant virtues: (i) pDNA is translated into the nucleus and mRNA is translated in the cytoplasm directly. The mRNA transfection is efficient even in quiescent cells, which is obviously different from pDNA transfection; (ii) the risk of insertional mutagenesis can be ignored by the nature of RNA. Hence, mRNA has a significant security compared to DNA in gene therapy for clinical applications; (iii) the immunogenic reaction of toll-like receptor-activated mRNA is weaker than the unmethylated CpG motifs of DNA recognized by TLR9; (iv) the mRNA transfection into host cells can be much easier because its construct is far smaller than pDNA. Furthermore, mRNA gene therapy circumvents the need for selecting a specific promoter, and thus the transfection process is relatively efficient and facile; (v) protein translation takes place almost immediately after mRNA transfection because of it's functionality in the cytoplasm without the need to enter into the nucleus (15, 21–24). Mainly because of the unstable structure and ubiquitous presence of RNase, the biggest concern about mRNA-based gene vehicle has been its stability and durability during its application. **Table 1** lists the comparisons between mRNA- and DNA-based gene carriers as regards to practical applications.

TABLE 1 | Comparisons between mRNA- and DNA-based gene carriers.

Immunogenicity	Low	High	(104)
Target cell type	Dividing and non-dividing cells	Dividing cells	(17)
Potential mutation	None	Possible	(25)
Cellular delivery	Much easier	More difficult	
Therapeutic action	Rapid (hours)	Delayed (3–5 days)	(25)
Production cost	High	Low	(26)
"Advanced therapy medicinal products" regulation required	No	Yes	(25)

IN VITRO SYNTHESIZATION OF TARGET GENE-BEARING mRNA

The structure of synthetic mRNA is the same as the structure of natural mRNA, containing a cap, 5′ and 3′ UTRs and a poly(A)-tail and the encoded gene of interest. Regardless of the application, the vital factor is bioavailability of the synthetic mRNA. In recent years, the cap structure of the eukaryotic mRNAs naturally occurring at the 5′end has been studied on the therapeutic use of mRNAs (22, 27, 28). The cap is involved in mRNA's maturation, nuclear export, initiation of translation, and their turnover through interacting with highly specialized cap-binding proteins (29, 30). Due to the existence of NTPs and a regular cap such as m7GpppGNpN, polymerase-mediated transcripts are highly capped in a reverse orientation (i.e., Gpppm7GpNpN) up to one-third to one-half of total transcripts (28, 31). Such reverse-capped transcripts significantly reduce the translational efficiency of mRNA. However, 3′-O-methyl, 3′-H, or 2′-O-methyl modified anti-reverse cap analogs (ARCAs) of the m7Guo can achieve 100% correct orientation, thereby resulting in higher translational efficiency of synthetic mRNAs (18, 32–34). It can also improve resistance to enzymatic degradation (35). ARCA is now widely used in *in vitro* synthesization of mRNA. 3′ UTR is another key regulator of intracellular kinetics of an mRNA molecule (36). The length of the 3′ UTR is a critical factor since the longer of the mRNAs 3′ UTRs the shorter of the half-life, meanwhile mRNAs with shorter 3′ UTRs are less efficiently translated (37, 38). Human globin 3′ UTRs are now being commonly used in mRNA synthesization, mainly based on the distinctive feature of human erythrocytes (17). Practically, the human 5′ UTR with Kozak sequence, standardized 3′ UTR sequence and ARCA cap analog are all commercially available. The presence and length of the 3′-poly(A)-tail in mRNA also have great importance for efficient translation and stability (39). Different administration route may result in diverse average half-life of protein production from transfected modified mRNA, it ranges from 50 h *in vitro* to 7–30 h *in vivo* (40). The majority of

Abbreviations: mRNA, messenger Ribonucleic Acid; GBM, Glioblastoma multiforme; WHO, World Health Organization; BBB, blood-brain barrier; BTB, brain-tumor barrier; pDNA, DNA-based plasmid; ARCA, anti-reverse cap analogs; PCR, Polymerase Chain Reaction; DOTAP, N-[1-(2,3-dioleoloxy)propyl]-N,N,N-trimethyl ammonium chloride; DCs, dendritic cells; HSC, hematopoietic stem cell; MSC, mesenchymal stem cell; NK, natural killer; CAR-T, chimeric antigen receptor T; TRAIL, tumor necrosis factor-related apoptosis inducing ligand.

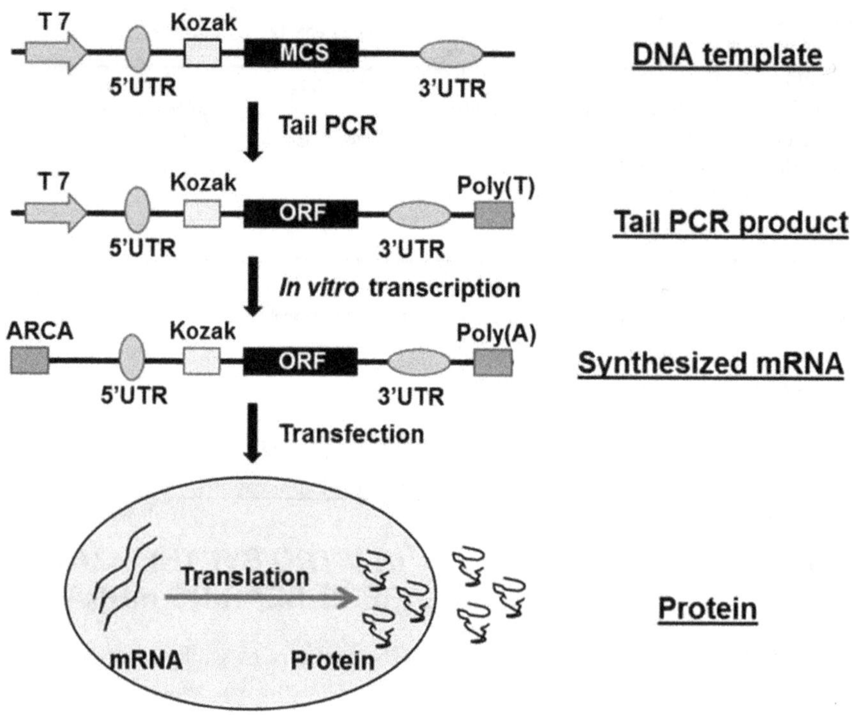

FIGURE 1 | Flow chat of mRNA synthesization *in vitro*. ARCA, anti-reverse cap analog; MCS, multiple cloning site; ORF, open reading frame; PCR, polymerase chain reaction; UTR, untranslated region. The flow chat was reproduced from Guo et al. (16).

mRNA decay are began with deadenylation of the poly(A)-tail total to ∼10 nucleotides (41, 42), so a poly (T_{120}) sequence was always introduced in the Tail PCR process in our previous studies (16, 20). The **Figure 1** shows the flow chart of mRNA synthesis *in vitro*.

DELIVERY OF SYNTHESIZED mRNA

Synthetic mRNAs have to be located in the cytoplasm of targeted cells to be translated into corresponding proteins using the host cell's machinery. As Kowalski et al. indicated, the delivery of exogenous synthetic mRNA is quite complex and requiring overcome numerous obstacles in extra- and intra-cellular to reach the cytoplasm exogenous synthetic mRNA delivery process is quite multifaceted and faces multiple extra- and intra-cellular barriers to reach the cytoplasm (43). Under most circumstances, the cell membrane is a major and formidable barrier for synthetic mRNA's intracellular delivery. The characteristics of mRNA and lipid bilayer components of the cell membrane are essential factors when we design an ideal method to deliver synthetic mRNAs to targeted cells. In general, the delivery of mRNA in intracellular is not as easy as small oligonucleotides, in part because of its larger size (300–5,000 kDa, up to 15 kb) and polyanionic feature, and it needs encapsulation into nanoparticle (43–45). The cell membrane is primarily made up of a lipid bilayer composed of zwitterionic and negatively charged phospholipids (43). The polar heads of the phospholipids point toward the aqueous environment and the hydrophobic tails form a hydrophobic core (43, 46). The ion channels and ion pumps mounted in the lipid bilayer maintain a negative potential (−40 to −80 mV) across the cell membrane, forming an electro-barrier for highly negatively charged mRNA molecules (47). Thus, appropriate supplementary measures are required to facilitate synthetic mRNA crossing the cell membrane. It is amazingly stable and sustained long time if the mRNA transferred into the cytoplasm (22). Since the relatively small size and single chain structure of mRNA, majority of the available delivery tools were shown to work better with mRNA which were well used for studying in plasmid DNA delivery (48, 49). After this, several mRNA delivery methods that are being utilized in preclinical and clinical studies are explicated and related pros and cons are also discussed.

Naked mRNA Delivery

The naked mRNA spontaneous uptake by cells is not satisfied, even though the transient expression was demonstrated in some studies (10, 50, 51). Some clinical trials using intratumoral injection of naked mRNA to encode tumor-associated antigens into patients with advanced melanoma and with liver cancer are currently being undertaken (43). Naked mRNAs can be passively transferred into cells of interest by electroporation, which is used on a certain type of cells in preclinical studies. When cells are treated with short high-field electric pulses, the difference of voltage along the cell membrane can cause temporary perforation, allowing mRNA molecules passively pass through the hole and spread into the cell. The electroporation-mediated delivery efficiency can be influenced by the electrical field, ionic strength of the medium, the cell type and other membrane permeability-related factors (22). Therefore, the electroporation conditions must be carefully balanced between the high uptake of synthetic mRNA and the high percentage of healthy cells. The earliest successful electroporation mRNA transfections were conducted on human hematopoietic cells and dendritic cells, which showed superior to spontaneous uptake and lipofection (48, 52). Later on, this method was also applied in other types of cells, such as stem cells and lymphocytes (53, 54). More recently, the high throughput electroporators were also successfully used to electroporate large volumes of cells (55, 56). Theoretically, electroporation and electroporator can be used in a variety of cells without special reagents, but expensive equipment is needed and more cells and mRNAs are required for each transfection. Because of the relatively high cell mortality rate, the electroporation conditions for each cell type need to be optimized to achieve the best results.

Lipoplex- and Polyplex-Mediated Transfection

Another method for synthetic mRNA delivery is the complexation of mRNA nucleic acids with cationic lipids or polymers forming lipoplexes and polyplexes through spontaneous charge interactions (57). The carrier materials bind nucleic acids and protect their cargo from degradation by forming tight particles containing PH-sensitive molecules that escape from the endosome and enter the cytoplasm after endocytosis (22, 58). Furthermore, these carriers can be functionalized for specific cell or tissue delivery of synthetic mRNA by modifying carrier's formulation (59). Now, lipoplex- and polyplex-mediated mRNA transfection is being commonly used in various preclinical studies. However, because cationic liposomes have relatively high cytotoxicity and may interfere with cell metabolism in different cells, cationic lipid-related carriers have been mainly limited to *in vitro* studies. In recent years, more complex mRNA vectors have been created, such as PH-reactive polymer nanoparticles, which can also be systematically delivered *in vivo* (60).

Inorganic Nanoparticle-Mediated Delivery

Although current mRNA delivery technologies are mainly concentrated on cationic polymers and liposomes, inorganic nanoparticles have also been developed. In 2009, Zohra et al. for the first time introduced that carbonate apatite inorganic nanoparticles bond with cationic liposomes of DOTAP (N-[1-(2,3-Dioleoloxy) propyl]-N, N, N-trimethyl ammonium chloride) could successfully generate high transfection efficiency of luciferase mRNA in both mitotic and non-mitotic cells (61). As an additional advantage, inorganic carbonate apatite combining with DOTAP could facilitate DOTAP-mediated mRNA expression (62). So, inorganic nanoparticle holds a promising potential to be widely used for synthetic mRNA delivery.

Polypeptide-Mediated Delivery

As another type of synthetic vehicles, precisely designed polypeptides are also used to deliver mRNA to the cell cytoplasm (63). Amphiphilic cationic feature of the polypeptide mainly determines the mRNA delivery function. As shown in Mastrobattista et al.'s recent study, the GALA peptide functionalized the target mRNA polyplexes (PPx-GALA) in dendritic cells (DCs), and the cellular uptake of mRNA that PPx-GALA complex is 18 times higher than lipofectamine without causing cytotoxicity (64). The conjugation of precisely designed peptide to mRNA polyplexes not only promotes the mRNA expression but also plays a significant role in targeting the specific type of cells or tissue.

Virus-Mediated Delivery

Synthetic mRNA can also be delivered into cells of interest by viral particles, which is different from conventional transfection. Such gene delivery-related viral infection requires cloning the target gene into a specific virus system and packaging specific cells to obtain the "modified" virus. Alphavirus, Sendai virus, and retrovirus have been utilized for mRNA delivery (65, 66). Retrovirus-mediated mRNA transfection can be delivered to the cytoplasm as a direct translation template for interest proteins, but the vector needs to be altered to prevent reverse translation (22). The advantage is that the infection efficiency is particularly high, especially some of the primary cells and living cells which are difficult to transfect. In addition, mRNA can avoid being degraded outside the cell by retroviral particle and the viral envelope may be modified for synthetic mRNA-transfer (67). Generally speaking, the virus system is time-consuming, expensive and complex, and may be potentially dangerous if it is improperly operated.

Cell- Mediated Delivery

Cell-mediated gene therapy has been extensively studied for decades. A variety of types of cells have been involved in this field, including hematopoietic stem cell (HSC) (68), mesenchymal stem cell (MSC) (69), dendritic cell (DC) (70), macrophage (71), natural killer (NK) cell (72), and chimeric antigen receptor T (CAR-T) cell (73). Anti-CD19 CAR-T cell products, the first FDA approved gene therapy for patients with pre-B cell acute lymphoblastic leukemia or B-cell lymphomas, have revolutionized anti-cancer therapy, giving a new treatment option for patients who have difficulty to receive standard treatment (74). DNA-based engineering strategies have been used in the majority of cell-mediated gene therapies. However, the advantage of mRNA transfection is that the rate and duration of target gene expression can be well-managed by adjusting the quantity of mRNA, which may avoid some DNA-engineered cell-induced adverse events, such as cytokine release syndrome following the infusion of CAR-expressing T cells. Recently, as an alternative modality, mRNA has been utilized for cell-mediated gene delivery. The studied cell type includes DC (75), NK cell (72), T cell (76), HSC (77), and MSC (16, 78, 79). The most notable advantage of using cell-mediated mRNA delivery lies in vehicle cell's homing capacity. The target mRNAs can be transfected into vehicle cells by preferred delivery method, such

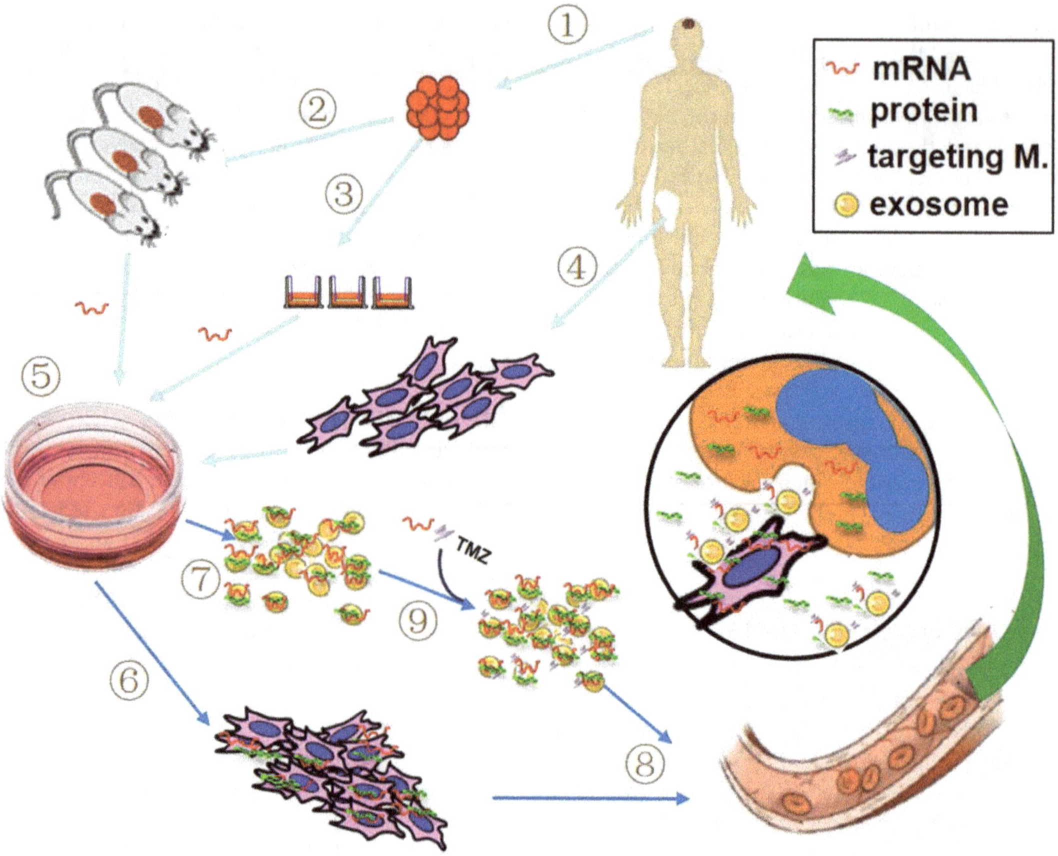

FIGURE 2 | Proposed patient-tailored glioblastoma treatment with mRNA-based therapeutic modality. If practical, the target mRNA is predetermined using resected tumor tissue (1) with patient-derived xenografted animal model (2) or real-time detection (3). Meanwhile, patient's own vehicle cells (like bone marrow-derived mesenchymal stem cells, MSCs) are prepared (4). The synthetic target mRNA is delivered into cultured vehicle cells by preferred transfection method (5) and the target mRNA-bearing cells (6) and associated exosomes (7) are collected for administration (8). If necessary, additional mRNA, specific targeting molecules and/or chemotherapeutics such as temozolomide (TMZ) can be directly loaded into the isolated exosomes prior to the administration (9). The insert picture illustrates the possible action modes of mRNA in the tumor site, including mRNA product (i.e., protein) from both vehicle cell and recipient cell, cell-to-cell contact, and exosome-mediated attack molecules.

as electroporation, viral or non-viral delivery. As illustrated in **Figure 2**, at the target site, mRNA-carried message can be transferred to recipient cells through several pathways: (1) cell-to-cell contact, such as DCs and CAR-T cell; (2) encoded protein produced in the vehicle cells, in the case of secreting protein or proteins containing transacting activator of transcription (TAT) segment; (3) parent cell-derived exosomes containing both mRNA and protein. Several clinical trials have been reported to use autologous DCs loaded with mRNA as a treatment of various cancers (22). In our recent work, the therapeutic efficacy of anticancer gene-engineered MSCs was also demonstrated in glioblastoma animal model (16).

Exosome-Mediated Delivery

As the key mediators for intercellular communications, exosomes play an important part in mRNA delivery. Exosomes are nanoscale membrane vesicles mainly composed of circular double-layer lipid membranes and intracapsular contents (80). During the biogenesis of exosomes, the vesicular membrane is formed through two steps of reverse invagination of the cellular plasma membrane, resulting in vesical membrane outside-facing-out. The biological significance of this property is 2-fold. Firstly, this membrane orientation is a necessary prerequisite for the application of exosomes to targeted cancer therapy due to the targeting molecules from mother cells are also exist in the exosomes (81). Secondly, the content of vesicles is closely connected with plasma membrane reverse invagination. Theoretically, anything in the cell cytoplasm can be inwrapped in exosomes (82, 83), including synthetic mRNA from transfected parent cells. Therefore, the delivered synthetic mRNA could exist inside of exosomes in two forms, mRNA and/or relevant protein (**Figure 2**). Furthermore, synthetic mRNA and chemotherapeutic drugs can also be directly loaded into isolated exosomes through conventional transfection technology (84). Isolated exosomes can be passively transmitted throughout the body, but their ability to target distribution depends primarily on the surface-derived targeting molecules form parent cells (84). In the recipient cells, exosomes are primarily absorbed into the cell by endocytosis, membrane fusion, or receptor-mediated internalization (85). Due to the cell-free nature and biological characteristics, exosomes replace cell-based modality (like CAR-T) and directly attack tumor cells. In regards to cancer therapy, exosomes have following advantages. First, exosomes can be used as "off-the-shelf" reagents so that the doses can be controlled according to the therapeutic condition. Second, their nanoscale size provides the possibility for solid tumor therapy such as GBM. Third, the combined and/or alternate use of cell-based and cell-free platforms will enhance the application value for cell-based cancer therapy (86).

THE THERAPEUTIC PROSPECTS OF MRNA-BASED GENE THERAPY FOR GLIOBLASTOMA

The reason why GBM is difficult to treat rests with its special biological characteristics, such as located in the brain and defended by both BBB and BTB, high heterogeneity, diffusing invasiveness, and capacity to resist conventional therapies. As mechanical barriers, BBB and BTB protect GBM from certain therapeutic agents. The high heterogeneity of GBM probably means that it cannot be well-cured by any single particular drug, especially biomarker-related agents. Its invasive growth property determines the highest recurrence rate after surgical resection, and its high capacity of drug resistance suggests that it cannot be efficiently treated by the sustained use of any specific drug. Taken together, an ideal anti-GBM strategy should adapt all challenges and meet the following requirements: (1) Anticancer actions are specifically confined to the tumor site; (2) personalized treatment plan according to the sensitivity of anticancer drugs predetermined; (3) multiple anticancer mechanisms can work simultaneously; and (4) the anticancer agents can be adaptively replaced. Of course, because GBM grows in a restricted intracranial environment, if practical, surgical resection is always the first treatment upon diagnosis, otherwise, the patients may die from some GBM-related complications, such as cerebral hernia, and we may not have the opportunity to provide any therapeutic intervention.

The Use of mRNA-Based Anticancer Gene Products as the Ultimate Attackers of the Tumor Has Special Superiority for GBM Treatment

As described earlier, nano-scaled target mRNA-bearing lipoplexes, polyplexes, liposomes and exosomes are all able to cross BBB and BTB in the brain (87, 88), overcoming the natural barriers. The rapid and transient expression nature of synthetic mRNA, which has been considered the biggest weakness of using mRNA for gene therapy, is just suitable for dealing with GBM's complexity and variability through its adaptive convertibility. It is also because of its short-term high-level expression, mRNA-based gene therapy has been intensively and almost exclusively focused on cancer treatment (89, 90). The selection of anti-oncogene depends mainly on the specific situation of each patient. If possible, predetermination should be performed using *in vitro* real-time detection of tumor cells or patient-derived xenografted animal model immediately after surgical resection (91, 92).

The Highly Specific Targeting Capability of mRNA-Based Modality Is Essential to Achieve the Most Effective Treatment of Cancer With Limited Side Effects

In this mRNA-based therapeutic modality, the GBM targeting can be achieved at least in three levels. (1) Cell level. The tumor-homing property has been verified in several types of cells, including NK cells, DCs, and MSCs (72, 93, 94). In addition to their ability of tumor-directed migration and incorporation, these types of cells are easy acquisition and fast *ex vivo* expansion. More importantly, they are feasible for autologous transplantation. These cells are also able to cross BBB especially under brain tumorous condition (95, 96). The targeting capacity of these cells can be further enhanced by transfecting specific targeting molecules (e.g., CAR-T). The therapeutic efficacy of GBM by cell-mediated and mRNA-based modality has heterogeneity in preclinical studies and a number of them are currently in different phases of clinical trials (16, 20, 96). (2) Exosome level. As aforementioned, anticancer mRNA-bearing exosomes are able to target tumor cells directed by the targeting molecules in their membrane, which originate from their parent cells. Furthermore, additional targeting molecules can be loaded into exosomes after their isolation. Several GBM-specific targeting peptides have been precisely investigated. These peptides act on a different part of the tumor cell through different mechanisms (97). (3) Molecular-level. Under certain circumstances, the ultimate attack molecules kill tumor cells in a tumor-specific manner. For example, tumor necrosis factor-related apoptosis inducing ligand (TRAIL) induces apoptosis specifically in tumor cells through binding with death receptors. This target specificity is determined by the differential expression of death receptors in tumor cells (98).

The Administration Route of mRNA Is a Patient-Tailored Selection

The selection of delivery routes of synthetic mRNA to GBM patients depends on the general evaluation of various parameters, including patient's glioma grade, stage, surgical, and chemotherapy history, as well as the available forms of synthetic mRNA carriers. In general, intravenous infusion is the safest and most practical administration method for various forms of synthetic mRNA. Other options include local injection, cerebrospinal fluid infusion, interventional infusion and administration through the nasopharyngeal pathway. However, it is worth noting that the alternate use and sometimes a combination of different mRNA content and different delivery method could be significantly beneficial for the patients with GBM. In our previous clinical trial, the combination of local application of MSCs during surgical operation and intravenous infusion of MSCs after surgery achieved an ideal outcome (99).

Although no clinical trials of mRNA-based GBM therapy have yet been completed, some are underway. A phase II randomized, blinded trial of CMV RNA-pulsed dendritic cells with tetanus-diphtheria toxoid vaccine in patients with newly-diagnosed glioblastoma is ongoing[1]. The mRNA-based therapy has not been widely adopted in treating GBM, but it had made great progress in other diseases. A phase 1 clinical trial showed that rabies vaccination based on mRNA encoding was safe and could produce functional antibodies (100). Martin Sebastian et al. reported a phase I/II a study of mRNA-based cancer immunotherapy on non-small cell lung cancer. The patients of this trial were well-tolerated and the antigen-specific immune responses were detected in 63% of assessable patients after five injections (101). The therapeutic prospects of mRNA-based gene therapy for GBM could proliferate when noted obstacles are overcome, such as the targeted delivery *in vivo*, rapid degradation, and short half-life. We also have to address the repetitive application and sufficient delivery efficiency in the brain.

CONCLUSIONS

The dissatisfactory outcome of GBM treatment has retained for decades. The reason why GBM is difficult to treat rests with its special biological characteristics such as high heterogeneity, diffusing invasiveness, and capacity to resist conventional therapies, as well as the existence of biological barriers, e.g., BBB and BTB. Compared with conventional DNA-based strategy, synthetic mRNA-mediated therapeutic modality holds many superior features including easy manipulation, rapid and transient expression, and adaptive convertibility without mutagenesis, which is suitable for dealing with glioblastoma's complexity and variability. Synthetic anticancer mRNAs carried by various vehicles, such as organic or inorganic nanoparticle-encapsulated complexes, patient-derived DCs or MSCs and their corresponding exosomes, act as the ultimate attackers of the tumor across biological barriers. In this mRNA-based therapeutic modality, specifically targeted GBM treatment can be guaranteed by adding targeting molecules at certain levels. The choice of mRNA-bearing vehicle and administration method is a fully patient-tailored selection. To date, mRNA has been used in preclinical clinical trials such as cancer immunotherapy, infectious disease control and regenerative medicine (24, 102, 103), but, anticancer treatment is the most developed application for mRNA (89, 104). The mRNA-based therapeutic modality holds a great promising potential to be efficiently utilized for the patients with GBM.

AUTHOR CONTRIBUTIONS

XT, LZ, and QC designed this research. RF, KH, and HP collected relevant literatures. XT and LD wrote and revised the manuscript. SZ helped to correct the language. All authors have read and approved the final manuscript.

REFERENCES

1. Weller M, Wick W, Aldape K, Brada M, Berger M, Pfister SM, et al. Glioma. *Nat Rev Dis Primers.* (2015) 1:15017. doi: 10.1038/nrdp.2015.17
2. Louis DN, Perry A, Reifenberger G, von Deimling A, Figarella-Branger D, Cavenee WK, et al. The 2016 World Health Organization Classification of Tumors of the Central Nervous System: a summary. *Acta Neuropathol.* (2016) 131:803–20. doi: 10.1007/s00401-016-1545-1
3. Holland EC. Glioblastoma multiforme: the terminator. *Proc Natl Acad Sci USA.* (2000) 97:6242–4. doi: 10.1073/pnas.97.12.6242
4. Philips A, Henshaw DL, Lamburn G, O'Carroll MJ. Brain tumours: rise in glioblastoma multiforme incidence in England 1995-2015 suggests an adverse environmental or lifestyle factor. *J Environ Public Health.* (2018) 2018:7910754. doi: 10.1155/2018/7910754
5. Walker EV, Davis FG, CBTR founding affiliates. Malignant primary brain and other central nervous system tumors diagnosed in Canada from 2009 to 2013. *Neuro Oncol.* (2019) 21:360–9. doi: 10.1093/neuonc/noy195
6. Jhanwar-Uniyal M, Labagnara M, Friedman M, Kwasnicki A, Murali R. Glioblastoma: molecular pathways, stem cells and therapeutic targets. *Cancers.* (2015) 7:538–55. doi: 10.3390/cancers7020538
7. Tomiyama A, Ichimura K. Signal transduction pathways and resistance to targeted therapies in glioma. *Semin Cancer Biol.* (2019) 58:118–29. doi: 10.1016/j.semcancer.2019.01.004
8. Agarwal S, Sane R, Oberoi R, Ohlfest JR, Elmquist WF. Delivery of molecularly targeted therapy to malignant glioma, a disease of the whole brain. *Expert Rev Mol Med.* (2011) 13:e17. doi: 10.1017/S1462399411001888
9. Westphal M, Lamszus K. The neurobiology of gliomas: from cell biology to the development of therapeutic approaches. *Nat Rev Neurosci.* (2011) 12:495–508. doi: 10.1038/nrn3060
10. Wolff JA, Malone RW, Williams P, Chong W, Acsadi G, Jani A, et al. Direct gene transfer into mouse muscle *in vivo*. *Science.* (1990) 247(4949 Pt 1):1465–8.
11. Caffery B, Lee JS, Alexander-Bryant AA. Vectors for glioblastoma gene therapy: viral & non-viral delivery strategies. *Nanomaterials.* (2019) 9:E105. doi: 10.3390/nano9010105
12. Rosenecker J, Huth S, Rudolph C. Gene therapy for cystic fibrosis lung disease: current status and future perspectives. *Curr Opin Mol Ther.* (2006) 8:439–45.
13. Hacein-Bey-Abina S, Hauer J, Lim A, Picard C, Wang GP, Berry CC, et al. Efficacy of gene therapy for X-linked severe combined immunodeficiency. *N Engl J Med.* (2010) 363:355–64. doi: 10.1056/NEJMoa1000164
14. Sanders N, Rudolph C, Braeckmans K, De Smedt SC, Demeester J. Extracellular barriers in respiratory gene therapy. *Adv Drug Deliv Rev.* (2009) 61:115–27. doi: 10.1016/j.addr.2008.09.011
15. Leonhardt C, Schwake G, Stogbauer TR, Rappl S, Kuhr JT, Ligon TS, et al. Single-cell mRNA transfection studies: delivery, kinetics and statistics by numbers. *Nanomedicine.* (2013) 10:679–88. doi: 10.1016/j.nano.2013.11.008
16. Guo XR, Yang ZS, Tang XJ, Zou DD, Gui H, Wang XL, et al. The application of mRNA-based gene transfer in mesenchymal stem cell-mediated cytotoxicity of glioma cells. *Oncotarget.* (2016) 7:55529–42. doi: 10.18632/oncotarget.10835
17. Orlandini von Niessen AG, Poleganov MA, Rechner C, Plaschke A, Kranz LM, Fesser S, et al. Improving mRNA-based therapeutic gene delivery by expression-augmenting 3' UTRs identified by cellular library screening. *Mol Ther.* (2018) 27:824–36. doi: 10.1016/j.ymthe.2018.12.011
18. Stepinski J, Waddell C, Stolarski R, Darzynkiewicz E, Rhoads RE. Synthesis and properties of mRNAs containing the novel "anti-reverse" cap analogs 7-methyl(3'-O-methyl)GpppG and 7-methyl (3'-deoxy)GpppG. *RNA.* (2001) 7:1486–95.
19. Jemielity J, Stepinski J, Jaremko M, Haber D, Stolarski R, Rhoads RE, et al. Synthesis of novel mRNA 5' cap-analogues: dinucleoside P1, P3-tri-, P1, P4-

tetra-, and P1, P5-pentaphosphates. *Nucleosides Nucleotides Nucleic Acids.* (2003) 22:691–4. doi: 10.1081/NCN-120022611

20. Guo XR, Hu QY, Yuan YH, Tang XJ, Yang ZS, Zou DD, et al. PTEN-mRNA engineered mesenchymal stem cell-mediated cytotoxic effects on U251 glioma cells. *Oncol Lett.* (2016) 11:2733–40. doi: 10.3892/ol.2016.4297
21. Bangel-Ruland N, Tomczak K, Fernandez Fernandez E, Leier G, Leciejewski B, Rudolph C, et al. Cystic fibrosis transmembrane conductance regulator-mRNA delivery: a novel alternative for cystic fibrosis gene therapy. *J Gene Med.* (2013) 15:414–26. doi: 10.1002/jgm.2748
22. Vallazza B, Petri S, Poleganov MA, Eberle F, Kuhn AN, Sahin U. Recombinant messenger RNA technology and its application in cancer immunotherapy, transcript replacement therapies, pluripotent stem cell induction, and beyond. *Wiley Interdiscip Rev RNA.* (2015) 6:471–99. doi: 10.1002/wrna.1288
23. Tavernier G, Andries O, Demeester J, Sanders NN, De Smedt SC, Rejman J. mRNA as gene therapeutic: how to control protein expression. *J Control Release.* (2011) 150:238–47. doi: 10.1016/j.jconrel.2010.10.020
24. Meng Z, O'Keeffe-Ahern J, Lyu J, Pierucci L, Zhou D, Wang W. A new developing class of gene delivery: messenger RNA-based therapeutics. *Biomater Sci.* (2017) 5:2381–92. doi: 10.1039/c7bm00712d
25. Berraondo P, Martini PGV, Avila MA, Fontanellas A. Messenger RNA therapy for rare genetic metabolic diseases. *Gut.* (2019) 68:1323–30. doi: 10.1136/gutjnl-2019-318269
26. Li B, Zhang X, Dong Y. Nanoscale platforms for messenger RNA delivery. *Wiley Interdiscip Rev Nanomed Nanobiotechnol.* (2019) 11:e1530. doi: 10.1002/wnan.1530
27. Grudzien-Nogalska E, Kowalska J, Su W, Kuhn AN, Slepenkov SV, Darzynkiewicz E, et al. Synthetic mRNAs with superior translation and stability properties. *Methods Mol Biol.* (2013) 969:55–72. doi: 10.1007/978-1-62703-260-5_4
28. Rhoads RE. Synthetic mRNA: production, introduction into cells, and physiological consequences. *Methods Mol Biol.* (2016) 1428:3–27. doi: 10.1007/978-1-4939-3625-0_1
29. Topisirovic I, Svitkin YV, Sonenberg N, Shatkin AJ. Cap and cap-binding proteins in the control of gene expression. *Wiley Interdiscip Rev RNA.* (2011) 2:277–98. doi: 10.1002/wrna.52
30. Furuichi Y. Discovery of m(7)G-cap in eukaryotic mRNAs. *Proc Jpn Acad Ser B Phys Biol Sci.* (2015) 91:394–409. doi: 10.2183/pjab.91.394
31. Pasquinelli AE, Dahlberg JE, Lund E. Reverse 5' caps in RNAs made *in vitro* by phage RNA polymerases. *RNA.* (1995) 1:957–67.
32. Kocmik I, Piecyk K, Rudzinska M, Niedzwiecka A, Darzynkiewicz E, Grzela R, et al. Modified ARCA analogs providing enhanced translational properties of capped mRNAs. *Cell Cycle.* (2018) 17:1624–36. doi: 10.1080/15384101.2018.1486164
33. Jemielity J, Fowler T, Zuberek J, Stepinski J, Lewdorowicz M, Niedzwiecka A, et al. Novel "anti-reverse" cap analogs with superior translational properties. *RNA.* (2003) 9:1108–22. doi: 10.1261/rna.5430403
34. Grudzien-Nogalska E, Stepinski J, Jemielity J, Zuberek J, Stolarski R, Rhoads RE, et al. Synthesis of anti-reverse cap analogs (ARCAs) and their applications in mRNA translation and stability. *Methods Enzymol.* (2007) 431:203–27. doi: 10.1016/S0076-6879(07)31011-2
35. Wojtczak BA, Sikorski PJ, Fac-Dabrowska K, Nowicka A, Warminski M, Kubacka D, et al. 5'-Phosphorothiolate dinucleotide cap analogues: reagents for messenger RNA modification and potent small-molecular inhibitors of decapping enzymes. *J Am Chem Soc.* (2018) 140:5987–99. doi: 10.1021/jacs.8b02597
36. Guhaniyogi J, Brewer G. Regulation of mRNA stability in mammalian cells. *Gene.* (2001) 265:11–23. doi: 10.1016/s0378-1119(01)00350-x
37. Schwanhausser B, Busse D, Li N, Dittmar G, Schuchhardt J, Wolf J, et al. Global quantification of mammalian gene expression control. *Nature.* (2011) 473:337–42. doi: 10.1038/nature10098
38. Tanguay RL, Gallie DR. Translational efficiency is regulated by the length of the 3' untranslated region. *Mol Cell Biol.* (1996) 16:146–56.
39. Sergeeva OV, Koteliansky VE, Zatsepin TS. mRNA-based therapeutics - Advances and perspectives. *Biochemistry.* (2016) 81:709–22. doi: 10.1134/S0006297916070075
40. Pardi N, Tuyishime S, Muramatsu H, Kariko K, Mui BL, Tam YK, et al. Expression kinetics of nucleoside-modified mRNA delivered in lipid nanoparticles to mice by various routes. *J Control Release.* (2015) 217:345–51. doi: 10.1016/j.jconrel.2015.08.007
41. Garneau NL, Wilusz J, Wilusz CJ. The highways and byways of mRNA decay. *Nat Rev Mol Cell Biol.* (2007) 8:113–26. doi: 10.1038/nrm2104
42. Chen CY, Shyu AB. Mechanisms of deadenylation-dependent decay. *Wiley Interdiscip Rev RNA.* (2011) 2:167–83. doi: 10.1002/wrna.40
43. Kowalski PS, Rudra A, Miao L, Anderson DG. Delivering the messenger: advances in technologies for therapeutic mRNA delivery. *Mol Ther.* (2019) 27:710–28. doi: 10.1016/j.ymthe.2019.02.012
44. Kauffman KJ, Dorkin JR, Yang JH, Heartlein MW, DeRosa F, Mir FF, et al. Optimization of lipid nanoparticle formulations for mRNA delivery *in vivo* with fractional factorial and definitive screening designs. *Nano Lett.* (2015) 15:7300–6. doi: 10.1021/acs.nanolett.5b02497
45. Fenton OS, Kauffman KJ, McClellan RL, Appel EA, Dorkin JR, Tibbitt MW, et al. Bioinspired alkenyl amino alcohol ionizable lipid materials for highly potent *in vivo* mRNA delivery. *Adv Mater.* (2016) 28:2939–43. doi: 10.1002/adma.201505822
46. Harayama T, Riezman H. Understanding the diversity of membrane lipid composition. *Nat Rev Mol Cell Biol.* (2018) 19:281–96. doi: 10.1038/nrm.2017.138
47. Flewelling RF, Hubbell WL.The membrane dipole potential in a total membrane potential model. Applications to hydrophobic ion interactions with membranes. *Biophys J.* (1986) 49:541–52. doi: 10.1016/S0006-3495(86)83664-5
48. Van Tendeloo VF, Ponsaerts P, Lardon F, Nijs G, Lenjou M, Van Broeckhoven C, et al. Highly efficient gene delivery by mRNA electroporation in human hematopoietic cells: superiority to lipofection and passive pulsing of mRNA and to electroporation of plasmid cDNA for tumor antigen loading of dendritic cells. *Blood.* (2001) 98:49–56. doi: 10.1182/blood.v98.1.49
49. Zou S, Scarfo K, Nantz MH, Hecker JG. Lipid-mediated delivery of RNA is more efficient than delivery of DNA in non-dividing cells. *Int J Pharm.* (2010) 389:232–43. doi: 10.1016/j.ijpharm.2010.01.019
50. Diken M, Kreiter S, Selmi A, Britten CM, Huber C, Tureci O, et al. Selective uptake of naked vaccine RNA by dendritic cells is driven by macropinocytosis and abrogated upon DC maturation. *Gene Ther.* (2011) 18:702–8. doi: 10.1038/gt.2011.17
51. Probst J, Weide B, Scheel B, Pichler BJ, Hoerr I, Rammensee HG, et al. Spontaneous cellular uptake of exogenous messenger RNA *in vivo* is nucleic acid-specific, saturable and ion dependent. *Gene Ther.* (2007) 14:1175–80. doi: 10.1038/sj.gt.3302964
52. Kalady MF, Onaitis MW, Padilla KM, Emani S, Tyler DS, Pruitt SK. Enhanced dendritic cell antigen presentation in RNA-based immunotherapy. *J Surg Res.* (2002) 105:17–24. doi: 10.1006/jsre.2002.6435
53. Smits E, Ponsaerts P, Lenjou M, Nijs G, Van Bockstaele DR, Berneman ZN, et al. RNA-based gene transfer for adult stem cells and T cells. *Leukemia.* (2004) 18:1898–902. doi: 10.1038/sj.leu.2403463
54. Rabinovich PM, Komarovskaya ME, Wrzesinski SH, Alderman JL, Budak-Alpdogan T, Karpikov A, et al. Chimeric receptor mRNA transfection as a tool to generate antineoplastic lymphocytes. *Hum Gene Ther.* (2009) 20:51–61. doi: 10.1089/hum.2008.068
55. Choi Y, Yuen C, Maiti SN, Olivares S, Gibbons H, Huls H, et al. A high throughput microelectroporation device to introduce a chimeric antigen receptor to redirect the specificity of human T cells. *Biomed Microdevices.* (2010) 12:855–63. doi: 10.1007/s10544-010-9440-3
56. Li L, Liu LN, Feller S, Allen C, Shivakumar R, Fratantoni J, et al. Expression of chimeric antigen receptors in natural killer cells with a regulatory-compliant non-viral method. *Cancer Gene Ther.* (2010) 17:147–54. doi: 10.1038/cgt.2009.61
57. Wasungu L, Hoekstra D. Cationic lipids, lipoplexes and intracellular delivery of genes. *J Control Release.* (2006) 116:255–64. doi: 10.1016/j.jconrel.2006.06.024
58. Midoux P, Pichon C, Yaouanc JJ, Jaffres PA. Chemical vectors for gene delivery: a current review on polymers, peptides and lipids containing histidine or imidazole as nucleic acids carriers. *Br J Pharmacol.* (2009) 157:166–78. doi: 10.1111/j.1476-5381.2009.00288.x
59. Pichon C, Midoux P. Mannosylated and histidylated LPR technology for

vaccination with tumor antigen mRNA. *Methods Mol Biol.* (2013) 969:247–74. doi: 10.1007/978-1-62703-260-5_16
60. Su X, Fricke J, Kavanagh DG, Irvine DJ. *In vitro* and *in vivo* mRNA delivery using lipid-enveloped pH-responsive polymer nanoparticles. *Mol Pharm.* (2011) 8:774–87. doi: 10.1021/mp100390w
61. Zohra FT, Chowdhury EH, Nagaoka M, Akaike T. High performance mRNA transfection through carbonate apatite-cationic liposome conjugates. *Biomaterials.* (2009) 30:4006–13. doi: 10.1016/j.biomaterials.2009.02.050
62. Zohra FT, Chowdhury EH, Nagaoka M, Akaike T. Drastic effect of nanoapatite particles on liposome-mediated mRNA delivery to mammalian cells. *Anal Biochem.* (2005) 345:164–6. doi: 10.1016/j.ab.2005.06.031
63. Ardejani MS, Orner BP. Materials science. Obey the peptide assembly rules. *Science.* (2013) 340:561–2. doi: 10.1126/science.1237708
64. Lou B, De Koker S, Lau CYJ, Hennink WE, Mastrobattista E. mRNA polyplexes with post-conjugated GALA peptides efficiently target, transfect, and activate antigen presenting cells. *Bioconjug Chem.* (2019). 30:461–75. doi: 10.1021/acs.bioconjchem.8b00524
65. Lundstrom K. Alphaviruses in gene therapy. *Viruses.* (2009) 1:13–25. doi: 10.3390/v1010013
66. Galla M, Schambach A, Baum C. Retrovirus-based mRNA transfer for transient cell manipulation. *Methods Mol Biol.* (2013) 969:139–61. doi: 10.1007/978-1-62703-260-5_10
67. Munch RC, Muhlebach MD, Schaser T, Kneissl S, Jost C, Pluckthun A, et al. DARPins: an efficient targeting domain for lentiviral vectors. *Mol Ther.* (2011) 19:686–93. doi: 10.1038/mt.2010.298
68. Naldini L. *Ex vivo* gene transfer and correction for cell-based therapies. *Nat Rev Genet.* (2011) 12:301–15. doi: 10.1038/nrg2985
69. Bianco P. "Mesenchymal" stem cells. *Annu Rev Cell Dev Biol.* (2014) 30:677–704. doi: 10.1146/annurev-cellbio-100913-013132
70. Lesterhuis WJ, de Vries IJ, Schreibelt G, Lambeck AJ, Aarntzen EH, Jacobs JF, et al. Route of administration modulates the induction of dendritic cell vaccine-induced antigen-specific T cells in advanced melanoma patients. *Clin Cancer Res.* (2011) 17:5725–35. doi: 10.1158/1078-0432.CCR-11-1261
71. Geissmann F, Manz MG, Jung S, Sieweke MH, Merad M, Ley K. Development of monocytes, macrophages, and dendritic cells. *Science.* (2010) 327:656–61. doi: 10.1126/science.1178331
72. Carlsten M, Levy E, Karambelkar A, Li L, Reger R, Berg M, et al. Efficient mRNA-based genetic engineering of human NK cells with high-affinity CD16 and CCR7 augments rituximab-induced ADCC against lymphoma and targets NK cell migration toward the lymph node-associated chemokine CCL19. *Front Immunol.* (2016) 7:105. doi: 10.3389/fimmu.2016.00105
73. Palucka K, Banchereau J. Cancer immunotherapy via dendritic cells. *Nat Rev Cancer.* (2012) 12:265–77. doi: 10.1038/nrc3258
74. Shah NN, Fry TJ. Mechanisms of resistance to CAR T cell therapy. *Nat Rev Clin Oncol.* (2019) 16:372–85. doi: 10.1038/s41571-019-0184-6
75. Fornaguera C, Guerra-Rebollo M, Angel Lazaro M, Castells-Sala C, Meca-Cortes O, Ramos-Perez V, et al. mRNA delivery system for targeting antigen-presenting cells *in vivo*. *Adv Healthc Mater.* (2018) 7:e1800335. doi: 10.1002/adhm.201800335
76. Eggers R, Philippi A, Altmeyer MO, Breinig F, Schmitt MJ. Primary T cells for mRNA-mediated immunotoxin delivery. *Gene Ther.* (2018) 25:47–53. doi: 10.1038/gt.2017.87
77. Antony JS, Latifi N, Haque A, Lamsfus-Calle A, Daniel-Moreno A, Graeter S, et al. Gene correction of HBB mutations in CD34(+) hematopoietic stem cells using Cas9 mRNA and ssODN donors. *Mol Cell Pediatr.* (2018) 5:9. doi: 10.1186/s40348-018-0086-1
78. Hamann A, Nguyen A, Pannier AK. Nucleic acid delivery to mesenchymal stem cells: a review of nonviral methods and applications. *J Biol Eng.* (2019) 13:7. doi: 10.1186/s13036-019-0140-0
79. Toh WS, Lai RC, Zhang B, Lim SK. MSC exosome works through a protein-based mechanism of action. *Biochem Soc Trans.* (2018) 46:843–53. doi: 10.1042/BST20180079
80. Robbins PD, Morelli AE. Regulation of immune responses by extracellular vesicles. *Nat Rev Immunol.* (2014) 14:195–208. doi: 10.1038/nri3622
81. Blanchard N, Lankar D, Faure F, Regnault A, Dumont C, Raposo G, et al. TCR activation of human T cells induces the production of exosomes bearing the TCR/CD3/ζ complex. *J Immunol.* (2002) 168:3235–41. doi: 10.4049/jimmunol.168.7.3235
82. Kim HS, Choi DY, Yun SJ, Choi SM, Kang JW, Jung JW, et al. Proteomic analysis of microvesicles derived from human mesenchymal stem cells. *J Proteome Res.* (2012) 11:839–49. doi: 10.1021/pr200682z
83. Mittelbrunn M, Gutierrez-Vazquez C, Villarroya-Beltri C, Gonzalez S, Sanchez-Cabo F, Gonzalez MA, et al. Unidirectional transfer of microRNA-loaded exosomes from T cells to antigen-presenting cells. *Nat Commun.* (2011) 2:282. doi: 10.1038/ncomms1285
84. Alvarez-Erviti L, Seow Y, Yin H, Betts C, Lakhal S, Wood MJ. Delivery of siRNA to the mouse brain by systemic injection of targeted exosomes. *Nat Biotechnol.* (2011) 29:341–5. doi: 10.1038/nbt.1807
85. Kourembanas S. Exosomes: vehicles of intercellular signaling, biomarkers, and vectors of cell therapy. *Annu Rev Physiol.* (2015) 77:13–27. doi: 10.1146/annurev-physiol-021014-071641
86. Tang XJ, Sun XY, Huang KM, Zhang L, Yang ZS, Zou DD, et al. Therapeutic potential of CAR-T cell-derived exosomes: a cell-free modality for targeted cancer therapy. *Oncotarget.* (2015) 6:44179–90. doi: 10.18632/oncotarget.6175
87. El Andaloussi S, Lakhal S, Mager I, Wood MJ. Exosomes for targeted siRNA delivery across biological barriers. *Adv Drug Deliv Rev.* (2013) 65:391–7. doi: 10.1016/j.addr.2012.08.008
88. Wood MJ, O'Loughlin AJ, Samira L. Exosomes and the blood-brain barrier: implications for neurological diseases. *Ther Deliv.* (2011) 2:1095–9. doi: 10.4155/tde.11.83
89. Van Tendeloo VF, Ponsaerts P, Berneman ZN. mRNA-based gene transfer as a tool for gene and cell therapy. *Curr Opin Mol Ther.* (2007) 9:423–31.
90. Uzgun S, Nica G, Pfeifer C, Bosinco M, Michaelis K, Lutz JF, et al. PEGylation improves nanoparticle formation and transfection efficiency of messenger RNA. *Pharm Res.* (2011) 28:2223–32. doi: 10.1007/s11095-011-0464-z
91. Luo J, Guo XR, Tang XJ, Sun XY, Yang ZS, Zhang Y, et al. Intravital biobank and personalized cancer therapy: the correlation with omics. *Int J Cancer.* (2014) 135:1511–6. doi: 10.1002/ijc.28632
92. Tuveson D, Hanahan D. Translational medicine: cancer lessons from mice to humans. *Nature.* (2011) 471:316–7. doi: 10.1038/471316a
93. Xie C, Yang Z, Suo Y, Chen Q, Wei D, Weng X, et al. Systemically infused mesenchymal stem cells show different homing profiles in healthy and tumor mouse models. *Stem Cells Transl Med.* (2017) 6:1120–31. doi: 10.1002/sctm.16-0204
94. Moniri MR, Sun XY, Rayat J, Dai D, Ao Z, He Z, et al. TRAIL-engineered pancreas-derived mesenchymal stem cells: characterization and cytotoxic effects on pancreatic cancer cells. *Cancer Gene Ther.* (2012) 19:652–8. doi: 10.1038/cgt.2012.46
95. Conaty P, Sherman LS, Naaldijk Y, Ulrich H, Stolzing A, Rameshwar P. Methods of mesenchymal stem cell homing to the blood-brain barrier. *Methods Mol Biol.* (2018) 1842:81–91. doi: 10.1007/978-1-4939-8697-2_6
96. Brown NF, Carter TJ, Ottaviani D, Mulholland P. Harnessing the immune system in glioblastoma. *Br J Cancer.* (2018) 119:1171–81. doi: 10.1038/s41416-018-0258-8
97. Raucher D. Tumor targeting peptides: novel therapeutic strategies in glioblastoma. *Curr Opin Pharmacol.* (2019) 47:14–9. doi: 10.1016/j.coph.2019.01.006
98. Dai LJ, Moniri MR, Zeng ZR, Zhou JX, Rayat J, Warnock GL. Potential implications of mesenchymal stem cells in cancer therapy. *Cancer Lett.* (2011) 305:8–20. doi: 10.1016/j.canlet.2011.02.012
99. Zhang ZX, Guan LX, Zhang K, Zhang Q, Dai LJ. A combined procedure to deliver autologous mesenchymal stromal cells to patients with traumatic brain injury. *Cytotherapy.* (2008) 10:134–9. doi: 10.1080/14653240701883061
100. Alberer M, Gnad-Vogt U, Hong HS, Mehr KT, Backert L, Finak G, et al. Safety and immunogenicity of a mRNA rabies vaccine in healthy adults: an open-label, non-randomised, prospective, first-in-human phase 1 clinical trial. *Lancet.* (2017) 390:1511–20. doi: 10.1016/S0140-6736(17)31665-3
101. Sebastian M, Schroder A, Scheel B, Hong HS, Muth A, von Boehmer L, et al. A phase I/IIa study of the mRNA-based cancer immunotherapy CV9201 in patients with stage IIIB/IV non-small cell lung cancer. *Cancer Immunol Immunother.* (2019) 68:799–812. doi: 10.1007/s00262-019-02315-x
102. Sahin U, Kariko K, Tureci O. mRNA-based therapeutics–developing a new class of drugs. *Nat Rev Drug Discov.* (2014) 13:759–80. doi: 10.1038/nrd4278

103. Van Lint S, Renmans D, Broos K, Dewitte H, Lentacker I, Heirman C, et al. The ReNAissanCe of mRNA-based cancer therapy. *Expert Rev Vaccines.* (2015) 14:235–51. doi: 10.1586/14760584.2015.957685

104. Phua KK, Staats HF, Leong KW, Nair SK. Intranasal mRNA nanoparticle vaccination induces prophylactic and therapeutic anti-tumor immunity. *Sci Rep.* (2014) 4:5128. doi: 10.1038/srep05128

16

The Clinical Significance of Soluble Programmed Cell Death-Ligand 1 (sPD-L1) in Patients with Gliomas

Shujun Liu [1,2], Yadi Zhu [1,2], Chenxi Zhang [1,2], Xiangrui Meng [1,2], Bo Sun [3], Guojun Zhang [1,2], Yubo Fan [3] and Xixiong Kang [1,2,3]*

[1] Laboratory Diagnosis Center, Beijing Tiantan Hospital, Capital Medical University, Beijing, China, [2] Beijing Engineering Research Center of Immunological Reagents and Clinical Research, Beijing, China, [3] Beijing Advanced Innovation Center for Biomedical Engineering, Beihang University, Beijing, China

Correspondence:
Xixiong Kang
kangxxtt@sina.com

Background: Soluble PD-L1 (sPD-L1) in the circulation has been documented to activate global immunosuppression and is considered a predictor of negative clinical outcomes in several malignances. However, the clinical significance of sPD-L1 in the peripheral blood and cerebrospinal fluid (CSF) of patients with glioma remains unclear.

Objective: The aim of this study was to detect the correlations of sPD-L1 with clinical features in brain tumors and assess the diagnostic value of this protein in gliomas.

Methods: Serum samples were obtained from 73 patients with glioma, 20 patients with meningioma, and 49 healthy controls (HCs) in this study. In total, 31 CSF samples were collected from the matched glioma patients, and seven samples were collected from the matched meningioma patients. The expression of serum sPD-L1 in the glioma cohort was followed for 20 days after surgery to examine the kinetics in the circulation. Inflammatory markers were evaluated based on preoperative blood parameters. The sPD-L1 levels in the serum and CSF were determined by enzyme-linked immunosorbent assay (ELISA). The logistic regression model was used to assess the independent associations of sPD-L1 with gliomas, including high-grade gliomas.

Results: Serum and CSF levels of sPD-L1 were significantly elevated in patients with gliomas compared to those with meningiomas and HCs. Additionally, increased levels of sPD-L1 were observed in relatively advanced tumors. sPD-L1 overexpression in the CSF appears to be more representative of aggressive tumor features than overexpression in the serum. For glioma diagnosis, both serum and CSF sPD-L1 showed significant value in the diagnosis and stratification of glioma, and the best diagnostic performance was obtained with serum sPD-L1 rather than blood-based inflammatory markers. In addition, a descending trend in the level of serum sPD-L1 was observed in postoperative patients.

Conclusion: In gliomas, elevated circulating and CSF sPD-L1 levels are associated with aggressive biological activities. The results of the current study suggest that sPD-L1 is a promising biomarker for gliomas that can be used in clinical practice.

Keywords: glioma, soluble programmed cell death-ligand 1, biomarker, cerebrospinal fluid, inflammatory markers

INTRODUCTION

Gliomas, which account for the majority of central nervous system (CNS) tumors, are correlated with high rates of recurrence and mortality (1). However, molecular information such as the mutational status of isocitrate dehydrogenase (IDH) genes and the combined deletion of chromosome arms 1p and 19q (1p/19q codeletion) is integral to the 2016 World Health Organization (WHO) criteria for gliomas (2). Thus, these updates have shifted treatment approaches from histological type-based therapy to genotype-based therapy (3). Despite some advances in neurosurgical resection and treatment regimens, the prognosis of patients with high-grade gliomas remains dismal (4). The current methods for diagnosing and monitoring gliomas are seriously dependent on invasive procedures such as biopsy or surgery, which create challenges in the management of cancer patients (5). Accordingly, identifying a reliable liquid-based biomarker that can be measured quickly and safely is an attractive clinical approach.

For liquid-based biomarkers, several blood-based inflammatory markers, such as the neutrophil-to-lymphocyte ratio (NLR), derived NLR (dNLR), and platelet-to-lymphocyte ratio (PLR), have been highlighted for their pivotal roles in the stratification and prognosis of gliomas (6, 7). Likewise, hematological biomarkers used for indicating nutritional and immunological statuses, such as the prognostic nutrition index (PNI) and albumin-to-globulin ratio (AGR), have been identified as predictive markers in advanced brain tumors (8, 9). In contrast, other reports concluded that these markers were prone to various biases (10).

Recently, the discovery of immune checkpoint molecules, such as programmed death-1 (PD-1) protein and its ligand, namely, programmed death-ligand 1 (PD-L1), has provided novel therapeutic targets. Considering the lack of effective treatments for gliomas, immunotherapy, especially anti-PD-1/PD-L1 antibodies, has brought hope for brain malignances (11, 12). In fact, PD-L1 expression on the surface of tumor cells, one of the potential indicators for checkpoint inhibitor use (13), was found to be detectable in a portion of glioma patients (14, 15). However, ample tumor tissue is still required for assessing PD-L1 expression in tumor cells and the tumor microenvironment (16). Appealingly, PD-L1 is expressed not only on the surface of cells but also in a soluble form in the circulation, which is thought to be released from PD-L1-positive cells (17).

Similar to membrane-binding PD-L1, soluble PD-L1 (sPD-L1) is currently thought to contribute to systemic immunosuppression (18, 19). Recently, a few published reports have shown that sPD-L1 is an indispensable predictor in various types of cancer (20–22), especially for checkpoint blockade treatments (23, 24). In addition, some studies have referred to circulating sPD-L1 as a surrogate marker for tumor PD-L1 expression (25). Given that both sPD-L1 and the previously mentioned blood markers have been regarded as indicators of the host immune state (21), we were interested in determining the associations between sPD-L1 measurements and peripheral blood markers in gliomas.

It is worth mentioning that our previous study showed that sPD-L1 in the peripheral blood was a potential predictor for the diagnosis and prognosis of preoperative patients with glioma. Nevertheless, blood is one of the easiest biofluids to obtain, but it is not the optimal fluid for collecting precise biomarkers derived from brain tumors due to the isolation established by the blood-brain barrier (BBB) (26). Instead, the cerebrospinal fluid (CSF) directly contacts the interstitial fluid in the CNS; thus, the CSF is considered to be the optimal source of markers for CNS tumors (27). It is still unclear whether the circulating sPD-L1 level can reflect the expression level in the CSF because insufficient findings on central and peripheral sPD-L1 measurements in gliomas have been reported.

As such, in this study, we aimed to elucidate these issues through the following clinical evaluations: (a) exploring the relationships of serum sPD-L1 with blood-based inflammatory markers; (b) detecting the concentration of sPD-L1 in the CSF and illustrating the relationship between sPD-L1 measurements in the serum and CSF; (c) determining the correlations of sPD-L1 levels with glioma classification, histological characteristics and molecular features; and (d) evaluating the predictive significance of sPD-L1 in gliomas. This report may provide new clues for developing and validating reliable and minimally invasive biomarkers for CNS tumors in future clinical practices.

METHODS

The study protocol was approved by the ethics committee of Beijing Tiantan Hospital.

Study Subjects

Patients with brain tumors who underwent magnetic resonance imaging (MRI) between January and April 2019 were consecutively followed. In total, 73 patients with histologically confirmed glioma were included in this study. Furthermore, 20 patients with meningioma were sex-matched with the glioma patients and enrolled in this study. All patients underwent maximal safe surgical resection and were diagnosed histologically based on the recent WHO classification guidelines. Molecular markers of glioma, such as the IDH1 genotype (IDH1 mutant or wild type), Ki-67 expression status and 1p/19q status (1p/19q codeleted or maintained), were recorded when possible. Immunohistochemistry (IHC) and direct gene sequencing were conducted by pathologists according to routine methods at Beijing Tiantan Hospital (28, 29). The histopathological examination results were verified independently by at least two pathology experts. Other clinical data were extracted from medical records. Corticosteroids such as dexamethasone and methylprednisolone were administered to patients to decrease tumor-associated edema.

Forty-three healthy volunteers, who were matched with the selected glioma patients in terms of sex and age, were included in the healthy control (HC) group.

Blood Sampling

Peripheral blood samples were obtained upon admission to the hospital before surgery, and clinical parameters [white blood cells (WBCs), neutrophil, lymphocyte, monocyte, and platelet counts, serum albumin and globulin levels] were part of the standard workup at the Laboratory Diagnosis Center of Beijing Tiantan Hospital. In addition, the preoperative NLR (ratio of the neutrophil count to the lymphocyte count), dNLR [ratio of (the WBC count—the neutrophil count) to the lymphocyte count], PLR (ratio of the platelet count to the lymphocyte count), AGR (ratio of the albumin level to the globulin level), and PNI [the albumin level (g/L) + the total lymphocyte count × 5] were calculated.

To assess the temporal dynamics of serum sPD-L1 in glioma patients, we performed monitoring every 3 days postoperatively. Collectively, we obtained postoperative samples as follows: 44 samples at 48 h, 34 samples on day 5, 27 samples on day 8, 9 samples on day 11, 5 samples on day 14 and 4 samples on day 20.

Serum was obtained from each subject during routine venipuncture. To remove blood cells, the serum tubes were centrifuged at 2,500×g for 10 min at room temperature. The separated serum samples were immediately stored at −80°C until analysis. Repeated cycles of freezing and thawing of the samples were avoided.

CSF Sampling

Thirty-one matched CSF samples from the glioma cohort and seven from the meningioma cohort were collected via lumbar puncture on days 3–6 after resection. The initial 2 mL of CSF was used for protein level measurements and cytology examination. CSF supernatants were transferred to cryotubes and stored at −80°C.

Measurement of sPD-L1

Both serum and CSF sPD-L1 were examined using a specific enzyme-linked immunosorbent assay (ELISA; PDCD1LG1 ELISA kit, USCN Life Science, Wuhan, China) according to the manufacturer's instructions. In brief, samples to be tested were added to the wells of microtiter plates and incubated for 1 h. Then, the biotinylated antibody was incubated for 1 h, followed by incubation with the avidin-peroxidase conjugate for 30 min. Finally, the substrate TMB was incubated for 15 min, after which the reaction was terminated using H_2SO_4. The OD was measured at 450 nm. All steps were run at 37°C. Each sample was tested in duplicate. The detection limit of the ELISA kit was 0.056 ng/mL.

Statistical Analysis

Continuous variables are presented as the means ± standard deviation (SD) or medians and the minimum-maximum range. Comparisons among different cohorts were performed using analysis of variance (ANOVA) with the Kruskal-Wallis test for nonnormally distributed variables (The *post-hoc* Bonferroni test was used for multiple comparisons). The differences between the two groups were calculated using the *t*-test or Mann-Whitney *U*-test according to the normality of the data. Categorical variables were analyzed and compared between two groups using the chi-squared test or Fisher's exact test. The association of the sPD-L1 with glioma and glioma grade was analyzed using multivariate logistic regression. For Pearson's correlation analysis, sPD-L1 data were log 10 transformed to obtain a more symmetric data distribution. For rank correlation analysis, Spearman's correlation coefficient (rho) was used. A receiver operating characteristic (ROC) curve was generated for each marker. The areas under the curves (AUCs) were assessed to evaluate the performance of each marker for predicting gliomas and distinguishing high- and low-grade gliomas. The dynamics of sPD-L1 in the serum were analyzed by the mixed-model approach. Statistical analysis was performed using SPSS (version 24.0, IBM, New York, USA) or GraphPad Prism 8 software (GraphPad Software Inc., San Diego, CA, USA).

RESULTS

Study Subjects

Seventy-three patients with glioma and 20 patients with meningioma were prospectively recruited. In addition, 49 healthy volunteers were included as the control (HC) group. The clinical and demographic features and hematological parameters of the study subjects are listed in **Table 1**.

The circulatory sPD-L1 protein levels exhibited the highest concentrations in the glioma cohort (median: 0.5594 ng/mL, range: 0–1.4235 ng/mL) compared with that in the meningioma (0.0688, 0.0454–1.4117; $p < 0.001$) and HC cohorts (0.1107, 0–0.5908; $p < 0.001$) (**Table 1** and **Figure 1A**).

As shown in **Table 1** and **Table S1**, patient age was higher in the meningioma cohort than in the glioma ($p = 0.001$) and HC cohorts ($p < 0.001$). However, when the correlation of serum PD-L1 levels with age was analyzed according to the different cohorts, we did not find any significant differences (**Table 2**).

Relationship of Serum sPD-L1 to Inflammatory Markers

First, we assessed the differences in peripheral blood markers among the study cohorts. Generally, **Table 1** indicates that significant differences were present for WBCs, neutrophils, monocytes, platelets, albumin, the NLR and the PNI.

By performing a *post-hoc* test, we observed significantly higher levels of WBCs, neutrophils, monocytes, and the NLR in the glioma patients than in the HCs (**Table S1**). Additionally, decreased levels of albumin and the PNI were present in the glioma group compare with that in HCs, although the differences did not reach significance. The levels of monocytes and platelets were increased in the glioma patients compared with meningioma patients (**Table S1**). Nevertheless, no significant differences were observed for lymphocytes, the dNLR, PLR, or the AGR (**Table 1**).

When the contributions to serum sPD-L1 levels were further assessed, the inflammatory markers failed to yield any significant associations with serum sPD-L1 in the glioma and meningioma cohorts. Notably, the monocyte count was found to be significantly associated with the sPD-L1 level in the peripheral blood, although the degree was weak ($r = 0.299$, $p = 0.037$) (**Table 2**).

To determine the association of sPD-L1 with glioma, the parameters that were notably different among the cohorts were further included into a multivariate logistic regression model. As indicated in **Table S2**, a significantly independent

TABLE 1 | Baseline epidemiological and hematological markers of study populations.

	Glioma	Meningioma	HC	*p*
n	73	20	49	
Age (years)	39.88 ± 16.66[§]	53.30 ± 15.73[#]	36.82 ± 10.78	<0.001*
Sex				
Male	46 (63.01%)	15 (75%)	31 (63.27%)	0.587
Female	27 (36.99%)	5 (25%)	18 (36.73%)	
sPD-L1 (ng/mL)	0.5594 (0–1.4235)	0.0688 (0.0454–1.4117)	0.1107 (0–0.5908)	<0.001*
Hematological markers				
WBC (10^9/L)	6.69 ± 1.76[#]	6.17 ± 1.67	5.51 ± 1.45	0.001*
Neutrophils (10^9/L)	4.25 ± 1.47[#]	4.08 ± 1.55[#]	3.17 ± 1.02	<0.001*
Lymphocytes (10^9/L)	1.92 ± 0.78	1.63 ± 0.59	1.84 ± 0.49	0.234
Monocytes (10^9/L)	0.38 ± 0.13[§#]	0.32 ± 0.08	0.31 ± 0.09	0.003*
Platelets (10^9/L)	242.49 ± 62.23[§]	198.80 ± 55.84	222.75 ± 49.97	0.011*
Albumin (g/L)	45.32 ± 3.03[§]	42.78 ± 5.31[#]	45.92 ± 2.36	0.019*
NLR	2.50 ± 1.22[#]	2.93 ± 1.71[#]	1.78 ± 0.55	<0.001*
dNLR	1.28 ± 0.11	1.31 ± 0.11	1.27 ± 0.15	0.688
PLR	141.93 ± 63.11	138.58 ± 66.56	131.96 ± 47.43	0.656
PNI	54.93 ± 5.02[§]	50.94 ± 6.90[#]	55.12 ± 3.49	0.027*
AGR	1.70 ± 0.25	1.61 ± 0.23	1.70 ± 0.23	0.278
Tumor characteristics				
Size (cm^3)	80.00 (1.20–439.28)	43.57 (3.75–741.66)	Na	0.055
Ki-67 (%)	10.0 (1.0–80.0)	5.5 (1.0–30.0)	Na	0.018*
WHO grade				
I–II	39 (53.43%)	19 (95%)	Na	<0.001*
III–IV	34 (46.57%)	1 (5%)	Na	
Steroid therapy[a]				
no	6 (8.2%)	2 (10%)	Na	0.258
≤3 days	16 (21.9%)	4 (20%)	Na	
3–7 days	33 (45.2%)	5 (25%)	Na	
≥7 days	18 (24.7%)	9 (45%)	Na	

Data are shown as the means ± SD, medians (range) or number (%).
An asterisk (*) indicates a significant difference.
[#]$P < 0.05$ vs. HC.
[§]$P < 0.05$ vs. meningioma.
[a]At a dose of 10 mg dexamethasone or 40 mg methylprednisolone per day.
WBC, white blood cell count; NLR, neutrophil-to-lymphocyte ratio; dNLR, derived NLR; PLR, platelet-to-lymphocyte ratio; PNI, prognostic nutritional index; AGR, albumin-to-globulin ratio; Na, not applicable.

correlation was identified between sPD-L1 and glioma (OR: 1.085, $p < 0.001$). Nevertheless, the other variables (age, WBC, neutrophils, monocytes, platelets, albumin, NLR, and PNI) were not significantly associated with glioma (**Table S2**).

Relationship of Serum sPD-L1 With Brain Tumor Features

As shown in **Table 1**, the median Ki-67 expression was discernably higher in the glioma cohorts (median: 10.0%, range: 1.0–80.0%) than in the meningioma cohorts (median: 5.5%, range: 1.0–30.0%; $p = 0.018$). Low-grade tumors were more frequently observed in the meningioma cohort vs. the glioma cohort ($p < 0.001$). However, the tumor size was not significantly different (**Table 1**).

Subsequently, we observed a positive relationship between Ki-67 and sPD-L1 in the glioma patients ($r = 0.246$, $p = 0.036$), and Spearman's rank correlation was markedly positive between the WHO grade and sPD-L1 level ($r = 0.387$, $p = 0.001$). In contrast, neither the Ki-67 index nor the WHO grade was significantly associated with serum sPD-L1 levels in meningioma (**Table 2**).

Association of Serum sPD-L1 With Glioma Grade

According to the WHO criteria (30), grade I–II gliomas were referred to as low-grade gliomas (LGGs), and grade III–IV gliomas were referred to as high-grade gliomas (HGGs). In our cohort, 39 patients were diagnosed with LGG, and 34 were diagnosed with HGG.

In the comparison between LGG and HGG patients, both the Ki-67 index and serum sPD-L1 levels were elevated in HGG patients vs. LGG patients ($p < 0.001$ and $p = 0.006$, respectively). Moreover, the age at the time of diagnosis was younger in LGG patients ($p = 0.004$, **Table 3**). Regarding the hematological parameters, the levels of neutrophils, monocytes, NLR, dNLR, and PLR were markedly upregulated in HGG patients, whereas notably increased levels of lymphocytes, PNI and AGR were present in LGG patients (**Table 3**).

However, similar to the results shown above, we did not find any significant correlations between blood-based markers and serum sPD-L1 with respect to the glioma grade (**Table S3**).

Next, the predictive value of these variables in high-grade glioma was assessed using a multivariate stepwise logistic regression analysis. The analysis revealed that sPD-L1 (OR: 1.030, $p = 0.013$) and NLR (OR: 2.850, $p = 0.001$) were independent factors for the prediction of HGGs, while the other parameters (age, neutrophils, lymphocytes, monocytes, dNLR, PLR, PNI, and AGR) were not independent predictors (**Table S4**).

Collectively, these results suggest that the occurrence of aggressive neoplasms in the brain may explain the elevated sPD-L1 levels in the serum.

Dynamics of sPD-L1 in the Serum of Glioma Patients

After 20 days of post-surgery surveillance, a decline in the sPD-L1 level was noted during the postoperative period. Notably, the level of sPD-L1 was dramatically decreased on the 5th day after resection. In addition, the lowest level was observed on the 14th day after surgery (**Figure 2A**).

In total, 67 glioma patients received concomitant antiedematous therapy during the perioperative period (**Table 1**). However, as depicted in **Figure 2B**, the sPD-L1 levels remained decreased after surgery in the six patients who did not receive steroid treatment (yellow curve in **Figure 2B**). A similar phenomenon was observed in other patients who were administered steroids for different periods of time (**Figure 2B**).

CSF sPD-L1 in Brain Tumor Patients

To complete the analysis of sPD-L1 in brain tumor patients, we further evaluated sPD-L1 expression in the CSF. Globally,

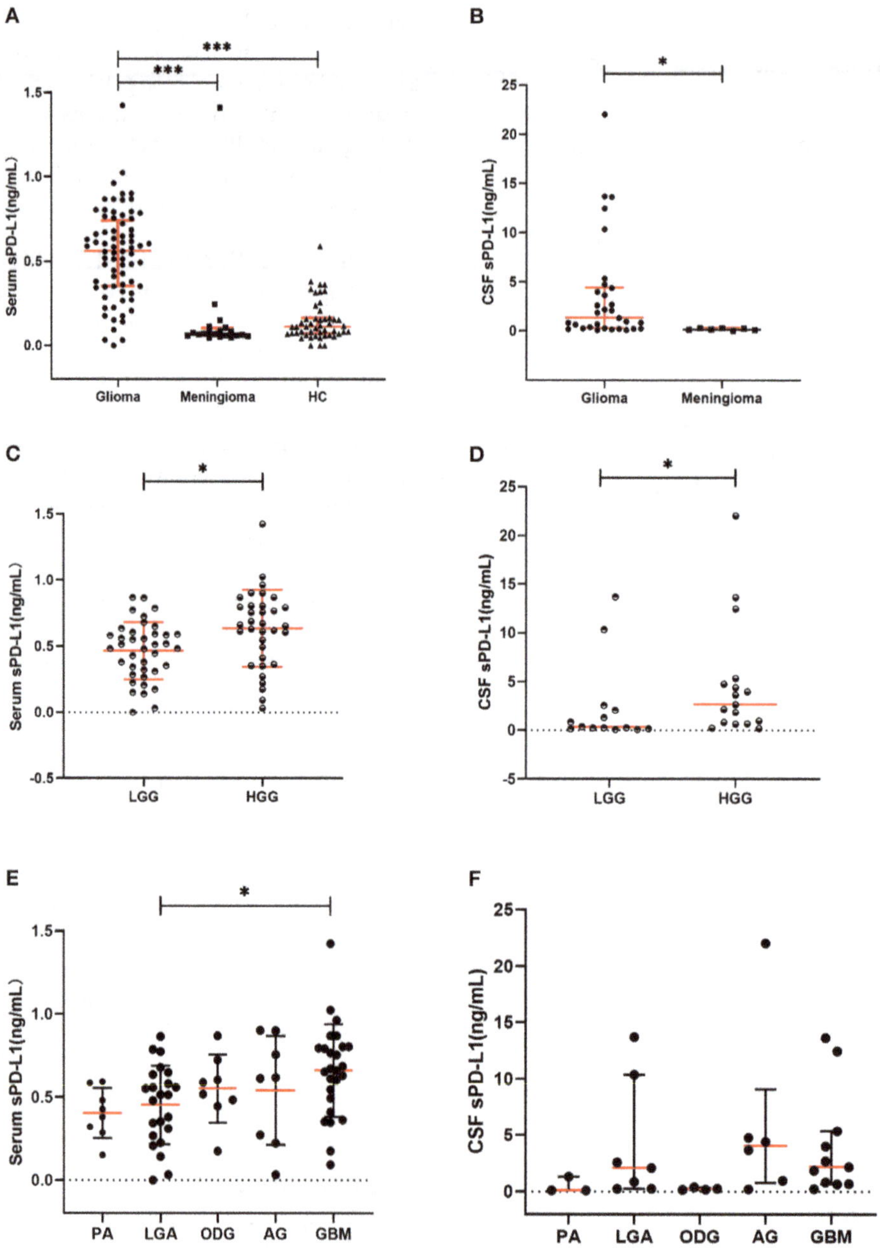

FIGURE 1 | Soluble PD-L1 measurements in study subjects. **(A)** sPD-L1 overexpression in the serum of patients with glioma compared with that of meningioma patients and HCs. **(B)** sPD-L1 levels in the CSF of patients with glioma or meningioma. **(C)** sPD-L1 measurements in the serum of patients with high- or low-grade glioma. **(D)** sPD-L1 measurements in the CSF of patients with high- or low-grade glioma. **(E)** sPD-L1 measurements in the serum of patients with different pathological types of glioma. **(F)** sPD-L1 measurements in the CSF of patients with different pathological types of glioma. For simplicity, only significant differences are shown. The red horizontal lines within the data signify the medians. Statistical significance was defined as $^{*}p < 0.05$ or $^{***}p < 0.001$.

38 matched CSF samples including 31 from glioma patients and seven from meningioma patients were obtained from brain tumor patients after resection. The characteristics of the CSF samples are shown in **Table 4**.

Increased levels of sPD-L1 were found in the CSF of glioma patients (1.3202 ng/mL, 0.0925–22.0392 ng/mL; $p = 0.003$) compared with that of meningioma patients (0.1538 ng/mL, 0.0475–0.3157 ng/mL) (**Table 4** and **Figure 1B**).

As shown in **Table 4**, a difference in the WBC count was observable between the glioma and meningioma CSF samples. In addition, PD-L1 expression appeared to be notably associated with the WBC count in the glioma CSF samples ($r = 0.577$, $p = 0.001$), but this relationship was not significant in the meningioma CSF samples ($r = 0.162, p > 0.05$).

Similar to the findings in the serum, elevated levels of sPD-L1 were observed in the CSF of patients with more advanced grade

TABLE 2 | Correlations between varied features and serum sPD-L1 concentrations in different cohorts.

	Glioma		Meningioma		HC	
	Correlation	*p*	Correlation	*p*	Correlation	*p*
Age	0.217	0.066	0.083	0.727	0.271	0.060
WBC	0.010	0.930	−0.180	0.448	0.086	0.555
NEU	0.050	0.675	−0.196	0.409	0.064	0.664
MONO	0.188	0.111	−0.365	0.114	0.299	0.037*
ALB	−0.055	0.647	−0.172	0.468	−0.192	0.186
PLT	−0.058	0.628	0.128	0.592	0.006	0.965
NLR	0.093	0.432	−0.294	0.208	0.039	0.793
PNI	−0.105	0.376	−0.025	0.917	−0.135	0.354
Ki-67	0.246	0.036*	−0.035	0.884	Na	Na
WHO grade	0.387	0.001*	−0.017	0.942	Na	Na

The relationships were assessed by Pearson's or Spearman's rank correlation.
An asterisk (*) indicates a significant difference.
WBC, white blood cell count; NEU, neutrophils; MONO, monocytes; ALB, albumin; PLT, platelets; NLR, neutrophil-to-lymphocyte ratio; PNI, prognostic nutritional index; Na, not applicable.

gliomas ($p = 0.029$) (**Table S5** and **Figure 1D**). Nevertheless, the other CSF parameters failed to show any significant variations between LGG patients and HGG patients (**Table S5**).

TABLE 3 | Demographic and hematological parameters between low-grade gliomas and high-grade gliomas.

	LGGs	HGGs	*P*
n	39	34	
Age (year)	34.72 ± 16.66	45.79 ± 14.78	0.004*
Sex (M/F)	26/13	20/14	0.489
Tumor size (cm^3)	76.95 (1.20–270.0)	98.00 (18.02–439.28)	0.075
Ki-67 (%)	5.0 (1.0–15.0)	35.0 (10.0–80.0)	<0.001*
sPD-L1 (ng/mL)	0.4623 ± 0.2166	0.6316 ± 0.2899	0.006*
Hematological markers			
WBC (10^9/L)	6.34 ± 1.57	7.09 ± 1.9	0.070
Neutrophils (10^9/L)	3.76 ± 1.2	4.81 ± 1.58	0.002*
Lymphocytes (10^9/L)	2.09 ± 0.87	1.73 ± 0.6	0.046*
Monocytes (10^9/L)	0.35 ± 0.11	0.42 ± 0.15	0.015*
Platelets (10^9/L)	233.44 ± 63.17	252.88 ± 60.4	0.185
Albumin (g/L)	45.95 ± 3.12	44.62 ± 2.82	0.062
NLR	2.00 ± 0.79	3.09 ± 1.37	<0.001*
dNLR	1.24 ± 0.08	1.33 ± 0.12	<0.001*
PLR	122.39 ± 46.45	164.34 ± 72.37	0.005*
PNI	56.39 ± 5.48	53.26 ± 3.89	0.007*
AGR	1.77 ± 0.24	1.63 ± 0.24	0.012*

An asterisk (*) indicates a significant difference.
NLR, neutrophil-to-lymphocyte ratio; dNLR, derived NLR; PLR, platelet-to-lymphocyte ratio; PNI, prognostic nutritional index; AGR, albumin-to-globulin ratio.

Association Between Serum and CSF PD-L1 Expression

The glioma cohort consisted of patients with different histopathological types of disease, including pilocytic astrocytoma (PA), low-grade astrocytoma (LAG), oligodendroglioma (ODG), anaplastic glioma (AG), and glioblastoma (GBM). The sPD-L1 levels in the serum and CSF for each disease type are shown in **Table 5**.

Associations of sPD-L1 Levels With Disease Features in Glioma

The differences among different pathological types were notable when serum sPD-L1 was used as a marker ($p = 0.036$). As indicated in **Figure 1E**, the serum sPD-L1 concentration was markedly higher in GBM than in LGA ($p = 0.043$). Similar to the PD-L1 expression pattern in the serum, the CSF PD-L1 level differed according to histological type ($p = 0.032$), but no significant differences were found between any two types (**Figure 1F**).

When the sPD-L1 level difference was analyzed according to tumor size, the difference in CSF sPD-L1 was significant, but the difference in serum sPD-L1 was not, suggesting that the effect of tumor size on CSF PD-L1 measurements was stronger than that on serum sPD-L1 measurements. In addition, samples with high Ki-67 expression had significantly higher sPD-L1 levels in both the serum and CSF than samples with low Ki-67 expression.

Overall, a higher sPD-L1 level might reflect more aggressive histopathological features in glioma.

Associations of sPD-L1 Levels With Molecular Characteristics

As shown in **Table 5**, we did not find any differences in serum sPD-L1 related to the IDH1 genotype or 1p/19q status. Next, we explored the associations between molecular subtypes and CSF sPD-L1. The glioma patients with mutated IDH-1 ($p = 0.042$) or 1p/19q codeletion ($p = 0.017$) were found to have relatively low levels of CSF sPD-L1.

Correlation Between Serum and CSF Measurements

Thirty-one glioma patients had both their serum and CSF sPD-L1 levels measured. As indicated in **Figure 3A**, the median CSF sPD-L1 concentration was 1.32 (0.09–22.04) ng/mL, which was significantly higher than the level in the serum (0.56 ng/mL, 0–1.42 ng/mL; $p = 0.002$).

The level in the serum appeared to positively correlate with the level in the CSF of the glioma patients ($r = 0.428$, $p = 0.016$, **Figure 3B**).

Evaluation of the Diagnostic Efficacy of Inflammatory Markers and sPD-L1 in Gliomas

As indicated in **Table 6**, AUCs generated by ROC analysis showed the diagnostic efficacy of different inflammatory markers in glioma patients. When blood-based biomarkers in glioma patients were compared with the corresponding markers in healthy volunteers and meningioma patients, we observed that serum sPD-L1 had the best value for the diagnosis of glioma [0.906 (0.850–0.962), **Figure 4A**]. In addition, the efficacy of CSF

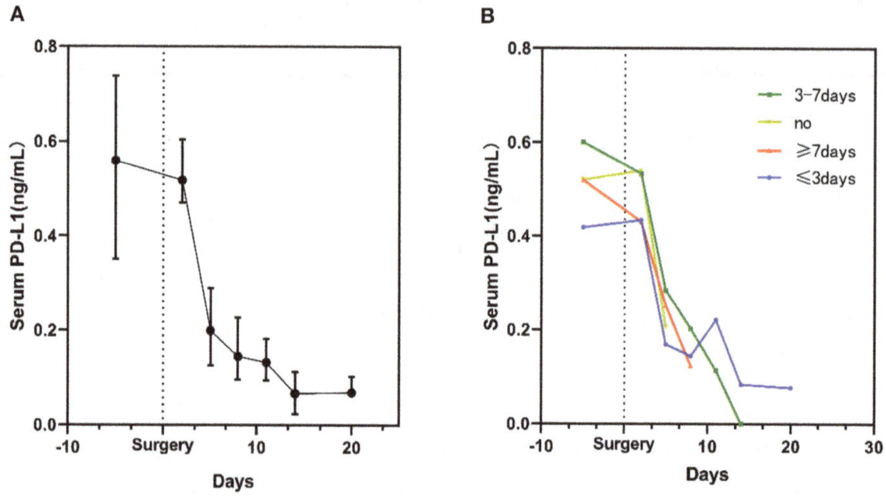

FIGURE 2 | Kinetic changes in serum sPD-L1 levels in glioma patients during the perioperative period. **(A)** Kinetic changes in all glioma patients. Dots display the medians, and whiskers represent the interquartile ranges. **(B)** Serum sPD-L1 levels in patients stratified by the time of exposure to steroids. The plots display the medians.

TABLE 4 | CSF features of brain tumors after resection.

	Glioma	Meningioma	*p*
N	31	7	–
CSF sPD-L1 (ng/mL)	1.3202 (0.0925–22.0392)	0.1538 (0.0475–0.3157)	0.004*
Characteristics			
Protein (mg/dL)	106.10 (25.40–3,213.00)	81.00 (28.30–134.20)	0.179
Nucleated cells (cells/mm^3)	5,266 (42–156,468)	6,747 (2–39,158)	0.658
WBC (cells/mm^3)	847 (7–10,376)	58 (2–3,311)	0.049*
PMN (cells/mm^3)	82.0 (0–96.4)	51.7 (0–90.6)	0.125
MN (cells/mm^3)	16.6 (0–80.5)	14.9 (0–48.7)	0.632

An asterisk (*) indicates a significant difference.
PMN, polymorphonuclear cells; MN, mononuclear cells; WBC, white blood cells.

sPD-L1 was demonstrated to be significant in distinguishing glioma from meningioma (**Figure 4A**).

Similarly, we investigated the diagnostic value of each marker for predicting HGG. As shown in **Table 6** and **Figure 4B**, both serum sPD-L1 and CSF sPD-L1 showed notable predictive value for HGG. Furthermore, a higher accuracy in distinguishing HGG from LGG was achieved with CSF sPD-L1 levels than with serum sPD-L1 levels [0.731 (0.545–0.917) vs. 0.702 (0.577–0.827), respectively, **Figure 4B**].

DISCUSSION

At present, the difficulties associated with performing biopsies hamper glioma diagnosis and therapeutic intervention, highlighting the need to discover non-invasive or minimally invasive biomarkers for early diagnosis and correct stratification (31). sPD-L1 can be detected in biofluids, providing a novel diagnostic test for a variety of tumors (32–34). In our previous study, elevated sPD-L1 levels in the serum were observed in preoperative patients with HGG. In this study, we endeavored to collect laboratory parameters and tumor characteristics to investigate the clinical significance of sPD-L1 in gliomas. Thus, we recruited patients with benign tumors as controls to test the potential role of sPD-L1 in malignant brain tumors.

Consistent with our previous results, overexpression of circulating sPD-L1 occurred in glioma patients (median: 0.5594 ng/mL, range: 0–1.4235 ng/mL), while the concentrations were notably lower in HCs (0.1107, 0–0.5908, $p < 0.001$) and meningioma patients (0.0688, 0.0454–1.4117, $p < 0.001$) (**Figure 1A**). Likewise, the enhanced level of serum sPD-L1 was reproducibly present in HGG (**Table 3**).

It has been documented that inflammation is involved in the pathogenesis and promotion of cancer (35). Therefore, blood components, such as WBCs, neutrophils, lymphocytes, monocytes, platelets and albumin, have been widely used for detecting the host inflammatory response in cancers (6, 36). Furthermore, inflammation-based scores derived from the abovementioned parameters, such as the NLR, PLR, dNLR, AGR, and PNI, have been demonstrated to be positively associated with glioma grade and negative outcomes (7–9, 37). Notably, these peripheral blood biomarkers have been recently adopted for predicting the outcomes of patients treated with checkpoint inhibitors (38–40). In addition, accumulating findings indicate that an elevated sPD-L1 level is a kind of sign of systematic inflammation provoked by neoplasms (21, 41). Given this aspect, we first investigated whether there are associations between serum sPD-L1 and inflammatory markers in preoperative gliomas. In agreement with the above results, we observed increased levels of WBCs, neutrophils, monocytes and the NLR in glioma patients, and relatively low levels of albumin and

TABLE 5 | Serum and CSF sPD-L1 levels in gliomas stratified by disease features.

	Serum			CSF		
	n	sPD-L1	*p*	*n*	sPD-L1	*p*
	73	0.5594 (0–1.4235)	–	31	1.3202 (0.0925–22.0392)	–
WHO grade						
LGG	39	0.4623 ± 0.2166	0.006*	14	0.325 (0.093–13.701)	0.029*
HGG	34	0.6316 ± 0.2899		17	2.676 (0.199–22.039)	
Pathology						
PA	8	0.4029 ± 0.1512	0.036*	3	0.099 (0.092–1.32)	0.032*
LGA	23	0.4521 ± 0.2370		7	1.470 (0.14–13.701)	
AG	8	0.5393 ± 0.3273		6	4.034 (0.20–22.04)	
ODG	8	0.5509 ± 0.2047		4	0.259 (0.18–0.39)	
GBM	26	0.6600 ± 0.2782		11	2.171 (0.23–13.63)	
Tumor size						
≤80 cm^3[a]	37	0.5710 ± 0.2448	0.333	14	0.454 (0.092–13.634)	0.010*
>80 cm^3	36	0.5104 ± 0.2855		17	2.581 (0.199–22.039)	
Ki-67						
≤10%[a]	37	0.4618 ± 0.2263	0.009*	14	0.325 (0.093–13.701)	0.029*
>10%	36	0.6227 ± 0.2809		17	2.676 (0.199–22.039)	
IDH-1 type						
Mutant	37	0.5509 ± 0.2973	0.595	18	0.823 (0.18–22.039)	0.042*
Wild type	22	0.5918 ± 0.2595		8	3.172 (0.15–10.36)	
1p19q status						
Codeleted	12	0.5349 ± 0.2341	0.672	7	0.259 (0.14–4.77)	0.017*
Maintained	47	0.5740 ± 0.2949		19	2.676 (0.23–22.039)	

An asterisk (*) indicates a significant difference.
[a] The median value in the glioma cohort.
PA, pilocytic astrocytoma; LGA, low-grade astrocytoma; ODG, oligodendroglioma; AG, anaplastic glioma; GBM, glioblastoma; IDH, isocitrate dehydrogenase.

the PNI were also expressed in the glioma patients (**Table 1**). In addition, the inflammation scores such as NLR, dNLR, and PLR were markedly upregulated in high-grade gliomas, which were consistent with the results of previous studies (6, 42, 43). Regardless, the serum sPD-L1 levels failed to yield any significant associations with systemic inflammatory markers in the glioma patients (**Tables 2, 3**).

The multivariate analysis revealed that sPD-L1 is independently associated with glioma after adjusting for age and the mentioned hematological markers (**Table S2**). For glioma diagnosis, the AUC obtained from the ROC curve was 0.906 (0.850–0.962) for serum sPD-L1, which was higher than that for the NLR [0.628 (0.535–0.720)], WBCs [0.667 (0.578–0.755)], neutrophils [0.672 (0.582–0.761)], and monocytes [0.657 (0.567–0.748)]. Accordingly, serum sPD-L1 showed better diagnostic performance than the abovementioned inflammatory markers. When the diagnostic power was further evaluated to distinguish HGGs from LGGs, the performance of circulatory sPD-L1 levels was significant (AUC: 0.702). Even after multivariate analysis, sPD-L1 retained its power to independently predict HGGs (OR: 1.030; 95% CI: 1.006–1.054, $p = 0.013$). Collectively, this observation has highlighted the potential role of sPD-L1 in glioma diagnosis and stratification.

Next, we attempted to uncover the perioperative dynamics of circulating sPD-L1 levels in glioma patients. The expression of sPD-L1 in the serum was prospectively evaluated after craniotomy for up to 20 days. In this context, the sPD-L1 levels in the circulation were observed to consistently decrease after tumor removal, which persisted regardless of the use of steroids (**Figure 2B**). The serum levels were markedly decreased on the 5th day after surgical resection. Some published studies assert that the sPD-L1 level after treatment may reflect the residual tumor burden (44, 45). Since all the glioma patients underwent maximal safe surgical resection, we speculated that the removal of the tumor might partly explain the decline in serum sPD-L1. However, it was reported that the low level of sPD-L1 indicated inflammation suppression (46). Taking into account the fact that most patients had received steroid therapy for edema (47), and the steroids are known to cause systemic immunosuppression (48), the decrease in the circulating sPD-L1 level might be affected by the use of steroids. Nevertheless, the correlation between serum sPD-L1 and steroids remains ambiguous. sPD-L1 is a dynamic marker, varying across time points; therefore, long-term studies are needed to examine the potential clinical relevance in the future.

Herein, an elevated serum sPD-L1 level was present in patients with relatively advanced brain tumors, as expected (**Tables 1, 3** and **Figure 1**). Combined with our unpublished results demonstrating that an elevated sPD-L1 level could predict reduced progression-free survival in patients with gliomas, we hypothesized that sPD-L1 is involved in the aggressive biological activities of tumors. Notably in this context, patients with high Ki-67 expression had significantly increased circulating sPD-L1 levels (**Table 5**). Ki-67 has been validated as a marker of proliferation in the initial phase of adult neurogenesis and is used clinically to assess tumor cell proliferative activity in diverse tumor types (49). Although the mechanistic link remains unclear, we suggest that sPD-L1 represents the PD-L1 expression in tumor tissue (25), which is accompanied by suppression of the immune response. In addition, the soluble form of PD-L1 is biologically activated in compromised antitumor immune responses (19). Both scenarios lead to immune tolerance; consequently, neoplastic cells would have no limits to proliferation. Therefore, abnormal expression of sPD-L1 may be an indicator of the occurrence and development of brain malignances. Furthermore, the serum sPD-L1 level could provide a tool for monitoring treatment response.

There are two ways for a brain protein to access the peripheral blood, that is, by CSF flow into the venous blood or by penetrating though the BBB (50). Given this information, we suspected that the high levels of sPD-L1 in the peripheral blood were due to molecules leaking from the CSF. To explore this relationship, we evaluated the expression of CSF sPD-L1 in matched patients. In our case series, we found excessive sPD-L1 expression in the CSF of glioma patients compared with that of meningioma patients (**Figure 1B**), suggesting that CSF sPD-L1 is released from a large number of tumor cells. Moreover, the expression of sPD-L1 was dramatically increased in the CSF

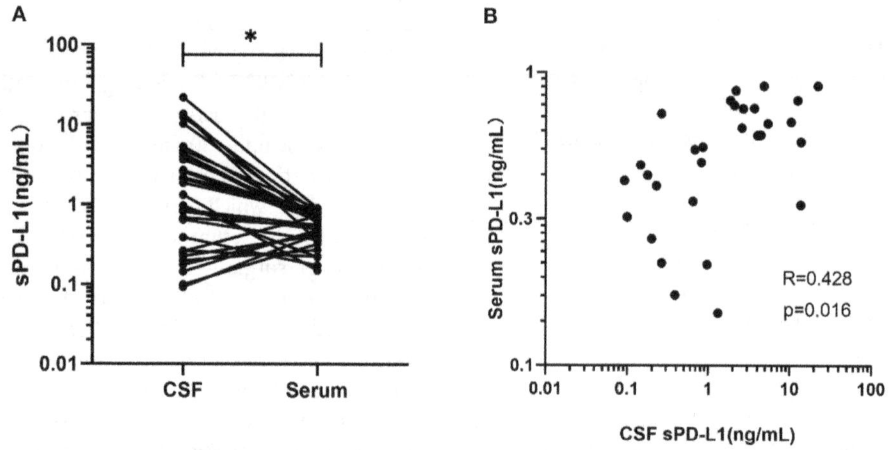

FIGURE 3 | Comparison and correlation between sPD-L1 in the serum and matched CSF of glioma patients. **(A)** sPD-L1 measurements in CSF and matched serum samples collected from 31 patients. **(B)** Correlation between serum and CSF sPD-L1 levels in individual patients with gliomas ($n = 31$). Pearson's correlation coefficients (R) and *P*-values are shown. Statistical significance was defined as $^*p < 0.05$.

TABLE 6 | Diagnostic value of inflammatory markers in gliomas.

Parameters	AUC (95% CI)	
	Glioma vs. other	**HGG vs. LGG**
Serum sPD-L1	0.906 (0.850–0.962)*	0.702 (0.577–0.827)*
CSF sPD-L1	0.853 (0.728–0.977)*	0.731 (0.545–0.917)*
WBC in the CSF	0.742 (0.538–0.946)*	0.571 (0.366–0.777)
NLR	0.628 (0.535–0.720)*	0.752 (0.636–0.868)*
dNLR	0.514 (0.418–0.609)	0.733 (0.616–0.849)*
NEU	0.672 (0.582–0.761)*	0.700 (0.578–0.821)*
WBC	0.667 (0.578–0.755)*	0.619 (0.488–0.750)
MONO	0.657 (0.567–0.748)*	0.654 (0.528–0.779)*
PLT	0.605 (0.511–0.698)*	0.602 (0.471–0.734)
LY	0.517 (0.421–0.612)	0.647 (0.518–0.777)*
ALB	0.494 (0.398–0.590)	0.656 (0.529–0.784)*
PLR	0.517 (0.421–0.613)	0.682 (0.556–0.804)*
PNI	0.491 (0.395–0.586)	0.689 (0.566–0.812)*
AGR	0.541 (0.446–0.636)	0.676 (0.552–0.800)*

Other includes healthy controls and patients with meningioma.
An asterisk (*) indicates a significant difference.
AUC, area under the curve; WBC, white blood cell count; LY, lymphocytes; dNLR, derived NLR; NEU, neutrophils; MONO, monocytes; ALB, albumin; PLT, platelets; NLR, neutrophil-to-lymphocyte ratio; PLR, platelet-to-lymphocyte ratio; AGR, albumin-to-globulin ratio; PNI, prognostic nutritional index.

compared with that in matched serum [1.3202 (0.0925–22.0392) vs. 0.5594 (0–1.4235), respectively, $p = 0.002$]. Subsequently, a positive correlation between serum and CSF PD-L1 levels was observed, although the degree of significance was mild ($r = 0.428$).

Another important purpose of this study was to investigate the roles of sPD-L1 in different biofluids for the diagnosis and prediction of gliomas. For this purpose, we evaluated the differences in the sPD-L1 levels in the serum and CSF according to varied clinicopathological features of gliomas. Similar to the expression in the serum, sPD-L1 expression in the CSF was higher in more advanced gliomas than in less advanced gliomas (**Table 5**). However, regarding tumor size and molecular markers, the differences remained statistically significant in the CSF but not in the serum. An explanation for the results may be that the CSF is in direct contact with the CNS (51), which indicates that CSF sPD-L1 may be more suitable for CNS malignancies than serum sPD-L1 in clinical practice.

Numerous published reports have declared that an IDH mutation or 1p/19q codeletion can affect the pathological behaviors of gliomas (52, 53). These molecular parameters were incorporated into the 2016 WHO classification schema for brain tumors and have paved the way for more precise drug therapies for gliomas (2). Several lines of evidence have demonstrated that mutation of IDH1 indicates enhanced chemosensitivity and is associated with an improved prognosis in glioma patients (54). Additionally, it has been reported that glioma with 1p/19q codeletion is sensitive to alkylating agents and tends to have prolonged survival (55). In this study, the upregulated CSF sPD-L1 levels tended to occur in the glioma patients with wild-type IDH-1 or maintained 1p/19q. This finding might partly explain why the enhanced sPD-L1 levels were related to unfavorable outcomes in the glioma patients in our previous study. On the other hand, the detection of CSF sPD-L1 could be adopted to help make decisions for postsurgical treatments at an early phase.

It is much more preferable to adopt CSF evaluation than peripheral blood evaluation for diagnostic analysis since the CSF directly contacts the CNS. Conversely, the AUC for serum sPD-L1 was markedly higher than that of CSF sPD-L1 for predicting gliomas [0.906 (0.850–0.962) vs. 0.853 (0.728–0.977), respectively] in this context. Moreover, the blood-based biomarkers such as NLR (AUC: 0.752) and dNLR (0.733) showed a better performance than CSF sPD-L1 (0.731) for the differentiation of gliomas. The lack of predictive power

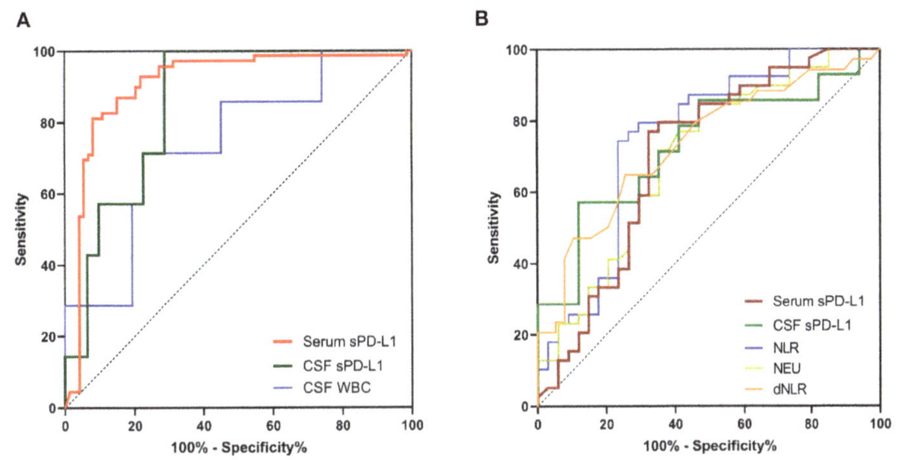

FIGURE 4 | The diagnostic value of inflammatory markers and sPD-L1 in gliomas. **(A)** ROC curves for predicting gliomas. **(B)** ROC curves for distinguishing high-grade gliomas from low-grade gliomas. For simplicity, only the ROC curves for which an AUC ≥ 0.70 are shown.

of CSF sPD-L1 might be due to the small number of CSF samples; therefore, further studies involving a larger cohort of patients might be needed to investigate the role of sPD-L1 in the CSF.

This study has several limitations. Although we detected upregulated levels of serum sPD-L1 among preoperative patients with glioma and observed a descending trend during the early postsurgical phase, it is not known whether sPD-L1 levels were affected by the concomitant therapy and whether sPD-L1 levels in serum fluctuate during tumor progression or remission. In addition, further investigation is required to determine whether sPD-L1 is robustly correlated with tumor activity, which would validate this soluble protein as a screening tool in future studies.

CONCLUSION

Our findings show the significant value of sPD-L1 in the serum and CSF for the diagnosis and discrimination of gliomas, providing the rationale to further study the role of sPD-L1 as a surrogated biomarker for the future clinical management of gliomas. Thus, the detection of sPD-L1 by intravenous or lumbar puncture rather than tumor tissue sampling could impact treatment decisions.

AUTHOR CONTRIBUTIONS

SL and YZ: study concept and design. SL, GZ, and CZ: methodology. SL, CZ, and XM: experiments. SL and BS: analysis and interpretation of data. SL: writing-original draft preparation. YF and XK: writing-review and editing. XK: supervision.

FUNDING

This work was supported by the National Science and Technology Major Project of China (2018ZX10307415-003).

ACKNOWLEDGMENTS

The authors wish to thank all the patients and healthy volunteers for providing blood samples.

REFERENCES

1. Wang Y, Jiang T. Understanding high grade glioma: molecular mechanism, therapy and comprehensive management. *Cancer Lett.* (2013) 331:139–46. doi: 10.1016/j.canlet.2012.12.024
2. Louis DN, Perry A, Reifenberger G, von Deimling A, Figarella-Branger D, Cavenee WK, et al. The 2016 World Health Organization classification of tumors of the central nervous system: a summary. *Acta Neuropathol.* (2016) 131:803–20. doi: 10.1007/s00401-016-1545-1
3. Barthel FP, Johnson KC, Wesseling P, Verhaak RGW. Evolving insights into the molecular neuropathology of diffuse gliomas in adults. *Neurol Clin.* (2018) 36:421–37. doi: 10.1016/j.ncl.2018.04.002
4. Stupp R, Taillibert S, Kanner A, Read W, Steinberg D, Lhermitte B, et al. Effect of tumor-treating fields plus maintenance temozolomide vs. maintenance temozolomide alone on survival in patients with glioblastoma: a randomized clinical trial. *JAMA.* (2017) 318:2306–16. doi: 10.1001/jama.2017.18718
5. Omuro A, DeAngelis LM. Glioblastoma and other malignant gliomas: a clinical review. *JAMA.* (2013) 310:1842–50. doi: 10.1001/jama.2013.280319
6. Zheng SH, Huang JL, Chen M, Wang BL, Ou QS, Huang SY. Diagnostic value of preoperative inflammatory markers in patients with glioma: a multicenter cohort study. *J Neurosurg.* (2018) 129:583–92. doi: 10.3171/2017.3.JNS161648
7. Lopes M, Carvalho B, Vaz R, Linhares P. Influence of neutrophil-lymphocyte ratio in prognosis of glioblastoma multiforme. *J Neurooncol.* (2018) 136:173–80. doi: 10.1007/s11060-017-2641-3
8. Wang PF, Meng Z, Song HW, Yao K, Duan ZJ, Yu CJ, et al. Preoperative changes in hematological markers and predictors of glioma grade and survival. *Front Pharmacol.* (2018) 9:886. doi: 10.3389/fphar.2018.00886
9. He ZQ, Ke C, Al-Nahari F, Duan H, Guo CC, Wang Y, et al. Low preoperative prognostic nutritional index predicts poor survival in patients with newly diagnosed high-grade gliomas. *J Neurooncol.* (2017) 132:239–47. doi: 10.1007/s11060-016-2361-0

10. Pierscianek D, Ahmadipour Y, Oppong MD, Rauschenbach L, Kebir S, Glas M, et al. Blood-based biomarkers in high grade gliomas: a systematic review. *Mol Neurobiol.* (2019) 56:6071–9. doi: 10.1007/s12035-019-1509-2
11. Reiss SN, Yerram P, Modelevsky L, Grommes C. Retrospective review of safety and efficacy of programmed cell death-1 inhibitors in refractory high grade gliomas. *J Immunother Cancer.* (2017) 5:99. doi: 10.1186/s40425-017-0302-x
12. Sampson JH, Maus MV, June CH. Immunotherapy for Brain Tumors. *J Clin Oncol.* (2017) 35:2450–6. doi: 10.1200/JCO.2017.72.8089
13. Duffy MJ, Crown J. Biomarkers for predicting response to immunotherapy with immune checkpoint inhibitors in cancer patients. *Clin Chem.* (2019) 65:1228–38. doi: 10.1373/clinchem.2019.303644
14. Berghoff AS, Kiesel B, Widhalm G, Rajky O, Ricken G, Wohrer A, et al. Programmed death ligand 1 expression and tumor-infiltrating lymphocytes in glioblastoma. *Neuro Oncol.* (2015) 17:1064–75. doi: 10.1093/neuonc/nou307
15. Nduom EK, Wei J, Yaghi NK, Huang N, Kong LY, Gabrusiewicz K, et al. PD-L1 expression and prognostic impact in glioblastoma. *Neuro Oncol.* (2016) 18:195–205. doi: 10.1093/neuonc/nov172
16. Antonios JP, Soto H, Everson RG, Moughon DL, Wang AC, Orpilla J, et al. Detection of immune responses after immunotherapy in glioblastoma using PET and MRI. *Proc Natl Acad Sci USA.* (2017) 114:10220–5. doi: 10.1073/pnas.1706689114
17. Chen Y, Wang Q, Shi B, Xu P, Hu Z, Bai L, et al. Development of a sandwich ELISA for evaluating soluble PD-L1 (CD274) in human sera of different ages as well as supernatants of PD-L1+ cell lines. *Cytokine.* (2011) 56:231–8. doi: 10.1016/j.cyto.2011.06.004
18. Dai S, Jia R, Zhang X, Fang Q, Huang L. The PD-1/PD-Ls pathway and autoimmune diseases. *Cell Immunol.* (2014) 290:72–9. doi: 10.1016/j.cellimm.2014.05.006
19. Frigola X, Inman BA, Lohse CM, Krco CJ, Cheville JC, Thompson RH, et al. Identification of a soluble form of B7-H1 that retains immunosuppressive activity and is associated with aggressive renal cell carcinoma. *Clin Cancer Res.* (2011) 17:1915–23. doi: 10.1158/1078-0432.CCR-10-0250
20. Shigemori T, Toiyama Y, Okugawa Y, Yamamoto A, Yin C, Narumi A, et al. Soluble PD-L1 expression in circulation as a predictive marker for recurrence and prognosis in gastric cancer: direct comparison of the clinical burden between tissue and serum PD-L1 expression. *Ann Surg Oncol.* (2018) 26:876–83. doi: 10.1245/s10434-018-07112-x
21. Kruger S, Legenstein ML, Rosgen V, Haas M, Modest DP, Westphalen CB, et al. Serum levels of soluble programmed death protein 1 (sPD-1) and soluble programmed death ligand 1 (sPD-L1) in advanced pancreatic cancer. *Oncoimmunology.* (2017) 6:e1310358. doi: 10.1080/2162402X.2017.1310358
22. Kushlinskii NE, Gershtein ES, Morozov AA, Goryacheva IO, Filipenko ML, Alferov AA, et al. Soluble ligand of the immune checkpoint receptor (sPD-L1) in blood serum of patients with renal cell carcinoma. *Bull Exp Biol Med.* (2019) 166:353–7. doi: 10.1007/s10517-019-04349-8
23. Zhou J, Mahoney KM, Giobbie-Hurder A, Zhao F, Lee S, Liao X, et al. Soluble PD-L1 as a biomarker in malignant melanoma treated with checkpoint blockade. *Cancer Immunol Res.* (2017) 5:480–92. doi: 10.1158/2326-6066.CIR-16-0329
24. Okuma Y, Wakui H, Utsumi H, Sagawa Y, Hosomi Y, Kuwano K, et al. Soluble programmed cell death ligand 1 as a novel biomarker for nivolumab therapy for non-small-cell lung cancer. *Clin Lung Cancer.* (2018) 19:410–7.e1. doi: 10.1016/j.cllc.2018.04.014
25. Shen H, Ji Y, Zhou D, Zhang Y, Wang W, Sun J, et al. Soluble programmed death-ligand 1 are highly expressed in peripheral T-cell lymphoma: a biomarker for prognosis. *Hematology.* (2019) 24:392–8. doi: 10.1080/16078454.2019.1590965
26. Aldape K, Brindle KM, Chesler L, Chopra R, Gajjar A, Gilbert MR, et al. Challenges to curing primary brain tumours. *Nat Rev Clin Oncol.* (2019) 16:509–20. doi: 10.1038/s41571-019-0177-5
27. Weston CL, Glantz MJ, Connor JR. Detection of cancer cells in the cerebrospinal fluid: current methods and future directions. *Fluids Barriers CNS.* (2011) 8:14. doi: 10.1186/2045-8118-8-14
28. You G, Sha Z-Y, Yan W, Zhang W, Wang Y-Z, Li S-W, et al. Seizure characteristics and outcomes in 508 Chinese adult patients undergoing primary resection of low-grade gliomas: a clinicopathological study. *Neuro Oncol.* (2011) 14:230–41. doi: 10.1093/neuonc/nor205
29. Capper D, Zentgraf H, Balss J, Hartmann C, von Deimling A. Monoclonal antibody specific for IDH1 R132H mutation. *Acta Neuropathol.* (2009) 118:599–601. doi: 10.1007/s00401-009-0595-z
30. Louis DN, Ohgaki H, Wiestler OD, Cavenee WK, Burger PC, Jouvet A, et al. The 2007 WHO classification of tumours of the central nervous system. *Acta Neuropathol.* (2007) 114:97–109. doi: 10.1007/s00401-007-0243-4
31. Saenz-Antonanzas A, Auzmendi-Iriarte J, Carrasco-Garcia E, Moreno-Cugnon L, Ruiz I, Villanua J, et al. Liquid biopsy in glioblastoma: opportunities, applications and challenges. *Cancers.* (2019) 11:E650. doi: 10.3390/cancers11070950
32. Amatatsu M, Arigami T, Uenosono Y, Yanagita S, Uchikado Y, Kijima Y, et al. Programmed death-ligand 1 is a promising blood marker for predicting tumor progression and prognosis in patients with gastric cancer. *Cancer Sci.* (2018) 109:814–20. doi: 10.1111/cas.13508
33. Xu J, Han X, Liu C, Gao N, Zhao J, Zhang X, et al. PD-L1 expression in pleural effusions of pulmonary adenocarcinoma and survival prediction: a controlled study by pleural biopsy. *Sci Rep.* (2018) 8:11206. doi: 10.1038/s41598-018-29156-5
34. Takada K, Toyokawa G, Shoji F, Okamoto T, Maehara Y. The significance of the PD-L1 expression in non-small-cell lung cancer: trenchant double swords as predictive and prognostic markers. *Clin Lung Cancer.* (2018) 19:120–9. doi: 10.1016/j.cllc.2017.10.014
35. Mantovani A, Allavena P, Sica A, Balkwill F. Cancer-related inflammation. *Nature.* (2008) 454:436–44. doi: 10.1038/nature07205
36. Huemer F, Lang D, Westphal T, Gampenrieder SP, Hutarew G, Weiss L, et al. Baseline absolute lymphocyte count and ECOG performance score are associated with survival in advanced non-small cell lung cancer undergoing PD-1/PD-L1 blockade. *J Clin Med.* (2019) 8:E1014. doi: 10.3390/jcm8071014
37. Zhang ZY, Zhan YB, Zhang FJ, Yu B, Ji YC, Zhou JQ, et al. Prognostic value of preoperative hematological markers combined with molecular pathology in patients with diffuse gliomas. *Aging.* (2019) 11:6252–72. doi: 10.18632/aging.102186
38. Soyano AE, Dholaria B, Marin-Acevedo JA, Diehl N, Hodge D, Luo Y, et al. Peripheral blood biomarkers correlate with outcomes in advanced non-small cell lung Cancer patients treated with anti-PD-1 antibodies. *J Immunother Cancer.* (2018) 6:129. doi: 10.1186/s40425-018-0447-2
39. Tanizaki J, Haratani K, Hayashi H, Chiba Y, Nakamura Y, Yonesaka K, et al. Peripheral blood biomarkers associated with clinical outcome in non-small cell lung cancer patients treated with Nivolumab. *J Thorac Oncol.* (2018) 13:97–105. doi: 10.1016/j.jtho.2017.10.030
40. Ferrucci PF, Ascierto PA, Pigozzo J, Del Vecchio M, Maio M, Antonini Cappellini GC, et al. Baseline neutrophils and derived neutrophil-to-lymphocyte ratio: prognostic relevance in metastatic melanoma patients receiving ipilimumab. *Ann Oncol.* (2016) 27:732–8. doi: 10.1093/annonc/mdw016
41. Zheng Z, Bu Z, Liu X, Zhang L, Li Z, Wu A, et al. Level of circulating PD-L1 expression in patients with advanced gastric cancer and its clinical implications. *Chin J Cancer Res.* (2014) 26:104–11. doi: 10.3978/j.issn.1000-9604.2014.02.08
42. Liang R, Li J, Tang X, Liu Y. The prognostic role of preoperative systemic immune-inflammation index and albumin/globulin ratio in patients with newly diagnosed high-grade glioma. *Clin Neurol Neurosurg.* (2019) 184:105397. doi: 10.1016/j.clineuro.2019.105397
43. Xu W, Wang D, Zheng X, Ou Q, Huang L. Sex-dependent association of preoperative hematologic markers with glioma grade and progression. *J Neurooncol.* (2018) 137:279–87. doi: 10.1007/s11060-017-2714-3
44. Buderath P, Schwich E, Jensen C, Horn PA, Kimmig R, Kasimir-Bauer S, et al. Soluble programmed death receptor ligands sPD-L1 and sPD-L2 as liquid biopsy markers for prognosis and platinum response in epithelial ovarian cancer. *Front Oncol.* (2019) 9:1015. doi: 10.3389/fonc.2019.01015
45. Ha H, Bang JH, Nam AR, Park JE, Jin MH, Bang YJ, et al. Dynamics of soluble programmed death-ligand 1 (sPDL1) during chemotherapy and its prognostic implications in cancer patients: biomarker development in immuno-oncology. *Cancer Res Treat.* (2019) 51:832–40. doi: 10.4143/crt.2018.311
46. Wasen C, Erlandsson MC, Bossios A, Ekerljung L, Malmhall C, Toyra Silfversward S, et al. Smoking is associated with low levels of soluble PD-L1 in rheumatoid arthritis. *Front Immunol.* (2018) 9:1677. doi: 10.3389/fimmu.2018.01677

47. Weller M, van den Bent M, Tonn JC, Stupp R, Preusser M, Cohen-Jonathan-Moyal E, et al. European Association for Neuro-Oncology (EANO) guideline on the diagnosis and treatment of adult astrocytic and oligodendroglial gliomas. *Lancet Oncol.* (2017) 18:e315–29. doi: 10.1016/S1470-2045(17)30194-8
48. Kostaras X, Cusano F, Kline GA, Roa W, Easaw J. Use of dexamethasone in patients with high-grade glioma: a clinical practice guideline. *Curr Oncol.* (2014) 21:e493–503. doi: 10.3747/co.21.1769
49. Kee N, Sivalingam S, Boonstra R, Wojtowicz JM. The utility of Ki-67 and BrdU as proliferative markers of adult neurogenesis. *J Neurosci Methods.* (2002) 115:97–105. doi: 10.1016/S0165-0270(02)00007-9
50. Strittmatter WJ. Bathing the brain. *J Clin Invest.* (2013) 123:1013–5. doi: 10.1172/JCI68241
51. Zorofchian S, Iqbal F, Rao M, Aung PP, Esquenazi Y, Ballester LY. Circulating tumour DNA, microRNA and metabolites in cerebrospinal fluid as biomarkers for central nervous system malignancies. *J Clin Pathol.* (2019) 72:271–80. doi: 10.1136/jclinpath-2018-205414
52. Eckel-Passow JE, Lachance DH, Molinaro AM, Walsh KM, Decker PA, Sicotte H, et al. Glioma groups based on 1p/19q, IDH, and TERT promoter mutations in tumors. *N Engl J Med.* (2015) 372:2499–508. doi: 10.1056/NEJMoa1407279
53. Reifenberger G, Wirsching H-G, Knobbe-Thomsen CB, Weller M. Advances in the molecular genetics of gliomas — implications for classification and therapy. *Nat Rev Clin Oncol.* (2016) 14:434. doi: 10.1038/nrclinonc.2016.204
54. Waitkus MS, Diplas BH, Yan H. Isocitrate dehydrogenase mutations in gliomas. *Neuro Oncol.* (2016) 18:16–26. doi: 10.1093/neuonc/nov136
55. Franceschi E, Tosoni A, De Biase D, Lamberti G, Danieli D, Pizzolitto S, et al. Postsurgical approaches in low-grade oligodendroglioma: is chemotherapy alone still an option? *Oncologist.* (2019) 24:664–70. doi: 10.1634/theoncologist.2018-0549

17

The Impact of Surgery in IDH 1 Wild Type Glioblastoma in Relation with the MGMT Deregulation

*Francesco Marchi[1], Nora Sahnane[2], Roberta Cerutti[2], Debora Cipriani[1], Jessica Barizzi[3], Federico Mattia Stefanini[4], Samantha Epistolio[3], Michele Cerati[2], Sergio Balbi[5], Luca Mazzucchelli[3], Fausto Sessa[2], Gianfranco Angelo Pesce[6], Michael Reinert[1,7] and Milo Frattini[3]**

[1] Service of Neurosurgery, Neurocenter of the Southern Switzerland, Regional Hospital of Lugano, Lugano, Switzerland, [2] Unit of Pathology, Department of Medicine and Surgery, University of Insubria-ASST Sette Laghi, Varese, Italy, [3] Institute of Pathology, Locarno, Switzerland, [4] Department of Statistics, Computer Science, Applications, University of Florence, Florence, Italy, [5] Division of Neurological Surgery, Department of Biotechnology and Life Sciences, University of Insubria-ASST Sette Laghi, Varese, Italy, [6] Radiation Oncology, Oncology Institute of Southern Switzerland, Bellinzona, Switzerland, [7] Faculty of Medicine, University of Bern, Bern, Switzerland

***Correspondence:**
Milo Frattini
milo.frattini@ti.ch

Object: The treatment of choice in glioblastoma (GBM) is the maximal surgical extent of resection (EOR) followed by adjuvant chemo-radiotherapy. Furthermore, methylguanine-DNA methyltransferase (MGMT) promoter methylation is associated with prolonged overall survival (OS) and progression free survival (PFS). The objective of the present study is correlate the biomolecular aspects in relation with EOR.

Materials and methods: We analyzed a series of 116 patients with IDH-1 wild type GBM and different EOR (Gross Total Resection—GTR-, Partial Resection—PR- and Biopsy), treated with adjuvant chemo-radiotherapy. The MGMT status was analyzed in terms of promoter methylation and protein expression.

Results: When GTR was possible, OS and PFS were significantly better compared to the other two groups ($p = 0.001$ and $p = 0.035$, respectively). MGMT methylation was significantly associated with better OS in the biopsy group ($p = 0.022$) and better OS and PFS in PR ($p = 0.02$ and $p = 0.012$, respectively), but not in the GTR group ($p = 0.252$ for OS, $p = 0.256$ for PFS) nor the PFS in the biopsy group ($p = 0.259$). MGMT protein expression levels do not show any association with OS and PFS, regardless of the type of surgery.

Conclusions: Our study confirms the positive association of a safe maximal EOR with better OS and PFS, and indicates a positive prognostic value of MGMT methylation status only in case of the presence of residual tumor tissue. MGMT protein expression seems not to play a clinical role in relation with the type of surgery.

Keywords: glioblastoma, extent of resection, MGMT, overall survival, progression free survival, temozolomide

INTRODUCTION

Glioblastoma (GBM) is the most common primary malignant brain tumor in adults (1). Currently, safe optimal surgical resection followed by adjuvant radiotherapy and chemotherapy is considered as the standard treatment approach for patients with GBM (2–4). However, despite advances in the last three decades and aggressive multimodal treatment, outcome remains poor for patients with GBM, with a median overall survival of 14–17 months from time at diagnosis (2, 3). Many studies have reported a positive correlation between the extent of resection (EOR) and the overall survival (OS) in patients with GBM, in particular for patients undergoing Gross Total Resection (GTR) with respect to whom receiving only a Subtotal Tumor Resection (STR) (5).

When GTR is not possible (due to several causes such as disease location and extension, general conditions of the patient), no clearly recognized criteria are proposed in the literature in order to stratify the STR group and, as a consequence, the threshold of EOR required for better prognosis remains controversial. Moreover, a recent observational retrospective study (6) has enrolled 38 patients who underwent PR and 78 biopsies and has pointed out that PR failed to improve OS and PFS compared with biopsy in patients with GBM ($p = 0.84$ and 0.48, respectively). Even the propensity score matching (PSM) between the PR and biopsy groups, according with this study, did not show any significant difference in OS and PFS between the groups ($p = 0.51$ and 0.75, respectively). The hazard ratios for OS and PFS of PR compared with biopsy were 0.98 and 0.73, respectively; however, the difference was not statistically significant ($p = 0.96$ and 0.39, respectively). Moreover, the surgical complication rate was higher in the PR group (14/32, 43.7%) than in the biopsy group (9/78, 11.5%) ($p < 0.01$). The cited study confirms that no significant association and benefit has been clearly yet demonstrated between the different degrees of PR and the biomolecular markers in regards of OS and PFS.

Methylguanine-DNA methyltransferase (MGMT) plays the pivotal role in the management of GBM patients: hypermethylation of MGMT promoter (causing absence of MGMT protein expression) leads to a higher response to temozolomide (TMZ), thus improving the patients' outcome (2, 7, 8). Furthermore, it has been discovered that additional mechanisms may decrease the MGMT expression. Approximately 20% of all patients with unmethylated GBM experiences an unexpected favorable outcome after chemoradiation, because mRNA expression was found to be unexpectedly low (9–11).

Only a few studies have investigated the influence of surgery on the clinical outcome in regards of the molecular markers (4, 12). Gessler et al. in their recent publication confirm that GTR is able to prolong PFS and OS when compared to incomplete resection, and the presence of methylation is a prognostic factor increasing significantly PFS and OS (4).

The aim of this study is to assess the relation between EOR and MGMT status (in terms of MGMT deregulation methylation and protein expression) by analyzing the clinical outcome (PFS and OS) of radio-chemotherapy treated IDH-1 wild type GBM patients, in correlation with the type of surgery.

Abbreviations: EOR, Extent of Resection; GBM, Glioblastoma; GTR, Gross Total Resection; IDH, Isocitrate Dehydrogenase; IHC, immunohistochemistry; MGMT, methylguanine-DNA methyltransferase; PFS, Progression Free Survival; PR, Partial Resection; OS, Overall Survival; STR, Subtotal Resection; TMZ, temozolomide.

MATERIALS AND METHODS

This bi-center retrospective cohort study included patients with newly diagnosed histologically reviewed GBM with IDH-1 wild type status from 2004 until 2013.

This work has been conducted in compliance with the protocol, the current version of the Declaration of Helsinki, the ICH-GCP or ISO EN 14155 (as far as applicable) as well as all national legal and regulatory requirements. Data and samples have been collected and analyzed for the study purpose only after the required authorizations from the competent Ethics Committees were obtained (Rif. CE 3086-2016-01108).

Inclusion criteria consist of age >18 years, histological diagnosis of IDH-1 wild type GBM (WHO IV), therapy with TMZ according with the Stupp scheme (60 Gray radiotherapy and concomitant chemotherapy with TMZ, followed by six cycles of maintenance TMZ), death caused by GBM, tissue availability for biomolecular analyses.

The OS (defined as the time from surgery to the date of death) and PFS (defined as the time from the first radio-chemotherapy treatment to the date of clinical or radiological progression according with the RANO criteria) were analyzed. Regarding the type of surgery, three groups were defined according with the post-op MRI performed in the first 72 h: GTR (with no contrast-enhancing residual tissue visible on T1 injected MRI sequences), incomplete Partial Resection (PR) (with evidence of contrast-enhancing residual tumor) and Biopsy.

Molecular Analyses

MGMT Promoter Methylation

Tissues for genomic DNA isolation were dissected manually from three 8-μm sections and DNA was obtained using automatic extraction (Maxwell, Promega, Madison, WI, USA). About 50–100 ng of DNA were subjected to bisulphite treatment using EZ DNA Methylation-Gold TM kit (Zymo Research, Irvine, CA, USA). Methylation status of six consecutive cytosines of MGMT promoter (chr10:131,265,507−131,265,556) was assessed by PCR-pyrosequencing of bisulphite-treated DNA by using MGMT Plus kit according to the recommended protocol (Diatech Pharmacogenetics, Jesi, Italy). A cut-off of 10% was set to score presence of promoter methylation. This value was determined calculating the limit of negative controls (DNA samples from 15 FFPE healthy brain tissues) for each cytosine (mean of methylation ratio adding 2× the Standard Deviation) assuming a Gaussian distribution of the raw signal from negative samples. The limit corresponded to 95% of the observed negative values.

MGMT Immunohistochemistry

Immunohistochemical reactions for MGMT protein were performed on whole tissue sections obtained from formalin-fixed, paraffin-embedded (FFPE) tumor blocks. Three -μm-thick sections were deparaffinized, rehydrated and pretreated with citrate buffer pH6 in microwave oven for 20 min. Monoclonal primary antibody anti-MGMT, clone MT3.1 (Chemicon International, Temecula, CA, USA) was used at a dilution of 1/400 and applied overnight at 4°C, followed by a polymeric detection system (Ultravision DAB Detection System, LabVision, Fremont, CA, USA) according to the manufacturer's protocol. According to the literature, immunohistochemical positivity was scored when more than 5% of neoplastic cells showed an intense nuclear staining (13, 14).

Statistical Analyses

Mean and median values were calculated at first to summarize results of each variable. The relative chi-square values were calculated on pairs of variables to describe the statistical association existing among variables: null hypothesis stating the lack of marginal association between pairs of variables (after discretization) was assessed through the chi-square test.

OS and PFS curves for censored data were obtained using the Kaplan-Meier estimator; comparisons of curves given different molecular characterizations were performed by logrank tests. PFS curves were also estimated and tested within strata defined by the variable of surgery.

All the analyses, graphs and reports were performed using the R software [R] and the following R packages: survival, bootstrap, rmarkdown, knitr (15–18).

RESULTS

The study includes 116 patients, 57 females (49.1%) and 59 males (50.9%). Among them, 81 underwent GTR of the tumor (69.8%), 18 PR (15.5%) while in 17 cases only biopsy was performed (14.7%). In 92 patients (corresponding to 79.3% of the whole cohort), we observed progression of the disease (PD), while the remaining 24 cases (20.7%) include both the six patients who are still alive ($N = 6$) and the 18 patients who deceased for other causes with no evidence of tumor progression.

Concerning the biomolecular aspects, 71 samples showed absence of MGMT promoter methylation tumors (61.2%), 41 methylation (35.3%) while in four samples the methylation status was not evaluable (3.4%). The immunohistochemical evaluation of the MGMT protein revealed a positive expression in 54 samples (46.5%) and a negative expression in 44 cases (37.9%), while in 18 cases (15.5%) the assay did not give evaluable results (**Table 1**). As for clinical data, OS was 15.5 months and PFS was 7 months.

We then analyzed the correlation between the type of surgery and the OS (**Figures 1A,B**). Patients who underwent a GTR had a significantly better OS (17 months) compared with those in whom a PR (14 months) or a biopsy (9 months) had been performed (Log-rank $p = 0.001$; GTR: HR = 0.3521, 95%CI: 0.1989, 0.6235; PR: HR = 0.3926, 95%CI: 0.1908, 0.8075) (**Figure 1A**). Analogously, grouping the patients who sustained PR and biopsy, we confirmed a significant longer OS for patients subjected to GTR (GTR = 17 months, PR + Biopsy = 11.5 months, Log-rank $p = 0.0333$; GTR: HR = 1.571, 95%CI: 1.0316, 2.3923) (**Figure 1B**). Similar results were obtained by comparing the type of surgery and PFS (**Figures 1C,D**). Indeed, the GTR group presented a longer PFS compared with the PR group and the biopsy group (GTR = 8.25 months, PR = 7.50 months, Biopsy = 4.00 months, Log-rank $p = 0.0352$; GTR: HR = 0.3681, 95%CI: 0.1738, 0.7799; PR: HR = 0.4444, 95%CI: 0.1877, 1.0522) (**Figure 1C**). On the contrary, GTR did not give a significant greater PFS compared with the value of the other two groups considered together (GTR = 8.25 months, PR + Biopsy = 7.00, Log-rank $p = 0.1187$; PR + biopsy: HR = 1.4774, 95%CI: 0.9211, 2.3698) (**Figure 1D**).

TABLE 1 | Synoptic overview of the patient population.

Patients	116	
IDH1 wild type GBM WHO IV	116	
Female	57	49.1%
Male	59	50.9%
GTR	81	69.8%
PR	18	15.5%
Biopsy	17	14.7%
Surgery + Radio-chemotherapy	116	
Deceased	110	94.8%
Alive	6	5.1%
Progression Disease (PD)	92	79.3%
Alive with no evidence of PD	6	5.1%
Deceased with no evidence of PD	18	15.5%
MGMT methylated	41	35.3%
MGMT non-methylated	71	61.2%
MGMT non definable	4	3.4%
MGMT protein expression positive	54	46.5%
MGMT protein expression negative	44	37.9%
MGMT expression not evaluable	18	15.5%

GBM, Glioblastoma; GTR, Gross Total Resection; MGMT, methylguanine-DNA methyltransferase; PR, Partial Resection.

Afterwards, the OS and the PFS were analyzed in relation with the MGMT promoter methylation and the protein expression evaluated by immunohistochemistry (IHC) (**Figures 2A–D**). The OS is significantly better in MGMT methylated GBMs than in MGMT unmethylathed ones (methylated: 19.5 months, unmethylathed: 14 months, Log-rank $p = 0.0056$; U: HR = 1.7653, 95%CI: 1.174, 2.6544) (**Figure 2A**). Same positive correlation, statistically significant, was found for PFS, with 9 months before progression in MGMT methylated patients and 7 months for MGMT unmethylated ones (Log-rank $p = 0.0347$; U: HR = 1.6014, 95%CI: 1.037, 2.473) (**Figure 2B**).

Regarding the levels of MGMT protein expression, patients who had low MGMT protein expression had a significantly improved OS compared with patients who had high MGMT protein expression (18 vs. 13 months; Log-rank $p = 0.0148$; Pos: HR = 1.6929, 95%CI: 1.1165, 2.567) (**Figure 2C**). On the contrary, no significant correlation was observed for MGMT

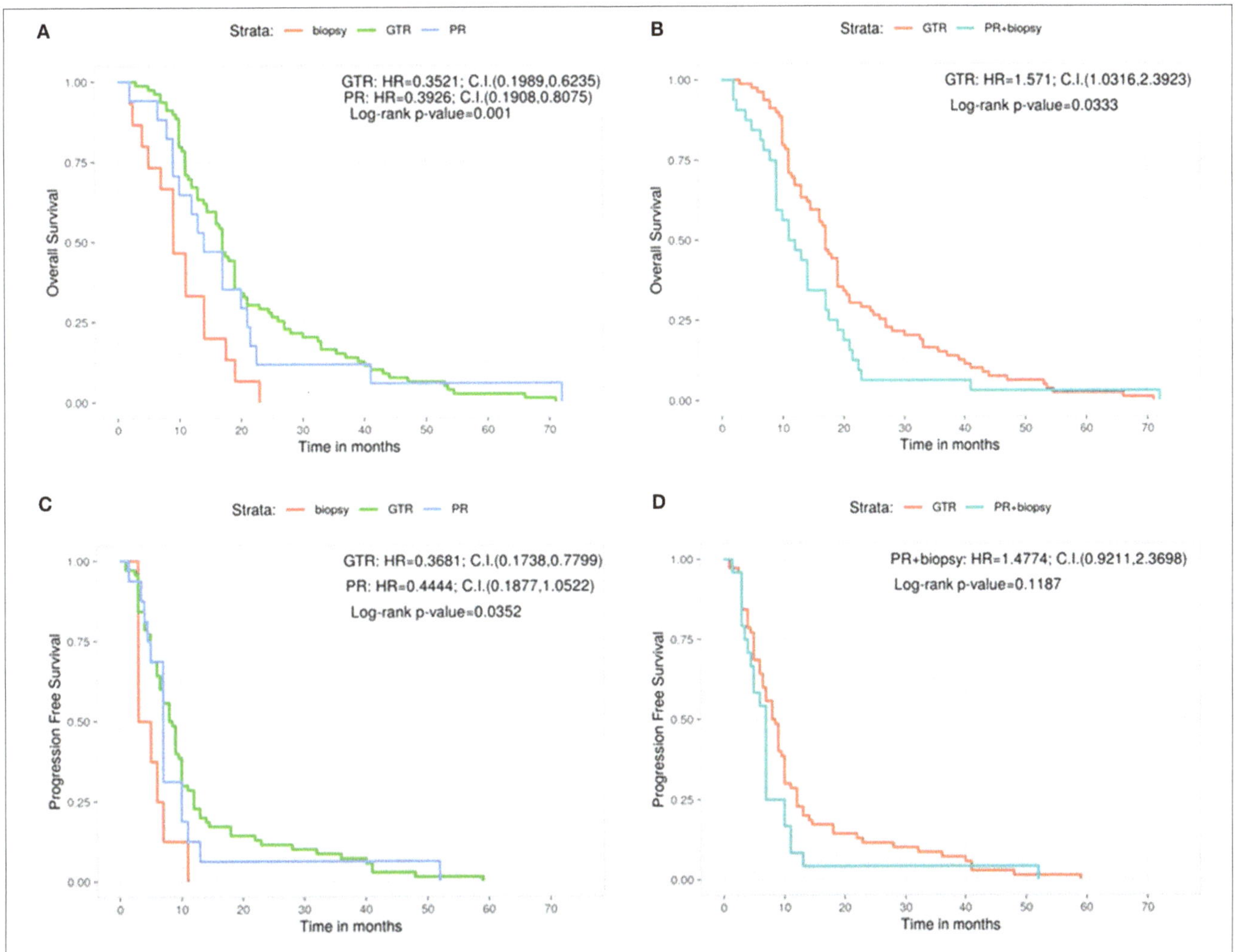

FIGURE 1 | Overall survival for each type of surgery **(A)** and grouping PR and biopsy groups **(B)**. Progression free survival for each type of surgery **(C)** and grouping PR and biopsy groups **(D)**. C.I., Confidence interval; GTR, gross total resection; H.R., hazard ratio; PR, partial resection.

protein expression in regards of PFS (8.75 months for GBMs showing low protein expression and 7 months for those with high protein expression, Log-rank $p = 0.3166$; Pos: HR = 1.2486, 95%CI: 0.8013, 1.9458) (**Figure 2D**).

Furthermore, we analyzed the outcome (in terms of both OS and PFS) subdividing the cohort on the basis of the three different types of surgery, in relation with the methylation status of the MGMT gene (**Figures 3A–F**). No significant correlation was found in patients with GTR between OS and methylation status (methylated = 19 months, unmethylated = 16 months, Log-rank $p = 0.252$; U: HR = 1.3125, 95%CI: 0.8277, 2.0813) (**Figure 3A**). A positive correlation was shown, instead, in the PR group, in which MGMT methylated patients had a better OS compared with the unmethylated ones (methylated = 31.8 months, unmethylated = 13.0 months, Log-rank $p = 0.0205$; U: HR = 8.5176, 95%CI: 1.0472, 69.2787) (**Figure 3B**). The same positive statistically significant correlation was observed in patients who underwent biopsy (methylated = 21 months, unmethylated = 9 months, Log-rank $p = 0.0226$; U: HR = undefined, 95%CI: 0, ∞) (**Figure 3C**).

As regards the PFS, patients who underwent a GTR and were MGMT methylated did not show a better outcome if compared with patients carrying MGMT unmethylated GBM (methylated = 9 months, unmethylated = 7 months, Log-rank $p = 0.256$; U: HR = 1.3215, 95%CI: 0.8134, 2.147) (**Figure 3D**). On the contrary, a statistically significant better PFS was noted in MGMT methylated patient with respect to MGMT unmethylated ones in the PR group (methylated = 13 months, unmethylated = 7 months, Log-rank $p = 0.0117$; U: HR = 9.0791, 95%CI: 1.141, 72.2475) (**Figure 3E**). Finally, absence of correlation between PFS and the methylation status was observed in the group of patients who underwent a biopsy (methylated = 5 months, unmethylated = 3 months, Log-rank $p = 0.2982$; U: HR = 2.5982, 95%CI: 0.2975, 22.6896) (**Figure 3F**).

Moreover, we analyzed the same variables (clinical outcome and EOR) on the light of the results of MGMT protein expression (**Figures 4A–F**). In terms of OS, patients who underwent a GTR with a low protein expression had a significant better outcome with respect to patients with high MGMT expression (low protein expression = 19.8 months, high protein

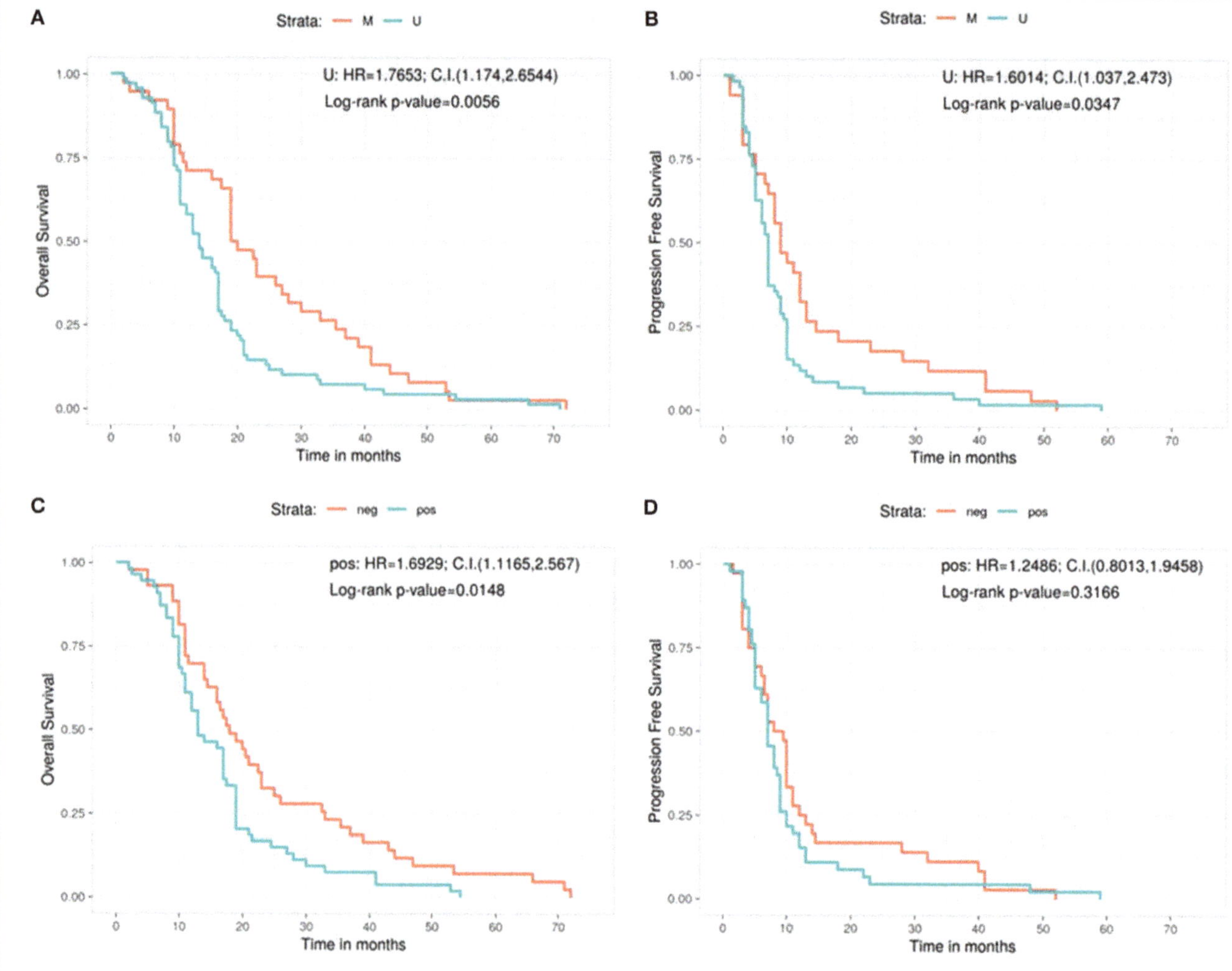

FIGURE 2 | Overall survival **(A)** and progression free survival **(B)** according with the MGMT methylation status. Overall survival **(C)** and progression free survival **(D)** according with the immunohistochemistry results. C.I., Confidence interval; H.R., hazard ratio; M, methylated; neg, IHC negative; pos, IHC positive; U, unmethylated.

expression = 16.5 months, Log-rank $p = 0.0476$; Pos: HR = 1.6592, 95%CI: 1.0144, 2.714) (**Figure 4A**). On the contrary, no significant correlations were found in the PR and in the biopsy groups regarding MGMT protein expression in terms of OS: 17 months for low protein expression patients vs. 12.5 months for those with high protein expression in the PR group (Log-rank $p = 0.3702$; Pos: HR = 1.6552, 95%CI: 0.5554, 4.9325) (**Figure 4B**), and 11 months in low protein expression patients vs. 8 months in patients with high MGMT expression in the biopsy group (Log-rank $p = 0.42$; Pos: HR = 1.596, 95%CI: 0.4772, 5.3374) (**Figure 4C**).

As regards PFS, IHC showed no significant relation between low and high protein expression patients in any group. In the GTR patients, the difference in PFS between low expressed and high expressed cases was 9.5 vs. 8 months (Log-rank $p = 0.6387$; Pos: HR = 1.1313, 95%CI: 0.6718, 1.905) (**Figure 4D**). In the PR group, PFS was 10 months for low protein expression patients vs. 7 months for patients with high MGMT protein levels (Log-rank $p = 0.3034$; Pos: HR = 1.8299, 95%CI: 0.5637, 5.9407) (**Figure 4E**). In the biopsy group, patients showing low protein expression level had a PFS of 5 months compared with 3 months of those with a high MGMT protein expression (Log-rank $p = 0.259$; Pos: HR = 2.3493, 95%CI: 0.3908, 14.1236) (**Figure 4F**).

DISCUSSION

Our paper presents a bicentric, retrospective study including a series of patients affected by IDH-1 wild type GBM treated with chemotherapy and radiotherapy after surgery.

Firstly, compared to the data in the literature, we tried to define three new unambiguous categories of surgical treatment: GTR, when no evidence of residual tumor on the T1 injected post-op sequences MRI; PR, if any enhancement is visible (independently of the residual volume); and biopsy, if only a small piece of tumor is taken for analysis. We think that this categorization is a novelty in literature considering the PR as the presence of residual tumor, regardless its volume. All the other

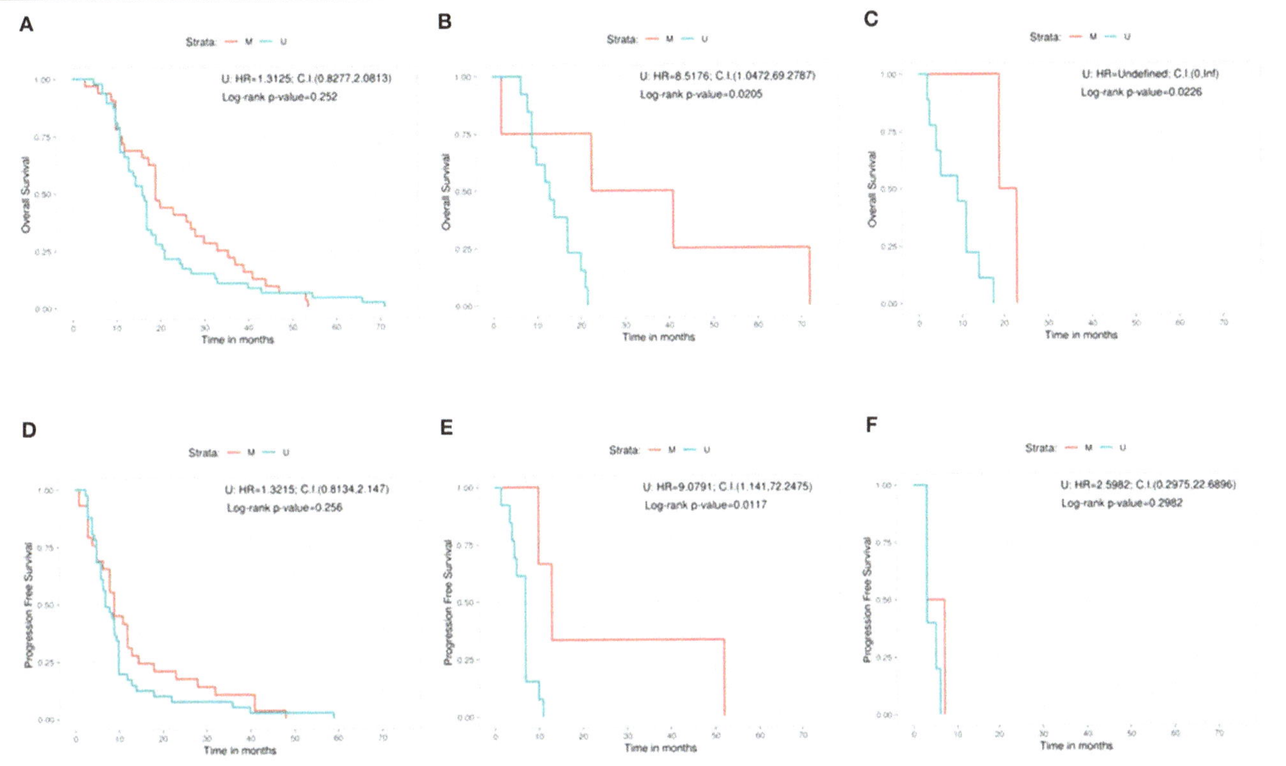

FIGURE 3 | Overall survival according with the MGMT methylation status for the gross total resection group **(A)**, the partial resection group **(B)**, and the biopsy group **(C)**. Progression free survival according with the MGMT methylation status for the gross total resection group **(D)**, the partial resection group **(E)**, and the biopsy group **(F)**. C.I., Confidence interval; H.R., hazard ratio; M, methylated; U, unmethylated.

studies, in fact, have defined the residual volume in a percentage that, in the majority of cases, may be subjective.

Our results confirm the well established statement for which, when feasible, GTR is the gold standard to achieve in the surgical treatment of GBMs with a longer term OS in this group of patients vs. both the PR group and the biopsy group (17 vs. 14 vs. 9 months for the different groups, respectively). Similar data are obtained comparing the GTR group with the PR + biopsy combined one (17 vs. 11.5, respectively). However, as stated above, the GTR in our work is the complete absence of residual tumor on the postop MRI and not, as in literature, the variable majority of tumor resected (>95 or >97%) considering the difficulty in the objective calculation of the percentage of the remnant tumor.

Regarding the PFS, we observed the same significant positive relation in favor of the GTR group compared with the PR and biopsy groups taken singularly (8.25 vs. 7.5 vs. 4, respectively) but not when the latter two (PR + biopsy) are assembled together. Also these data confirm the already published ones but, differently, in our work, the PR is considered any enhancement of any size visible on the postoperative MRI.

In respect of the MGMT methylated status and the better outcome, our results are in line with the main series published in literature (7, 19) with a median OS of 19.5 months for patients with a MGMT methylated GBM vs. 14 months for patients with an MGMT unmethylated GBM and 2 months more of PFS between the two groups. However, while the better prognosis in terms of OS was confirmed by protein expression levels assessed by IHC, no significant correlation between the two groups (low and high MGMT protein expression) was shown for the PFS with this analysis. Therefore, our study confirms the lower diagnostic value of IHC as compared to the evaluation of the MGMT methylation status.

The most interesting results have been obtained matching the MGMT status and the EOR. While we observed that the MGMT status is positively and significantly correlated to the clinical outcome in the PR group (OS of 31.8 months for patients with MGMT methylated GBM with respect to only 13 months for MGMT unmethylated GBM, PFS of 13 vs. 7 months, respectively), in the group of patients who underwent a GTR we did not observe any significant association between OS or PFS and the methylation status of MGMT gene. Likewise, the simple biopsy did not change significantly the outcome in terms of PFS in methylated vs. unmethylated patients with only 2 months achieved before disease progression. However, in terms of OS, patients characterized by an MGMT methylated GBM have an advantage of 12 months with respect to patients with an MGMT unmethylated tumor. Our results confirm those recently published but using clearly, objective and widely applicable categories of EOR (4, 12). Therefore, we can postulate that the identification of MGMT promoter methylation may identify a group of GBM patients who are correlated with a better

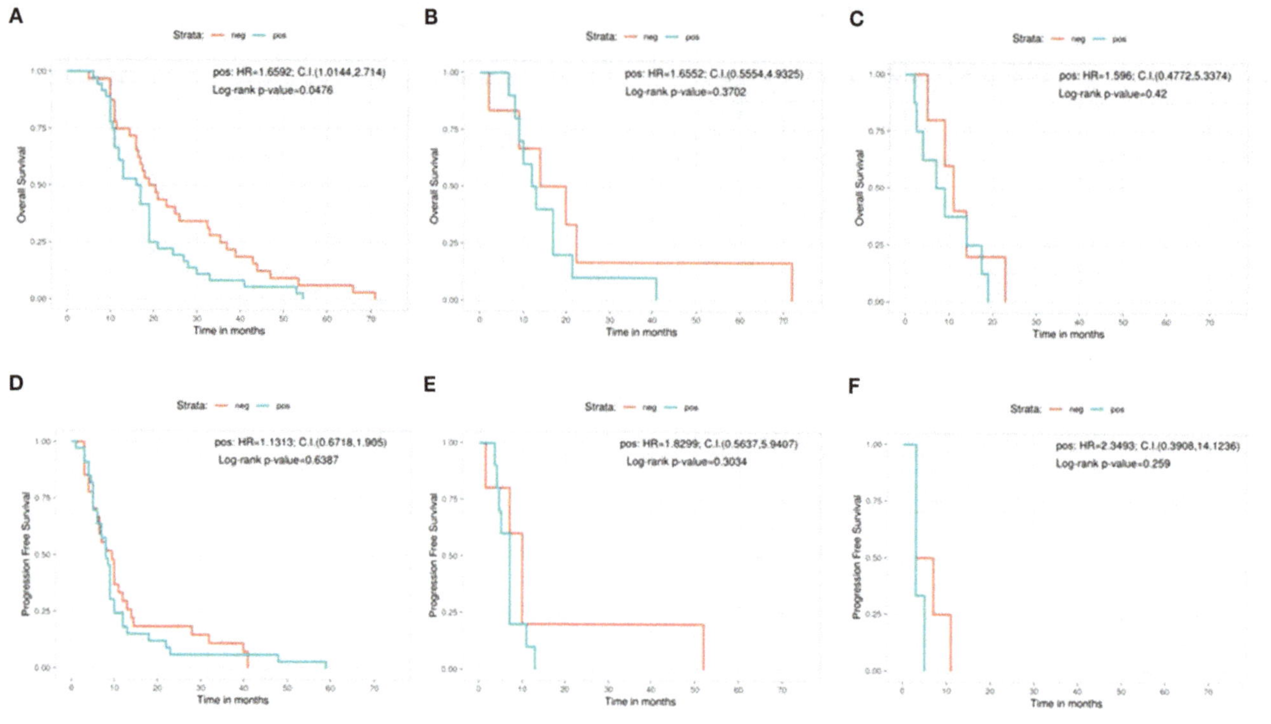

FIGURE 4 | Overall survival according with the protein expression in immunohistochemistry for the gross total resection group **(A)**, the partial resection group **(B)**, and the biopsy group **(C)**. Progression free survival according with the protein expression in immunohistochemistry for the gross total resection group **(D)**, the partial resection group **(E)**, and the biopsy group **(F)**. C.I., Confidence interval; H.R., hazard ratio; neg, IHC negative; pos, IHC positive.

response to the combined chemo-radiotherapy treatment only if the neoplastic tissue is still present. On the contrary, patients who are *bona fide* radically resected, will experience the same follow-up with respect to the combined chemo-radiation therapy.

IHC represents the classic worldwide used method for the detection of protein expression. However, especially for MGMT protein (as for other proteins located in cell nucleus), it can be sometimes hard to be evaluated, leading to the conclusion that MGMT promoter methylation should be the preferred method for assessing MGMT deregulation instead of IHC. In fact, literature reports that sometimes there is no correlation between MGMT expression and its promoter methylation (20). Also in our series IHC does not confirm the expected significant correlation between low protein expression and better clinical outcome in PR and biopsy groups. Indeed, the only favorable significant correlation (borderline, $p = 0.047$) for the low protein expression was noted in the OS for the patients who underwent GTR: they presented almost 20 months of survival vs. 16.5 months of those with samples expressing high levels of MGMT protein. Neither the GTR nor the PR or the biopsy group showed a significant relation between IHC and PFS.

Beside IHC limits, also the definition of MGMT promoter methylation is sometimes challenging, however literature reports some cut-off values that can be used to define a sample as positive for MGMT methylation (21). In our work we applied a cut-off of 10% that was decided on the bases of an internal control evaluation of a cohort of negative (healthy tissues) samples.

Our study present some limitations, such as the number of patients included in the analysis is small if compared to other series, even if not inferior to the majority of studies published. For this reason, the results of the present work are in line with those in the literature and seem to be not innovative. However, several aspects are not exhaustively treated in literature and some features can be helpful in everyday practice as, for example, the simple classification between GTR and PR or the importance of radio-chemotherapy in case of residual enhancement on the postoperative images.

To conclude, the present study confirms the better outcome in patients with GBM who sustained a GTR: maximal EOR in surgery seems to be confirmed as the most important prognostic value for OS and PFS in the treatment of GBM patients, thus indicating that, whenever possible, this is the goal that must be pursued by clinicians. Under these conditions, the most relevant biomarker, MGMT, does not seem to play any prognostic role. Theoretically and provocatively, the present study states that chemo-radiotherapy, in presence of complete resection, could not influence significantly OS and PFS, playing a substantial role only in case of residual tumor. When surgery is not possible, the MGMT methylated status is proven to be a favorable marker for OS and PFS in patients with remnant tumor after an incomplete tumor resection (in both PR and biopsied patients). On the contrary, IHC expression does not correlate with different OS or PFS in relation with the type of surgery, thus confirming the discrepancy between protein expression and MGMT methylation status evaluation and suggesting a superior predictive role of the latter.

We think that the current study, to the best of our knowledge, is one of the few studies which correlates biological aspects and different type of surgery in GBM patients treated with a combined chemo-radiotherapy. However, considering the continuous changes in the field of brain tumors, further studies are needed in order to confirm our data and to identify other possible correlations between the newest biological markers, the clinical outcome and the surgical treatment in patients with GBM.

AUTHOR CONTRIBUTIONS

FM and NS collected all clinical data and wrote the first draft of the manuscript. FM, DC, FS, GP, MR, and MF selected the cohort for the analyses. JB, MC, LM, FS, and GP selected all the specimens at histologic level. NS, RC, SE, and SB performed all the molecular characterization. SE, RC, and MF evaluated MGMT results. JB, MC, LM, FS, and GP evaluated IHC experiments. FMS was responsible for all the statistical analyses. FM, NS, and SE prepared the final version of the manuscript. FM, FS, GP, MR, and MF supervised the whole project.

FUNDING

This study was supported by Fondazione Ticinese contro il Cancro.

REFERENCES

1. Louis DN, Perry A, Reifenberger G, Von Deimling A, Figarella-Branger D, Cavenee WK, et al. The 2016 World Health Organization classification of tumors of the central nervous system: a summary. *Acta Neuropathol.* (2016) 131:803–20. doi: 10.1007/s00401-016-1545-1
2. Stupp R, Mason WP, van den Bent MJ, Weller M, Fisher B, Taphoorn MJB, et al. Radiotherapy plus concomitant and adjuvant temozolomide for glioblastoma. *N Engl J Med.* (2005) 352:987–96. doi: 10.1056/NEJMoa043330
3. Weller M, van den Bent M, Hopkins K, Tonn JC, Stupp R, Falini A, et al. EANO guideline for the diagnosis and treatment of anaplastic gliomas and glioblastoma. *Lancet Oncol.* (2014) 15:e395–403. doi: 10.1016/S1470-2045(14)70011-7
4. Gessler F, Bernstock JD, Braczynski A, Lescher S, Baumgarten P, Harter PN, et al. Surgery for glioblastoma in light of molecular markers: impact of resection and MGMT promoter methylation in newly diagnosed IDH-1 wild-type glioblastomas. *Neurosurgery.* (2018) 84:190–7. doi: 10.1093/neuros/nyy049
5. Brown TJ, Brennan MC, Li M, Church EW, Brandmeir NJ, Rakszawski KL, et al. Association of the extent of resection with survival in glioblastoma: a systematic review and meta-analysis. *JAMA Oncol.* (2016) 2:1460–9. doi: 10.1001/jamaoncol.2016.1373
6. Byun J, Kim YH, Nam SJ, Park JE, Cho YH, Kim HS, et al. Comparison of survival outcomes between partial resection and biopsy for primary glioblastoma: a propensity score-matched study. *World Neurosurg.* (2019) 121:e858–66. doi: 10.1016/j.wneu.2018.09.237
7. Hegi ME, Diserens AC, Gorlia T, Hamou MF, de Tribolet N, Weller M, et al. MGMT gene silencing and benefit from temozolomide in glioblastoma. *N Engl J Med.* (2005) 352:997–1003. doi: 10.1056/NEJMoa043331
8. Esteller M, Hamilton SR, Burger PC, Baylin SB, Herman JG. Inactivation of the DNA repair gene O6-methylguanine-DNA methyltransferase by promoter hypermethylation is a common event in primary human neoplasia. *Cancer Res.* (1999) 59:793–7.
9. Everhard S, Tost J, El Abdalaoui H, Crinière E, Busato F, Marie Y, et al. Identification of regions correlating MGMT promoter methylation and gene expression in glioblastomas. *Neuro Oncol.* (2009) 11:348–56. doi: 10.1215/15228517-2009-001
10. Ramakrishnan V, Kushwaha D, Koay DC, Reddy H, Mao Y, Zhou L, et al. Post-transcriptional regulation of O(6)-methylguanine-DNA methyltransferase MGMT in glioblastomas. *Cancer Biomark.* (2011) 10:185–93. doi: 10.3233/CBM-2012-0245
11. Kreth S, Limbeck E, Hinske LC, Schütz SV, Thon N, Hoefig K, et al. In human glioblastomas transcript elongation by alternative polyadenylation and miRNA targeting is a potent mechanism of MGMT silencing. *Acta Neuropathol.* (2013) 125:671–81. doi: 10.1007/s00401-013-1081-1
12. Kreth FW, Thon N, Simon M, Westphal M, Schackert G, Nikkhah G, et al. Gross total but not incomplete resection of glioblastoma prolongs survival in the era of radiochemotherapy. *Ann Oncol.* (2013) 24:3117–23. doi: 10.1093/annonc/mdt388
13. Brell M, Tortosa A, Verger E, Gil JM, Viñolas N, Villá S, et al. Prognostic significance of O6-methylguanine-DNA methyltransferase determined by promoter hypermethylation and immunohistochemical expression in anaplastic gliomas. *Clin Cancer Res.* (2005) 11:5167–74. doi: 10.1158/1078-0432.CCR-05-0230
14. Cao VT, Jung TY, Jung S, Jin SG, Moon KS, Kim IY, et al. The correlation and prognostic significance of MGMT promoter methylation and MGMT protein in glioblastomas. *Neurosurgery.* (2009) 65:866–75. doi: 10.1227/01.NEU.0000357325.90347.A1
15. Xie Y. *A Comprehensive Tool for Reproducible Research in R. Implementing Reproducible Computational Research.* New York, NY: CRC Press Group (2014).
16. Therneau T. *A Package for Survival Analysis in S_. Version.* (2015). Available online at: https://cran.r-project.org/package=survival (accessed December 11, 2018).
17. Allaire J. *Dynamic Documents for R. R Package Version 1.11.* (2018). Available online at: https://rmarkdown.rstudio.com/ (accessed December 11, 2018).
18. Team RC. *A Language and Environment for Statistical Computing.* (2018). Available online at: https://www.r-project.org/ (accessed December 11, 2018).
19. Stupp R, van den Bent MJ, Hegi ME. Optimal role of temozolomide in the treatment of malignant gliomas. *Curr Neurol Neurosci Rep.* (2005) 5:198–206. doi: 10.1007/s11910-005-0047-7
20. Rodriguez FJ, Thibodeau SN, Jenkins RB, Schowalter KV, Caron BL, O'Neill BP, et al. MGMT immunohistochemical expression and promoter methylation in human glioblastoma. *Appl Immunohistochem Mol Morphol.* (2008) 16:59–65. doi: 10.1097/PAI.0b013e31802fac2f
21. Brigliadori G, Foca F, Dall'Agata M, Rengucci C, Melegari E, Cerasoli, et al. Defining the cutoff value of MGMT gene promoter methylation and its predictive capacity in glioblastoma. *J Neurooncol.* (2016) 128:333–9. doi: 10.1007/s11060-016-2116-y

18

A Potential Mechanism of Temozolomide Resistance in Glioma–Ferroptosis

Zhifang Hu [1†], *Yajing Mi* [1†], *Huiming Qian* [2†], *Na Guo* [1], *Aili Yan* [1], *Yuelin Zhang* [2*] and *Xingchun Gao* [1,2*]

[1] *Shaanxi Key Laboratory of Brain Disorders, School of Basic Medical Science, Xi'an Medical University, Xi'an, China,*
[2] *Shaanxi Key Laboratory of Ischemic Cardiovascular Disease, Institute of Basic and Translational Medicine, Xi'an Medical University, Xi'an, China*

Correspondence:
Yuelin Zhang
zhangyuelin68@163.com
Xingchun Gao
gxc199281003@163.com

† These authors have contributed equally to this work

Temozolomide (TMZ) is the first-line chemotherapy drug that has been used to treat glioma for over a decade, but the benefits are limited by half of the treated patients who acquired resistance. Studies have shown that glioma TMZ resistance is a complex process with multiple factors, which has not been fully elucidated. Ferroptosis, which is a new type of cell death discovered in recent years, has been reported to play an important role in tumor drug resistance. The present study reviews the relationship between ferroptosis and glioma TMZ resistance, and highlights the role of ferroptosis in glioma TMZ resistance. Finally, the investigators discussed the future orientation for ferroptosis in glioma TMZ resistance, in order to promote the clinical use of ferroptosis induction in glioma treatment.

Keywords: ferroptosis, glioma, temozolomide, GPX4, drug resistance

INTRODUCTION

Gliomas originate in the neuroectodermal layer, and are the most common CNS tumors in clinic. This accounts for more than 30% of all primary intracranial tumors, and 74.6% of these are malignant gliomas (1). The present treatment of gliomas is based on surgical treatment, combined with radiotherapy and chemotherapy. Due to the specificity of the anatomical locations of gliomas and the characteristics of invasive growth, and the toilless relapse after an operation, the median survival of high-grade glioma patients is only 12–15 months, and the 5-year survival rate is <5% (2).

Clinical practice has proven that chemotherapy can effectively improve the survival time and rate of glioma patients in the comprehensive treatment of glioma. Among the first-line chemotherapeutic drugs of gliomas, temozolomide (TMZ) has been considered to be the most effective treatment drug for glioma due to its advantages, such as oral administration, easy penetration through the blood-brain barrier, acidic environment stability, and no toxicity of superposition with other drugs. Studies have shown that postoperative adjuvant TMZ chemotherapy can increase the survival period from 12.1 months to 14.6 months in high-grade glioma patients (3). This 2.5-month survival period extension is a huge improvement in treatment. However, in clinical applications, the efficacy of TMZ was found to be only 46%, and this was even lower in recurrent glioma patients (4). The glioma resistance to TMZ is the most important cause of chemotherapy failure. Studies have shown that glioma TMZ resistance is the result of multiple factors, and the molecular mechanisms are very complex.

In 2012, Dixon et al. (5) investigated the mechanism of selective killing of RAS-mutated tumor cells through the antitumor drug erastin. Then, they discovered and reported a new cell death mode-ferroptosis, which has great differences in morphology, biochemistry and genetic aspects with the presently known apoptosis, necrosis, and autophagic cell death. A number of studies have revealed that ferroptosis plays an important role in cancer development and drug resistance (6, 7). A clear understanding of ferroptosis in glioma TMZ resistance would benefit the clinical practice of applying ferroptosis to glioma therapy. The present review summarizes the mechanisms of ferroptosis, and the signaling pathways involved in ferroptosis and glioma TMZ resistance.

FERROPTOSIS

Ferroptosis is distinct from other forms of regulated cell death, such as apoptosis, autophagy, necroptosis, and pyroptosis (8). The typical signs of ferroptosis are the increase in cellular lipid reactive oxygen, shrunken mitochondria, and the increase in mitochondrial membrane density (5). Studies have found that iron-dependent Fenton reaction and glutathione (GSH) loss, which lead to reactive oxygen species (ROS) accumulation in cells, are the direct causes of ferroptosis. When the iron homeostasis in tissue cells is disrupted, the excess iron would be converted to H_2O_2 and lipid peroxides would be converted into ROS via the Fenton reaction, which induces ferroptosis. However, this can be specifically reversed by iron chelators (9). Cysteine (Cys) is the rate-limiting substrate for GSH synthesis. The Cys uptake in cells is regulated by the cystine/glutamate reverse transporter functional subunit Solute Carrier Family 7 Member 11 (SLC7A11). Ferroptosis inducer erastin induces ferroptosis by inhibiting SLC7A11 from blocking Cys absorption, and reducing GSH synthesis to promote ROS accumulation (5). The decrease in GSH content in cells can also inhibit the activity of Glutathione peroxidase 4 (GPX4), resulting in the decrease in cell antioxidant capacity and lipid reactive oxygen increase, and eventually causing ferroptosis (10, 11). Recently, researchers have found that ferroptosis suppressor protein 1 (FSP1) (previously known as apoptosis-inducing factor mitochondrial 2 [AIFM2]) is a potent ferroptosis resistance factor, which has a protective effect on GPX4 deletion-induced ferroptosis (12, 13). Studies conducted over the past decade have defined core regulators that regulated cell ferroptosis, including GPX4, nuclear factor erythroid 2-related factor 2 (nrf2), SLC7A11, Activated transcription factor 4 (ATF4), p53 (especially acetylation-defective mutant p53) (**Figure 1**), and FSP1. All these regulators also play an important role in glioma TMZ resistance. The present study will review the relationship between ferroptosis and glioma TMZ resistance, and highlight the role of ferroptosis in glioma TMZ resistance.

TEMOZOLOMIDE RESISTANCE IN GLIOMA

The chemical name of TMZ is 3-methyl-4-oxoimidazo[5,1-d](1–3, 5)tetrazine-8-carboxamide. This is an oral alkylating agent, and its antitumor activity was first discovered in 1987 (14). This became the effective first-line chemotherapeutic agent for the treatment of glioma patients since the FDA approved its efficacy in 2005 (15, 16). TMZ elicits cytotoxicity through the methylation of DNA guanine residues at the O6 and N7 positions, and adenine at the N3 position (17). The alkylation of the O6 site on guanine leads to its subsequent nucleotide mispairing with thymine instead of cytosine during the subsequent DNA replication (18). Then, the mismatched lethal base pairs would cause single- and double-strand DNA breaks, induce cell cycle arrest at the G2/M, and eventually lead to cell death (19, 20). As it is known, the methylated DNA can be repaired by methyltransferase, and O6-methylguanine methyltransferase (MGMT) can reverse methylation of the O6 position of guanine. Hence, many studies have proven that glioma patients with high MGMT expression are naturally resistant to TMZ (21, 22). In addition to the natural TMZ resistance, glioma patients can obtain TMZ resistance through a variety of mechanisms when treated with TMZ. Recent advances in the understanding glioma TMZ resistance have introduced presented many novel independent mechanisms, such as epigenetic regulation for transcription, including miRNA (23), histone modification (24, 25), and DNA methylation (26). Autophagy is a mechanism to maintain cell homeostasis, which is activated in tumor cells through radiation and chemotherapeutic agents (27, 28). Furthermore, a number of studies have found that TMZ treatment could induce autophagy to help glioma cells resist the TMZ treatment (16, 29). Apoptosis is the final common pathway triggered by TMZ cytotoxicity (30), and the caspase and Bcl-2 family members all regulate glioma TMZ resistance (30–32). In addition, autophagy also takes part in the TMZ-induced cytotoxicity for glioma cells, and targeting autophagy can be sensitive to TMZ treatment (29). Evidence suggests that glioma stem cells (GSC) is a subpopulation of glioblastoma cells, which are capable of self-renewal, tumorigenesis, radio-resistance, and chemo-resistance (including TMZ) (33–35). Recent studies have shown that ferroptosis takes part in glioma TMZ resistance, which may be a new potential mechanism for TMZ resistance in glioma. This will be discussed in detail below.

FERROPTOSIS AND GLIOMA TEMOZOLOMIDE RESISTANCE

The Role of Iron Metabolism in Ferroptosis and TMZ Resistance

Ferroptosis is an iron dependent form of programmed cell death, and the excess iron contributes to ferroptosis by producing ROS through Fenton reaction (36). Iron is an inorganic element for cell basic function, and is especially highly required for cancer cells (37). The iron metabolism is a complex network of iron absorption, storage, and export. Transferrin receptor (TfR1) binds ferric iron ($Fe3+$) in circulation, and binds to the membrane protein transferrin receptor (TfR). Then, the Tf-Fe-TfR conjugate enters the cell through clathrin-mediated endocytosis (38). Cytoplasmic iron is stored in ferritin, which is an iron storage protein complex that consists of ferritin light

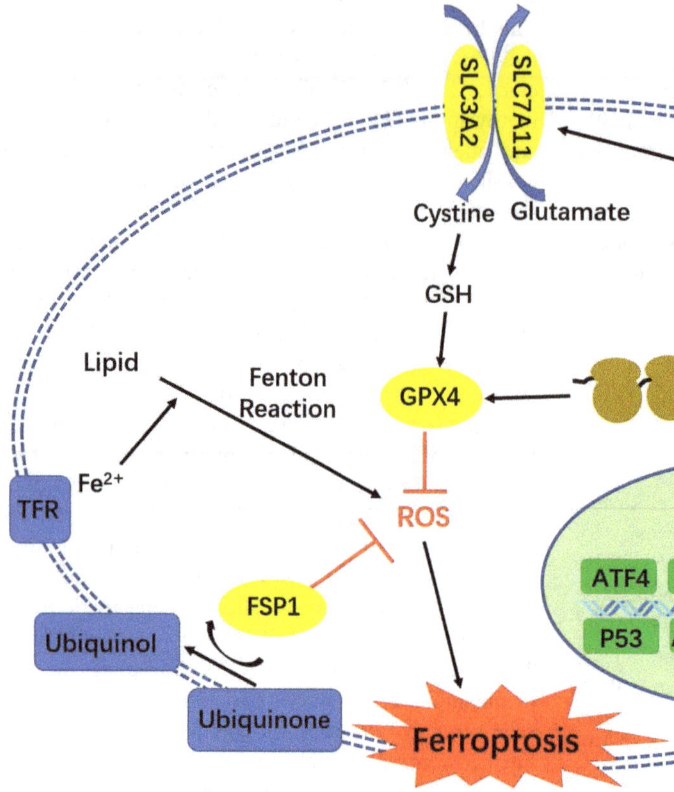

FIGURE 1 | The regulatory network of ferroptosis.

chain (FTL) and ferritin heavy chain 1 (FTH1). Finally, the excess iron is exported by the membrane protein ferroportin (an iron efflux pump, also termed as SLC11A3) (39).

Many studies have shown that iron is an essential element for drug-resistant cells. Hence, ferroptosis, which is an iron-related cell death, also plays an important role in cancer drug-resistance. Schonberg et al. (40) reported that the expression of transferrin is upregulated in GSC, and that the iron uptake promoted the GSC proliferation, while disrupting the iron metabolism in GSCs could reduce the GSC cell growth (41). Multiple studies have revealed that the expression of TfR1 and TfR2 are upregulated in proliferating and malignant cells, including GBM (42, 43). The study conducted by Calzolari et al. has proven that TfR2 expression is inversely correlated with tumor histologic grade, and is associated with the sensitivity to TMZ of glioma cells (43, 44). Feng et al. (45) reported that TfR is a specific ferroptosis maker. These results show that iron metabolism is involved in glioma TMZ resistance and ferroptosis. Furthermore, the study conducted by Chen et al. (46) has proven that erastin (ferroptosis inducer) sensitizes glioma cells to TMZ. Iron-chelating agents (ferroptosis inhibitor), which are used to remove excess iron by binding free iron, can enhance the TMZ cytotoxicity in glioma cells. The study conducted by Alexiou et al. (47) has proven that deferiprone (DFP), which is an orally administered iron chelator, can significantly reduce glioma cell viability combination with TMZ. It has been reported that curcumin, which is a biologically active iron chelator (48, 49), can sensitizes glioma to TMZ by simultaneously generating ROS and disrupting the AKT/mTOR signaling (50). Recently, Chen et al. (51) reported that ALZ003, which is a curcumin analog, induces ferroptosis by blocking the AR-mediated GPX4 expression, inhibiting TMZ–resistant glioblastoma.

ROS in Ferroptosis and TMZ Resistance

ROS is produced by metabolic pathways, and play important roles in tissue homeostasis and cell signaling (52, 53). The iron-dependent accumulation of ROS is the characteristic of ferroptosis (54). Furthermore, ROS-induced lipid peroxidation is not only a critical role in ferroptosis, but also affects the apoptosis, autophagy, and TMZ resistance in glioma cells (53, 55, 56). Biochemically, the intracellular GSH depletion, which inhibits anti-peroxidant defense and iron, involved in the Fenton reaction would result to the accumulation of lipid peroxidation, promoting ferroptosis. The present study will summarize the lipid peroxidation regulating mechanism between ferroptosis and glioma TMZ resistance.

SLC7A11 Regulates Ferroptosis in Glioma TMZ Resistance

SLC7A11, which is also known as xCT, encodes 12 transmembrane domains, and is a functional subunit that constitutes the cystine/glutamate counter transporter (System

Xc-) that regulates the intracellular glutamate and extracellular cystine exchange. Cysteine is the rate-limiting substrate for the synthesis of biological antioxidant glutathione (GSH). Sufficient cystine can ensure the synthesis of intracellular GSH, and the level of GSH in cells plays an important role in glioma drug resistance (57). Chen et al. reported that highly expressed SLC7A11 in gliomas can regulate the resistance of TMZ. However, suppressing the SLC7A11 expression can enhance the sensitivity of gliomas to TMZ using siRNA (46). Polewski et al. (58) also confirmed that the inhibition of SLC7A11 expression in gliomas can reduce the level of GSH in cells, and increase the sensitivity to TMZ.

The latest research shows that SLC7A11 plays an important role in the regulation of ferroptosis. SLC7A11 can participate in ferroptosis by regulating the synthesis of GSH, affecting the level of ROS in cells, and the accumulation of lipid peroxides. Studies have shown that salicylic acid sulfapyridine (SAS) inhibits SLC7A11 activity, which can cause ferroptosis and increase the cystine intake using β-mercaptoethanol, in order to reverse the ferroptosis inducer erastin-induced ferroptosis in HT1080 cells (5). Jiang et al. (59) reported that the overexpression of SLC7A11 in tumor cells inhibits ROS-induced ferroptosis, and weakens the inhibitory effect of p53 3KR on tumor growth. In the SLC7A11 knockout mouse model, SLCA11 was confirmed to inhibit the cell ferroptosis induced by iron overload (60). The toxicity of TMZ to glioma cells is correlated to the expression of SLC7A11, and ferroptosis would enhance this effect of TMZ (61). These findings suggest that SLC7A11 may play an important role in the TMZ resistance of glioma by regulating ferroptosis.

The Effect of GPX4 in Ferroptosis and TMZ Resistance

GPX4 is a powerful antioxidant enzyme in the body. GSH is used as a substrate to reduce lipid oxidation products, and suppress the ferroptosis. The ferroptosis inducer RSL3 mainly induces ferroptosis by inhibiting the activity of GPX4. The expression of GPX4 in gliomas increases with the increasing grades of gliomas, and the expression of GPX suppressed by siRNA can inhibit the proliferation and migration of glioma cells (62). Further studies have found that GPX4 plays an important role in tumor resistance. Inhibiting the activity of GPX4 can enhance the ferroptosis of drug-resistant cells, and thereby enhance the sensitivity to chemotherapeutics (63). The treatment of glioma cells with the GPX4 inhibitor RSL3 can enhance the ferroptosis of cells (64). All these studies suggest that GPX4 may play an important role in the resistance of tumor cells by regulating ferroptosis, including glioma TMZ resistance, but the regulatory mechanisms need further study.

The Effect of ACSL4 in Ferroptosis and TMZ Resistance

Yang et al. (65) reported that polyunsaturated fatty acids (PUFAs) are the most susceptible lipids to ROS damage in the course of ferroptosis, when compared to other the classes of lipids by lipidomics analysis. Acyl-CoA synthetase long-chain family member 4 (ACSL4) is a member of the long chain family of acyl-CoA synthetase proteins, and an enzyme responsible for esterifying polyunsaturated fatty acids (PUFA) into acyl CoA, which is a necessary step to form PUFA-containing phospholipids (66, 67). Yuan et al. (67) reported that ACSL4 contributes to ferroptosis by producing of 5-hydroxyeicosatetraenoic acid (5-HETE). The study conducted by Doll et al. has also proven that the inhibition of ACSL4 expression could decrease the oxidization of a number of sensitive fatty acids (arachidonic acid [AA] and AdA-containing PE species) in the membrane, as critical determinants of sensitivity to ferroptosis. Furthermore, the pharmacological inhibition of ACSL4 (such as thiazolidinediones [TZD]) could prevent ferroptosis (66). Recently, Cheng et al. reported that the expression of ACSL4 was downregulated in human glioma tissues and cells. The overexpression of ACSL4 decreased the expression of GPX4, increased the levels of 5-HETE, and induced a reduction in cell viability. The siRNA-mediated silencing of ACSL4 promoted the proliferation in glioma cells via the decrease in ferroptosis through the enhancement of GPX4 expression. All these results suggest that ACSL4 inhibition directly affects the expression of GPx4, which finally promotes glioma cell proliferation by inhibiting ferroptosis (68). As mentioned above, GPX4 plays an important role in the resistance of tumor cells by regulating ferroptosis. Therefore, ACSL4 may also regulate TMZ resistance in gliomas by affecting the GPX4 expression. However, the study of its resistance to TMZ in gliomas has not been reported at present.

Other Pathways Regulate Ferroptosis and Glioma TMZ Resistance

Nrf2 Regulates Ferroptosis in Glioma TMZ Resistance

Nrf2 is an important transcription factor that regulates the antioxidant stress response in cells, and is mainly combined with the antioxidant response element (ARE) to regulate downstream antioxidant protein expression, and respond to oxidative stress. In Nrf2 knockout mice, it was found that Nrf2 appears with two different effects on the occurrence and development of tumors: under physiological conditions, it can protect normal cells and suppress tumorigenesis; however, it has a "dark" side in the pathophysiological process of tumorigenesis and development. Nrf2 and its downstream genes are highly expressed in many tumor cells (including gliomas) or tissues, and it has a role in promoting tumor growth, proliferation, and drug resistance (69–72). Numerous studies have shown that Nrf2 also plays an important role in TMZ resistance in gliomas (73–75). The treatment of glioma cells with TMZ would induce high expression of Nrf2, and the inhibition of Nrf2 expression can increase the sensitivity of glioma cells to TMZ (73–75).

Many researches have shown that Nrf2 also plays an important role in the regulation of ferroptosis. Kerins et al. reported that several genes (FTL/FTH1, FPN1, and GPX4) involved in iron storage and iron ion export are regulated by Nrf2. Hence, Nrf2 can affect cell iron stability and regulate iron-dependent cell death-ferroptosis (76). Another study further pointed out that Nrf2 is a negative regulator of ferroptosis, and that the ferroptosis inducer erastin can inhibit the degradation of Nrf2 by regulating the p62-Keap1-NRF2 signal pathway, thereby inhibiting the occurrence of ferroptosis in hepatoma cells (77). The inhibition of the Nrf2-ARE pathway could reverse the resistance to drugs and ferroptosis in head-neck cancer cells (78). Patients with highly expressed Nrf2 in gliomas have poor prognosis and a short survival time (64). The overexpression of Nrf2 can promote the proliferation of glioma cells. Further studies have found that Nrf2 can regulate the expression of SLC7A11 to resist ferroptosis (64). Wang et al. also demonstrated that iron can regulates SLC7A11 transcription through ROS-Nrf2-ARE, thereby affecting the occurrence of ferroptosis in liver cells (60). These above findings indicate that Nrf2 can resist ferroptosis by regulating the expression of SLC7A11, which could affect the TMZ resistance of glioma by regulating ferroptosis.

ATF4 Regulates Ferroptosis in Glioma TMZ Resistance

Activated transcription factor 4 (ATF4) is a basic leucine zipper transcription factor that belongs to the cAMP response element binding protein (CREB) family, which is also known as cAMP-response element binding protein2 (CREB2). This regulates the downstream gene transcription by binding an amino acid response element (AARE) in the promoter of the target gene. ATF4 is involved in regulating a variety of physiological and pathological processes, such as the regulation of hematopoiesis, osteoblast differentiation, endoplasmic reticulum stress, and tumor growth. Previous studies have reported that the promoter region of SLC7A11 contains two AARE elements, which is a direct downstream gene of ATF4. ATF4 in bladder cancer cells can regulate the expression of SLC7A11 (79). Studies have shown that glioma patients with a high expression of ATF4 have a shorter survival time, and ATF4 can inhibit the ferroptosis of glioma cells by regulating the expression of the downstream gene SLC7A11, in order to promote tumor proliferation and angiogenesis (80). More recently, Chen et al. (81) reported that Dihydroartemisinin (DHA) could induce ferroptosis in glioma cells through the PERK/ATF4/HSPA5 pathway. Further research has revealed that the TMZ treatment of glioma cells led to the increase in ATF4 expression, the overexpression of ATF4 can enhance the glioma cells resistance to TMZ, and the inhibition of ATF4 expression can increase the sensitivity of glioma cells to TMZ. Furthermore, the ATF4 promotion to glioma TMZ resistance was achieved by enhancing the expression of SLC7A11 (82). In brief, these findings indicate that ATF4 can affect glioma ferroptosis and TMZ resistance by regulating the expression of SLC7A11.

Effect of P53 in Ferroptosis and TMZ Resistance

P53 is one of the most extensively studied tumor suppressor gene, and was named for encoding a 53 KD protein. Normal P53 in cells can regulate cell proliferation, DNA damage repair, senescence, and apoptosis, etc. When P53 mutated, it loses the function of regulation of cell growth, and becomes an oncogene. Studies have shown that P53 also plays an important role in TMZ resistance in gliomas. Lee et al. reported that the effect of TMZ and chloroquine in the treatment of gliomas depend on the p53 condition, and that the combination therapy can inhibit the proliferation of P53-positive glioma cells and the promotion of apoptosis. However, this has no effect on glioma cells with mutant P53 (83). Further studies have found that mutations and deletions in the P53 gene frequently occur in gliomas. Another research revealed that 28% of glioma patients had P53 mutations (84), while P53 mutations are considered to have a negative influence on glioma radiotherapy and TMZ therapy (85, 86). P53 mutation is closely correlated to the poor prognosis of patients with glioblastoma, and may reduce the sensitivity of glioblastoma to TMZ by increasing the expression of drug resistance gene MGMT (87).

Recent studies have shown that P53 also plays an important role in the regulation of ferroptosis. P53 directly targets SLC7A11, and reduces the cell uptake of cystine by inhibiting the transcription of SLC7A11, thereby limiting the production of GSH in cells, significantly increasing the sensitivity of ferroptosis, and further discovering an acetylation defect p53 3KR mutant. Hence, this loses its ability to induce cell cycle arrest, apoptosis, and aging, but retains the ability to inhibit ferroptosis through the suppression of SLC7A11 (59). P53 can slow down the consumption of GSH in cells and reduce ROS production by regulating the p53-p21 axis, and inhibit ferroptosis due to the metabolic pressure (88). The above-mentioned researches indicate that P53 plays an important role in both TMZ resistance and ferroptosis in gliomas, but the specific regulatory mechanisms still need further studies and elucidation.

The Relationship Among Ferroptosis, Autophagy, Apoptosis, and Glioma TMZ Resistance

As mentioned above, autophagy and apoptosis also play important role in glioma TMZ resistance. An original study reported that ferroptosis is distinct from other regulated cell deaths (RCDs), including autophagy, apoptosis, and necrosis (5). However, recently, numerous studies have revealed that there is a complex relationship between ferroptosis and other types of cell death, including autophagy and apoptosis (89). Hou et al. (90) reported that the activation of the autophagy pathway promotes ferroptosis through the degradation of ferritin. Torii et al. (91) suggested that autophagy contributes to erastin-induced ferroptosis through the generation of lysosomal ROS. Yang et al. (92) reported that autophagy promotes ferroptosis by regulating the novel ARNTL-EGLN1-HIF1A pathway. All these suggest that the activation of the autophagic machinery can trigger ferroptosis, and ferroptosis inducers enhance the cell death by activating the autophagy (89, 93). Considering that autophagy also takes part in glioma TMZ resistance (20), the inhibition of autophagy can enhance the TMZ cytotoxicity to glioma cells (94). These suggest that ferroptosis may play an important role in glioma TMZ resistance. Consistently, a recent study also revealed that the inhibition of autophagy could increase the susceptibility of GSC to TMZ by igniting ferroptosis (95).

Many researches have shown that glioma cells undergo apoptosis after treatment with TMZ (30). Recently, researchers found an interrelationship between ferroptosis and apoptosis, and that ferroptosis may occur while sharing common signals or regulators with apoptosis. Zheng et al. (96) reported that nanomaterial MON-p53 can eradicate cancer cells by switching apoptosis to ferroptosis. Hong et al. suggested that ferroptotic agent-induced ER stress response plays an important role in the cross-talk between ferroptosis and apoptosis (97, 98). Furthermore, lipid peroxidation not only leads to ferroptosis, but also stimulates the activation of both the intrinsic and extrinsic apoptotic signaling pathways (53). All these suggest that ferroptosis may regulate glioma TMZ resistance by affecting the autophagy or apoptosis. However, the mechanism needs further research.

CONCLUSION AND PERSPECTIVE

The mechanism of gliomas drug resistance to TMZ is very complex, and is not fully understood. The present understanding cannot explain all drug resistance phenomena, and the present status of TMZ drug resistance has not improved in clinical gliomas. Ferroptosis is a newly discovered death mode, which plays an important role in the TMZ resistance of gliomas, and ferroptosis resistance may be a new mechanism of TMZ resistance in gliomas. Targeted ferroptosis can be used as one of the potential therapies to reverse TMZ resistance. This would be the multi-cytotoxic strategy, in which ferroptosis inducers or xCT inhibitors combination with TMZ are used to treat glioma patients. As a chemo-sensitizer by ferroptosis-induction, erastin could sensitize glioblastoma cells to temozolomide (46). A curcumin analog (ALZ003) could induce the TMZ-resistant glioma cell growth ferroptosis by disrupting the GPX4-Mediated redox homeostasis (51). This suggests that GPX4 and alter ROS could be novel targets for developing anti-cancer drugs. Although the advantages of ferroptosis are promising in cancer treatment, there are still details that needs to be formally addressed in the pre-clinical setting and clinical achievability, and this is partly due to the complexity observed in different contexts, such as P53 or Ras-mutant cancer cells (8). Hence, further studies on ferroptosis mechanism in the TMZ resistance of gliomas would provide new ideas and new targets for the clinical reversal of drug resistance in glioma TMZ chemotherapy.

AUTHOR CONTRIBUTIONS

ZH and HQ produced the manuscript. YZ and XG conceived and designed framework of this article. ZH and NG collected and analyzed the literature. All authors contributed to the article and approved the submitted version.

FUNDING

This work was supported by the National Natural Science Foundation of China (Nos. 81873740 and 81601376), the Shaanxi Youth Talents Project, Scientific Research program Funded by Shaanxi Provincial Education Department (No. 19JS057), the Xi'an Medical University Key Disciplines of Molecular Immunology and the Foundation of Xi'an Medical University (2018PT08, 2018PT10, and 2018DXS1-10), and the Youth Innovation Team of Shaanxi University.

ACKNOWLEDGMENTS

The authors appreciate the valuable suggestions from the other members of their laboratories.

REFERENCES

1. Ostrom QT, Gittleman H, Xu J, Kromer C, Wolinsky Y, Kruchko C, et al. CBTRUS statistical report: primary brain and other central nervous system tumors diagnosed in the United States in 2009-2013. *Neuro Oncol.* (2016) 18:v1–v75. doi: 10.1093/neuonc/now207
2. Khasraw M, Lassman AB. Advances in the treatment of malignant gliomas. *Curr Oncol Rep.* (2010) 1:26–33. doi: 10.1007/s11912-009-0077-4
3. Thomas AA, Brennan CW, DeAngelis LM, Omuro AM. Emerging therapies for glioblastoma. *JAMA Neurol.* (2014) 11:1437–44. doi: 10.1001/jamaneurol.2014.1701
4. Garcia M, Clopes A, Bruna J, Martinez M, Fort E, Gil M. Critical appraisal of temozolomide formulations in the treatment of primary brain tumors: patient considerations. *Cancer Manage Res.* (2009) 2009:137–150. doi: 10.2147/CMAR.S5598
5. Dixon SJ, Lemberg KM, Lamprecht MR, Skouta R, Zaitsev EM, Gleason CE, et al. Ferroptosis: an iron-dependent form of nonapoptotic cell death. *Cell.* (2012) 5:1060–72. doi: 10.1016/j.cell.2012.03.042
6. Friedmann Angeli JP, Krysko DV, Conrad M. Ferroptosis at the crossroads of cancer-acquired drug resistance and immune evasion. *Nat Rev Cancer.* (2019) 7:405–14. doi: 10.1038/s41568-019-0149-1
7. Gao X, Guo N, Xu H, Pan T, Lei H, Yan A, et al. Ibuprofen induces ferroptosis of glioblastoma cells via downregulation of nuclear factor erythroid 2-related factor 2 signaling pathway. *Anticancer Drugs.* (2020) 31:27–34. doi: 10.1097/CAD.0000000000000825
8. Mou Y, Wang J, Wu J, He D, Zhang C, Duan C, et al. Ferroptosis, a new form of cell death: opportunities and challenges in cancer. *J Hematol Oncol.* (2019) 1:34. doi: 10.1186/s13045-019-0720-y
9. Xie Y, Hou W, Song X, Yu Y, Huang J, Sun X, et al. Ferroptosis: process and function. *Cell Death Differ.* (2016) 3:369–79. doi: 10.1038/cdd.2015.158
10. Yang WS, Sri Ramaratnam R, Welsch ME, Shimada K, Skouta R, Viswanathan VS, et al. Regulation of ferroptotic cancer cell death by GPX4. *Cell.* (2014) 1-2:317–31. doi: 10.1016/j.cell.2013.12.010
11. Dixon SJ, Stockwell BR. The hallmarks of ferroptosis. *Annu Rev Canc Biol.* (2019) 3:35–54. doi: 10.1146/annurev-cancerbio-030518-055844
12. Bersuker K, Hendricks JM, Li Z, Magtanong L, Ford B, Tang PH, et al. The CoQ oxidoreductase FSP1 acts parallel to GPX4 to inhibit ferroptosis. *Nature.* (2019) 7784:688–92. doi: 10.1038/s41586-019-1705-2
13. Doll S, Freitas FP, Shah R, Aldrovandi M, da Silva MC, Ingold I, et al. FSP1 is a glutathione-independent ferroptosis suppressor. *Nature.* (2019) 7784:693–8. doi: 10.1038/s41586-019-1707-0
14. Stevens MF, Hickman JA, Langdon SP, Chubb D, Vickers L, Stone R, et al. Antitumor activity and pharmacokinetics in mice of 8-carbamoyl-3-methyl-imidazo[5,1-d]-1,2,3,5-tetrazin-4(3H)-one (CCRG 81045; M & B 39831), a novel drug with potential as an alternative to dacarbazine. *Cancer Res.* (1987) 22:5846–52.
15. Stupp R, Mason WP, van den Bent MJ, Weller M, Fisher B, Taphoorn MJ, et al. Radiotherapy plus concomitant and adjuvant temozolomide for glioblastoma. *N Engl J Med.* (2005) 10:987–96. doi: 10.1056/NEJMoa043330

16. Jiapaer S, Furuta T, Tanaka S, Kitabayashi T, Nakada M. Potential strategies overcoming the temozolomide resistance for glioblastoma. *Neurol Med Chir (Tokyo).* (2018) 10:405–21. doi: 10.2176/nmc.ra.2018-0141
17. Denny BJ, Wheelhouse RT, Stevens MF, Tsang LL, Slack JA. NMR and molecular modeling investigation of the mechanism of activation of the antitumor drug temozolomide and its interaction with DNA. *Biochemistry.* (1994) 31:9045–51. doi: 10.1021/bi00197a003
18. Kanzawa T, Bedwell J, Kondo Y, Kondo S, Germano IM. Inhibition of DNA repair for sensitizing resistant glioma cells to temozolomide. *J Neurosurg.* (2003) 6:1047–52. doi: 10.3171/jns.2003.99.6.1047
19. Lee SY. Temozolomide resistance in glioblastoma multiforme. *Genes Dis.* (2016) 3:198–210. doi: 10.1016/j.gendis.2016.04.007
20. Kanzawa T, Germano IM, Komata T, Ito H, Kondo Y, Kondo S. Role of autophagy in temozolomide-induced cytotoxicity for malignant glioma cells. *Cell Death Differ.* (2004) 4:448–57. doi: 10.1038/sj.cdd.4401359
21. van Nifterik KA, van den Berg J, van der Meide WF, Ameziane N, Wedekind LE, Steenbergen RDM, et al. Absence of the MGMT protein as well as methylation of the MGMT promoter predict the sensitivity for temozolomide. *Br J Cancer.* (2010) 1:29–35. doi: 10.1038/sj.bjc.6605712
22. Donson AM, Addo-Yobo SO, Handler MH, Gore L, Foreman NK. MGMT promoter methylation correlates with survival benefit and sensitivity to temozolomide in pediatric glioblastoma. *Pediatr Blood Cancer.* (2007) 4:403–7. doi: 10.1002/pbc.20803
23. Li Y, Liu Y, Ren J, Deng S, Yi G, Guo M, et al. miR-1268a regulates ABCC1 expression to mediate temozolomide resistance in glioblastoma. *J Neuro Oncol.* (2018) 3:499–508. doi: 10.1007/s11060-018-2835-3
24. Banelli B, Carra E, Barbieri F, Wurth R, Parodi F, Pattarozzi A, et al. The histone demethylase KDM5A is a key factor for the resistance to temozolomide in glioblastoma. *Cell Cycle.* (2015) 21:3418–29. doi: 10.1080/15384101.2015.1090063
25. Abe H, Natsumeda M, Kanemaru Y, Watanabe J, Tsukamoto Y, Okada M, et al. MGMT expression contributes to temozolomide resistance in H3K27M-mutant diffuse midline gliomas and MGMT silencing to temozolomide sensitivity in IDH-mutant gliomas. *Neurol Med Chir.* (2018) 7:290–5. doi: 10.2176/nmc.ra.2018-0044
26. Chai RC, Chang YZ, Wang QW, Zhang KN, Li JJ, Huang H, et al. A novel DNA methylation-based signature can predict the responses of MGMT promoter unmethylated glioblastomas to temozolomide. *Front Genet.* (2019) 10:910. doi: 10.3389/fgene.2019.00910
27. Sui X, Chen R, Wang Z, Huang Z, Kong N, Zhang M, et al. Autophagy and chemotherapy resistance: a promising therapeutic target for cancer treatment. *Cell Death Dis.* (2013) 4:e838. doi: 10.1038/cddis.2013.350
28. Gewirtz DA. The challenge of developing autophagy inhibition as a therapeutic strategy. *Cancer Res.* (2016) 19:5610–4. doi: 10.1158/0008-5472.CAN-16-0722
29. Yan Y, Xu Z, Dai S, Qian L, Sun L, Gong Z. Targeting autophagy to sensitive glioma to temozolomide treatment. *J Exp Clin Cancer Res.* (2016) 35:23. doi: 10.1186/s13046-016-0303-5
30. Roos WP, Batista LF, Naumann SC, Wick W, Weller M, Menck CF, et al. Apoptosis in malignant glioma cells triggered by the temozolomide-induced DNA lesion O6-methylguanine. *Oncogene.* (2007) 2:186–97. doi: 10.1038/sj.onc.1209785
31. Li G, Zhang H, Liu Y, Kong L, Guo Q, Jin F. Effect of temozolomide on livin and caspase-3 in U251 glioma stem cells. *Exp Ther Med.* (2015) 3:744–50. doi: 10.3892/etm.2014.2144
32. Gratas C, Sery Q, Rabe M, Oliver L, Vallette FM. Bak and Mcl-1 are essential for Temozolomide induced cell death in human glioma. *Oncotarget.* (2014) 9:2428–35. doi: 10.18632/oncotarget.1642
33. Bao S, Wu Q, McLendon RE, Hao Y, Shi Q, Hjelmeland AB, et al. Glioma stem cells promote radioresistance by preferential activation of the DNA damage response. *Nature.* (2006) 7120:756–60. doi: 10.1038/nature05236
34. Lathia JD, Mack SC, Mulkearns-Hubert EE, Valentim CL, Rich JN. Cancer stem cells in glioblastoma. *Genes Dev.* (2015) 12:1203–17. doi: 10.1101/gad.261982.115
35. Fukushima T, Takeshima H, Kataoka H. Anti-glioma therapy with temozolomide and status of the DNA-repair gene MGMT. *Anticancer Res.* (2009) 11:4845–54.
36. Wang S, Luo J, Zhang Z, Dong D, Shen Y, Fang Y, et al. Iron and magnetic: new research direction of the ferroptosis-based cancer therapy. *Am J Cancer Res.* (2018) 10:1933–46.
37. Wang Y, Yu L, Ding J, Chen Y. Iron metabolism in cancer. *Int J Mol Sci.* (2019) 20:95. doi: 10.3390/ijms20010095
38. Mayle KM, Le AM, Kamei DT. The intracellular trafficking pathway of transferrin. *Biochim Biophys Acta.* (2012) 3:264–81. doi: 10.1016/j.bbagen.2011.09.009
39. Kazan HH, Urfali-Mamatoglu C, Gunduz U. Iron metabolism and drug resistance in cancer. *Biometals.* (2017) 5:629–41. doi: 10.1007/s10534-017-0037-7
40. Schonberg DL, Miller TE, Wu Q, Flavahan WA, Das NK, Hale JS, et al. Preferential iron trafficking characterizes glioblastoma stem-like cells. *Cancer Cell.* (2015) 4:441–55. doi: 10.1016/j.ccell.2015.09.002
41. Legendre C, Garcion E. Iron metabolism: a double-edged sword in the resistance of glioblastoma to therapies. *Trends Endocrinol Metab.* (2015) 6:322–31. doi: 10.1016/j.tem.2015.03.008
42. Recht L, Torres CO, Smith TW, Raso V, Griffin TW. Transferrin receptor in normal and neoplastic brain tissue: implications for brain-tumor immunotherapy. *J Neurosurg.* (1990) 6:941–5. doi: 10.3171/jns.1990.72.6.0941
43. Voth B, Nagasawa DT, Pelargos PE, Chung LK, Ung N, Gopen Q, et al. Transferrin receptors and glioblastoma multiforme: current findings and potential for treatment. *J Clin Neurosci.* (2015) 7:1071–6. doi: 10.1016/j.jocn.2015.02.002
44. Calzolari A, Larocca LM, Deaglio S, Finisguerra V, Boe A, Raggi C, et al. Transferrin receptor 2 is frequently and highly expressed in glioblastomas. *Transl Oncol.* (2010) 2:123–34. doi: 10.1593/tlo.09274
45. Feng H, Schorpp K, Jin J, Yozwiak CE, Hoffstrom BG, Decker AM, et al. Transferrin receptor is a specific ferroptosis marker. *Cell Rep.* (2020) 10:3411–23.e3417. doi: 10.1016/j.celrep.2020.02.049
46. Chen L, Li X, Liu L, Yu B, Xue Y, Liu Y. Erastin sensitizes glioblastoma cells to temozolomide by restraining xCT and cystathionine-gamma-lyase function. *Oncol Rep.* (2015) 3:1465–74. doi: 10.3892/or.2015.3712
47. Alexiou GA, Gerogianni P, Vartholomatos E, Kyritsis AP. Deferiprone enhances temozolomide cytotoxicity in glioma cells. *Cancer Invest.* (2016) 10:489–95. doi: 10.1080/07357907.2016.1233424
48. Jiao Y, Wilkinson J 4th, Di X, Wang W, Hatcher H, Kock ND, et al. Curcumin, a cancer chemopreventive and chemotherapeutic agent, is a biologically active iron chelator. *Blood.* (2009) 2:462–9. doi: 10.1182/blood-2008-05-155952
49. Jiao Y, Wilkinson J 4th, Christine Pietsch E, Buss JL, Wang W, Planalp R, et al. Iron chelation in the biological activity of curcumin. *Free Radic Biol Med.* (2006) 7:1152–60. doi: 10.1016/j.freeradbiomed.2005.11.003
50. Yin H, Zhou Y, Wen C, Zhou C, Zhang W, Hu X, et al. Curcumin sensitizes glioblastoma to temozolomide by simultaneously generating ROS and disrupting AKT/mTOR signaling. *Oncol Rep.* (2014) 4:1610–6. doi: 10.3892/or.2014.3342
51. Chen TC, Chuang JY, Ko CY, Kao TJ, Yang PY, Yu CH, et al. AR ubiquitination induced by the curcumin analog suppresses growth of temozolomide-resistant glioblastoma through disrupting GPX4-Mediated redox homeostasis. *Redox Biol.* (2020) 30:101413. doi: 10.1016/j.redox.2019.101413
52. Ferreira CA, Ni D, Rosenkrans ZT, Cai W. Scavenging of reactive oxygen and nitrogen species with nanomaterials. *Nano Res.* (2018) 10:4955–84. doi: 10.1007/s12274-018-2092-y
53. Su LJ, Zhang JH, Gomez H, Murugan R, Hong X, Xu D, et al. Reactive oxygen species-induced lipid peroxidation in apoptosis, autophagy, and ferroptosis. *Oxid Med Cell Longev.* (2019) 2019:5080843. doi: 10.1155/2019/5080843
54. Sui X, Zhang R, Liu S, Duan T, Zhai L, Zhang M, et al. RSL3 drives ferroptosis through GPX4 inactivation and ROS production in colorectal cancer. *Front Pharmacol.* (2018) 9:1371. doi: 10.3389/fphar.2018.01371
55. Wu W, Wu Y, Mayer K, von Rosenstiel C, Schecker J, Baur S, et al. Lipid peroxidation plays an important role in chemotherapeutic effects of temozolomide and the development of therapy resistance in human glioblastoma. *Transl Oncol.* (2020) 3:100748. doi: 10.1016/j.tranon.2020.100748

56. Lo Dico A, Salvatore D, Martelli C, Ronchi D, Diceglie C, Lucignani G, et al. Intracellular redox-balance involvement in temozolomide resistance-related molecular mechanisms in glioblastoma. *Cells.* (2019) 8:1315. doi: 10.3390/cells8111315
57. Zhu ZL, Du SS, Du YB, Ren J, Ying GG, Yan Z. Glutathione reductase mediates drug resistance in glioblastoma cells by regulating redox homeostasis. *J Neurochem.* (2018) 1:93–104. doi: 10.1111/jnc.14250
58. Polewski MD, Reveron-Thornton RF, Cherryholmes GA, Marinov GK, Cassady K, Aboody KS. Increased expression of system xc- in glioblastoma confers an altered metabolic state and temozolomide resistance. *Mol Cancer Res.* (2016) 12:1229–42. doi: 10.1158/1541-7786.MCR-16-0028
59. Jiang L, Kon N, Li TY, Wang SJ, Su T, Hibshoosh H, et al. Ferroptosis as a p53-mediated activity during tumour suppression. *Nature.* (2015) 7545:57–62. doi: 10.1038/nature14344
60. Wang H, An P, Xie E, Wu Q, Fang X, Gao H, et al. Characterization of ferroptosis in murine models of hemochromatosis. *Hepatology.* (2017) 2:449–65. doi: 10.1002/hep.29117
61. Sehm T, Rauh M, Wiendieck K, Buchfelder M, Eyupoglu IY, Savaskan NE. Temozolomide toxicity operates in a xCT/SLC7a11 dependent manner and is fostered by ferroptosis. *Oncotarget.* (2016) 46:74630–47. doi: 10.18632/oncotarget.11858
62. Zhao HY, Ji B, Chen JG, Huang QF, Lu XG. Gpx 4 is involved in the proliferation, migration and apoptosis of glioma cells. *Pathol Res Pract.* (2017) 6:626–33. doi: 10.1016/j.prp.2017.04.025
63. Hangauer MJ, Viswanathan VS, Ryan MJ, Bole D, Eaton JK, Matov A, et al. Drug-tolerant persister cancer cells are vulnerable to GPX4 inhibition. *Nature.* (2017) 7679:247–50. doi: 10.1038/nature24297
64. Fan Z, Wirth AK, Chen D, Wruck CJ, Rauh M, Buchfelder M, et al. Nrf2-Keap1 pathway promotes cell proliferation and diminishes ferroptosis. *Oncogenesis.* (2017) 8:e371. doi: 10.1038/oncsis.2017.65
65. Yang WS, Kim KJ, Gaschler MM, Patel M, Shchepinov MS, Stockwell BR. Peroxidation of polyunsaturated fatty acids by lipoxygenases drives ferroptosis. *Proc Natl Acad Sci U S A.* (2016) 34:E4966–4975. doi: 10.1073/pnas.1603244113
66. Doll S, Proneth B, Tyurina YY, Panzilius E, Kobayashi S, Ingold I, et al. ACSL4 dictates ferroptosis sensitivity by shaping cellular lipid composition. *Nat Chem Biol.* (2017) 1:91–8. doi: 10.1038/nchembio.2239
67. Yuan H, Li X, Zhang X, Kang R, Tang D. Identification of ACSL4 as a biomarker and contributor of ferroptosis. *Biochem Biophys Res Commun.* (2016) 3:1338–43. doi: 10.1016/j.bbrc.2016.08.124
68. Cheng J, Fan YQ, Liu BH, Zhou H, Wang JM, Chen QX. ACSL4 suppresses glioma cells proliferation via activating ferroptosis. *Oncol Rep.* (2020) 1:147–58. doi: 10.3892/or.2019.7419
69. Jung BJ, Yoo HS, Shin S, Park YJ, Jeon SM. Dysregulation of NRF2 in cancer: from molecular mechanisms to therapeutic opportunities. *Biomol Ther (Seoul).* (2018) 1:57–68. doi: 10.4062/biomolther.2017.195
70. Taguchi K, Yamamoto M. The KEAP1-NRF2 system in cancer. *Front Oncol.* (2017) 7:85. doi: 10.3389/fonc.2017.00085
71. Xia M, Yu H, Gu S, Xu Y, Su J, Li H, et al. p62/SQSTM1 is involved in cisplatin resistance in human ovarian cancer cells via the Keap1-Nrf2-ARE system. *Int J Oncol.* (2014) 6:2341–8. doi: 10.3892/ijo.2014.2669
72. Zhu J, Wang H, Fan Y, Lin Y, Zhang L, Ji X, et al. Targeting the NF-E2-related factor 2 pathway: a novel strategy for glioblastoma (review). *Oncol Rep.* (2014) 2:443–50. doi: 10.3892/or.2014.3259
73. Rocha CR, Kajitani GS, Quinet A, Fortunato RS, Menck CF. NRF2 and glutathione are key resistance mediators to temozolomide in glioma and melanoma cells. *Oncotarget.* (2016) 30:48081–92. doi: 10.18632/oncotarget.10129
74. Shi L, Li H, Zhan Y. All-trans retinoic acid enhances temozolomide-induced autophagy in human glioma cells U251 via targeting Keap1/Nrf2/ARE signaling pathway. *Oncol Lett.* (2017) 3:2709–14. doi: 10.3892/ol.2017.6482
75. Zhang L, Wang H. FTY720 inhibits the Nrf2/ARE pathway in human glioblastoma cell lines and sensitizes glioblastoma cells to temozolomide. *Pharmacol Rep.* (2017) 6:1186–93. doi: 10.1016/j.pharep.2017.07.003
76. Kerins MJ, Ooi A. The roles of NRF2 in modulating cellular iron homeostasis. *Antioxid Redox Signal.* (2018) 29:1756–73. doi: 10.1089/ars.2017.7176
77. Sun X, Ou Z, Chen R, Niu X, Chen D, Kang R, et al. Activation of the p62-Keap1-NRF2 pathway protects against ferroptosis in hepatocellular carcinoma cells. *Hepatology.* (2016) 1:173–84. doi: 10.1002/hep.28251
78. Roh JL, Kim EH, Jang H, Shin D. Nrf2 inhibition reverses the resistance of cisplatin-resistant head and neck cancer cells to artesunate-induced ferroptosis. *Redox Biol.* (2017) 11:254–62. doi: 10.1016/j.redox.2016.12.010
79. Ye P, Mimura J, Okada T, Sato H, Liu T, Maruyama A, et al. Nrf2- and ATF4-dependent upregulation of xCT modulates the sensitivity of T24 bladder carcinoma cells to proteasome inhibition. *Mol Cell Biol.* (2014) 18:3421–34. doi: 10.1128/MCB.00221-14
80. Chen D, Rauh M, Buchfelder M, Eyupoglu IY, Savaskan N. The oxido-metabolic driver ATF4 enhances temozolamide chemo-resistance in human gliomas. *Oncotarget.* (2017) 31:51164–76. doi: 10.18632/oncotarget.17737
81. Chen Y, Mi Y, Zhang X, Ma Q, Song Y, Zhang L, et al. Dihydroartemisinin-induced unfolded protein response feedback attenuates ferroptosis via PERK/ATF4/HSPA5 pathway in glioma cells. *J Exp Clin Cancer Res.* (2019) 1:402. doi: 10.1186/s13046-019-1413-7
82. Chen D, Fan Z, Rauh M, Buchfelder M, Eyupoglu IY, Savaskan N. ATF4 promotes angiogenesis and neuronal cell death and confers ferroptosis in a xCT-dependent manner. *Oncogene.* (2017) 40:5593–608. doi: 10.1038/onc.2017.146
83. Lee SW, Kim HK, Lee NH, Yi HY, Kim HS, Hong SH, et al. The synergistic effect of combination temozolomide and chloroquine treatment is dependent on autophagy formation and p53 status in glioma cells. *Cancer Lett.* (2015) 2:195–204. doi: 10.1016/j.canlet.2015.02.012
84. Shajani-Yi Z, de Abreu FB, Peterson JD, Tsongalis GJ. Frequency of somatic TP53 mutations in combination with known pathogenic mutations in colon adenocarcinoma, non-small cell lung carcinoma, and gliomas as identified by next-generation sequencing. *Neoplasia.* (2018) 3:256–62. doi: 10.1016/j.neo.2017.12.005
85. Blough MD, Beauchamp DC, Westgate MR, Kelly JJ, Cairncross JG. Effect of aberrant p53 function on temozolomide sensitivity of glioma cell lines and brain tumor initiating cells from glioblastoma. *J Neuro Oncol.* (2011) 1:1–7. doi: 10.1007/s11060-010-0283-9
86. Chiang MF, Chou PY, Wang WJ, Sze CI, Chang NS. Tumor suppressor WWOX and p53 alterations and drug resistance in glioblastomas. *Front Oncol.* (2013) 3:43. doi: 10.3389/fonc.2013.00043
87. Wang X, Chen JX, Liu JP, You C, Liu YH, Mao Q. Gain of function of mutant TP53 in glioblastoma: prognosis and response to temozolomide. *Ann Surg Oncol.* (2014) 4:1337–44. doi: 10.1245/s10434-013-3380-0
88. Tarangelo A, Magtanong L, Bieging-Rolett KT, Li Y, Ye J, Attardi LD, et al. p53 Suppresses metabolic stress-induced ferroptosis in cancer cells. *Cell Rep.* (2018) 3:569–75. doi: 10.1016/j.celrep.2017.12.077
89. Zhou B, Liu J, Kang R, Klionsky DJ, Kroemer G, Tang D. Ferroptosis is a type of autophagy-dependent cell death. *Semin Cancer Biol.* (2019). doi: 10.1016/j.semcancer.2019.03.002. [Epub ahead of print].
90. Hou W, Xie Y, Song X, Sun X, Lotze MT, Zeh HJ, et al. Autophagy promotes ferroptosis by degradation of ferritin. *Autophagy.* (2016) 8:1425–8. doi: 10.1080/15548627.2016.1187366
91. Torii S, Shintoku R, Kubota C, Yaegashi M, Torii R, Sasaki M, et al. An essential role for functional lysosomes in ferroptosis of cancer cells. *Biochem J.* (2016) 6:769–77. doi: 10.1042/BJ20150658
92. Yang M, Chen P, Liu J, Zhu S, Kroemer G, Klionsky DJ, et al. Clockophagy is a novel selective autophagy process favoring ferroptosis. *Sci Adv.* (2019) 7:eaaw2238. doi: 10.1126/sciadv.aaw2238
93. Liu J, Kuang F, Kroemer G, Klionsky DJ, Kang R, Tang D. Autophagy-dependent ferroptosis: machinery and regulation. *Cell Chem Biol.* (2020) 27:420–35. doi: 10.1016/j.chembiol.2020.02.005
94. Knizhnik AV, Roos WP, Nikolova T, Quiros S, Tomaszowski KH, Christmann M, et al. Survival and death strategies in glioma cells: autophagy, senescence and apoptosis triggered by a single type of temozolomide-induced DNA damage. *PLoS One.* (2013) 1:e55665. doi: 10.1371/journal.pone.0055665

95. Buccarelli M, Marconi M, Pacioni S, De Pascalis I, D'Alessandris QG, Martini M, et al. Inhibition of autophagy increases susceptibility of glioblastoma stem cells to temozolomide by igniting ferroptosis. *Cell Death Dis.* (2018) 8:841. doi: 10.1038/s41419-018-0864-7
96. Zheng DW, Lei Q, Zhu JY, Fan JX, Li CX, Li C, et al. Switching apoptosis to ferroptosis: metal-organic network for high-efficiency anticancer therapy. *Nano Lett.* (2017) 1:284–291. doi: 10.1021/acs.nanolett.6b04060
97. Lee YS, Lee DH, Choudry HA, Bartlett DL, Lee YJ. Ferroptosis-induced endoplasmic reticulum stress: cross-talk between ferroptosis and apoptosis. *Mol Cancer Res.* (2018) 7:1073–6. doi: 10.1158/1541-7786.MCR-18-0055
98. Hong SH, Lee DH, Lee YS, Jo MJ, Jeong YA, Kwon WT, et al. Molecular crosstalk between ferroptosis and apoptosis: emerging role of ER stress-induced p53-independent PUMA expression. *Oncotarget.* (2017) 70:115164–78. doi: 10.18632/oncotarget.23046

19

Fingolimod Augments Monomethylfumarate Killing of GBM Cells

Paul Dent[1*], *Laurence Booth*[1*], *Jane L. Roberts*[1], *Andrew Poklepovic*[2] *and John F. Hancock*[3]

[1] Departments of Biochemistry and Molecular Biology, Virginia Commonwealth University, Richmond, VA, United States, [2] Departments of Medicine, Virginia Commonwealth University, Richmond, VA, United States, [3] Department of Integrative Biology and Pharmacology, University of Texas Health Science Center, Houston, TX, United States

***Correspondence:**
Paul Dent
paul.dent@vcuhealth.org
Laurence Booth
laurence.booth@vcuhealth.org

Previously we demonstrated that the multiple sclerosis drug dimethyl fumarate (DMF) and its plasma breakdown product MMF could interact with chemotherapeutic agents to kill both GBM cells and activated microglia. The trial NCT02337426 demonstrated the safety of DMF in newly diagnosed GBM patients when combined with the standard of care Stupp protocol. We hypothesized that another multiple sclerosis drug, fingolimod (FTY720) would synergize with MMF to kill GBM cells. MMF and fingolimod interacted in a greater than additive fashion to kill PDX GBM isolates. MMF and fingolimod radiosensitized glioma cells and enhanced the lethality of temozolomide. Exposure to [MMF + fingolimod] activated an ATM-dependent toxic autophagy pathway, enhanced protective endoplasmic reticulum stress signaling, and inactivated protective PI3K, STAT, and YAP function. The drug combination reduced the expression of protective c-FLIP-s, MCL-1, BCL-XL, and in parallel caused cell-surface clustering of the death receptor CD95. Knock down of CD95 or over-expression of c-FLIP-s or BCL-XL suppressed killing. Fingolimod and MMF interacted in a greater than additive fashion to rapidly enhance reactive oxygen species production and over-expression of either thioredoxin or super-oxide dismutase two significantly reduced the drug-induced phosphorylation of ATM, autophagosome formation and [MMF + fingolimod] lethality. In contrast, the production of ROS was only marginally reduced in cells lacking ATM, CD95, or Beclin1. Collectively, our data demonstrate that the primary generation of ROS by [MMF + fingolimod] plays a key role, via the induction of toxic autophagy and death receptor signaling, in the killing of GBM cells.

Keywords: fingolimod, dimethyl fumarate, Gilenya, Tecfidera, RAS, glioblastoma, microglia

INTRODUCTION

Glioblastoma multiforme (GBM) remains an incurable malignancy, with a median survival of ~14 months from initial presentation (1). There are several issues with developing new effective GBM therapeutics; e.g., the blood brain barrier often prevents the full therapeutic dose of many drugs reaching a brain-localized tumor; the brain is also an immunologically privileged environment that results both in a lack of checkpoint immunotherapy efficacy but also in an environment that contains activated brain associated macrophages, the microglia, which promote the growth, invasion, and survival of GBM cells (2–6). In the specific instance of brain tumors, whether metastatic disease or GBMs, activated microglia have a symbiotic relationship with tumor cells, each producing growth factors and cytokines that reinforces the malignant phenotype of the tumor cells (7, 8). Thus, one approach to treat tumors localized in the brain would be to break the symbiotic positive relationship between the microglia and the tumor cells.

Multiple sclerosis is a disease in which brain and spinal cord axons undergo demyelination in part due to the actions of an auto-immune disease (9, 10). Activated T cells can enter the CNS where they cause inflammation that promotes additional demyelination, that in turn attracts macrophages that enhance the inflammatory response. In the past 10 years two novel therapeutic agents have been approved for the treatment of relapsing remitting MS: Gilenya® (fingolimod, FTY720) and Tecfidera® (dimethyl-fumarate, DMF) (11, 12). Both drugs are administered orally (PO). Fingolimod is an analog of sphingosine-1-phosphate (S1P), with a plasma C max of ~150 nM. Fingolimod is taken up and phosphorylated before it then acts in an autocrine fashion to activate S1P receptors; receptor activation results in receptor internalization and its proteolytic destruction (13, 14). This results in reactive T cells not migrating to the site of CNS inflammation, and a reduction in disease sequelae. DMF is rapidly metabolized in the plasma of patients to monomethyl-fumarate (MMF) and has a C max in plasma of ~15 μM, with an approximate steady state tissue and plasma concentration of 5 μM. Most laboratory-based oncology studies have used DMF, not MMF, and in over 90% of all publications have used the drug above the clinically relevant range, and the range recommended by the drug makers, Biogen (15, 16). Thus, very little is known about the "real" biology of MMF. For example, high concentrations of DMF, e.g., 30–100 μM, can rapidly increase expression of the anti-oxidant enzymes NRF2 and HO-1 in tumor cells (17, 18). However, in our hands, using MMF at a clinically relevant concentration of 5 μM, no alterations in NRF2 or HO-1 expression were observed in a genetically diverse set of primary human GBM cells. At supra-physiologic concentrations DMF can suppress the inflammatory biology of microglia and astrocytes (19).

The present studies were performed to determine whether the multiple sclerosis medications fingolimod and MMF interact to kill GBM cells and to determine some of the molecular mechanisms by which killing occurs. Our data strongly argue that ATM-AMPK, CD95-caspase 8, and reactive oxygen species signaling play key roles in the killing efficacy of the drug combination.

Abbreviations: ERK, extracellular regulated kinase; PI3K, phosphatidyl inositol 3 kinase; ca, constitutively active; dn, dominant negative; ER, endoplasmic reticulum; AIF, apoptosis inducing factor; AMPK, AMP-dependent protein kinase; mTOR, mammalian target of rapamycin; JAK, Janus Kinase; STAT, Signal Transducers and Activators of Transcription; MAPK, mitogen activated protein kinase; PTEN, phosphatase and tensin homolog on chromosome ten; ROS, reactive oxygen species; CMV, empty vector plasmid or virus; si, small interfering; SCR, scrambled; IP, immunoprecipitation; VEH, vehicle; DMF, dimethyl fumarate; MMF, monomethyl fumarate; FTY, FTY720, also known as fingolimod and Gilenya; HDAC, histone deacetylase; GBM, glioblastoma multiforme.

MATERIALS AND METHODS

Materials

MMF was purchased from Selleckchem (Houston, TX). Neratinib was kindly supplied by Puma Biotechnology Inc. (Los Angeles, CA). Fingolimod (FTY720) was purchased from Sigma-Aldrich (St. Louis MO). Trypsin-EDTA, DMEM, RPMI, penicillin-streptomycin were purchased from GIBCOBRL (GIBCOBRL Life Technologies, Grand Island, NY). Other reagents and performance of experimental procedures were as described (15, 20–24). Antibodies used: AIF (5318), BAX (5023), BAK (12105), BAD (9239), BIM (2933), BAK1 (12105), Beclin1 (3495), cathepsin B (31718), CD95 (8023), FADD (2782), eIF2α (5324), P-eIF2α S51 (3398), ULK-1 (8054), P-ULK-1 S757 (14202), P-AMPK S51 (2535), AMPKα (2532), P-ATM S1981 (13050), ATM (2873), ATG5 (12994), mTOR (2983), P-mTOR S2448 (5536), P-mTOR S2481 (2974), ATG13 (13468), MCL-1 (94296), BCL-XL (2764), P-AKT T308 (13038), P-ERK1/2 (5726), P-STAT3 Y705 (9145), P-p65 S536 (3033), p62 (23214), LAMP2 (49067) all from Cell Signaling Technology; P-ULK-1 S317 (3803a) from Abgent; P-ATG13 S318 (19127) from Novus Biologicals.

Methods

Culture, Transfection and *in vitro* Exposure of Cells to Drugs

Primary human GBM isolates were grown in bulk in the flanks of NRG mice; multiple tumor isolates were used throughout the studies in this manuscript. Briefly, tumors were isolated, mechanically macerated, filtered and plated in flasks. Initially, cells were cultured at 37°C (5% (v/v CO_2) *in vitro* using RPMI supplemented with 0.5% (v/v) fetal calf serum and 10% (v/v) Non-essential amino acids. After ~2 weeks of growth and several passages to remove contaminating mouse fibroblasts, GBM cells were grown in RPMI supplemented with 2.0% (v/v) fetal calf serum and 10% (v/v) Non-essential amino acids. Cells were frozen down in bulk and each vial grown/utilized for a maximum of four weeks of *in vitro* culture. Stem cell variants of the PDX GBM isolates were prepared as described (15, 25–27). Freshly isolated GBM cells and activated microglia directly from the operating room were separated and grown in RPMI supplemented with 2.0% (v/v) fetal calf serum and 10% (v/v) Non-essential amino acids for 6 h, followed by drug exposure and viability assessments made the following day (15, 25–27). Cells were transfected with siRNA molecules or plasmids as described in prior manuscripts (20–24). Cells were transfected with a plasmid to express GFP-K-RAS V12 (0.1 μg) using lipofectamine 2000. Twenty-four hours after transfection, cells were used in assays examining their staining for GFP and RFP.

Detection of Cell Viability, Protein Expression, and Protein Phosphorylation by Immuno-Fluorescence Using a Hermes WiScan Machine [https://www.idea-bio.com/ (20–24)]

The text below discussing the Methods we use with the Hermes microscope is reproduced from text published in these review articles (28–30). "The Hermes machine combines high quality optics with a high-quality computer driven microscope stage, and with dedicated software, e.g., to analyze the immunofluorescent staining intensity of individual cells, i.e., *true* in-cell western blotting. A typical experiment: three independent cultures of a particular tumor cell type are sub-cultured into individual 96-well plates. Twenty-four h after plating, the cells are transfected with a control plasmid or a control siRNA, or with plasmids to express various proteins or validated siRNA molecules to knock down the expression of various proteins. After another 24 h, the cells are ready for drug exposure(s). At various time-points after the initiation of drug exposure, cells are fixed in place with permeabilization. Standard immunofluorescent blocking procedures are employed, followed by incubation of different wells with a variety of validated primary antibodies. The next morning, after washing, fluorescent-tagged secondary antibodies are added to each well; in general, we have found that using more than two tagged antibodies in each well-results in poorer data/image quality. After 3 h of incubation, the secondary antibody is removed, the cells washed again, and are hydrated with phosphate buffered saline prior to microscopic examination. Based on the experiment, cells are visualized at either 10X magnification for bulk assessments of immunofluorescent staining intensity or at 60X magnification for assessments of protein or protein-protein co-localization (**Supplemental Figure 1**)."

"For studies at 10X magnification, the operator selects which fluorescent antibody will be assessed first, i.e., in the red or green channel, and then focuses the microscope in a vehicle control transfection control well. The operator then outlines for the computer controlling the microscope "what is a cell." In other words, the operator manually inputs the criteria for each specific tumor cell line segregating away detection of what is obvious debris or a staining artifact. The operator then sets how many cells per well are to be assessed for their immunofluorescent staining intensity; we initially selected 40 cells per well but have now moved to assessing 100. The computer/microscope then determines the background fluorescence in the well and in parallel randomly determines the mean fluorescent intensity of those 100 cells; the operator is provided with this mean intensity value. Of note for scientific rigor is that the operator does not personally manipulate the microscope to examine specific cells; the entire fluorescent accrual method is independent of the operator. Once the entire plate has been scanned for one of the secondary antibodies, the second secondary antibody with a different fluorescence range can similarly be used to define the mean intensity value in each well. Once data from the first set of plated cells has been obtained, the second and third sets of plated cells can be processed through the machine. Thus, we obtain three independent sets of fluorescence data from the three individual cultures, with 300 cells under each condition being assessed. Typically, the total expression of a particular protein will be assessed alongside additional staining to define the levels of different phosphorylation sites within the protein, e.g., total ULK1, P-ULK1 S317, P-ULK1 S757. Within these analyses it is also essential to include wells to define invariant protein loading controls, such as the expression level of ERK2 or AKT. For phospho-proteins, data can be presented in two ways, either bar graphs where the total protein expression/loading is presented alongside changes in phospho-protein levels, or with just bars for the phospho-protein fluorescence data corrected for the amount of protein expression, i.e., the stoichiometry of protein phosphorylation. For proteins whose total expression changes after drug exposure, the use of invariant total ERK2 or total AKT expression is used instead as a loading control. Usually, alongside our numeric bar graph data, we also present images of stained cells, taken at 60X magnification, which visually reveal the extent of protein over-expression or of protein knock down. The Hermes microscope has also proved very useful at examining protein-protein interactions at 60X magnification. Three to four images of cells stained in the red and green fluorescence channels are taken for each treatment/transfection/condition. Images are ~4 MB sized files. Images are merged using Adobe Photoshop. The image intensity and contrast is then *post-hoc* altered in an identical fashion inclusive for each group of images/treatments/conditions, so that the image with the weakest intensity is still visible to the naked eye for publication purposes but also that the image with the highest intensity is still within the dynamic range, i.e., not over-saturated."

"At present, many laboratories still utilize traditional western blotting with secondary antibodies conjugated to luciferase, with enhanced chemiluminescence and X-ray film as a read-out; this approach has a limited dynamic range and for the 21st Century lacks sufficient rigor. Other laboratories with access to fluorescent imagers such as the Odyssey system use SDS PAGE with fluorescent tagged secondary antibodies, and these systems have a 5- to 6-log dynamic range. The Odyssey system can, at a gross level, also perform in-cell immunoblotting including co-staining in the red and green fluorescence channels. All of the above procedures require a considerable amount of operator input, including the isolation, lysis, clarification, and loading of proteins onto an SDS PAGE gel, followed by transfer to immobilon. This creates inherent errors in defining small drug-induced alterations to expression and phosphorylation; these are all processing stages where the rigor of the experiment can be compromised. Our use of the Hermes system abolishes all of the intermediate steps as cells are fixed *in situ*. Furthermore, unlike traditional SDS PAGE, the proteins retain their native conformations which for a number of proteins, e.g., detecting changes in chaperone conformation cause by drug exposures, presented data that could not have been obtained using traditional SDS PAGE. Thus, the in-cell assessments of altered phosphorylation or expression using the Hermes microscope provide data with more rigor and a much lower standard deviation difference, permitting changes of 20–30% intensity to be assessed for statistical significance."

"An additional benefit of using the Hermes system is that it promotes a greater level of rigorous non-manipulatable data. As mentioned earlier, the cells are fixed in place and stained, and then once the machine has been set to recognize the morphology of any specific tumor cell type, the role of the operator has ended. Data is obtained by the machine in a random fashion examining cell staining intensities wherever it detects cells; the operator cannot skew their data by plating more cells in one well-compared to another, or by picking certain cells to scan, leaving other cells out. We believe that our approach using the Hermes WiScan microscope, or with similar computer-controlled microscope products, should become the standard of approach for immunoblotting/immunofluorescence work."

Assessment of ROS

"Cells were treated with the drugs and 15 min prior to the indicated time point the media was removed and cells incubated with diacetate dihydro-DCF-DA (5 μM) (20–24). Fluorescence measurements were obtained 15 min after DCFH-DA addition with a Vector 3 plate reader. Data are presented corrected for basal fluorescence of vehicle-treated cells at each time point and expressed as the arbitrary units provided by the plate reader/the increase in ROS levels."

Animal Studies

Studies were performed under VCU IACUC protocol AD20008. Animals, $n = 3$ per group, were treated for 14 days with vehicle control (cremophore QD Days 1–14) or with [fingolimod, FTY 0.6 mg/kg + DMF, 75 mg/kg]. For both drugs, this represents an approximate 3-fold higher dosing than would occur in a human multiple sclerosis patient. Five-micron sections of normal tissues were obtained, and H&E staining performed to detect any changes in tissue morphology. No alteration in animal body mass was observed comparing vehicle control treated and [FTY + DMF] treated mice (not shown).

Data Analysis

Comparison of the effects of various treatments (in triplicate three times) was using one-way ANOVA and a two tailed Student's *t*-test. Statistical examination of *in vivo* animal survival data utilized a two tailed Student's *t*-test and log rank statistical analyses between the different treatment groups. Differences with a $p < 0.05$ were considered statistically significant. Experiments are the means of multiple individual points from multiple experiments (± SEM).

RESULTS

The Mayo clinic-derived and characterized PDX GBM cells are grown in bulk *in vivo* to maintain their tumorigenic biology and invasive characteristics, and the present studies used multiple isolates from different GBM5, GBM6, GBM12, and GBM14 tumors/mice *in vitro*. Fingolimod and MMF at physiologic concentrations interacted in an additive to greater than additive fashion to kill a genetically diverse group of primary and established GBM isolates and GBM stem cells (**Figure 1A**). Similar killing data were obtained using colony formation assays (**Figure 1B**). The combination of [MMF + fingolimod] enhanced the lethality of the standard of care drug temozolomide against GBM cells, and also against a fresh primary GBM isolate with its associated activated microglia (**Figure 1C**). Prior studies have demonstrated that the [MMF + fingolimod] combination could kill other primary GBM isolates, TNBC breast cancer cell lines, NSCLC isolates, ovarian isolates and sarcoma isolates (15). Both MMF and fingolimod radiosensitized our GBM isolates (**Figure 1D**). We next determined whether animals exposed to fingolimod and MMF in combination would exhibit any normal tissue toxicities. Animals were treated daily for 14 days with drug doses ∼3 times higher than those of either drug in multiple sclerosis patients. Supra-physiologic doses of the drugs *in vivo* did not cause damage to "normal tissues" in the mouse (**Figure 1E**). This finding argues that the [MMF + fingolimod] drug combination will likely be "safe" in a human cancer patient.

We selected the PDX models GBM6 and GBM14 for further in-depth analyses. The GBM6 isolate expresses the truncated constitutively active ERBB1 vIII and the GBM14 isolate lacks PTEN expression. In many prior experimental therapeutics studies, we have performed agnostic screening analyses following exposure of cancer cells to drugs using the Hermes wide-field microscope. Using fluorescence intensity imaging of individual cells, we define the changes in the expression and phosphorylation of multiple signal transduction proteins (20, 21, 24, 31). Signaling by ERK1/2, AKT, mTOR, p70 S6K, STAT3, and STAT5 was assessed, as was signaling by ATM, the AMPK and eIF2 alpha. Studies also closely examined the regulation of autophagy, measuring the levels of Beclin1, ATG5 and the phosphorylation of ULK1 and ATG13. The levels of multiple cytoprotective proteins were assessed including MCL-1, BCL-XL, and c-FLIP-s.

In GBM6, but not GBM14, the drugs combined to further activate ATM and AMPK; in several prior studies using different drug combinations we have delineated an ATM-AMPK-ULK1-ATG13 pathway that promotes autophagosome formation (**Figures 2A,B**) (20, 21, 24, 31). In GBM14 cells, fingolimod as a single agent strongly activated ATM-AMPK signaling. In both cell lines FTY720 and MMF interacted to promote ULK-1 S317 phosphorylation; S317 is a site targeted by the AMPK and elevated S317 phosphorylation equates to ULK-1 kinase activation. This was associated with enhanced ATG13 S318 phosphorylation; elevated S318 phosphorylation is a key trigger event to initiate autophagosome formation. The [MMF + fingolimod] combination rapidly inactivated mTORC1, mTORC2, AKT, ERK1/2, p70 S6K, STAT3/5, and NFκB. Inactivation of mTORC1 and mTORC2 results in ULK-1 S757 dephosphorylation that also promotes ULK-1 kinase activity. In both GBM6 and GBM14 cells, the drugs interacted to reduce STAT5 Y694 phosphorylation and in one of the isolates STAT3 Y705 phosphorylation. In one isolate, the drugs also interacted to reduce NFκB S536 phosphorylation. As judged by elevated PKR-like endoplasmic reticulum kinase (PERK) phosphorylation and elevated eIF2α S51 phosphorylation, FTY720 caused a strong endoplasmic reticulum stress response. In both isolates, the drug combination also reduced the expression of the caspase 8/10 inhibitor c-FLIP-s, that potentially could facilitate death receptor signaling.

We have recently demonstrated that the irreversible ERBB1/2/4 inhibitor neratinib could down-regulate the expression of RAS proteins, and based on this data and the fact that phosphorylated fingolimod causes sphingosine-1-phosphate receptor 1 internalization and degradation, we wished to determine whether this drug could act upon RAS proteins in GBM cells, in a manner similar to neratinib (20, 21, 24, 31). In GBM6 cells, that express an NH2-terminal truncated active ERBB1 vIII [fingolimod + MMF], caused intracellular clustering

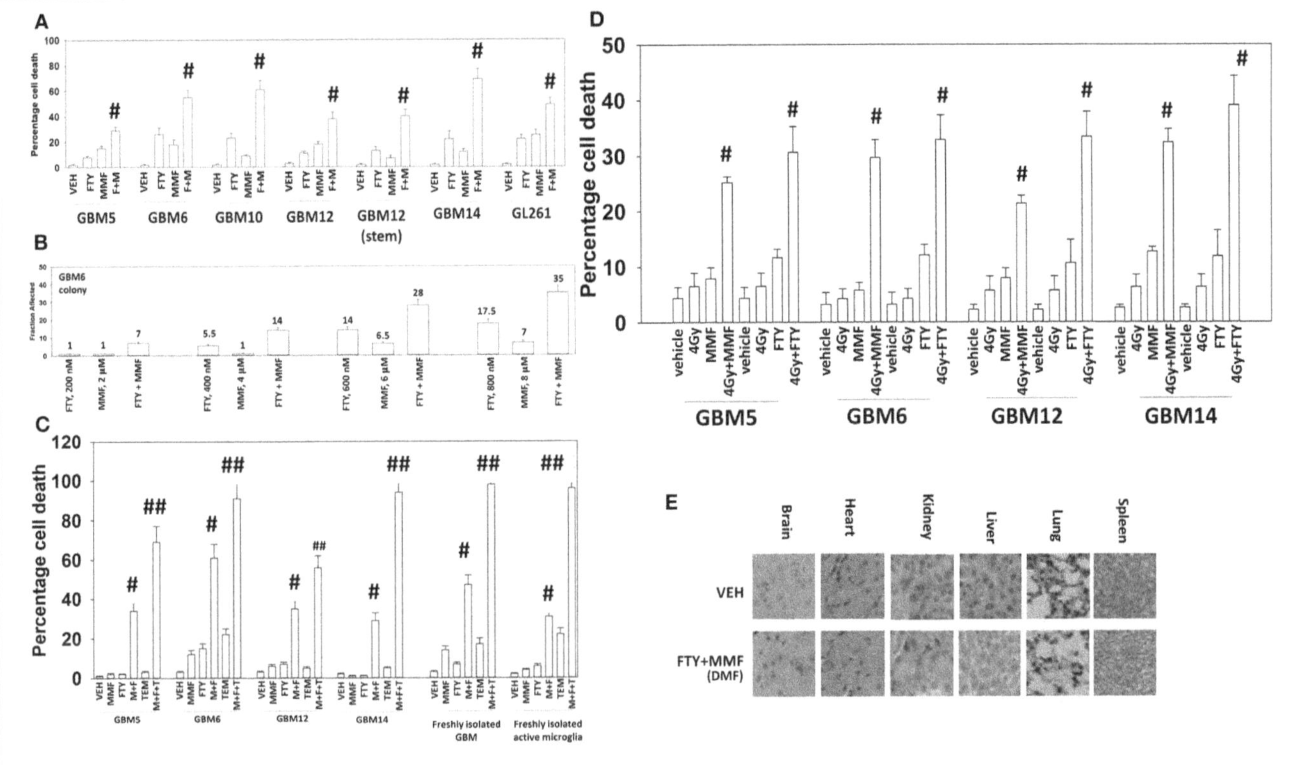

FIGURE 1 | Gilenya and Tecfidera interact to kill GBM cells. **(A)** GBM cells were treated with vehicle control (VEH), fingolimod (FTY, 100 nM), MMF (5 μM), or the drugs in combination for 24 h. Cells were isolated, and viability determined by trypan blue exclusion assay (n = 3 ± SD) #$p < 0.05$ greater than fingolimod alone. **(B)** GBM6 cells were plated as single cells 250/500 cells per 60 mm dish. Twelve hours after plating, cells were treated with vehicle control, fingolimod (200–800 nM), MMF (2–8 μM), or the drugs in combination at a fixed dose ratio for 24 h. After 24 h, the media was removed, the cells washed with warm drug-free media, and then incubated in drug-free media for an additional 9 days. Cells/colonies were fixed in place and stained with crystal violet. Colonies of >50 cells were counted, and the fraction affected determined ($n = 6$ plates per-condition ± SD). **(C)** GBM cells and fresh activated microglia were treated with vehicle control [FTY, 100 nM + MMF, 5 μM], temozolomide (TMZ, 1 μM), or the drugs in combination for 24 h. Cells were isolated, and viability determined by trypan blue exclusion assay ($n = 3 \pm$ SD) #$p < 0.05$ greater than vehicle control; ##$p < 0.05$ greater than [FTY + MMF] value. **(D)** GBM cells were treated with vehicle control [FTY, 100 nM + MMF, 5 μM], ionizing radiation (4 Gy), or the drugs in combination for 24 h. Cells were isolated, and viability determined by trypan blue exclusion assay (n = 3 ± SD) # greater than radiation single agent value. **(E)** Mice were treated for 14 days QD and PO with vehicle control (cremophore) or with [fingolimod, FTY 0.6 mg/kg + DMF, 75 mg/kg]. Five-micron sections of normal tissues were obtained, and H&E staining performed to detect any changes in tissue morphology. No alteration in animal body mass was observed comparing vehicle control treated and [FTY + DMF] treated mice (not shown).

of the receptor; unlike fingolimod, our positive control neratinib increased clustering followed later by reduced expression of the receptor (**Figure 3A**). In GBM6 cells, fingolimod as a single agent could reduce the total expression of both wild type K- and N-RAS proteins (**Figure 3B**). To confirm this finding via a different approach, we transfected GBM6 cells with a plasmid to express K-RAS V12–GFP. In a manner similar to the data for ERBB1 vIII in Panel A, fingolimod caused intracellular vesicularization of K-RAS V12–GFP, that was maintained for 8 h (**Figure 3C**). In contrast, the positive control neratinib initially caused RAS vesicularization but at later times reduced the levels of GFP+ fluorescence. Finally, we wished to determine whether the effect of fingolimod on RAS vesicularization was specific only in GBM cells. PANC1 pancreatic cancer cells express a mutant K-RAS protein. PANC1 cells were transfected with plasmids to express K-RAS V12–GFP and K-RAS V12–RFP. In these cells, fingolimod appeared to cause greater levels of RAS vesicularization than were observed in the GBM cells (**Figure 3D**). In contrast to data from GBM cells, after 8 h of drug exposure, fingolimod reduced GFP+ and RFP+ fluorescence levels.

Additional descriptive studies were performed to further delineate the responses of GBM cells to [MMF + fingolimod]. After drug exposure, the expression of proteins generally considered to be protective against toxic stresses including MCL-1, BCL-XL, c-FLIP-s declined whereas the expression of proteins that facilitated autophagosome formation, ATG5 and Beclin1, increased (**Figures 2A,B, 4A**). The expression of β-catenin declined. High non-physiologic concentrations of DMF (>5 μM) have been proposed to increase the expression of NRF2 and HO-1 that are proteins which in a broad sense will act to suppress reactive oxygen species (ROS) production. ROS production is essential for the activation and activities of many different types of immune cell. Reactive oxygen also activates cytosolic ATM (32). Lower concentrations of MMF rapidly enhanced the production of ROS in GBM cells that

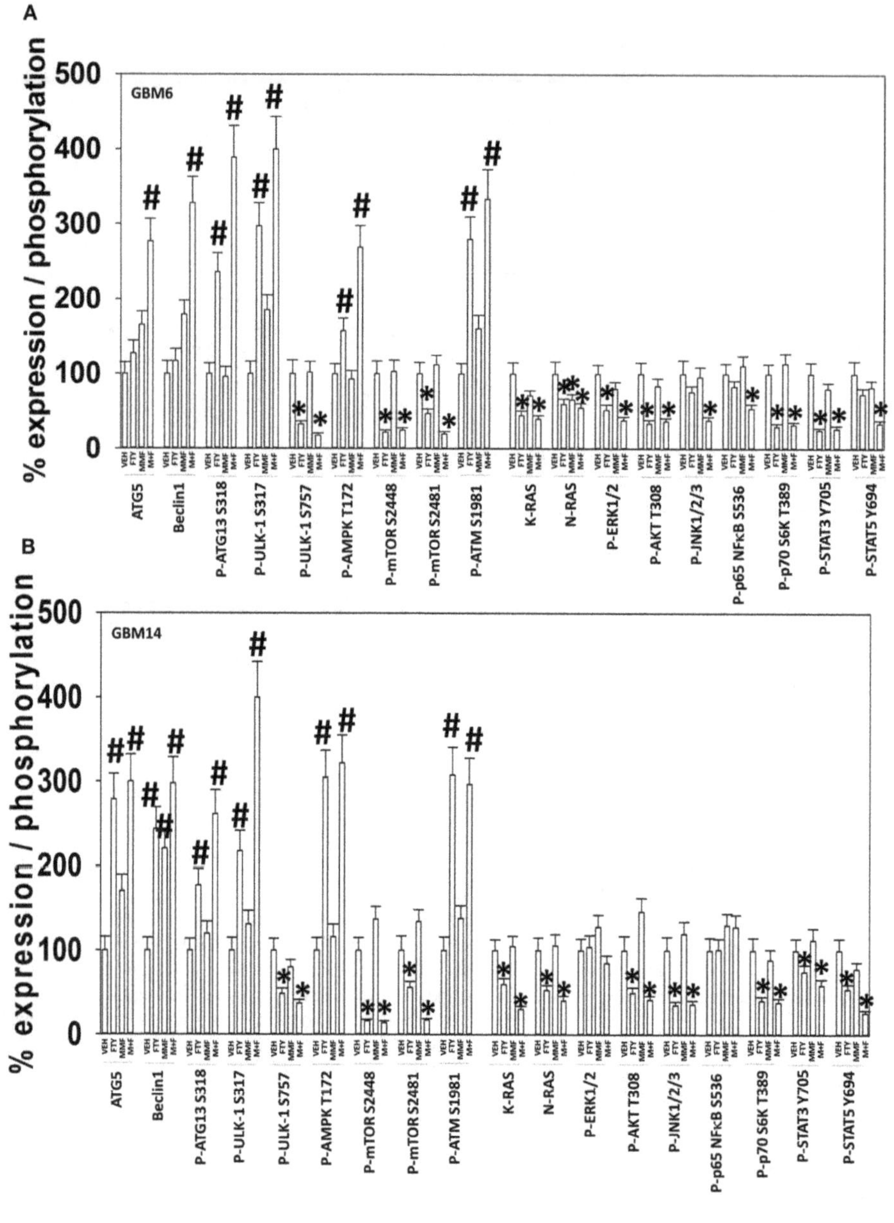

FIGURE 2 | [FTY + MMF] exposure enhances ER stress signaling, causes DNA damage, and inactivates multiple protective signaling pathways. **(A)** GBM6 and **(B)** GBM14 cells were treated with vehicle control (VEH), fingolimod (FTY, 100 nM), MMF (5 μM), or the drugs in combination for 6 h. Cells were fixed in place and immuno-staining performed to detect the total expression and phosphorylation of the noted proteins. Analyses for densitometric scanning of fluorescence intensity were performed at 10X magnification on >120 cells per condition, in a random fashion in a Hermes WiScan machine ($n = 3 \pm$ SD) $^{*}p < 0.05$ less than exposure in vehicle control; #$p < 0.05$ greater than exposure in vehicle control.

remained constant for almost 4 h (**Figure 4B**). As a single agent fingolimod, also at a clinically relevant concentration (100 nM), modestly and transiently increased ROS production. When the drugs were combined, fingolimod significantly enhanced the ability of MMF to generate ROS over the 4-h time course. Over-expression of thioredoxin (TRX) or superoxide dismutase 2 (SOD2) quenched ROS production and significantly reduced [MMF + fingolimod] lethality, as did expression of activated MEK1, dominant negative IκB S32A S36A, and treatment with the JNK inhibitory peptide (**Figure 4C**, not shown). In cells treated with [MMF + fingolimod], despite exhibiting elevated ROS levels, no compensatory survival alterations in the expression of NRF2 or HO-1 were observed (not shown).

In **Figure 2** we observed that [MMF + fingolimod] inactivated mTOR and increased the phosphorylation of ATG13, all strongly suggesting that the drug combination was promoting autophagosome formation. GBM cells were transfected to express the fusion protein LC3-GFP-RFP which permits the

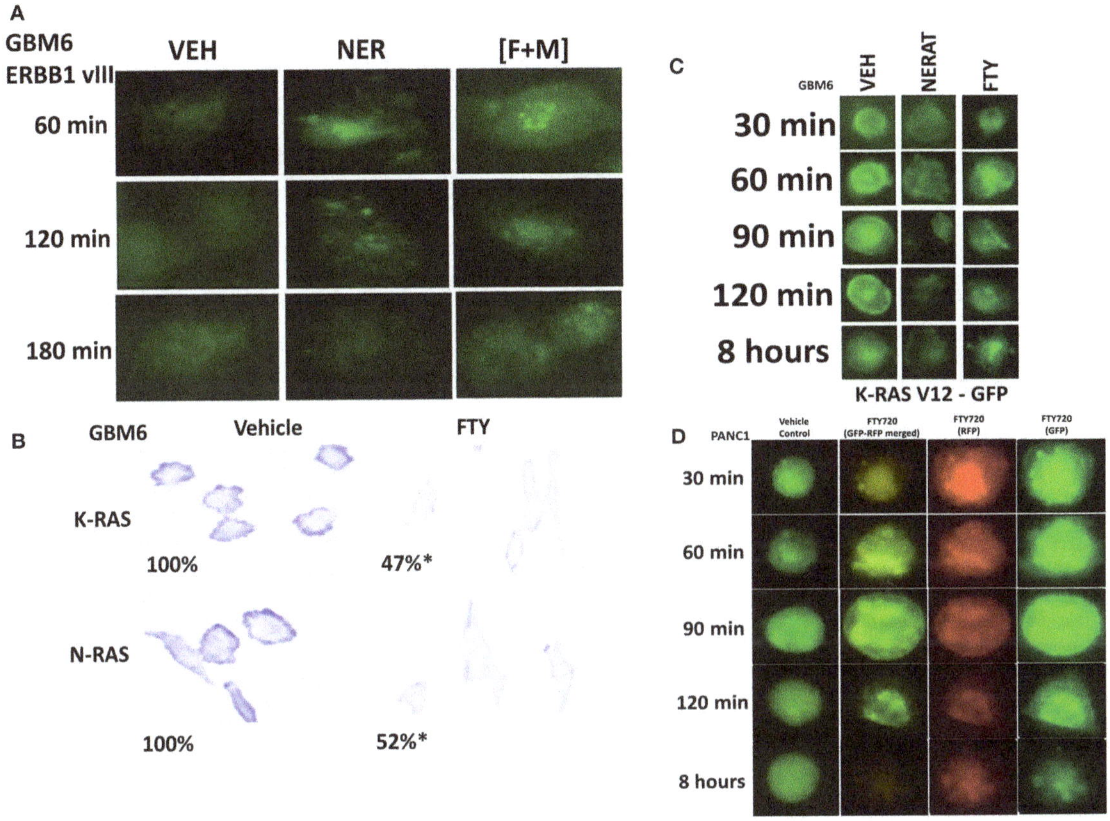

FIGURE 3 | [FTY + MMF] exposure causes intracellular clustering of ERBB1 vIII and the degradation of RAS proteins. **(A)** GBM6 cells that express ERBB1 vIII were treated with vehicle control (VEH), neratinib (100 nM), or [fingolimod (FTY, 100 nM) + MMF (5 μM)] in combination. Cells were fixed in place at the indicated time points and the localization of ERBB1 vIII determined using an antibody raised against the COOH terminal portion of ERBB1. **(B)** GBM6 cells were treated with vehicle control (VEH) or with fingolimod (FTY, 100 nM) for 6 h. Cells were fixed in place and immuno-staining performed to detect the expression and localization of K-RAS and N-RAS. Analyses for densitometric scanning of fluorescence intensity were performed at 10X magnification on >120 cells per condition ($n = 3 \pm$ SD) $^*p < 0.05$ less than exposure in vehicle control. **(C)** GBM6 cells were transfected with a plasmid to express K-RAS V12–GFP. Twenty-four hours later, cells were treated with vehicle control (VEH), fingolimod (FTY, 100 nM) or with the irreversible ERBB1/2/4 inhibitor neratinib (100 nM) for 0.5–8 h. Cells were imaged at 60X magnification and representative images from each condition at each time point are presented. **(D)** PANC1 pancreatic cancer cells that express an endogenous mutant K-RAS were transfected with plasmids to express K-RAS V12–GFP and K-RAS V12–RFP. Twenty-four h after transfection cells were treated with vehicle control or with fingolimod (FTY720, 100 nM) for the indicated time points. Cells were imaged at 60X magnification in the Hermes WiScan microscope and images were merged in Photoshop CS5.

detection over a time course of autophagosomes (GFP+ RFP+) and autolysosomes (RFP+); i.e., autophagic flux. Treatment of cells with [MMF + Fingolimod] increased the levels of autophagosomes followed temporally later by the formation of autolysosomes, arguing that the drug combination was stimulating autophagic flux (**Figures 5A,B**). Over-expression of TRX or SOD2 to quench reactive oxygen species or a mutant active form of mTOR to inactivate the kinase upstream of ATG13, ULK1, significantly reduced the drug-stimulated elevations in the levels of autophagosomes and autolysosomes.

ATM in the cytosol can be activated by reactive oxygen species whereas ATM associated with DNA in the nucleus can be activated by DNA damage (32). **Figure 2** demonstrated that fingolimod activated ATM but data in **Figure 4** demonstrated that fingolimod weakly elevated reactive oxygen species levels. This suggests fingolimod may be causing a DNA damage-induced activation of ATM. And, as an HDAC inhibitor, fingolimod has the potential to cause DNA damage. Knock down of ATM or AMPKα modestly, though significantly, reduced amount of ROS generated by MMF and by [MMF + fingolimod] 2 h after exposure, each by ~20% (**Figure 6A**). Knock down of ATM or AMPKα significantly reduced the ability of the drug combination to stimulate autophagosome formation after 4 h by 45–90% (**Figures 6B,C**). Although evidence from **Figures 2**, **4** would argue that reactive oxygen species plays a secondary role in the regulation of ATM activity, over-expression of TRX or SOD2 significantly reduced the drug combination-stimulated phosphorylation of ATM S1981 ~50–60% (**Figure 6D**). Collectively, the data in **Figures 2–6** demonstrate that the initial sharp increase in ROS generation caused by [MMF + fingolimod] exposure is essential for robust ATM activation and for autophagosome formation, and that ROS generation is upstream of ATM activation and autophagy. Future studies will be required to explore the

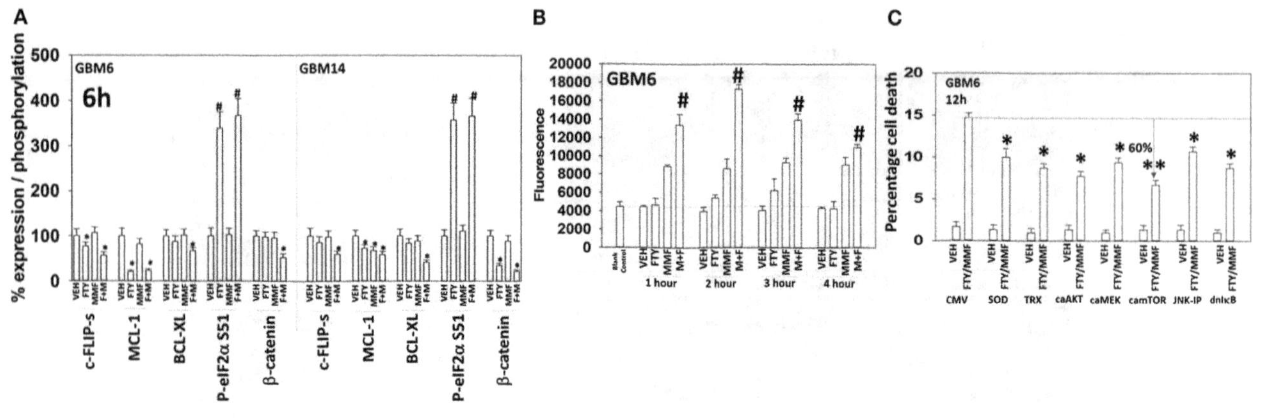

FIGURE 4 | [FTY + MMF] exposure reduces the expression of c-FLIP-s, MCL-1, BCL-XL, and β-catenin and elevates reactive oxygen species levels. **(A)** GBM6 and GBM14 cells were treated with vehicle control (VEH), fingolimod (FTY, 100 nM), MMF (5 μM), or the drugs in combination for 6 h. Cells were fixed in place and immuno-staining performed to detect the total expression and phosphorylation of the noted proteins. Analyses for densitometric scanning of fluorescence intensity were performed at 10X magnification on >120 cells per condition ($n = 3 \pm$ SD). **(B)** GBM6 cells were treated with vehicle control, fingolimod (FTY, 100 nM), MMF (5 μM), or the drugs in combination. Fifteen min prior to the indicated time point the media was removed and cells incubated with diacetate dihydro-DCF-DA (5 μM). Fluorescence measurements were obtained 15 min after DCFH-DA addition with a Vector 3 plate reader. Data are presented corrected for basal fluorescence of vehicle-treated cells at each time point and expressed as the arbitrary units provided by the plate reader/the increase in ROS levels ($n = 3 \pm$ SD). **(C)** GBM6 cells were transfected with an empty vector control plasmid (CMV) or with plasmids to express SOD2, TRX, activated AKT, activated MEK1, activated mTOR, or IκB S32A S36A. The JNK-IP (10 μM) was added to a CMV transfected cell 30 min before any drug exposure. Twenty-four h after transfection, cells were treated with vehicle control or [fingolimod (FTY, 100 nM) + MMF (5 μM)] in combination for 12 h. Cells were isolated, and viability determined by trypan blue exclusion assay ($n = 3 \pm$ SD). $^{\#}p < 0.05$ greater than corresponding VEH value; $^{*}p < 0.05$ less than corresponding VEH value; $^{**}p < 0.01$ less than corresponding VEH value.

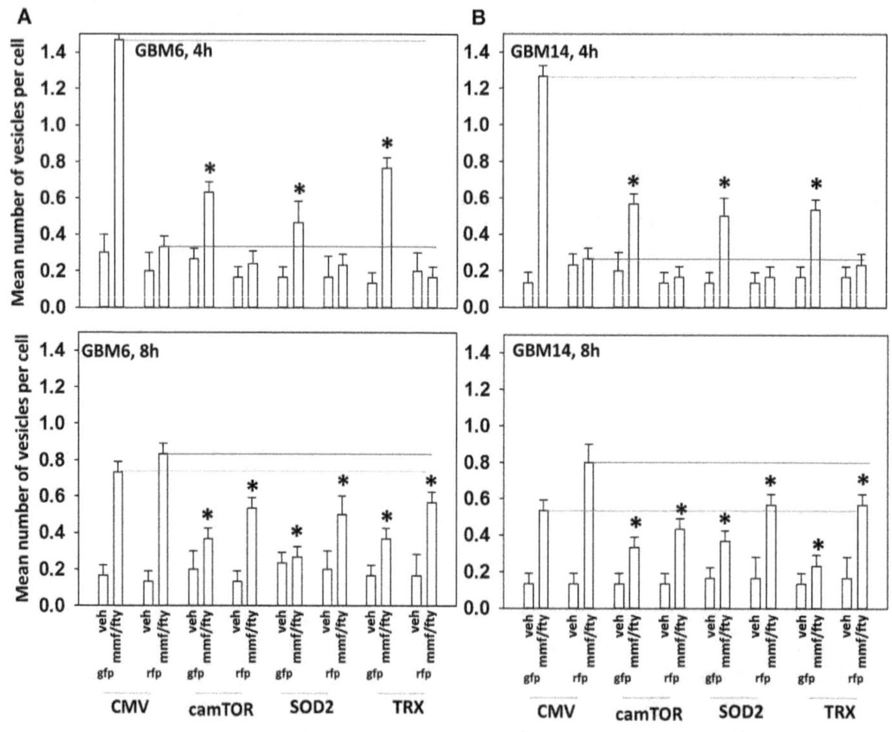

FIGURE 5 | ROS production after [FTY + MMF] exposure is essential for autophagosome and autolysosome formation. **(A,B)** GBM6 and GBM14 cells were transfected with a plasmid to express LC3-GFP-RFP in parallel with an empty vector plasmid (CMV), a plasmid to express activated mTOR, or with plasmids to express superoxide dismutase 2 (SOD2) or thioredoxin (TRX). Twenty-four h afterwards, cells were treated with vehicle control (VEH) or with [fingolimod (FTY, 100 nM), MMF (5 μM)] in combination for 4 or 8 h. Cells were imaged at 60X magnification; at least 40 cells per condition in independent triplicate were examined and the mean number of vesicles per cell presented ($n = 3 \pm$ SD). $^{*}p < 0.05$ less that corresponding value in CMV transfected cells.

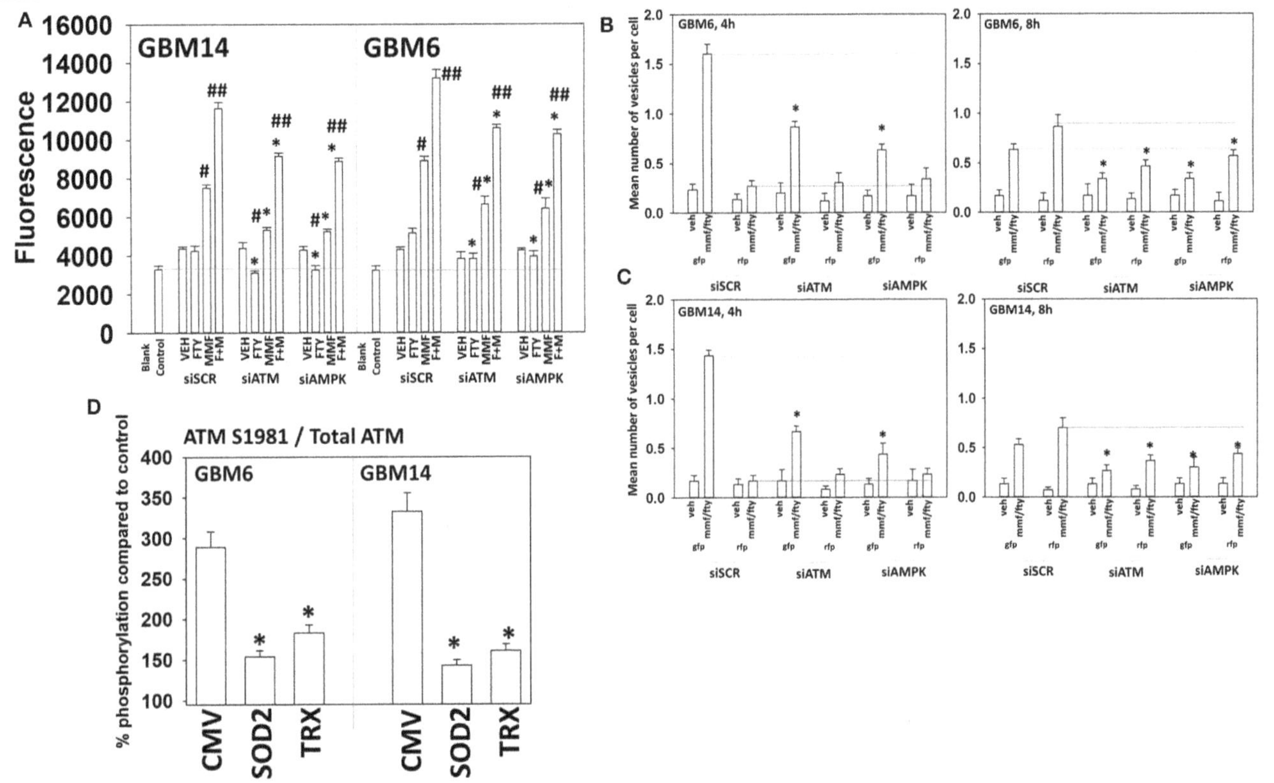

FIGURE 6 | Activation of ATM and the induction of autophagy by [FTY + MMF] requires ATM-AMPK signaling. **(A)** GBM6 and GBM14 cells were transfected with a scrambled control siRNA (siSCR) or with siRNA molecules to knock down ATM or AMPKα. Twenty-four hours later, cells were treated with vehicle control or with [fingolimod (FTY, 100 nM) and MMF (5 μM)] in combination. Fifteen minutes prior to the indicated time point the media was removed and cells incubated with diacetate dihydro-DCF-DA (5 μM). Fluorescence measurements were obtained 15 min after DCFH-DA addition with a Vector 3 plate reader. Data are presented corrected for basal fluorescence of vehicle-treated cells at each time point and expressed as the arbitrary units provided by the plate reader/the increase in ROS levels ($n = 3 \pm$ SD) #$p < 0.05$ greater than corresponding vehicle control value; ##$p < 0.05$ greater than corresponding MMF value; *$p < 0.05$ less than corresponding value in siSCR cells. **(B,C)** GBM6 and GBM14 cells were transfected with a plasmid to express LC3-GFP-RFP in parallel with scrambled siRNA control (siSCR) or with siRNA molecules to knock down the expression of ATM or AMPKα. Twenty-four h later, cells were treated with vehicle control (VEH) or with [fingolimod (FTY, 100 nM), MMF (5 μM)] in combination for 4 or 8 h. Cells were imaged at 60X magnification; at least 40 cells per condition in independent triplicate were examined and the mean number of vesicles per cell presented ($n = 3 \pm$ SD). *$p < 0.05$ less that corresponding value in siSCR transfected cells. **(D)** GBM6 and GBM14 cells were transfected with an empty vector plasmid (CMV) or with plasmids to express superoxide dismutase 2 (SOD2) or thioredoxin (TRX). Twenty-four hours afterwards, cells were treated with vehicle control (VEH) or with [fingolimod (FTY, 100 nM), MMF (5 μM)] in combination for 6 h. Cells were fixed in place and immuno-staining performed to detect the total expression and phosphorylation of ATM S1981. Analyses for densitometric scanning of fluorescence intensity were performed at 10X magnification on >120 cells per condition ($n = 3 \pm$ SD) *$p < 0.05$ less than exposure in vehicle control; #$p < 0.05$ greater than exposure in vehicle control.

role of nuclear DNA damage in the activation of ATM after drug exposure.

Based on the data in **Figures 1–6**, using molecular tools, we next performed additional semi-descriptive studies designed ultimately to define the key protein regulators/pathways of viability after [MMF + fingolimod] exposure. Cell killing deliberately measured after only 12 h, i.e., the numeric values of percentage cell death are relatively low but are performed at this time point so as to define those key proteins/pathways who play a *primary* role in the killing processes. Proteins that were congruent in both PDX isolates for regulating tumor cell killing by the drug combination were: [BAX, BAK, BAD; MCL-1, BCL-XL] that could be considered as a mitochondrial apoptosis regulatory pathway; [ATM, AMPK, ULK-1, ATG5, Beclin1, Cathepsin B] that could considered as an autophagy/lysosomal pathway; [CD95, c-FLIP-s] as a death receptor pathway feeding into the apoptosis pathway; and enhanced [PERK, eIF2α] ER stress signaling that promotes cell survival (**Figures 7A,B**). With respect to death receptor signaling, fingolimod, but not MMF, caused plasma membrane clustering of CD95, indicative of death receptor activation (**Figure 7C**). Over-expression of the reactive oxygen species quenching enzymes TRX or SOD2 modestly, though significantly, reduced CD95 plasma membrane levels (**Figure 7D**). Tyrosine phosphorylation of CD95 is known to play a key role in its activation (33). Tyrosine phosphatases are potently inhibited by reactive oxygen species and thus inhibition of PTPases by ROS may represent a mechanism of CD95 activation.

As presented in **Figure 2**, knock down of PERK or eIF2α enhanced [MMF + fingolimod] lethality, implying endoplasmic reticulum stress signaling was protective. Hence, we next determined whether other endoplasmic reticulum

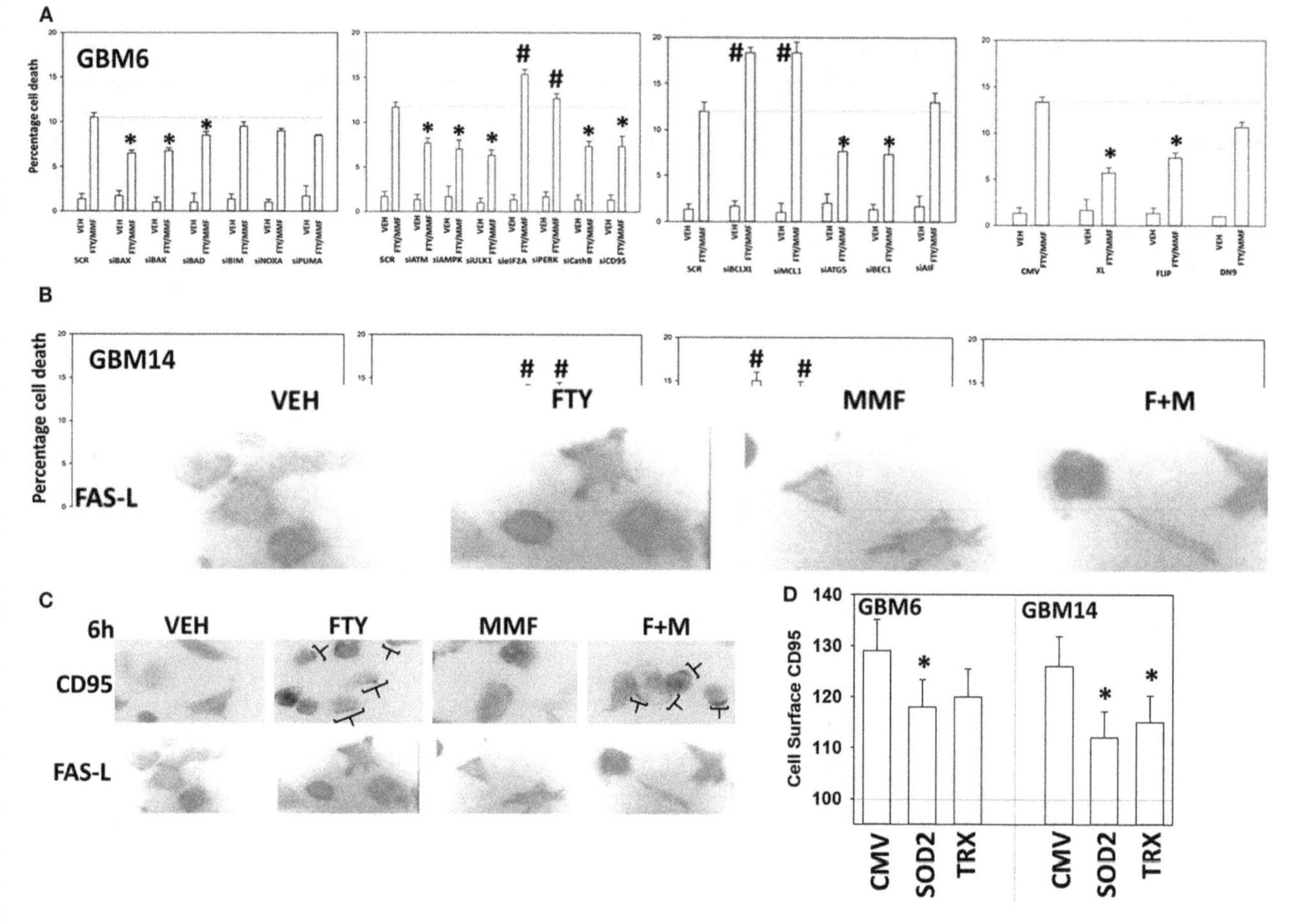

FIGURE 7 | Knock down of CD95, ATM, AMPK, ULK1, ATG5, Beclin1, cathepsin B, BAX, and BAK suppressed [fingolimod + MMF] lethality whereas knock down of PERK, eIF2α, MCL-1, and BCL-XL promoted death. **(A,B)** GBM6 and GBM14 cells were transfected with a scrambled control siRNA (SCR) or with the siRNA molecules noted in the graph panels. In parallel, other portions of cells were transfected with an empty vector control plasmid (CMV) or with plasmids to express c-FLIP-s, BCL-XL, or dominant negative caspase 9. Twenty-four hours after transfection, cells were treated with vehicle control or [fingolimod (FTY, 100 nM) + MMF (5 μM)] in combination for 12 h. Cells were isolated, and viability determined by trypan blue exclusion assay ($n = 3 \pm$ SD). $^{*}p < 0.05$ less killing than the corresponding value in both GBM6 and GBM14 cells; $^{\#}p < 0.05$ greater killing than the corresponding value in both GBM6 and GBM14 cells. **(C)** GBM6 cells were treated with vehicle control, fingolimod (FTY, 100 nM), MMF (5 μM), or the drugs in combination for 6 h. Cells were fixed in place and immune-staining performed with validated antibodies to detect the total expression of CD95 and FAS-L. Cells were imaged at 60X magnification; areas in brackets indicate CD95 clustering on the plasma membrane. **(D)** GBM6 and GBM14 cells were transfected with an empty vector plasmid (CMV) or with plasmids to express superoxide dismutase 2 (SOD2) or thioredoxin (TRX). Twenty-four hours afterwards, cells were treated with vehicle control (VEH) or with [fingolimod (FTY, 100 nM), MMF (5 μM)] in combination for 6 h. Cells were fixed in place without permeabilization and immunostaining performed to detect CD95 cell surface localization. Cells were imaged at 60X magnification; at least 120 cells per condition in independent triplicate were examined and the mean number of vesicles per cell presented ($n = 3 \pm$ SD); $^{*}p < 0.05$ less that corresponding value in CMV transfected cells.

stress pathways regulated the survival response to [MMF + fingolimod] treatment. Knock down of the IRE1-XBP1 pathway or the ATF6 pathway, in a manner like knock down of the PERK-eIF2α pathway, enhanced killing GBM6 and GBM14 cells (**Figure 8**). In GBM6 cells, knock down of the ER stress pathways enhanced MMF lethality, whereas in GBM14 no enhancement occurred. In GBM6 cells, fingolimod lethality was not altered by knock down of the ER stress pathways whereas in the GBM14 cells, killing was modestly enhanced. Whether PTEN functionality (GBM14) or ERBB1 vIII expression (GBM6) specifically alters the role of ER stress signaling in survival will require studies beyond the scope of the present manuscript.

Glioblastoma is a highly invasive tumor type, and one signaling pathway that can interact with ERBB1-RAS signaling to promote tumor cell migration and invasion is the Hippo Pathway (34). The downstream effectors of this pathway, YAP and TAZ, are active when dephosphorylated, and in the nucleus where they act as co-transcription factors (35). Treatment of GBM6 and GBM14 cells caused a bi-phasic regulation of YAP and TAZ phosphorylation, as well as of their upstream kinases LATS1/2 and of docking

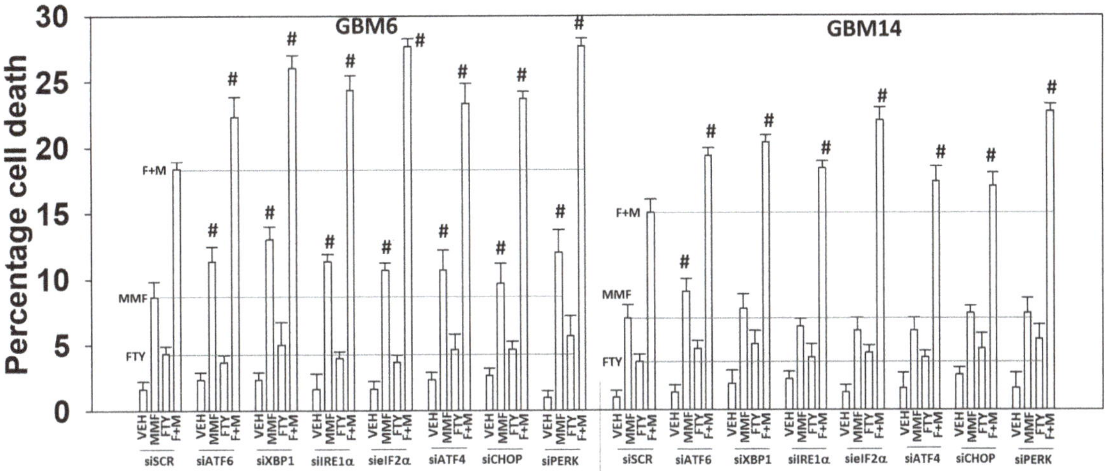

FIGURE 8 | Endoplasmic reticulum stress signaling plays a protective role against [MMF + fingolimod] exposure. GBM6 and GBM14 cells were transfected with a scrambled siRNA control (siSCR) or with the indicated siRNA molecules to knock down the expression of proteins that regulate ER stress pathways. Twenty-four hours after transfection, cells were treated with vehicle control, MMF (5 μM), fingolimod (100 nM), or the drugs in combination for 12 h. Cells were isolated, and viability determined by trypan blue exclusion assay ($n = 3 \pm$ SD). #$p < 0.05$ greater than corresponding value in siSCR cells.

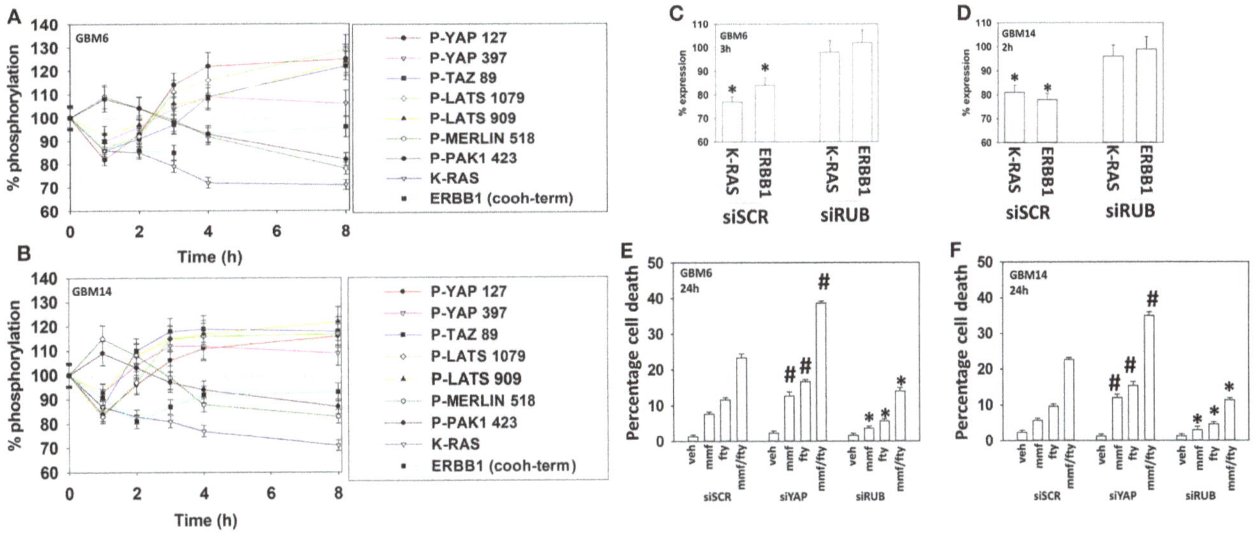

FIGURE 9 | Fingolimod causes bi-phasic activation followed by inactivation of YAP and TAZ. **(A,B)** GBM6 and GBM14 cells were treated with vehicle control or with fingolimod (100 nM). At each time point over the 0–8 h time course cells were fixed in place and immunostaining performed to determine the fluorescence intensity levels of: total YAP, total TAZ; total Merlin; total PAK1; total LATS1; P-YAP S127; P-YAP S397; P-TAZ S89; P-LATS T1079; P-LATS S909; P-Merlin S518; P-PAK1 T423; total ERBB1; and total K-RAS from 10X magnification images (120 cells per condition, $n = 3 \pm$ SD). **(C,D)** GBM6 and GBM14 cells were transfected with a scrambled control siRNA (siSCR) or with an siRNA to knock down the expression of Rubicon. Twenty-four h after transfection cells were treated with vehicle control or with fingolimod (100 nM). At each time point over the 0–8 h time course cells were fixed in place and immunostaining performed to determine the fluorescence intensity levels of: total ERBB1; total K-RAS from 10X magnification images (120 cells per condition, $n = 3 \pm$ SD). *$p < 0.05$ less than vehicle control. **(E,F)** GBM6 and GBM14 cells were transfected with a scrambled control siRNA (siSCR) or with an siRNA to knock down the expression of Rubicon or the expression of YAP. Twenty-four h after transfection cells were treated with vehicle control, fingolimod (100 nM), MMF (5 μM), or the drugs in combination for 24 h. Cells were isolated, and viability determined by trypan blue exclusion assay ($n = 3 \pm$ SD). *$p < 0.05$ less than corresponding value in siSCR cells; #$p < 0.05$ greater than corresponding value in siSCR cells.

proteins Merlin and PAK1 (**Figures 9A,B**). In both cell types, fingolimod within the first 2 h of exposure initially caused dephosphorylation of YAP, TAZ, and LATS1/2 and increased the phosphorylation of Merlin and PAK1. These events facilitate the co-transcription factor activities of YAP and TAZ, with Merlin acting to regulate complex formation and downstream signaling from small GTP binding proteins (36). At later times, 3–8 h after exposure, fingolimod caused the phosphorylation of YAP, TAZ, LATS1/2, and caused the dephosphorylation of Merlin and PAK1. Reduced Merlin phosphorylation enhances the ability of Merlin to act as a docking/chaperone protein bringing LATS1/2 into a closer association with YAP/TAZ, which enhances YAP/TAZ phosphorylation, thereby reducing YAP/TAZ activity (37).

One mechanism of plasma membrane internalization and subsequent protein digestion is called LC3-associated phagocytosis (LAP) (37). Key regulatory proteins in this process include Rubicon and Beclin1; our prior data demonstrated Beclin1 knock down protected cells from [MMF + fingolimod] lethality. Knock down of Rubicon prevented fingolimod from reducing the protein levels of K-RAS and ERBB1 (**Figures 9C,D**) (38). Knock down of Rubicon reduced the lethality of fingolimod, MMF and the drug combination (**Figures 9E,F**). In contrast, knock down of YAP enhanced killing by the drugs alone or in combination. These findings argue that reduced YAP phosphorylation caused by fingolimod leads to enhanced killing by the drug and that in cells incapable of LAP-dependent K-RAS/ERBB1 destruction, fingolimod lethality is significantly reduced.

DISCUSSION

The recognized actions of fingolimod and of DMF are to suppress immune system activity such that the host's auto-immune actions against demyelinated nerves, i.e., multiple sclerosis, are reduced. Although both drugs act to reduce the reactivity of the immune system, they do so through different mechanisms. Glioblastoma, for its overall malignancy and its invasion and privileged environment, relies heavily on its symbiotic relationship with activated/reactive microglia. As such, we hypothesized that a combination of the CNS-permeant drugs fingolimod and DMF/MMF could have therapeutic potential in this disease. Prior studies demonstrated that MMF reduced GBM cell invasiveness and enhanced the toxicity of temozolomide and ionizing radiation (15). MMF killed freshly isolated activated human microglia which correlated with reduced IL-6, TGFβ, and TNFα production. The MMF and fingolimod combination further reduced, below either agent individually, both GBM and activated microglia viability and their production of cytokines. In animals treated with DMF and fingolimod for 14 continuous days, no obvious damage to normal tissues was observed.

We demonstrated that the drug combination enhanced ATM/AMPK/ULK-1 signaling that corresponded with enhanced ATG13 S318 phosphorylation, as observed in prior therapeutics studies; in one isolate knock down of ATG5 and Beclin1 was protective against drug lethality whereas in the other it was not. Both isolates required the lysosomal protease cathepsin B for complete execution of the tumor cells. The drug combination reduced the protein levels of cytoprotective proteins such as ERBB1 vIII, K-RAS, N-RAS, c-FLIP-s, MCL-1, and BCL-XL. Knock down of CD95 or FADD, or over-expression of c-FLIP-s reduced drug combination killing arguing that the extrinsic pathway played a partial role in the killing process. Knock down of MCL-1 or BCL-XL enhanced tumor cell death whereas over-expression of BCL-XL was protective as was knock down of BAX, BAK and BAD. This data more definitively supports the drug combination causing mitochondrial dysfunction as a key component of the killing process. Knock down of apoptosis inducing factor significantly protected cells whereas expression of dominant negative caspase 9, i.e., "classic" apoptosis via caspase 3, did not. Alongside the role of cathepsin B, these findings demonstrate that the [MMF + fingolimod] combination kills through non-apoptotic processes.

At non-physiologic DMF/MMF concentrations, an order of magnitude higher than used herein, the drug has been shown to modulate the anti-oxidant response in cells, increasing the expression of NRF2 and HO-1. Because of this data linking DMF/MMF to the anti-oxidant response, we investigated whether MMF and fingolimod interacted to alter ROS levels and whether ROS generation play any role in tumor cell killing. MMF enhanced the production of ROS in GBM cells that was significantly enhanced in a greater than additive fashion by fingolimod. Over-expression of thioredoxin or superoxide dismutase 2 suppressed ROS production and drug combination lethality, yet the drug combination altered neither the levels of TRX and SOD2 expression, nor the levels of NRF2 and HO-1. Over-expression of either TRX or SOD2 significantly reduced the drug-induced phosphorylation of ATM, autophagosome formation and [MMF + fingolimod] lethality whereas the production of ROS was only marginally reduced in cells lacking ATM, CD95, or Beclin1. Thus, the greater than additive induction of ROS by the combination of MMF and fingolimod represents a key primary step in the initiation of the killing process. Further work will be required to define the source(s) of ROS production, e.g., mitochondria.

In many previous manuscripts we have demonstrated that a diverse set of compounds, and chemotherapeutic drug combinations, activate the death receptor CD95. For example, in primary hepatocytes, bile acid-induced CD95 activation can under certain circumstances enhance growth or, alternatively, cell death (39). In tumor cells, CD95 activation appears to only promote cell death. HDAC inhibitors, and fingolimod is an HDAC inhibitor, can increase the expression of CD95 and FAS-Ligand, and whilst [MMF + fingolimod] did not enhance CD95 and FAS-L levels, the drug combination did cause "capping" of CD95 on the cell surface. Genetically manipulated over-expression of TRX or SOD2 only partially reduced the plasma membrane clustering of CD95, arguing that other mechanisms play a more essential role in the process. Additional research will be required to fully define the molecular mechanisms of CD95 activation.

The molecular mechanisms by which [MMF + fingolimod] reduce the expression levels of K-RAS are poorly understood. Our data argued that the drugs reduced K-RAS and ERBB1 levels via Rubicon-dependent LAP followed by autophagic digestion. Clathrin-coated pits and caveolae are also two major endocytic structures which could play roles in RAS/ERBB1 destruction (40). Cholesterol, whose levels are regulated by AMPK signaling via inhibition of acetyl CoA carboxylase, an effect that also will lower the levels of farnesyl- and geranylgeranyl prenylation substrates, could impact K-RAS prenylation of K-RAS.

Fingolimod exposure initially "activated" YAP and TAZ by causing their dephosphorylation, followed later by enhancing their phosphorylation above baseline, i.e., reducing YAP/TAZ co-transcription factor activity. After fingolimod enters a cell it is phosphorylated where-after it acts in an autocrine fashion binding to S1P receptors. Initially, fingolimod causes receptor activation which is rapidly followed by receptor internalization and receptor degradation. S1P has been shown to reduce YAP phosphorylation and promote invasion, which is congruent with our findings (41, 42). However, when fingolimod has caused destruction of the S1P receptors, we observe increased YAP phosphorylation above basal levels. This suggests there may be a dynamic balance of S1P-dependent regulation of YAP in GBM cells which controls migration and invasion.

A considerable number of studies have used "modern" drug modulators of signal transduction processes in the hope of discovering a new approach to prolong survival of GBM patients. However, the median survival for GBM patients has only marginally improved over the past two decades when these drugs have been available. Checkpoint inhibitory and cellular immunotherapies have yet to exhibit any significant alteration in progression free or overall survival (43, 44). If we cannot enhance the immune system to attack GBM tumor cells, we reasoned, our initial conceptual approach became instead to attack the immune cell-rich soil in which the GBM tumor cells require to grow, thereby suppressing tumor cell growth and invasion, and with the hope that this will also enhance the lethality of standard of care therapeutics.

Our *in vitro* data has confirmed that the [MMF + fingolimod] drug combination acts to suppress the cytokine production and viability of freshly isolated activated human microglia. To our pleasant surprise, this drug combination also effectively killed multiple PDX isolates of human GBM cells, and both MMF and fingolimod enhance the lethality of temozolomide and of ionizing radiation. In addition to these observations was that this drug combination promoted the degradation of RAS proteins and oncogenic receptors such as ERBB1 vIII. Furthermore, the drugs inactivated YAP/TAZ signaling which further reduced viability. Future studies will be required to understand whether [MMF + fingolimod] can suppress GBM tumor growth *in vivo* in parallel with the combination altering cytokine production and modifying reactive microglia biology, without causing normal tissue toxicity.

AUTHOR CONTRIBUTIONS

PD wrote the manuscript. JH edited the manuscript and provided essential reagents. PD and AP conceptualized the experiments. LB and JR performed the experiments.

FUNDING

Support for the present study was funded from philanthropic funding from Massey Cancer Center, the Universal Inc. Chair in Signal Transduction Research and PHS R01-CA192613 (PD).

ACKNOWLEDGMENTS

Thanks to Dr. J. Martinez (NIEHS, Research Triangle, NC); Dr. H. F. Young and the Betts Family Fund for support in the purchase of the Hermes Wiscan instrument.

DEDICATION

This manuscript is dedicated to the corresponding author's wife who for the past 6 years, daily, has had to take Gilenya.

REFERENCES

1. Wick W, Osswald M, Wick A, Winkler F. Treatment of glioblastoma in adults. *Ther Adv Neurol Disord.* (2018) 11:1756286418790452. doi: 10.1177/1756286418790452
2. Balça-Silva J, Matias D, Carmo AD, Sarmento-Ribeiro AB, Lopes MC, Moura-Neto V. Cellular and molecular mechanisms of glioblastoma malignancy: implications in resistance and therapeutic strategies. *Semin Cancer Biol.* (2019) 58:130–41. doi: 10.1016/j.semcancer.2018.09.007
3. Razpotnik R, Novak N, Curin Šerbec V, Rajcevic U. Targeting malignant brain tumors with antibodies. *Front Immunol.* (2017) 8:1181. doi: 10.3389/fimmu.2017.01181
4. Roesch S, Rapp C, Dettling S, Herold-Mende C. When immune cells turn bad-tumor-associated microglia/macrophages in glioma. *Int J Mol Sci.* (2018) 19:E436. doi: 10.3390/ijms19020436
5. Schiffer D, Mellai M, Bovio E, Annovazzi L. The neuropathological basis to the functional role of microglia/macrophages in gliomas. *Neurol Sci.* (2017) 38:1571–7. doi: 10.1007/s10072-017-3002-x
6. Poon CC, Sarkar S, Yong VW, Kelly JJP. Glioblastoma-associated microglia and macrophages: targets for therapies to improve prognosis. *Brain.* (2017) 140:1548–60. doi: 10.1093/brain/aww355
7. Ahmed S, Gull A, Khuroo T, Aqil M, Sultana Y. Glial cell: a potential target for cellular and drug based therapy in various CNS diseases. *Curr Pharm Des.* (2017) 23:2389–99. doi: 10.2174/1381612823666170316124500
8. Quail DF, Joyce JA. The microenvironmental landscape of brain tumors. *Cancer Cell.* (2017) 31:326–41. doi: 10.1016/j.ccell.2017.02.009
9. Gupta N, Shyamasundar S, Patnala R, Karthikeyan A, Arumugam TV, Ling EA, et al. Recent progress in therapeutic strategies for microglia-mediated neuroinflammation in neuropathologies. *Expert Opin Ther Targets.* (2018) 22:765–81. doi: 10.1080/14728222.2018.1515917
10. Baecher-Allan C, Kaskow BJ, Weiner HL. Multiple sclerosis: mechanisms and immunotherapy. *Neuron.* (2018) 97:742–68. doi: 10.1016/j.neuron.2018.01.021
11. Pitteri M, Magliozzi R, Bajrami A, Camera V, Calabrese M. Potential neuroprotective effect of Fingolimod in multiple sclerosis and its association with clinical variables. *Expert Opin Pharmacother.* (2018) 19:387–95. doi: 10.1080/14656566.2018.1434143
12. von Glehn F, Dias-Carneiro RPC, Moraes AS, Farias AS, Silva VAPG, Oliveira FTM, et al. Dimethyl fumarate downregulates the immune response through the HCA2/GPR109A pathway: implications for the treatment of multiple sclerosis. *Mult Scler Relat Disord.* (2018) 23:46–50. doi: 10.1016/j.msard.2018.04.016

13. Edmonds Y, Milstien S, Spiegel S. Development of small-molecule inhibitors of sphingosine-1-phosphate signaling. *Pharmacol Ther.* (2011) 132:352–60. doi: 10.1016/j.pharmthera.2011.08.004
14. Payne SG, Milstien S, Barbour SE, Spiegel S. Modulation of adaptive immune responses by sphingosine-1-phosphate. *Semin Cell Dev Biol.* (2004) 15:521–7. doi: 10.1016/j.semcdb.2004.05.008
15. Booth L, Cruickshanks N, Tavallai S, Roberts JL, Peery M, Poklepovic A, et al. Regulation of dimethyl-fumarate toxicity by proteasome inhibitors. *Cancer Biol Ther.* (2014) 15:1646–57. doi: 10.4161/15384047.2014.967992
16. Bennett Saidu NE, Bretagne M, Mansuet AL, Just PA, Leroy K, Cerles O, et al. Dimethyl fumarate is highly cytotoxic in KRAS mutated cancer cells but spares non-tumorigenic cells. *Oncotarget.* (2018) 9:9088–99. doi: 10.18632/oncotarget.24144
17. Georgakopoulos ND, Frison M, Alvarez MS, Bertrand H, Wells G, Campanella M. Reversible Keap1 inhibitors are preferential pharmacological tools to modulate cellular mitophagy. *Sci Rep.* (2017) 7:10303. doi: 10.1038/s41598-017-07679-7
18. Gillard GO, Collette B, Anderson J, Chao J, Scannevin RH, Huss DJ, et al. DMF, but not other fumarates, inhibits NF-κB activity *in vitro* in an Nrf2-independent manner. *J Neuroimmunol.* (2015) 283:74–85. doi: 10.1016/j.jneuroim.2015.04.006
19. Peng H, Li H, Sheehy A, Cullen P, Allaire N, Scannevin RH. Dimethyl fumarate alters microglia phenotype and protects neurons against proinflammatory toxic microenvironments. *J Neuroimmunol.* (2016) 299:35–44. doi: 10.1016/j.jneuroim.2016.08.006
20. Booth L, Roberts JL, Poklepovic A, Avogadri-Connors F, Cutler RE, Lalani AS, et al. HDAC inhibitors enhance neratinib activity and when combined enhance the actions of an anti-PD-1 immunomodulatory antibody *in vivo.* *Oncotarget.* (2017) 8:90262–77. doi: 10.18632/oncotarget.21660
21. Booth L, Roberts JL, Poklepovic A, Kirkwood J, Sander C, Avogadri-Connors F, et al. The levels of mutant K-RAS and mutant N-RAS are rapidly reduced in a Beclin1/ATG5 -dependent fashion by the irreversible ERBB1/2/4 inhibitor neratinib. *Cancer Biol Ther.* (2018) 19:132–7. doi: 10.1080/15384047.2017.1394556
22. Booth L, Roberts JL, Rais R, Kirkwood J, Avogadri-Connors F, Cutler RE Jr, et al. [Neratinib + Valproate] exposure permanently reduces ERBB1 and RAS expression in 4T1 mammary tumors and enhances M1 macrophage infiltration. *Oncotarget.* (2017) 9:6062–74. doi: 10.18632/oncotarget.23681
23. Booth L, Roberts JL, Rais R, Cutler RE Jr, Diala I, Lalani AS, et al. Palbociclib augments Neratinib killing of tumor cells that is further enhanced by HDAC inhibition. *Cancer Biol Ther.* (2018) 5:1–12. doi: 10.1080/15384047.2018.1507665
24. Booth L, Roberts JL, Rais R, Cutler RE Jr, Diala I, Lalani AS, et al. Neratinib augments the lethality of [regorafenib + sildenafil]. *J Cell Physiol.* (2019). 234:4874–87. doi: 10.1002/jcp.27276
25. Booth L, Roberts JL, Cruickshanks N, Grant S, Poklepovic A, Dent P. Regulation of OSU-03012 toxicity by ER stress proteins and ER stress-inducing drugs. *Mol Cancer Ther.* (2014) 13:2384–98. doi: 10.1158/1535-7163.MCT-14-0172
26. Booth L, Roberts JL, Cruickshanks N, Tavallai S, Webb T, Samuel P, et al. PDE5 inhibitors enhance celecoxib killing in multiple tumor types. *J Cell Physiol.* (2015) 230:1115–27. doi: 10.1002/jcp.24843
27. Yacoub A, Mitchell C, Hong Y, Gopalkrishnan RV, Su ZZ, Gupta P, et al. MDA-7 regulates cell growth and radiosensitivity *in vitro* of primary (non-established) human glioma cells. *Cancer Biol Ther.* (2004) 3:739–51. doi: 10.4161/cbt.3.8.968
28. Dent P, Booth L, Poklepovic A, Hancock JF. Signaling alterations caused by drugs and autophagy. *Cell Signal.* (2019) 64:109416. doi: 10.1016/j.cellsig.2019.109416
29. Booth LA, Roberts JL, Dent P. The role of cell signaling in the crosstalk between autophagy and apoptosis in the regulation of tumor cell survival in response to sorafenib and neratinib. *Semin Cancer Biol.* (2019). doi: 10.1016/j.semcancer.2019.10.013. [Epub ahead of print].
30. Booth L, Poklepovic A, Dent P. Not the comfy chair! Cancer drugs that act against multiple active sites. *Expert Opin Ther Targets.* (2019) 23:893–901. doi: 10.1080/14728222.2019.1691526
31. Dent P, Booth L, Roberts JL, Liu J, Poklepovic A, Lalani AS, et al. Neratinib inhibits Hippo/YAP signaling, reduces mutant K-RAS expression, and kills pancreatic and blood cancer cells. *Oncogene.* (2019) 38:5890–904. doi: 10.1038/s41388-019-0849-8
32. Tripathi DN, Chowdhury R, Trudel LJ, Tee AR, Slack RS, Walker CL, et al. Reactive nitrogen species regulate autophagy through ATM-AMPK-TSC2-mediated suppression of mTORC1. *Proc Natl Acad Sci USA.* (2013) 110:E2950–7. doi: 10.1073/pnas.1307736110
33. Park MA, Mitchell C, Zhang G, Yacoub A, Allegood J, Häussinger D, et al. Vorinostat and sorafenib increase CD95 activation in gastrointestinal tumor cells through a Ca(2+)-*de novo* ceramide-PP2A-reactive oxygen species-dependent signaling pathway. *Cancer Res.* (2010) 70:6313–24. doi: 10.1158/0008-5472.CAN-10-0999
34. Guichet PO, Masliantsev K, Tachon G, Petropoulos C, Godet J, Larrieu D, et al. Fatal correlation between YAP1 expression and glioma aggressiveness: clinical and molecular evidence. *J Pathol.* (2018) 246:205–16. doi: 10.1002/path.5133
35. Artinian N, Cloninger C, Holmes B, Benavides-Serrato A, Bashir T, Gera J. Phosphorylation of the hippo pathway component AMOTL2 by the mTORC2 kinase promotes YAP signaling, resulting in enhanced glioblastoma growth and invasiveness. *J Biol Chem.* (2015) 290:19387–401. doi: 10.1074/jbc.M115.656587
36. Lee H, Hwang SJ, Kim HR, Shin CH, Choi KH, Joung JG, et al. Neurofibromatosis 2 (NF2) controls the invasiveness of glioblastoma through YAP-dependent expression of CYR61/CCN1 and miR-296-3p. *Biochim Biophys Acta.* (2016) 1859:599–611. doi: 10.1016/j.bbagrm.2016.02.010
37. Wong SW, Sil P, Martinez J. Rubicon: LC3-associated phagocytosis and beyond. *FEBS J.* (2018) 285:1379–88. doi: 10.1111/febs.14354
38. Martinez J, Malireddi RK, Lu Q, Cunha LD, Pelletier S, Gingras S, et al. Molecular characterization of LC3-associated phagocytosis reveals distinct roles for Rubicon, NOX2 and autophagy proteins. *Nat Cell Biol.* (2015) 17:893–906. doi: 10.1038/ncb3192
39. Qiao L, Studer E, Leach K, McKinstry R, Gupta S, Decker R, et al. Deoxycholic acid (DCA) causes ligand-independent activation of epidermal growth factor receptor (EGFR) and FAS receptor in primary hepatocytes: inhibition of EGFR/mitogen-activated protein kinase-signaling module enhances DCA-induced apoptosis. *Mol Biol Cell.* (2001) 12:2629–45. doi: 10.1091/mbc.12.9.2629
40. Delos Santos RC, Garay C, Antonescu CN. Charming neighborhoods on the cell surface: plasma membrane microdomains regulate receptor tyrosine kinase signaling. *Cell Signal.* (2015) 27:1963–76. doi: 10.1016/j.cellsig.2015.07.004
41. Yu FX, Zhao B, Panupinthu N, Jewell JL, Lian I, Wang LH, et al. Regulation of the Hippo-YAP pathway by G-protein-coupled receptor signaling. *Cell.* (2012) 150:780–91. doi: 10.1016/j.cell.2012.06.037
42. Cheng JC, Wang EY, Yi Y, Thakur A, Tsai SH, Hoodless PA. S1P stimulates proliferation by upregulating CTGF expression through S1PR2-mediated YAP activation. *Mol Cancer Res.* (2018) 16:1543–55. doi: 10.1158/1541-7786.MCR-17-0681
43. Buchroithner J, Erhart F, Pichler J, Widhalm G, Preusser M, Stockhammer G, et al. Audencel immunotherapy based on dendritic cells has no effect on overall and progression-free survival in newly diagnosed glioblastoma: a phase II randomized trial. *Cancers.* (2018) 10:E372. doi: 10.3390/cancers10100372
44. Reznik E, Smith AW, Taube S, Mann J, Yondorf MZ, Parashar B, et al. Radiation and immunotherapy in high-grade gliomas: where do we stand? *Am J Clin Oncol.* (2018) 41:197–212. doi: 10.1097/COC.0000000000000406

Permissions

All chapters in this book were first published by Frontiers; hereby published with permission under the Creative Commons Attribution License or equivalent. Every chapter published in this book has been scrutinized by our experts. Their significance has been extensively debated. The topics covered herein carry significant findings which will fuel the growth of the discipline. They may even be implemented as practical applications or may be referred to as a beginning point for another development.

The contributors of this book come from diverse backgrounds, making this book a truly international effort. This book will bring forth new frontiers with its revolutionizing research information and detailed analysis of the nascent developments around the world.

We would like to thank all the contributing authors for lending their expertise to make the book truly unique. They have played a crucial role in the development of this book. Without their invaluable contributions this book wouldn't have been possible. They have made vital efforts to compile up to date information on the varied aspects of this subject to make this book a valuable addition to the collection of many professionals and students.

This book was conceptualized with the vision of imparting up-to-date information and advanced data in this field. To ensure the same, a matchless editorial board was set up. Every individual on the board went through rigorous rounds of assessment to prove their worth. After which they invested a large part of their time researching and compiling the most relevant data for our readers.

The editorial board has been involved in producing this book since its inception. They have spent rigorous hours researching and exploring the diverse topics which have resulted in the successful publishing of this book. They have passed on their knowledge of decades through this book. To expedite this challenging task, the publisher supported the team at every step. A small team of assistant editors was also appointed to further simplify the editing procedure and attain best results for the readers.

Apart from the editorial board, the designing team has also invested a significant amount of their time in understanding the subject and creating the most relevant covers. They scrutinized every image to scout for the most suitable representation of the subject and create an appropriate cover for the book.

The publishing team has been an ardent support to the editorial, designing and production team. Their endless efforts to recruit the best for this project, has resulted in the accomplishment of this book. They are a veteran in the field of academics and their pool of knowledge is as vast as their experience in printing. Their expertise and guidance has proved useful at every step. Their uncompromising quality standards have made this book an exceptional effort. Their encouragement from time to time has been an inspiration for everyone.

The publisher and the editorial board hope that this book will prove to be a valuable piece of knowledge for researchers, students, practitioners and scholars across the globe.

List of Contributors

Yu-Qing Liu, Fan Wu, Jing-Jun Li, Yang-Fang Li, Xing Liu and Rui-Chao Chai
Department of Molecular Neuropathology, Beijing Neurosurgical Institute, Beijing, China
Chinese Glioma Genome Atlas Network, Beijing, China

Zheng Wang
Chinese Glioma Genome Atlas Network, Beijing, China
Department of Neurosurgery, Beijing Tiantan Hospital, Capital Medical University, Beijing, China

Yulin Wang and Minghua Zhuang
Department of Neurosurgery, The First Affiliated Hospital of Shantou University Medical College, Shantou, China

Xin Liu
Department of Stomatology, The First Affiliated Hospital of Shantou University Medical College, Shantou, China

Weijiang Zhao
Center for Neuroscience, Shantou University Medical College, Shantou, China

Lu-yang Zhang, Qing Guo, Ge-fei Guan, Wen Cheng and Peng Cheng
Department of Neurosurgery, The First Hospital of China Medical University, Shenyang, China

An-hua Wu
Department of Neurosurgery, The First Hospital of China Medical University, Shenyang, China
College of Applied Technology, China Medical University, Shenyang, China

Chao Zhang, An-bin Chen, Zhong Yao, Wei-guo Li, Shu-jun Xu and Xiang-yu Ma
Department of Neurosurgery, Qilu Hospital, Shandong University, Jinan, China
Brain Science Research Institute, Shandong University, Jinan, China

Cheng-fen Liu
Department of Neurosurgery, Qilu Hospital, Shandong University, Jinan, China

Kazutaka Fukumura
Department of Translational Molecular Pathology, The University of Texas MD Anderson Cancer Center, Houston, TX, United States

Wei Yu, Lili Zhang and Qichun Wei
Department of Radiation Oncology, The Second Affiliated Hospital, Zhejiang University School of Medicine, Hangzhou, China
Cancer Institute (Ministry of Education Key Laboratory of Cancer Prevention and Intervention), Zhejiang University Cancer Institute, Hangzhou, China

Anwen Shao
Department of Neurosurgery, The Second Affiliated Hospital, Zhejiang University School of Medicine, Hangzhou, China

Evan D. H. Gates
Department of Imaging Physics, The University of Texas MD Anderson Cancer Center, Houston, TX, United States
Graduate School of Biomedical Sciences, The University of Texas MD Anderson Cancer Center UTHealth, Houston, TX, United States

Jie Yang
Graduate School of Biomedical Sciences, The University of Texas MD Anderson Cancer Center UTHealth, Houston, TX, United States
Department of Radiation Oncology, NYU Langone School of Medicine, New York, NY, United States

Jonathan S. Lin
Department of Imaging Physics, The University of Texas MD Anderson Cancer Center, Houston, TX, United States
Medical Scientist Training Program, Baylor College of Medicine, Houston, TX, United States
Department of Bioengineering, Rice University, Houston, TX, United States

Jeffrey S. Weinberg and Sujit S. Prabhu
Department of Neurosurgery, The University of Texas MD Anderson Cancer Center, Houston, TX, United States

Lihong Long
Department of Radiation Oncology, The University of Texas MD Anderson Cancer Center, Houston, TX, United States

David Fuentes
Department of Imaging Physics, The University of Texas MD Anderson Cancer Center, Houston, TX, United States

Erik P. Sulman
Department of Radiation Oncology, NYU Langone School of Medicine, New York, United States

Jason T. Huse
Department of Translational Molecular Pathology, The University of Texas MD Anderson Cancer Center, Houston, TX, United States
Department of Pathology, The University of Texas MD Anderson Cancer Center, Houston, TX, United States

Dawid Schellingerhout
Departments of Neuroradiology and Cancer Systems Imaging, University of Texas MD Anderson Cancer Center, Houston, TX, United State

Tao Jin
The National Key Clinical Specialty, Guangdong Provincial Key Laboratory on Brain Function Repair and Regeneration, Department of Neurosurgery, The Engineering Technology Research Center of Education Ministry of China, Zhujiang Hospital, Southern Medical University, Guangzhou, China
Department of Neurosurgery, Shantou Central Hospital, Affiliated Shantou Hospital of Sun Yat-sen University, Shantou, China

Mingfa Liu, Yan Liu and Zhennan Xu
Department of Neurosurgery, Shantou Central Hospital, Affiliated Shantou Hospital of Sun Yat-sen University, Shantou, China

Yuanzhi Li
Department of Neurosurgery, Affiliated Hengyang Hospital of Southern Medical University (Hengyang Central Hospital), Hengyang, China

Haoqi He, Jie Liu and Yuxuan Zhang
The National Key Clinical Specialty, Guangdong Provincial Key Laboratory on Brain Function Repair and Regeneration, Department of Neurosurgery, The Engineering Technology Research Center of Education Ministry of China, Zhujiang Hospital, Southern Medical University, Guangzhou, China

Yiquan Ke
The National Key Clinical Specialty, Guangdong Provincial Key Laboratory on Brain Function Repair and Regeneration, Department of Neurosurgery, The Engineering Technology Research Center of Education Ministry of China, Zhujiang Hospital, Southern Medical University, Guangzhou, China
Key Laboratory of Mental Health of the Ministry of Education, Guangdong-Hong Kong-Macao Greater Bay Area Center for Brain Science and Brain-Inspired Intelligence, Southern Medical University, Guangzhou, China

Edie Zusman
NorthBay Medical Center, Fairfield, CA, United States

Maxim Sidorov, Eric Singer, Michelle Chen, Pierre-Yves Desprez, Sean McAllister and Liliana Soroceanu
California Pacific Medical Center (CPMC) Research Institute, San Francisco, CA, United States

Alexandria Ayala, Jimmin Chang, Gautam Prasad, Tyler Kang and Lawrence Dickinson
Pacific Brain and Spine Medical Group, Eden Medical Center-Sutter Research, Castro Valley, CA, United States

Nathan Salomonis and Kashish Chetal
Cincinnati Children's Hospital Medical Center (CCHMC) Biomedical Informatics, Cincinnati, OH, United States

Joseph Mark
NICO Corporation, Indianapolis, IN, United States

Xiangyang Deng, Dongdong Lin, Xiaojia Zhang, Zelin Yang, Xuchao Shen, Liang Yang, Xiangqi Lu, Hansong Sheng, Bo Yin, Nu Zhang and Jian Lin
Department of Neurosurgery, The Second Affiliated Hospital and Yuying Children's Hospital of Wenzhou Medical University, Wenzhou, China

Bo Chen
The Second Clinical Medical College, Wenzhou Medical University, Wenzhou, China

Xingxing Xu
School of Basic Medical Sciences, Wenzhou Medical University, Wenzhou, China

Hui-Chi Hung
Department of Pharmacology, College of Medicine, National Cheng-Kung University, Tainan, Taiwan

Chan-Chuan Liu
Institute of Basic Medical Sciences, College of Medicine, National Cheng-Kung University, Tainan, Taiwan

Jian-Ying Chuang
Graduate Institute of Neural Regenerative Medicine, College of Medical Science and Technology, Taipei Medical University, Taipei, Taiwan

Po-Wu Gean
Department of Pharmacology, College of Medicine, National Cheng-Kung University, Tainan, Taiwan
Institute of Basic Medical Sciences, College of Medicine, National Cheng-Kung University, Tainan, Taiwan
Department of Biotechnology and Bioindustry Sciences, National Cheng-Kung University, Tainan, Taiwan

Biao Yang, Yan-Bin Ma and Sheng-Hua Chu
Department of Neurosurgery, Shanghai Ninth People's Hospital Affiliated to Shanghai Jiao Tong University School of Medicine, Shanghai, China

Yuan-Bo Pan
Department of Neurosurgery, Second Affiliated Hospital, School of Medicine, Zhejiang University, Hangzhou, China

Hongbo Zhang and Shizhong Zhang
Department of Neurosurgery, Zhujiang Hospital, Southern Medical University, Guangzhou, China
Guangdong Provincial Key Laboratory on Brain Function Repair and Regeneration, The National Key Clinic Specialty, The Engineering Technology Research Center of Education Ministry of China, The Neurosurgery Institute of Guangdong Province, Southern Medical University, Guangzhou, China

Yuntao Li
Department of Neurosurgery, Renmin Hospital of Wuhan University, Wuhan, China
Department of Neurosurgery, Huzhou Central Hospital, Zhejiang University School of Medicine, Huzhou, China

Yinqiu Tan, Shuting Jiang, Dongyuan Liu and Qianxue Chen
Department of Neurosurgery, Renmin Hospital of Wuhan University, Wuhan, China

Qi Liu
Department of Rheumatology, The Third Affiliated Hospital of Sun Yat-sen University, Guangzhou, China

Jun Su, Wenyong Long, Changwu Wu, Mei Luo, Xiangyu Wang, Kai Xiao, Yang Li, Qun Xiao, Chi Zhang and Haoyu Li
Department of Neurosurgery, Xiangya Hospital, Central South University, Changsha, China

Qianquan Ma
Department of Neurosurgery, Peking University Third Hospital, Peking University, Beijing, China

Hailin Tang
Sun Yat-sen University Cancer Center, State Key Laboratory of Oncology in South China, Collaborative Innovation Center for Cancer Medicine, Guangzhou, China

Qing Liu
Department of Neurosurgery, Xiangya Hospital, Central South University, Changsha, China
Institute of Skull Base Surgery & Neuro-oncology at Hunan, Changsha, China

Jingfang Zheng, Qingping Lin, Hongli Liu and Yanlong Wang
Department of Gynecology, Women and Children's Hospital, School of Medicine, Xiamen University, Xiamen, China

Zhiying Su
Department of Reproductive Medicine, Women and Children's Hospital, School of Medicine, Xiamen University, Xiamen, China

Yang Kong and Jian Wang
Department of Neurosurgery, Qilu Hospital of Shandong University and Institute of Brain and Brain-Inspired Science, Shandong University, Jinan, China
Translational Cancer Research Group, Department of Biomedicine, University of Bergen, Bergen, Norway

Xiangjun Tang
Department of Neurosurgery, Renmin Hospital of Wuhan University, Wuhan, China
Department of Neurosurgery, Taihe Hospital, Hubei University of Medicine, Shiyan, China
Department of Neurosurgery, Affiliated Hospital of Xi'an Jiaotong, University Health Science Center, Xi'an, China

Shenqi Zhang and Qianxue Chen
Department of Neurosurgery, Renmin Hospital of Wuhan University, Wuhan, China

Longjun Dai
Department of Neurosurgery, Taihe Hospital, Hubei University of Medicine, Shiyan, China
Department of Surgery, University of British Columbia, Vancouver, BC, Canada

Shujun Liu, Yadi Zhu, Chenxi Zhang, Xiangrui Meng and Guojun Zhang
Laboratory Diagnosis Center, Beijing Tiantan Hospital, Capital Medical University, Beijing, China
Beijing Engineering Research Center of Immunological Reagents and Clinical Research, Beijing, China

Bo Sun and Yubo Fan
Beijing Advanced Innovation Center for Biomedical Engineering, Beihang University, Beijing, China

Xixiong Kang
Laboratory Diagnosis Center, Beijing Tiantan Hospital, Capital Medical University, Beijing, China
Beijing Engineering Research Center of Immunological Reagents and Clinical Research, Beijing, China
Beijing Advanced Innovation Center for Biomedical Engineering, Beihang University, Beijing, China

Rui Fu, Li Zhang, Kuanming Huang and Hao Peng
Department of Neurosurgery, Taihe Hospital, Hubei University of Medicine, Shiyan, China

Francesco Marchi and Debora Cipriani
Service of Neurosurgery, Neurocenter of the Southern Switzerland, Regional Hospital of Lugano, Lugano, Switzerland

Nora Sahnane, Roberta Cerutti, Michele Cerati and Fausto Sessa
Unit of Pathology, Department of Medicine and Surgery, University of Insubria-ASST Sette Laghi, Varese, Italy

Jessica Barizzi, Samantha Epistolio, Luca Mazzucchelli and Milo Frattini
Institute of Pathology, Locarno, Switzerland

Federico Mattia Stefanini
Department of Statistics, Computer Science, Applications, University of Florence, Florence, Italy

Andrew Poklepovic
Departments of Medicine, Virginia Commonwealth University, Richmond, VA, United States

Gianfranco Angelo Pesce
Radiation Oncology, Oncology Institute of Southern Switzerland, Bellinzona, Switzerland

Sergio Balbi
Division of Neurological Surgery, Department of Biotechnology and Life Sciences, University of Insubria-ASST Sette Laghi, Varese, Italy

Michael Reinert
Service of Neurosurgery, Neurocenter of the Southern Switzerland, Regional Hospital of Lugano, Lugano, Switzerland
Faculty of Medicine, University of Bern, Bern, Switzerland

Zhifang Hu, Yajing Mi, Na Guo and Aili Yan
Shaanxi Key Laboratory of Brain Disorders, School of Basic Medical Science, Xi'an Medical University, Xi'an, China

Huiming Qian and Yuelin Zhang
Shaanxi Key Laboratory of Ischemic Cardiovascular Disease, Institute of Basic and Translational Medicine, Xi'an Medical University, Xi'an, China

Xingchun Gao
Shaanxi Key Laboratory of Brain Disorders, School of Basic Medical Science, Xi'an Medical University, Xi'an, China
Shaanxi Key Laboratory of Ischemic Cardiovascular Disease, Institute of Basic and Translational Medicine, Xi'an Medical University, Xi'an, China

Paul Dent, Laurence Booth and Jane L. Roberts
Departments of Biochemistry and Molecular Biology, Virginia Commonwealth University, Richmond, VA, United States

John F. Hancock
Department of Integrative Biology and Pharmacology, University of Texas Health Science Center, Houston, TX, United States

Index